Causes, Diagnosis and Treatment of Alzheimer's Disease

Causes, Diagnosis and Treatment of Alzheimer's Disease

Editor: Trevor Cornfield

AMERICAN
MEDICAL PUBLISHERS
www.americanmedicalpublishers.com

AMERICAN
MEDICAL PUBLISHERS
www.americanmedicalpublishers.com

Cataloging-in-Publication Data

Causes, diagnosis and treatment of Alzheimer's disease / edited by Trevor Cornfield.
p. cm.
Includes bibliographical references and index.
ISBN 978-1-63927-865-7
1. Alzheimer's disease. 2. Alzheimer's disease--Etiology. 3. Alzheimer's disease--Treatment.
4. Alzheimer's disease--Diagnosis. I. Cornfield, Trevor.
RC523 .C38 2023
616.831--dc23

American Medical Publishers,
41 Flatbush Avenue,
1st Floor, New York,
NY 11217, USA

ISBN 978-1-63927-865-7 (Hardback)

Contents

Preface ... VII

Chapter 1 **Prebiotic Effect of Fructooligosaccharides from *Morinda officinalis* on Alzheimer's Disease in Rodent Models by Targeting the Microbiota-Gut-Brain Axis** ... 1
Diling Chen, Xin Yang, Jian Yang, Guoxiao Lai, Tianqiao Yong, Xiaocui Tang, Ou Shuai, Gailian Zhou, Yizhen Xie and Qingping Wu

Chapter 2 **Differential Roles of Environmental Enrichment in Alzheimer's Type of Neurodegeneration and Physiological Aging** ... 29
Vladimir V. Salmin, Yulia K. Komleva, Natalia V. Kuvacheva, Andrey V. Morgun, Elena D. Khilazheva, Olga L. Lopatina, Elena A. Pozhilenkova, Konstantin A. Shapovalov, Yulia A. Uspenskaya and Alla B. Salmina

Chapter 3 **Cognitive Function and Brain Atrophy Predict Non-Pharmacological Efficacy in Dementia: The Mihama-Kiho Scan Project2** ... 41
Ken-ichi Tabei, Masayuki Satoh, Jun-ichi Ogawa, Tomoko Tokita, Noriko Nakaguchi, Koji Nakao, Hirotaka Kida and Hidekazu Tomimoto

Chapter 4 **Challenges for Alzheimer's Disease Therapy: Insights from Novel Mechanisms Beyond Memory Defects** ... 48
Rudimar L. Frozza, Mychael V. Lourenco and Fernanda G. De Felice

Chapter 5 **On the Extraction and Analysis of Graphs from Resting-State fMRI to Support a Correct and Robust Diagnostic Tool for Alzheimer's Disease.** ... 61
Claudia Bachmann, Heidi I. L. Jacobs, PierGianLuca Porta Mana, Kim Dillen, Nils Richter, Boris von Reutern, Julian Dronse, Oezguer A. Onur, Karl-Josef Langen, Gereon R. Fink, Juraj Kukolja and Abigail Morrison

Chapter 6 **Use of Peptides for the Management of Alzheimer's Disease: Diagnosis and Inhibition** ... 85
Mohammad H. Baig, Khurshid Ahmad, Gulam Rabbani and Inho Choi

Chapter 7 **Analyzing the Behavior of Neuronal Pathways in Alzheimer's Disease Using Petri Net Modeling Approach** ... 91
Javaria Ashraf, Jamil Ahmad, Amjad Ali and Zaheer Ul-Haq

Chapter 8 **The Role of Fluoxetine in Activating Wnt/β-Catenin Signaling and Repressing β-Amyloid Production in an Alzheimer Mouse Model** ... 116
Min Huang, Yubin Liang, Hongda Chen, Binchu Xu, Cuicui Chai and Pengfei Xing

Chapter 9 **A Novel Early Diagnosis System for Mild Cognitive Impairment Based on Local Region Analysis** ... 129
Fatma E. A. El-Gamal, Mohammed M. Elmogy, Mohammed Ghazal, Ahmed Atwan, Manuel F. Casanova, Gregory N. Barnes, Robert Keynton, Ayman S. El-Baz and Ashraf Khalil

Chapter 10 **Decreased Bilateral FDG-PET Uptake and Inter-Hemispheric Connectivity in Multi-Domain Amnestic Mild Cognitive Impairment Patients....139**
Xiao Luo, Kaicheng Li, Qingze Zeng, Peiyu Huang, Yeerfan Jiaerken, Tiantian Qiu, Xiaojun Xu, Jiong Zhou, Jingjing Xu and Minming Zhang

Chapter 11 **Investigation of Gal-3 Expression Pattern in Serum and Cerebrospinal Fluid of Patients Suffering from Neurodegenerative Disorders....152**
Ghulam M. Ashraf and Saleh S. Baeesa

Chapter 12 **A Brainnetome Atlas Based Mild Cognitive Impairment Identification Using Hurst Exponent....160**
Zhuqing Long, Bin Jing, Ru Guo, Bo Li, Feiyi Cui, Tingting Wang and Hongwen Chen

Chapter 13 **The Histamine H3 Receptor Antagonist DL77 Ameliorates MK801-Induced Memory Deficits in Rats....168**
Nermin Eissa, Nadia Khan, Shreesh K. Ojha, Dorota Łazewska, Katarzyna Kieć-Kononowicz and Bassem Sadek

Chapter 14 **An Algorithm for Preclinical Diagnosis of Alzheimer's Disease....179**
Tapan K. Khan

Chapter 15 **Identification of a Novel Hemizygous SQSTM1 Nonsense Mutation in Atypical Behavioral Variant Frontotemporal Dementia....192**
Lin Sun, Zhouyi Rong, Wei Li, Honghua Zheng, Shifu Xiao and Xia Li

Chapter 16 **Analysis of Alzheimer's Disease Based on the Random Neural Network Cluster in fMRI....199**
Xia-an Bi, Qin Jiang, Qi Sun, Qing Shu and Yingchao Liu

Chapter 17 **Royal Jelly Reduces Cholesterol Levels, Ameliorates Aβ Pathology and Enhances Neuronal Metabolic Activities in a Rabbit Model of Alzheimer's Disease....209**
Yongming Pan, Jianqin Xu, Cheng Chen, Fangming Chen, Ping Jin, Keyan Zhu, Chenyue W. Hu, Mengmeng You, Minli Chen and Fuliang Hu

Permissions

List of Contributors

Index

Preface

Alzheimer's disease is one of the most common neurodegenerative diseases, and it is characterized by abnormal protein deposition in the brain. It is the most prevalent type of dementia. It has two primary causes. It may be caused by the extracellular accumulation of abnormal amounts of amyloid beta (Aβ) proteins which lead to accumulation of amyloid plaques. This disease may also occur due to intracellular accumulation of neurofibrillary tangles. In both these cases, the plaques and tangles formed by these proteins disrupt brain nerve cell transmission and affect the neuronal functioning and connectivity which leads to loss of brain function. Alzheimer's disease affects memory and thinking abilities of a person. Significant behavioral and psychological symptoms such as sleep changes are also observed. The current treatments available for this disease focus on improving symptoms of memory loss and problems with thinking and reasoning. This book is a valuable compilation of topics, ranging from the basic to the most complex advancements related to the causes, diagnosis and treatment of Alzheimer's disease. It aims to shed light on some of the unexplored aspects and recent researches on this disease. This book will serve as a valuable source of reference for students, researchers and medical practitioners.

The researches compiled throughout the book are authentic and of high quality, combining several disciplines and from very diverse regions from around the world. Drawing on the contributions of many researchers from diverse countries, the book's objective is to provide the readers with the latest achievements in the area of research. This book will surely be a source of knowledge to all interested and researching the field.

In the end, I would like to express my deep sense of gratitude to all the authors for meeting the set deadlines in completing and submitting their research chapters. I would also like to thank the publisher for the support offered to us throughout the course of the book. Finally, I extend my sincere thanks to my family for being a constant source of inspiration and encouragement.

Editor

1

Prebiotic Effect of Fructooligosaccharides from *Morinda officinalis* on Alzheimer's Disease in Rodent Models by Targeting the Microbiota-Gut-Brain Axis

Diling Chen[1], Xin Yang[2], Jian Yang[1], Guoxiao Lai[1,3], Tianqiao Yong[1], Xiaocui Tang[1], Ou Shuai[1,4], Gailian Zhou[3], Yizhen Xie[1,4*] and Qingping Wu[1]*

[1] State Key Laboratory of Applied Microbiology Southern China, Guangdong Provincial Key Laboratory of Microbial Culture Collection and Application, Guangdong Open Laboratory of Applied Microbiology, Guangdong Institute of Microbiology, Chinese Academy of Sciences, Guangzhou, China, [2] Department of Pharmacy, The Fifth Affiliated Hospital of Guangzhou Medical University, Guangzhou, China, [3] Guangxi University of Chinese Medicine, Nanning, China, [4] Guangdong Yuewei Edible Fungi Technology Co., Ltd., Guangzhou, China

***Correspondence:**
Diling Chen
diling1983@163.com
Yizhen Xie
xieyizhen@126.com

Gut microbiota influences the central nervous system disorders such as Alzheimer's disease (AD). The prebiotics and probiotics can improve the host cognition. A previous study demonstrated that fructooligosaccharides from *Morinda officinalis* (OMO) exert effective memory improvements in AD-like animals, thereby considered as potential prebiotics; however, the underlying mechanism still remains enigma. Thus, the present study investigated whether OMO is effective in alleviating AD by targeting the microbiota-gut-brain axis. OMO was administered in rats with AD-like symptoms (D-galactose- and $A\beta_{1-42}$-induced deficient rats). Significant and systematic deterioration in AD-like animals were identified, including learning and memory abilities, histological changes, production of cytokines, and microbial community shifts. Behavioral experiments demonstrated that OMO administration can ameliorate the learning and memory abilities in both AD-like animals significantly. AD parameters showed that OMO administration cannot only improve oxidative stress and inflammation disorder, but also regulate the synthesis and secretion of neurotransmitter. Histological changes indicated that OMO administration ameliorates the swelling of brain tissues, neuronal apoptosis, and down-regulation of the expression of AD intracellular markers (Tau and $A\beta_{1-42}$). 16S rRNA sequencing of gut microbiota indicated that OMO administration maintains the diversity and stability of the microbial community. In addition, OMO regulated the composition and metabolism of gut microbiota in inflammatory bowel disease (IBD) mice model treated by overdosed antibiotics and thus showed the prebiotic potential. Moreover, gut microbiota plays a major role in neurodevelopment, leading to alterations in gene expression in critical brain and intestinal regions, thereby resulting in perturbation to the programming of normal cognitive behaviors. Taken together, our findings suggest that the therapeutic effect of the traditional medicine, *M. officinalis*, on various neurological diseases such as AD, is at least partially contributed by its naturally occurring chemical constituent, OMO, via modulating the interaction between gut ecology and brain physiology.

Keywords: fructooligosaccharides, prebiotics, Alzheimer's disease, behavior, microbiota-gut-brain axis

INTRODUCTION

Gut microbiota is associated with several diseases, including neurodegenerative diseases such as Parkinson's disease (PD) and Alzheimer's disease (AD) (Petra et al., 2015; Jiang et al., 2017). Notably, the microbiota-gut-brain axis is a bi-directional communication system that is not fully understood; however, it is known to include neural, immune, endocrine, and metabolic pathways. Studies in germ-free animals and those exposed to pathogenic microbial infections, antibiotics, probiotics, or fecal microbiota transplantation suggest the link of gut microbiota with host cognition or AD-related pathogenesis (Pistollato et al., 2016; Harach et al., 2017; Liu et al., 2017; Rieder et al., 2017; Russo et al., 2017).

Several studies have supported the theory of the occurrence of a pathway of communication between the gut and the brain, modulated by gut microbiota (Gareau, 2014; Mayer et al., 2014). It has been speculated that targeting the microbiota can affect the behavior and modulate brain plasticity and cognitive functions while aging (Leung and Thuret, 2015). Some studies demonstrated that gut-targeted intervention by consuming *lactic acid bacteria* such as those in yogurt, could improve or delay the onset of cognitive decline associated with aging (Jung et al., 2012; Choi et al., 2015; Scott et al., 2017). Therefore, using probiotics for ameliorating the cognitive and behavioral disorders could be a potential treatment.

The hypothesis that the microbiota-gut-brain axis (Rhee et al., 2009) plays a critical role in health and disease, including neuropsychiatric disorders (Liu et al., 2017), is rapidly progressing. Nurturing a beneficial gut microbiome with prebiotics, such as fructooligosaccharides and inulin, is an appealing but under-investigated microbiota-induced manipulation. A previous study showed that the prebiotic treatment could modify the behavior across domains relevant to anxiety, depression, cognition, stress response, and social behavior (Burokas et al., 2017). Previous findings strengthened the evidence supporting the therapeutic targeting of gut microbiota in brain-gut axis disorders, thereby opening new prospects in the field of nutritional neuropsychopharmacology. Thus, it is imperative to develop novel and effective drugs or foods with prebiotic effects from natural resources.

Morinda officinalis How. (*M. officinalis*), as a Chinese traditional natural herbal medicine, contains a number of active components. Reportedly, the content of saccharides in *M. officinalis* radix is 49.79–58.25%, which is highly composed of oligosaccharides, such as inulin-type hexasaccharide exerting antidepressant effects in the model systems (Cai et al., 1996; Li et al., 2001). This phenomenon can be effectuated by up-regulating the expression of neurotrophic factors and/or down-regulating the $[Ca^{2+}]_i$ overloading (Li et al., 2004). Bajijiasu, another oligosaccharide, protects PC12 cells from $A\beta_{25-35}$-induced neurotoxicity (Chen et al., 2013), ameliorates the cognitive deficits induced by D-galactose in mice, and protects against ischemia-induced neuronal damage or death (Tan et al., 2000a,b). Our previous study suggested that oligosaccharide extracted from *M. officinalis* (OMO) might inhibit the oxidative stress and neuronal apoptosis, restore normal energy metabolism, as well as, increase the cell viability and mitochondrial membrane potential in AD animal models significantly (Chen et al., 2014a). However, the underlying mechanism is yet to be elucidated.

Alzheimer's disease is the most common neurodegenerative disorder, affecting approximately >5% of the worldwide population aged >65 years, annually. AD is a chronic neurodegenerative disease that frequently exhibits a slow progression accompanied by a greater recession of the disease over a period. Although the cause of AD is poorly understood, among various biochemical and morphological events, the presence of neurofibrillary tangles, senile plaques, and neuronal and synaptic loss are considerably noted (Chen et al., 2017). Several pieces of evidence have confirmed that the accumulation of intracellular β-amyloid (Aβ) may be an early event in the development of AD. Aβ is a peptide comprised of 36–43 amino acids formed by a large transmembrane glycoprotein, such as amyloid precursor protein (APP), expressed on the cell. Aβ may activate the inflammatory and neurotoxic processes, including the excessive generation of free radicals and oxidative damage among intracellular proteins and other macromolecules (Abbott, 2011). D-galactose can form advanced glycation end products (AGEs). The administration of D-galactose to human populations can induce cognitive deficits and disruptions in the synaptic communication. Thus, D-galactose-treated rats with synaptic disruption and memory impairment have been extensively used as model rodents (Zhan et al., 2014; Gao et al., 2016; Huang et al., 2016; Li et al., 2016). In our previous, we have used these two models to screen the effective compounds for curing the AD (Chen et al., 2014b, 2017). Thus, in this study, the two AD-like models were induced by D-galactose and Aβ, respectively.

Herein, we investigated whether OMO is effective in alleviating AD by targeting the microbiota-gut-brain axis. OMO was administered in rats exhibiting AD-like symptoms induced by D-galactose and $A\beta_{1-42}$, respectively. Some indexes and histological deterioration, including learning and memory abilities, histological alterations, production of cytokines, microbial communities, and transcriptome in small intestine and brain, were identified in AD-like animals. And the prebiotics were directly evaluated in an overdose antibiotics-treated trinitro-benzene-sulfonic acid (TNBS)-induced mice model.

MATERIALS AND METHODS

Animal Models and Treatments

Adult male Sprague–Dawley rats (180–220 g) and C57 mice (18–22 g, 10-moth-old) obtained from the Center of Laboratory Animal of Guangdong Province, SCXK [Yue] 2008-0020, SYXK [Yue] 2008-0085) were pair-housed in plastic cages in a temperature-controlled (25°C) colony room at a 12/12 h light/dark cycle. Food and water were available *ad libitum*. All experimental protocols were approved by the Center of Laboratory Animals of the Guangdong Institute of Microbiology (GT-IACUC20160426). All efforts were made to minimize the number of animals used.

D-Galactose-Induced Deficient Rats and Treatment

The rats were randomly divided into four groups as follows: control group received distilled water orally, model group received intraperitoneal injection (i.p.) of 100 mg/kg/d D-galactose (Zhong et al., 2016; Chen et al., 2017; Liang et al., 2017), low-dose group was administered D-galactose (100 mg/kg/d) by i.p. and gavage at a dosage of 50 mg/[kg·d] OMO, and high-dose group received D-galactose (100 mg/kg/d) by i.p. and gavage at a dosage of 100 mg/[kg·d] OMO daily in the morning. Every group consisted of eight animals, and the duration of the procedure was 8 weeks.

$A\beta_{1-42}$-Induced Deficient Rats and Treatment

The procedures were similar to those described previously (Chen et al., 2014b). Rats were anesthetized using 30 g/L pentobarbital sodium (40 mg/kg, i.p.; Sigma–Aldrich) and placed in a stereotaxic frame (RWD Life Science Co., Ltd., Shenzhen, China). The hair was shaved, scalp opened, and holes drilled with an electric dental drill (brushless motor, 30,000 rpm) according to the mouse brain atlas (AP-3.6 mm, ML ± 2.5 mm, DV3.0 mm). Then, 5 μL (10 μg) $A\beta_{1-42}$ in a fibrillar state (Chen et al., 2013) was slowly injected into the CA1 region of the hippocampus over a 5-min period in one hole, and the needle was retained inside for an additional 5 min. Subsequently, the wound was sutured, and penicillin (30 U/kg) was injected intramuscularly to protect against infection. Finally, the rats were isolated in a warm box until consciousness was recovered.

After 15 days, the rats were screened with water maze tests to identify the animals that were appropriate models, followed by random categorization into four groups as follows: control group (received saline and distilled water orally), model group (received $A\beta_{1-42}$ and distilled water orally), low-dose group (received $A\beta_{1-42}$ and OMO 50 mg/[kg·d] orally), high-dose group (received $A\beta_{1-42}$ and OMO 100 mg/[kg·d] orally). Every group consisted of seven animals, and the duration of the experiments was 28 days.

Water Maze Tests

The spatial learning and memory abilities of the rats were tested using the Morris water maze (MWM, DMS-2, Chinese Academy of Medical Sciences Institute of Medicine). The MWM consisted of a circular opaque fiberglass pool (200 cm diameter) filled with water (25 ± 1°C). The pool was surrounded by light blue curtains, and three distal visual cues were fixed on the curtains. A total of four floor light sources of equal power provided uniform illumination to the pool and testing room. A CCD camera was placed above the center of the pool in order to record the swim paths of the animals. The video output was digitized by an EthoVision tracking system (Noldus, Leesburg, VA, United States). The tests included three periods: initial spatial training, spatial reversal training, and the probe test; the procedures were same as those described previously (Chen et al., 2014b).

Evaluation of AD Parameters

The appearance, behavior, and fur color of the animals were observed and documented daily. The weights of the animals were measured every 3 days during the period of drug administration. Following the MWM, the blood and serum were acquired, and the brains of the animals were dissected. Routine index and cytokines (Wang et al., 2016), including the production of cytokines interleukins [(1L)-1α, 1L-2, 1L-8, 1L-10, 1L-11, IL-12], tumor necrosis factor (TNF)-γ, TNF-α, vascular endothelial growth factor (VGEF), human macrophage inflammatory protein-1α (MIP-α), and macrophage colony-stimulating factor (M-CSF), activities of malondialdehyde (MDA), total superoxide dismutase (T-SOD), catalase (CAT), glutathione reductase (GSH-Px), and levels of acetylcholine (ACh), acetylcholinesterase (AChE), and Na^+/K^+-ATPase, and some monoamine neurotransmitters, were measured.

A total of three brains, small intestine, and other tissues from each group were fixed in 4% paraformaldehyde and prepared as paraffin sections that were stained with hematoxylin-eosin (H&E) and immunohistochemistry (IHC) before examining under light microscopy (Zeng et al., 2013; Chen et al., 2014b).

Evaluation of Prebiotic Effects of OMO in TNBS-Induced Mice

After 24 h fasting, the mice were anesthetized by intraperitoneal injection of 2% sodium pentobarbital (0.2 ml/100 g), followed by intubation (latex tubing of 2 mm diameter, lubricated with edible oil before usage) from the anus, gently inserted into the lumen about 4.0 cm. Subsequently, 150 mg/kg of TNBS (Sigma–Aldrich, St. Louis, MO, United States, solubilized in 50% ethanol) solution was injected through the latex tubing, the rats were hanged upside down for 30 s to ensure complete seepage of the mixture into the lumen without leakage (Wei et al., 2017). Then, the animals were randomly divided into nine groups ($n = 9$): control, model, model and high-dose antibiotics, OMO (100 mg/kg/d), *Bifidobacterium*, OMO and high-dose antibiotics, OMO and *Bifidobacterium*, *Bifidobacterium* and high-dose antibiotics, OMO and *Bifidobacterium* and high-dose antibiotics. All the antibiotics were administered for 4 days, then inflammatory bowel disease (IBD) was induced with TNBS, followed 7-day drug treatments and TNBS induction, followed by an additional 4-day drug treatments.

Consequently, the mice were anesthetized by intraperitoneal injection of 2% sodium pentobarbital (0.25 ml/100 g). The blood plasma was collected by abdominal aortic method and serum by centrifugation (1500 r/min, 10 min). Then, the serum was assessed for the production of cytokines GM-CSF (granulocyte-macrophage colony-stimulating factor), TNF-γ, 1L-10, IL-12, 1L-17α, 1L-4, TNF-α, and VGEF. The colon and spleen obtained from the rats were fixed in 4% paraformaldehyde at pH 7.4 for further pathological observations, and the cecum contents were collected for 16S rRNA gene-based analysis.

Microbiome Analysis

Fresh fecal samples were collected before fasting of the rats and stored at −80°C. Frozen microbial DNA was isolated from mice cecal sample with total mass ranging from 1.2 to 20.0 ng and preserved at −20°C. The microbial 16S rRNA genes were amplified using the forward primer 5′-CCTAYGGGRBGCASCAG-3′ and reverse primer 5′-GGACTACNNGGGTATCTAAT-3′ for rats. Each amplified product was concentrated via solid-phase reversible immobilization and quantified by electrophoresis using an Agilent 2100 Bioanalyzer (Agilent, United States). After quantification of DNA concentration by NanoDrop, each sample was diluted to 1×10^9 molecules/μL in TE buffer and pooled. Subsequently, 20 μL of the pooled mixture was used for sequencing on Illumina MiSeq sequencing platform according to the manufacturer's instructions. The resulting reads were analyzed as described previously (Ling et al., 2014).

Transcriptome Analysis

The RNA-seq transcriptome library was prepared using the TruSeq™ RNA Sample Preparation Kit (Illumina, San Diego, CA, United States). *De novo* assembly and annotation identified the differentially expressed genes (DEGs) between different treatments; the expression level of each transcript was measured according to the fragments/kb of exon per million mapped reads method. RSEM[1] was used to quantify the abundance of genes and isoforms. The R statistical package software EdgeR[2] was used for the analysis of differential expression. Functional enrichment analysis was performed to identify the DEGs enriched significantly in Gene Ontology (GO) and metabolic pathways at Bonferroni-corrected *p*-value ≤ 0.05 as compared to the whole- transcriptome background. GO functional enrichment and KEGG pathway analyses were performed using Goatools[3] and KOBAS[4], respectively (Wang et al., 2010; Cabili et al., 2011; Sun et al., 2013; Trapnell et al., 2013).

Statistical Analysis

All data are described as the means ± standard deviations (SD) of at least three independent experiments. The significant differences between treatments were analyzed by one-way analysis of variance (ANOVA) test at $p < 0.05$ using statistical package for the social sciences (SPSS, Abacus Concepts, Berkeley, CA, United States) and Prism5 (GraphPad, San Diego, CA, United States) software.

[1]http://deweylab.biostat.wisc.edu/rsem/

[2]http://www.bioconductor.org/packages/2.12/bioc/html/edgeR.html

[3]https://github.com/tanghaibao/Goatools

[4]http://kobas.cbi.pku.edu.cn

RESULTS

Effects of OMO in D-Galactose-Induced Deficient Rats

Antioxidative and Neuroprotective Effects, Activation of Energy Metabolism and Regulation of Acetylcholine Esterase by OMO in D-Galactose-Induced Deficient Rats

The fur of the treated animals was much smoother than that of the model group. The average weight between the treated and the model groups did not differ significantly ($p > 0.05$); the animals weighed approximately 320 g at the beginning and 500 g at the end of the experiment (**Figure 1A**).

Compared to the model group, the incubation period for each OMO-treated group was significantly shorter. The incubation period for the low-dose OMO group was (86.37 ± 11.46 s) and that for the high-dose group was (82.00 ± 19.44 s) on the 1st day. Compared to the model group, the differences were significant ($p < 0.01$). On the 4th day, the incubation period for the low-dose OMO group was (39.30 ± 5.63 s) and that for the high-dose group was 30.74 ± 3.69 s; the differences were significant as compared to the model group ($p < 0.01$; **Figure 1B**). These results demonstrated that OMO administration could ameliorate D-galactose-induced learning and memory dysfunction in rats.

Probe test results did not reveal any significant differences ($p > 0.05$) among the groups with respect to total swimming distance or speed. The swimming time of the control group in the NW quadrant (28.00 ± 0.81 s) was significantly longer than that in the other three quadrants (24.36 ± 0.40, 24.21 ± 1.33, and 25.43 ± 1.465 s; $p < 0.01$). The swimming time in the NW quadrant of the model group was 25.23 ± 1.04 s, which was significantly shorter than the control group ($p < 0.01$), suggesting that the rats remembered the location of the placement of the platform. The swimming durations of the low- and high-dose OMO groups were 27.13 ± 0.85 and 29.00 ± 1.08 s, respectively, which were significantly longer than the model group. Compared to the model group, the differences were significant ($p < 0.01$; **Figure 1C**).

As shown in **Figure 1D**, the SOD levels in the low- and high-dose OMO groups were 95.05 ± 1.21, and 97.70 ± 1.43 (% of control), respectively, as compared to 90.45 ± 2.17 in the model groups. The differences were significant as compared to the model group ($p < 0.05$). In addition, the levels of GSH-Px and CAT showed similar trends, while that of the MDA showed opposite trends, suggesting that OMO encouraged SOD, MDA, CAT, and inhibited MDA production, thereby indicating that OMO administration can enhance the antioxidative activities in the D-galactose-induced deficient rats.

To evaluate the protective efficacy of OMO on the energy metabolism in D-galactose-treated rats, we measured the

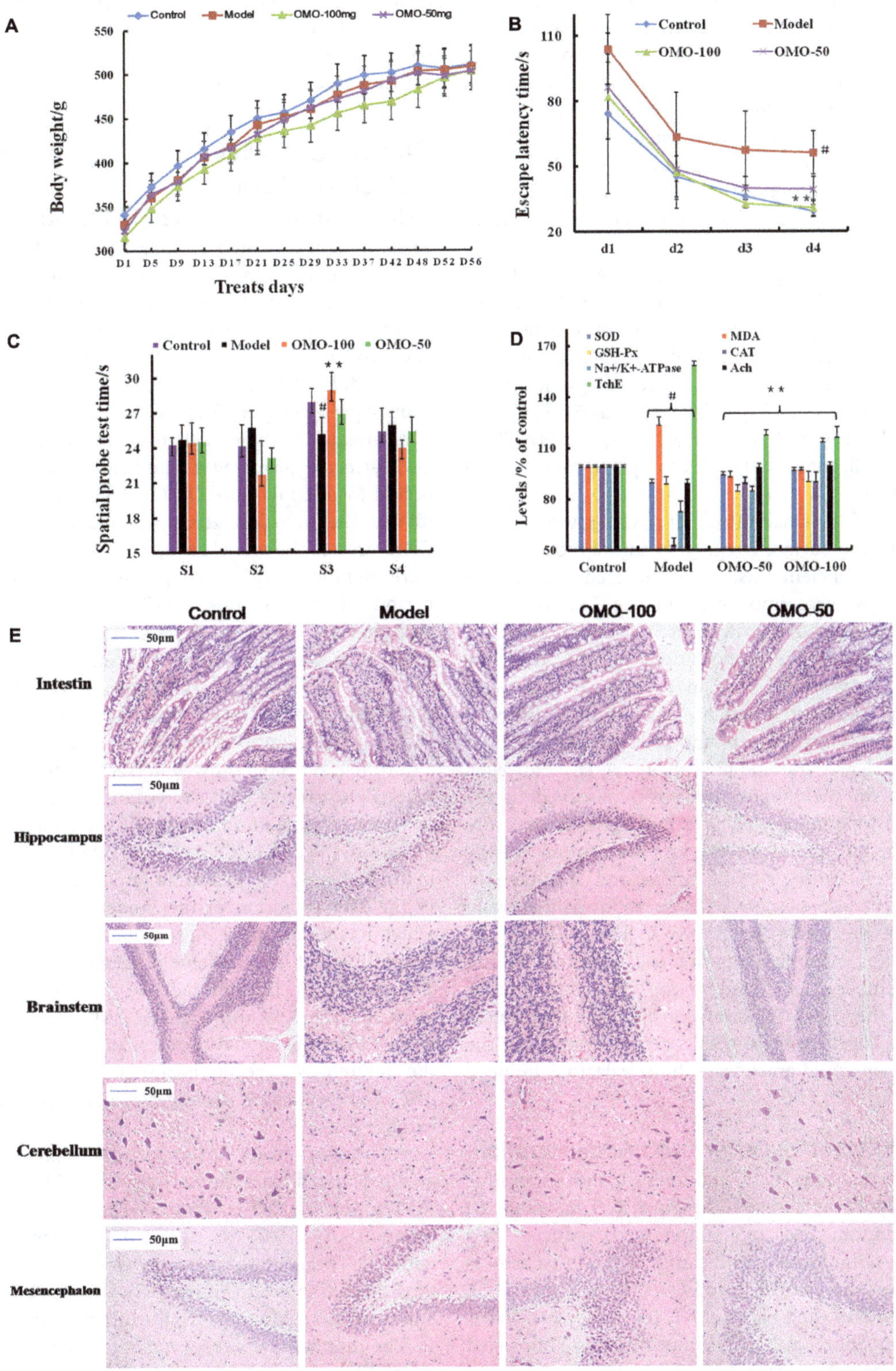

FIGURE 1 | Effect of OMO in D-galactose-induced deficient rats. **(A)** Body weight changes during the treatments time. **(B)** Escape latency in the MWM. **(C)** Swimming time in the platform quadrant during the spatial probe test. **(D)** Effect on SOD, MDA, CAT, GSH-Px TchE, Ach, and Na^+/K^+-ATPase levels. **(E)** Histopathological changes in the intestine and brain. The graph Control, control group; Model, model group; OMO-50 mg, low-dose group that received D-galactose (100 mg/kg/d) by i.p. and gavage at a dosage of 50 mg/[kg·d] in OMO; OMO-100 mg, high-dose group that received D-galactose (100 mg/kg/d) i.p. and gavage at a dosage of 100 mg/[kg·d] in OMO. Values are represented as mean ± SD (n = 6) and expressed as the percentage of the control group, $^{\#}p < 0.01$ vs. control group, $^{*}p < 0.05$ vs. model group, $^{**}p < 0.01$ vs. model group.

Na^+/K^+-ATPase levels in brain tissue. As shown in **Figure 1D**, the levels of Na^+/K^+-ATPase were significantly lower in the model group (73.53 ± 5.17% of control) as compared to the control group ($p < 0.05$). The levels of all the OMO-treated groups (90.15 ± 2.08 for low-dose, 90.83 ± 1.64 for high-dose) were increased significantly, and the differences were significantly different as compared to the model group ($p < 0.05$). These levels were based on the concentration-dependent activities; however, the specific underlying mechanism necessitates further studies.

Cholinergic system damage and abnormal ACh levels are observed in AD patients. The results are illustrated in **Figure 1D**. As compared to the model group (89.85 ± 1.93% of control), after treatment with different concentrations (50 and 100mg/[kg·d]) of OMO, the ACh levels of the model rats increased significantly to 99.22 ± 1.49 and 99.98 ± 1.52, respectively, ($p < 0.05$). The AchE decreased to 118.39 ± 1.93 and 116.70 ± 5.47, respectively. These differences were significant ($p < 0.05$) as compared to the model group (159.37 ± 4.15).

The HE staining of the small intestinal tissues revealed crypt atrophy, distortion, and surface irregularity in the model group D-galactose-induced deficient rats, while those changes in the OMO-treated groups were improved (**Figure 1E**, intestine). Moreover, the staining did not demonstrate any remarkable neuronal abnormalities in the hippocampus of the rats in the control group. The pyramidal cells in the CA1 region were arranged precisely and tightly, and no cell loss was observed. Additionally, in the control group, the cells were round and intact with stained clear, dark blue nuclei (**Figure 1E**). However, noticeable damage in the hippocampus was observed in the model groups by histopathology. The pyramidal layered structure was disintegrated, and the neuronal loss was found in the CA1 region. Neurons with pyknotic nuclei and shrunken or irregular shape were also observed. These abnormalities were attenuated by the treatment with OMO. The cells in the OMO-treated groups exhibited superior cell morphology and were more in number than those in the untreated groups, especially those in the OMO-100 treated group were superior to the control group. Together, these results demonstrated that the OMO administration could ameliorate the D-galactose-induced deficient rats.

Changes in Gut Microbiota after OMO Administration

Operational taxonomic unit (OTU) abundance and taxonomic profiles were analyzed as shown in **Figure 2**. The values of Chao1, ACE, Shannon, and npShannon were reduced, and that of Simpson was increased significantly in the D-galactose-induced group than the normal group ($p < 0.05$, **Figure 2A**). After treatment with 100 mg/kg/d OMO, the values of Chao1, ACE, Shannon, npShannon, and Simpson were improved to resemble the normal (**Figure 2A**). All the treated groups could be clustered using the principal component analysis (PCA) (**Figure 2B**); Bray-Curtis distance was shown at the phylum level in **Figure 2C** (*Verrucomicrotia*, *Proteobacteria*, *Firmicutes*, and *Bacteroidetes*), genus level in **Figure 2D** (left) (*Prevotella*, *Oscillospira*, *Lactobacillus*, *Bacteroides*, *Parabacteroides*, *Sutterella*, *Akkermansia*), and beta diversity at the genus level in **Figure 2D** (right). Our results indicated that OMO administration could maintain the abundance of gut microbiota in D-galactose-induced deficient rats, although additional studies are warranted.

Effects of OMO on $A\beta_{1-42}$-Induced Deficient Rats

Indexes Improvements by OMO Administration

The fur of the treated animals was much smoother than that of the model group. The average weight of model groups was found to be higher than that of the control group ($p < 0.05$), and we found that the rats in the model group present constipation and swollen belly. Moreover, the weight records of OMO-treated groups did not alter significantly ($p > 0.05$) as compared to the control group (**Figure 3A**).

Compared to the model group, the incubation period for each OMO-treated group was significantly shorter. The incubation period for the low-dose OMO group was 86.49 ± 11.64 s, while that for the high-dose group was 82.06 ± 19.44 s on the 1st day. Compared to the model group (113.75 ± 16.11 s), the differences were significant ($p < 0.01$). On the 4th day, the incubation period of the low-dose OMO group was 37.19 ± 5.36 s, and that for the high-dose group was 28.27 ± 3.96 s; the differences were significant as compared to the model group (56.29 ± 9.69 s, $p < 0.01$; **Figure 3Ba**). These results showed that OMO administration could ameliorate the $A\beta_{1-42}$-induced learning and memory dysfunction in rats.

Probe test results showed no significant differences ($p > 0.05$) among the groups with respect to the total swimming distance or speed. The swimming time of the control group in the NW quadrant (26.63 ± 3.83 s) was significantly longer than that in the other three quadrants ($p < 0.01$). The swimming time in the NW quadrant of the model group was 20.77 ± 2.36 s, which was significantly shorter than the control group ($p < 0.01$), suggesting that the rats remembered the location of the platform. The swimming time of the low- and high-dose OMO groups were 26.50 ± 3.59 and 27.36 ± 2.51 s, which were significantly longer than the model group. Compared to the model group, the differences were significant ($p < 0.01$), as shown in **Figure 3Bc**. The swimming distances did not differ among all groups (**Figure 3Bb**).

All the cytokines' levels in the serum of $A\beta_{1-42}$-induced group deviated from the normal; GM-CSF, TNF-γ, 1L-10, IL-12, 1L-17α, 1L-4, TNF-α, and VGEF were secreted significantly different ($p < 0.05$ or $p < 0.01$; **Figure 3C**). When treated with OMO, all these cytokines were strikingly recovered close to the baseline level (**Figure 3C**), thereby indicating that OMO administration can improve the inflammatory environment.

The monoamine neurotransmitter levels in right brain tissue were dissected from 4 rats in each group, according to the methods described previously (Chen et al., 2014b). **Figure 3D** showed that the levels of norepinephrine (NE), dopamine (DA), 5-hydroxytryptamine (5-HT), and 5-hydroxyindole acetic acid (5-HIAA) were reduced in $A\beta_{1-42}$-induced groups as compared to the control group, and the OMO administration can promote the secretion of some monoamine neurotransmitters (NE, DA,

A

Sequencing data summary at 97% similarity

Group	Label	Chao	Ace	Shannon	Npshannon	Simpson	Coverage
Model	0.03	12534 ± 2129[#]	22848 ± 4820	4.6015 ± 0.2331[#]	4.7236 ± 0.2399	0.0337 ± 0.0083[#]	0.9703 ± 0.0045
OMO-100	0.03	20851 ± 3266[*]	38967 ± 5280[*]	5.2774 ± 0.1225[*]	5.4313 ± 0.1441[*]	0.0197 ± 0.0035[*]	0.9565 ± 0.0072
Normal	0.03	23523 ± 2253	44079 ± 4056	5.6098 ± 0.2683	5.7747 ± 0.2074	0.0174 ± 0.0052	0.9472 ± 0.0192

The richness estimators (ACE and Chao), diversity indices (Shannon and Simpson), and Coverage were calculated using the Mothur software. Values given are the mean±SD, [#]$p<0.05$ *vs* normal, [*]$p<0.05$ *vs* model

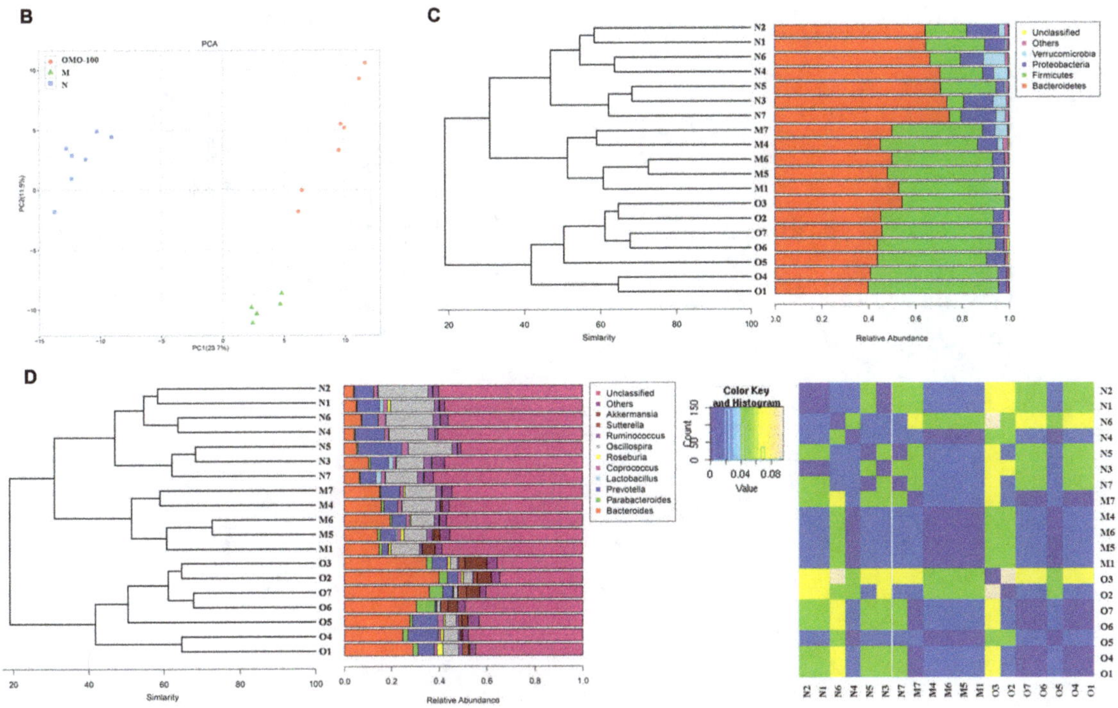

FIGURE 2 | Effects of OMO on gut microbiota in D-galactose-induced deficient rats. **(A)** Sequencing data summary at 97% similarity. **(B)** Results of PCA. **(C)** Classification and abundance of cecal contents at the phylum level. **(D)** Classification and abundance of cecal contents at the genus level, and the beta diversity. The graph N is normal group; M is model group; O is OMO-100 mg, high-dose group that received D-galactose (100 mg/kg/d) i.p., and gavage at a dosage of 100 mg/[kg·d] in OMO. Values are the means of six independent experiments ($n \geq 5$).

5-HT, and 5-HIAA) in a concentration-dependent manner (**Figure 3D**).

The HE staining of small intestinal tissues revealed crypt branching, atrophy, distortion, and surface irregularity in the model group $A\beta_{1-42}$-induced deficient rats, while those changes in the OMO-treated groups were improved (**Figure 3E**, intestine). The injury to the atrial tissues in the $A\beta_{1-42}$-induced group was more severe than that in the normal and OMO-treated groups. Furthermore, the HE staining did not reveal any remarkable neuronal abnormalities in the hippocampus of rats in the control group (**Figure 3E**). However, the obvious hippocampal histopathological damage was observed in the model groups. The pyramidal layered structure was disintegrated, and neuronal loss was found in the CA1 region. These abnormalities were attenuated by OMO treatment. The cells in OMO-treated groups exhibited better cell morphology and were more in number than those in the untreated groups, especially those in the OMO-100 treated group were superior to the control group. Compared to the normal group, the proportion of $A\beta_{1-42}$ and Tau-positive cells in rats in the model group was significantly higher than that in the normal group ($p < 0.05$), while the OMO administration down-regulated the expression of $A\beta_{1-42}$ and Tau proteins (**Figure 3E**).

The Gut Structure of the Microbiota Was Altered Significantly by OMO

OTU abundance and taxonomic profiles were analyzed as shown in **Figure 4**. Compared to the normal group, the diversity of the microbial communities in $A\beta_{1-42}$-induced (injected 10 or 20 μg fibrillar state of $A\beta_{1-42}$ into the CA1 region, **Figure 4D**) group was reduced and negatively related with the doses of $A\beta_{1-42}$ (**Figure 4A**); All the $A\beta_{1-42}$-induced groups were clustered as

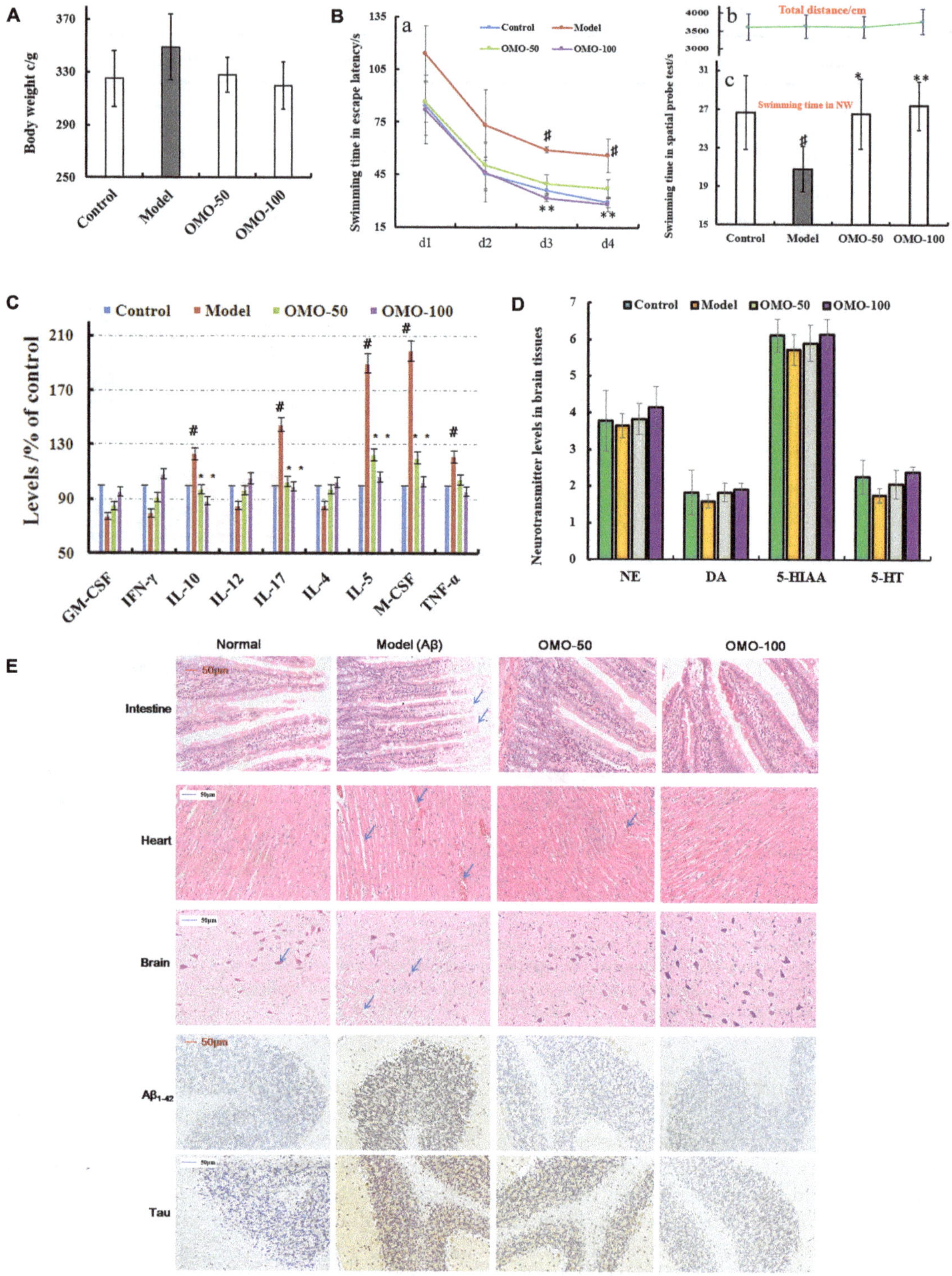

FIGURE 3 | Effect of OMO in $A\beta_{1-42}$-induced deficient rats. **(A)** Body weight changes during the treatments time. **(B-a)** Escape latency in the MWM. **(B-b)** Swimming distance. **(B-c)** Swimming time in the platform quadrant during the spatial probe test. **(C)** Level of cytokines GM-CSF, TNF-γ, 1L-10, IL-12, 1L-17α, 1L-4, TNF-α, and VGEF-α in the serum. **(D)** Levels of monoamine neurotransmitters (NE, DA, 5-HT, and 5-HIAA) in the brain tissue. **(E)** Histopathological changes in the intestine, heart, and brain, and the expressions of $A\beta_{1-42}$ and Tau proteins in brain tissues by immunohistochemistry. The graph Control, control group; Model, model group; OMO-50 mg, low-dose group that received D-galactose (100 mg/kg/d) i.p. and gavage at a dosage of 50 mg/[kg·d] in OMO; OMO-100 mg, high-dose group that received D-galactose (100 mg/kg/d) i.p. and gavage at a dosage of 100 mg/[kg·d] in OMO. Values are represented as mean ± SD (n = 6) and expressed as the percentage of the control group, $^{\#}p < 0.01$ vs. control group, $^{*}p < 0.05$ vs. model group, $^{**}p < 0.01$ vs. model group.

expected using PCA (**Figure 4B**), which indicated that the Aβ not only influences the brain but also changes the gut microbiota. After treatment with 50 mg/(kg·d) or 100 mg/(kg·d) OMO, the diversity of the microbial communities was improved similarly as that of the normal (**Figure 4C**).

Analysis revealed the difference of taxonomic abundance between different groups (**Figure 4E**). Some bacteria in the fecal samples changed considerably at the phylum level: for instance, *Verrucomicrotia, Proteobacteria, Firmicutes*, and *Bacteroidetes*. Moreover, at the genus level, the $A\beta_{1-42}$-induced rats exhibited the enrichment of potentially proinflammatory microbes, such as *Corynebacterium, Staphylococcus, Ruminococcus, Roseburia, Dorea*, and *Sutterella*, and the reduction of potentially anti-inflammatory microbes, such as *Bacteroides, Bifidobacterium, Prevotella, Parabacteroides, Coprococcus, Desulfovibrio*, and *Lactobacillus*, in comparison with the normal group (**Figure 4F**). However, the treatment with the OMO exhibited a reduction in proinflammatory microbes and enrichment of anti-inflammatory microbes. Thus, our results indicated that the OMO administration had the potential to regulate the structure of the gut microbiota.

We also constructed and visualized a taxonomic tree of the predominant taxa (**Figure 4G**), which showed that *Firmicutes, Bacteroidetes, Clostridia, Bacteroidia, Bacilli, Clostridiales, Lactobacillales, Bacteroidales, Lactobacillaceae*, and *Lactobacillus* were the predominant taxa. The altered details of the predominant taxa (**Figure 4H**) showed that the abundance of *Clostridia* and *Clostridiales* in $A\beta_{1-42}$-induced groups was increased sharply, while the aforementioned taxa as *Firmicutes, Bacteroidetes, Bacteroidia, Bacilli, Lactobacillales, Bacteroidales, Lactobacillaceae*, and *Lactobacillus* were reduced ($p < 0.05$ vs. normal group). On the other hand, the OMO-treated groups can reverse those changes, especially the probiotic *Lactobacillus* increased obviously, which indicated that OMO administration might have a prebiotic role in intestinal dysbacteriosis in AD animals as induced by $A\beta_{1-42}$.

Prebiotic Effect of OMO on TNBS-Induced Mice

The Tissue Damages and Inflammation Induced by TNBS Combined Antibiotics Were Relieved

In order to ensure the prebiotic role of OMO, we established an IBD mice model after a broad spectrum antibiotics treatment. Compared to the control group, post treatment with TNBS by enema, a majority of the mice presented diarrhea and the weight gain declined relatively (**Figure 5A**). All the cytokines' levels were deviated from the normal, as some anti-inflammatory cytokines of GM-CSF, TNF-γ, 1L-10, IL-12, 1L-17α, 1L-4, TNF-α, and VGEF were secreted differently ($p < 0.05$ or $p < 0.01$; **Figure 5C**). Simultaneously, we found that the content of lipopolysaccharide (LPS) (**Figure 5B**) was higher than that in the control group; the colon tissues (**Figure 5D**) and splenic tissues (**Figure 5E**) were severely damaged. Also, immunohistochemistry staining showed that the expressions of Foxp3 (**Figure 6A**), IL-17 (**Figure 6B**), NF-κB (**Figure 6C**), and TNF-α (**Figure 6D**) deviated from the control, especially the additional broad spectrum and overdose antibiotics groups. After treatment with OMO, all the deviated parameters returned to the baselines, especially the OMO + *Bifidobacterium*-treated group (**Figures 5, 6**). Cumulatively, our results suggested that OMO and *Bifidobacterium* exert anti-inflammatory effects in IBD, synergistically; however, the underlying mechanism needs further studies.

Promotion of the Engraftment Ability of *Bifidobacterium*

To clarify the synergistical action between OMO and *Bifidobacterium*, OTU abundance and taxonomic profiles were analyzed as shown in **Figure 7**. Compared to the normal group, the diversity of the microbial community in TNBS and TNBS and antibiotics-induced groups was reduced (**Figure 7A**). OMO can ameliorate this dysbacteriosis; the bacterial compositions at the phylum (**Figure 7C**) and family level (**Figure 7D**) encompassed *Verrucomicrotia, Proteobacteria, Firmicutes, Bacteroidetes, Lactobacillaceae*, and *Lachnospiraceae*. Our results showed that the relative abundance of *Bifidobacterium* was increased remarkably ($p < 0.05$, **Figure 5**), and the other probiotics *Lactobacillaceae* were also abundant in the microbial community with stable structures. We also constructed and visualized a taxonomic tree of the predominant taxa (**Figure 7B**), which showed that the *Firmicutes, Bacteroidetes, Clostridia, Bacteroidia, Bacilli, Clostridiales, Lactobacillales, Bacteroidales, Lactobacillaceae*, and *Lactobacillus* were the predominant taxa.

Influence of Aβ Levels on Microbiota-Gut-Brain Axis

In order to explore whether Aβ can influence the gut microbiota by targeting the microbiota-gut-brain axis, we injected 10 and 20 μg $A\beta_{1-42}$ into the CA1 region, respectively. Then, the fecal samples were collected once a week and the last 4 weeks, followed by microbiome analysis using the 16S rRNA genes. We also monitored the transcriptome of the small intestine and brain tissues at the 5th week after injection of $A\beta_{1-42}$.

Dynamic Variations of Gut Microbiota and KEGG Pathway Analysis in the $A\beta_{1-42}$-Induced Deficient Rats

The dynamic variations of gut microbiota showed that the diversity in the $A\beta_{1-42}$-induced microbial community (injected 10 or 20 μg fibrillar state of $A\beta_{1-42}$ into the CA1 region) group was reduced in the 4th week (L3, H3) than that in the 2nd and 3rd week (L1, L2 and H1, H2), as shown in **Figures 8B,C**, thereby indicating that such a diversity was reduced with the progression of the disease. **Figures 8D–F** showed that the diversity of the microbial community changed with the levels of $A\beta_{1-42}$, which revealed that the levels of $A\beta_{1-42}$ in the brain influenced the composition of the gut microbiota significantly. We also constructed and visualized a taxonomic tree of the predominant taxa (**Figure 8G**), which displayed that the *Firmicutes, Bacteroidetes, Clostridia, Bacteroidia, Bacilli, Clostridiales, Lactobacillales, Bacteroidales, Lactobacillaceae*, and *Lactobacillus* were the predominant taxa. The changes in the details of predominant taxa (**Figure 8H**), along with the

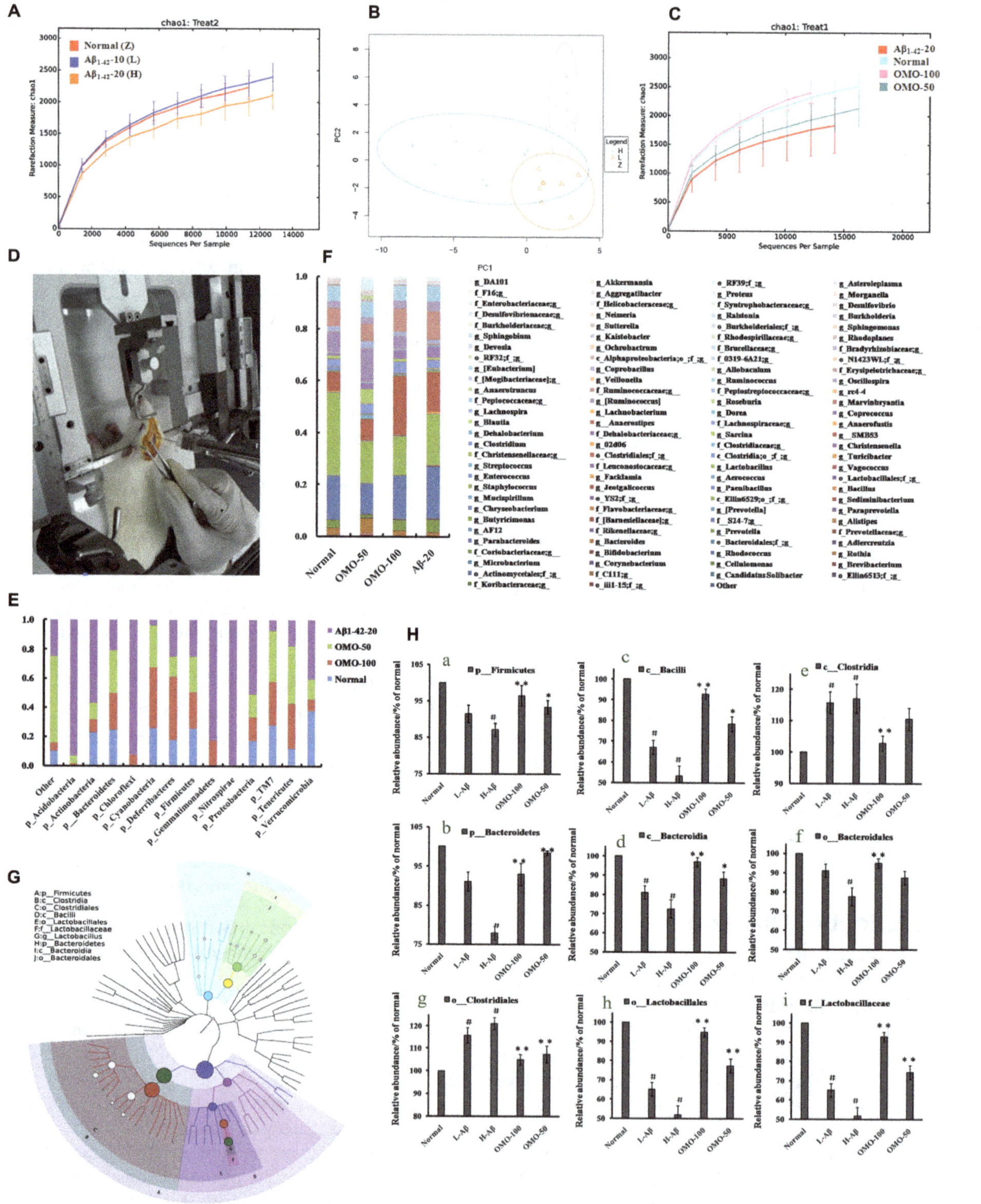

FIGURE 4 | Effects of OMO on gut microbiota in $A\beta_{1-42}$-induced deficient rats. **(A)** Rarefaction curve and **(B)** PCA results of different concentrations of $A\beta_{1-42}$-induced groups, H (20 μg of $A\beta_{1-42}$), L (20 μg of $A\beta_{1-42}$), Z (normal rats with vehicle). **(C)** Rarefaction curve. **(D)** Operation schematic diagram. **(E)** Classification and abundance of cecal contents at the phylum level. **(F)** Classification and abundance of cecal contents at the genus level. **(G)** The dominant species classification tree. **(H)** The relative abundance of the dominant microorganism. Values are the means of six independent experiments.

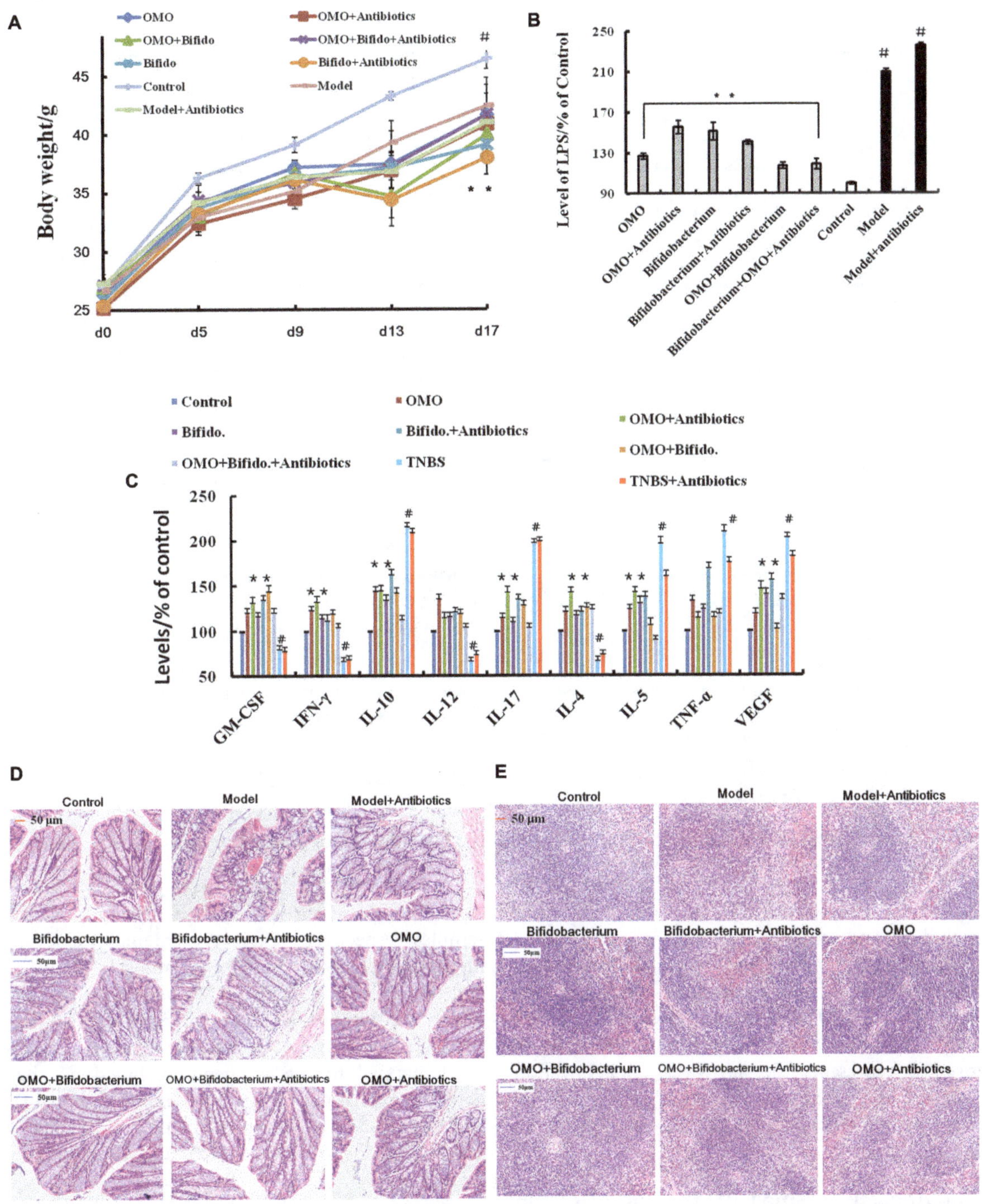

FIGURE 5 | OMO improves the pathological parameters of the high-dose broad spectrum antibiotics and TNBS-induced inflammatory bowel disease (IBD) mice. **(A)** Body weight changes. **(B)** Levels of LPS in serum. **(C)** The levels of cytokines (GM-CSF, TNF-γ, 1L-10, IL-12, 1L-17α, 1L-4, TNF-α, and VGEF-α) in serum. **(D)** The histopathological changes in colon. **(E)** The histopathological changes in spleen. Control is the normal group; model is the TNBS-induced group; model and high-dose antibiotics, HEP3 (100 mg/kg/d), *Bifidobacterium*, HEP3 and high-dose antibiotics, HEP3 and *Bifidobacterium*, *Bifidobacterium* and high-dose antibiotics, HEP3, *Bifidobacterium*, and high-dose antibiotics.

abundance of *Lactobacillaceae*, were negatively correlated with the dose of $A\beta_{1-42}$.

The KEGG pathway analysis showed that the metabolism of xenobiotics biodegradation, nucleotide metabolism, metabolism of terpenoids and polyketides, metabolism of other amino acids, metabolism of cofactors and vitamins, lipid metabolism, glycan biosynthesis and metabolism, enzyme families, energy metabolism, carbohydrate metabolism, biosynthesis of other

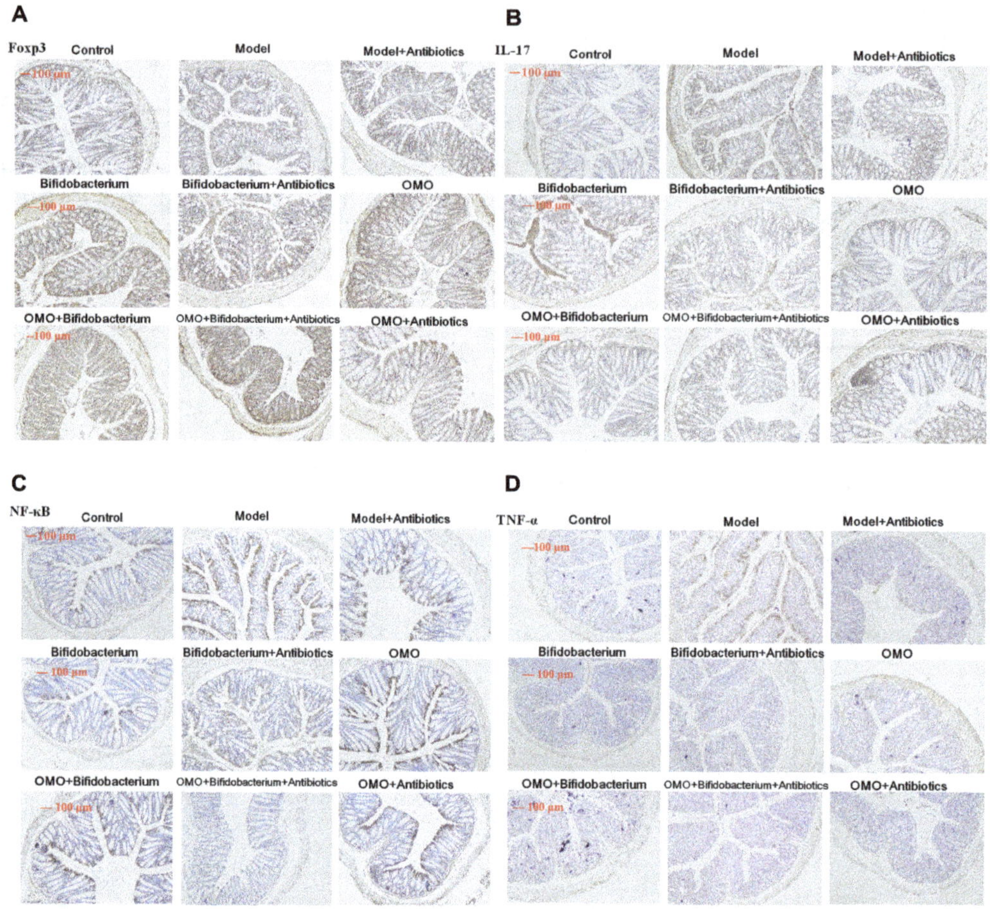

FIGURE 6 | Immunohistochemistry staining of Foxp3 **(A)**, IL-17 **(B)**, NF-κB p65 **(C)**, and TNF-α **(D)** in the colons of different experimental groups in high-dose broad spectrum antibiotics and TNBS-induced IBD mice after treatment with OMO.

secondary metabolites, and amino acid metabolism were altered according to the gut microbiota in the two AD-like rodent models. Additionally, many of these metabolisms were improved by the administration of OMO (**Figure 9A**) showed the dynamic variations in the 2nd, 3rd, and 4th week after injection of $A\beta_{1-42}$. **Figure 9B** represents the 5th week after injection of $A\beta_{1-42}$, all of which showed that the metabolism of gut microbiota was influenced by the levels of $A\beta_{1-42}$ in hippocampus.

Transcriptome Analysis in Small Intestine and Brain in Deficient Rats Post $A\beta_{1-42}$ Injection

Small intestine transcriptome analysis

After injection of $A\beta_{1-42}$ for 4 weeks, the rats were sacrificed, and the intestinal tissues were dissected and frozen in liquid nitrogen for RNA extraction and high-throughput RNA-sequencing. To obtain an overview of the gene expression profile of the intestine in AD model rats, three cDNA samples were generated from each group, mixed, and subjected to sequencing by the Illumina NextSeq 500 platform. Approximately 45,323,472, 55,358,634, and 45,134,740 raw reads with a length of 2 × 150 bp were generated for the $A\beta_{1-42}$-20, $A\beta_{1-42}$-10, and control group samples, respectively. After stringent quality assessment and data filtering, 44,973,944, 54,933,060, and 44,770,698 clean paired-end sequence reads with a Q20 percentage (those with a base quality > 20) over 99% were obtained from the differently treated samples, respectively. Of all the reads, approximately 86.0% were mapped to the rat genome. Based on the normalized data, the expression of 21933 genes was detected (**Figure 10A**), and the relative expressions of DEGs in all the three treated groups ($A\beta_{1-42}$-10, $A\beta_{1-42}$-20, and control) were shown in **Table 1**.

The general chi-squared test was used for the selection of significant DEGs. Based on the criteria of twofold or greater change and Q of $p < 0.05$, 349 unigenes were identified as significant DEGs between $A\beta_{1-42}$-10 and control group samples and 420 unigenes between $A\beta_{1-42}$-20 and control group samples (**Figure 10B**). To elucidate the DEGs in different contents of $A\beta_{1-42}$-induced groups, we used the gene expression profiling. As illustrated in the Venn diagram (**Figure 10C**), the number of genes, as well as the relationships among the overlap between the different groups, were shown in **Figures 10B,D**, indicating that $A\beta_{1-42}$ level in the brain can influence the transcriptome of the intestine.

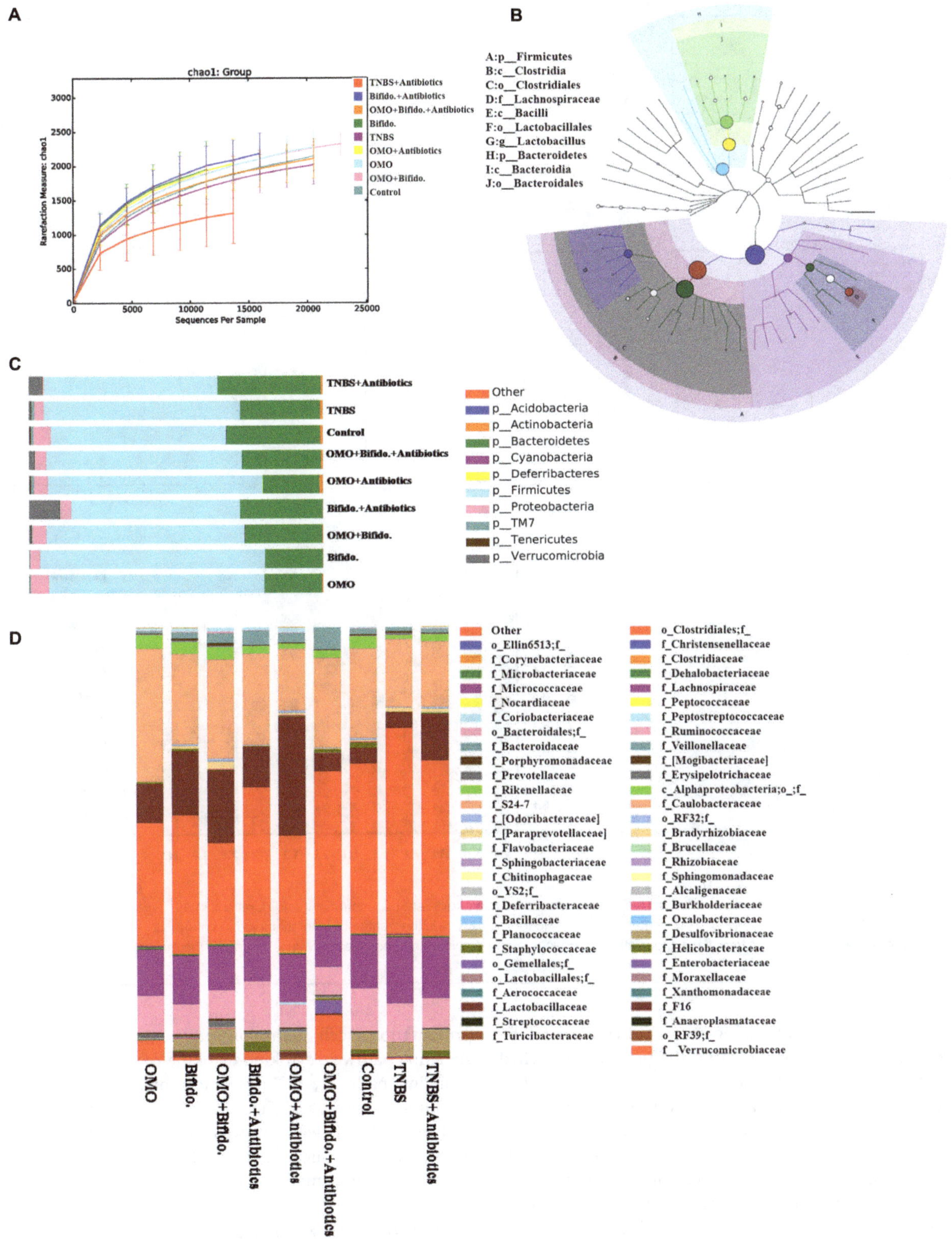

FIGURE 7 | Effects of OMO on the microbiota of cecal contents in high-dose broad spectrum antibiotics and TNBS-induced IBD mice. **(A)** The graph represents the rarefaction curve. **(B)** The dominant species classification tree. **(C)** The classification and abundance of cecal contents at the phylum level. **(D)** The classification and abundance of cecal contents at the family level. Values are the means of six independent experiments.

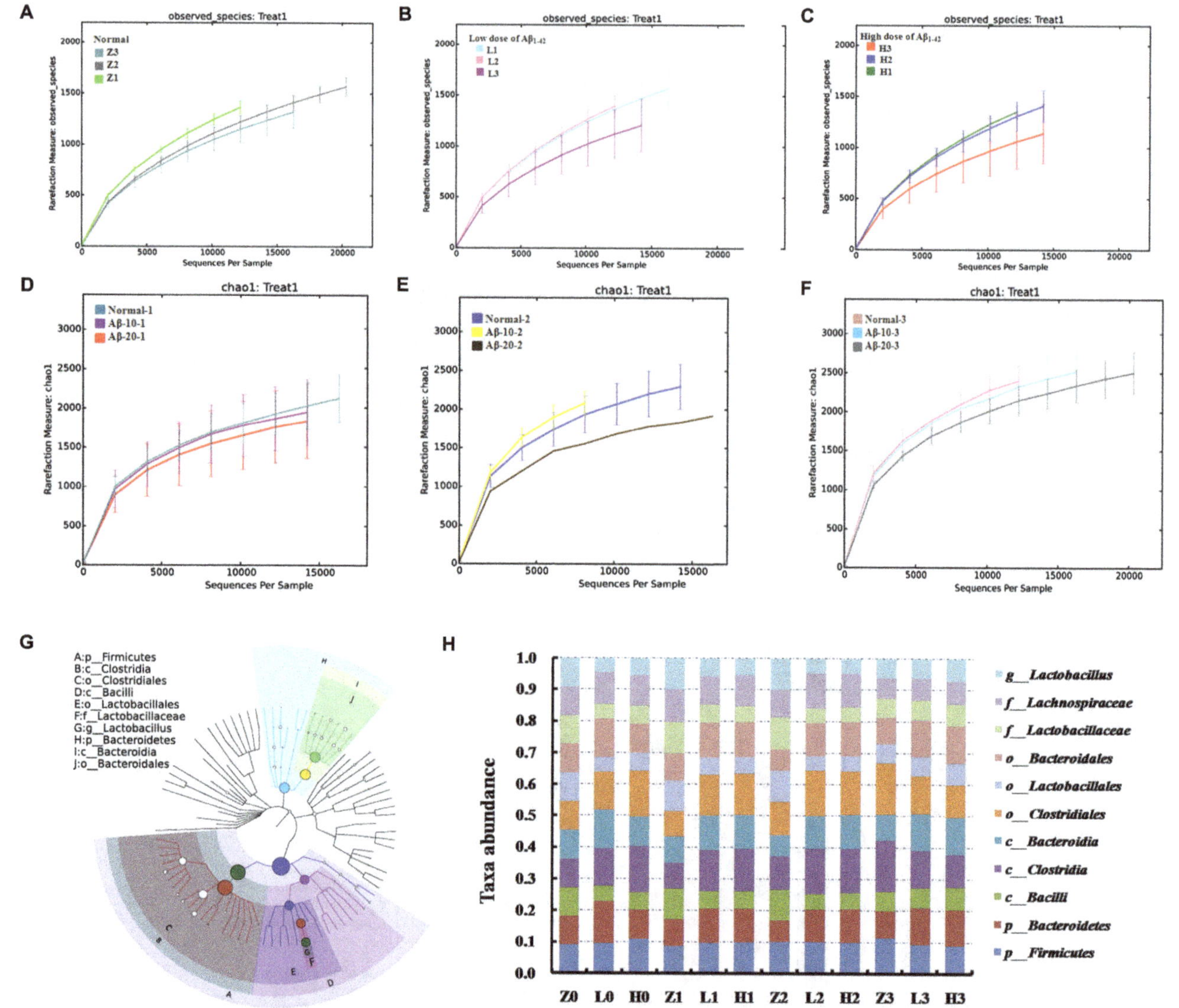

FIGURE 8 | Effects of $A\beta_{1-42}$ on gut microbiota in rats. **(A–F)** The rarefaction curve of different concentrations and durations in $A\beta_{1-42}$-induced groups, H (20 μg of $A\beta_{1-42}$), L (20 μg of $A\beta_{1-42}$), Z (normal rats with vehicle); H1, H2, and H3 (or L1, L2, L3) is the treatment time after injection of $A\beta_{1-42}$ at 2nd, 3rd, and 4th weeks; **(G)** is the dominant species classification tree; **(H)** is the relative abundance of the dominant microorganism. Values represent the means of six independent experiments.

To gain insights into the physiological processes regulated by the different $A\beta_{1-42}$ levels and identify the processes enriched in significant DEGs, we subjected significant DEGs to GO term enrichment analysis and KEGG pathway enrichment, a tool developed to represent the common and basic biological information in the annotation. The GO term enrichment results showed that the immune system, extracellular environment, and antigen reaction (Supplementary Tables S1-1–S1-3) altered in different $A\beta_{1-42}$ levels treated groups, which indicated that the inflammatory response of the gut is activated, the variations in the gut microbiota induced by $A\beta_{1-42}$ primarily influences the immune or inflammatory response in the gut.

The KEGG pathway results showed that the DEGs were mainly enriched in phagosome, antigen processing, and presentation, cell adhesion molecules (CAMs), PI3K-Akt signaling pathway, cytokine-cytokine receptor interaction, PPAR signaling pathway, ECM-receptor interaction, B cell receptor signaling pathway, and chemokine signaling pathway (**Figure 11**, and more details were showed in Supplementary Tables S2-1–S2-3), thereby indicating that $A\beta_{1-42}$ levels in the brain can influence the intestinal functions.

Brain transcriptome analysis

After injection of $A\beta_{1-42}$ for 4 weeks, the rats were sacrificed, and the brain tissues dissected and frozen in liquid nitrogen for RNA extraction and high-throughput RNA-sequencing. The overview of the brain gene expression profile in AD model rats was shown in **Figure 12**. The profiling analysis revealed the number

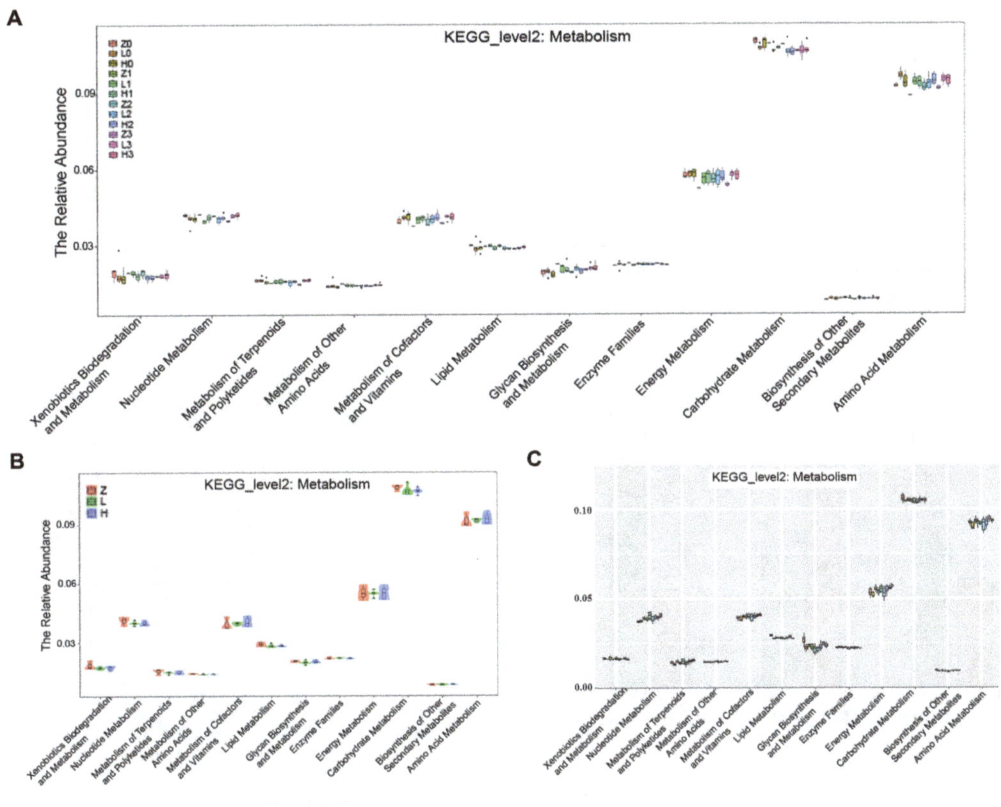

FIGURE 9 | The KEGG pathway enrichment of gut microbiota in the metabolism system. **(A)** The dynamic variations in the 2nd, 3rd, and 4th week after injection of $A\beta_{1-42}$ in rats. **(B)** The 4th week after injection of $A\beta_{1-42}$ in rats. **(C)** The high dose broad spectrum antibiotics and TNBS-induced IBD mice.

of genes (**Figures 12A-a,b**), the DEGs in **Figure 12B**, Venn diagram (**Figure 12C**), as well as, the relationships among the overlap between the different groups in **Figure 12D**; the relative expressions of DEGs in all the three treated groups ($A\beta_{1-42}$-10, $A\beta_{1-42}$-20, and control) were shown in **Table 2**, which indicated that the $A\beta_{1-42}$ levels could significantly influence the brain transcriptome.

The GO term enrichment results revealed that the single-multicellular organism process (GO:0044707), nervous system development (GO:0007399), system development (GO:0048731), single-organism developmental process (GO:0044767), multicellular organism development (GO:0007275), developmental process (GO:0032502), generation of neurons (GO:0048699), neurogenesis (GO:0022008), neuron differentiation (GO:0030182), and cell differentiation (GO:0030154) (Supplementary Tables S3-1–S3-3) were influenced after treatment with $A\beta_{1-42}$. In the $A\beta_{1-42}$-20 group, the synapse (GO:0045202), synaptic signaling (GO:0099536), synaptic transmission (GO:0007268), trans-synaptic signaling (GO:0099537), synapse part (GO:0044456), central nervous system development (GO:0007417), and behavior (GO:0007610) were changed more than that in the $A\beta_{1-42}$-10 group, which indicated that the occurrence of AD is dependent on the cumulative amount of $A\beta_{1-42}$. The KEGG pathway results showed that the DEGs were enriched mainly in neuroactive ligand-receptor interaction, cAMP signaling pathway, calcium signaling pathway, serotonergic synapse, PI3K-Akt signaling pathway, dopaminergic synapse, and ECM-receptor interaction (**Figure 13**, additional details were shown in Supplementary Tables S4-1–S4-3), all which indicated that the $A\beta_{1-42}$ levels can significantly influence the brain function.

DISCUSSION

Increasing evidence suggests that the microbiota-gut-brain axis plays a key role in regulating brain functions, and prebiotics are widely considered to have potential as modulators of brain dysfunctions; however, only limited studies are yet available. Herein, we reported that fructooligosaccharides from *M. officinalis* could markedly modify the behavior, improve oxidative stress and inflammation disorder, regulate the synthesis and secretion of neurotransmitter, ameliorate the swelling of brain tissues, and reduce neuronal apoptosis. We also reported that OMO administration alters the diversity and stability of the microbial community, the expression of the genes of AD intracellular markers such as Tau and $A\beta_{1-42}$. In addition, OMO administration exerted an adequate prebiotic role in regulating the composition and metabolism of gut microbiota in an overdose antibiotics-treated IBD mice model.

Gut microbiota plays a major role in maintaining normal physiological functions in the host. The changes in gut

A

A. Statistics of $A\beta_{1-42}$-induced deficits rat intestine transcriptome sequences

Sample	Useful Reads	Map events count	Total Mapped		Multiple Mapped		Uniquely Mapped	
			Reads	%	Reads	%	Reads	%
$A\beta_{1-42}$-20	54,933,060	55,788,025	47,162,606	85.85	3,019,287	6.40	44,143,319	93.60
$A\beta_{1-42}$-10	44,973,944	42,538,143	38,913,479	86.52	1,862,179	4.79	37,051,300	95.21
Control	44,770,698	43,515,860	38,469,828	85.93	2,078,474	5.40	36,391,354	94.60

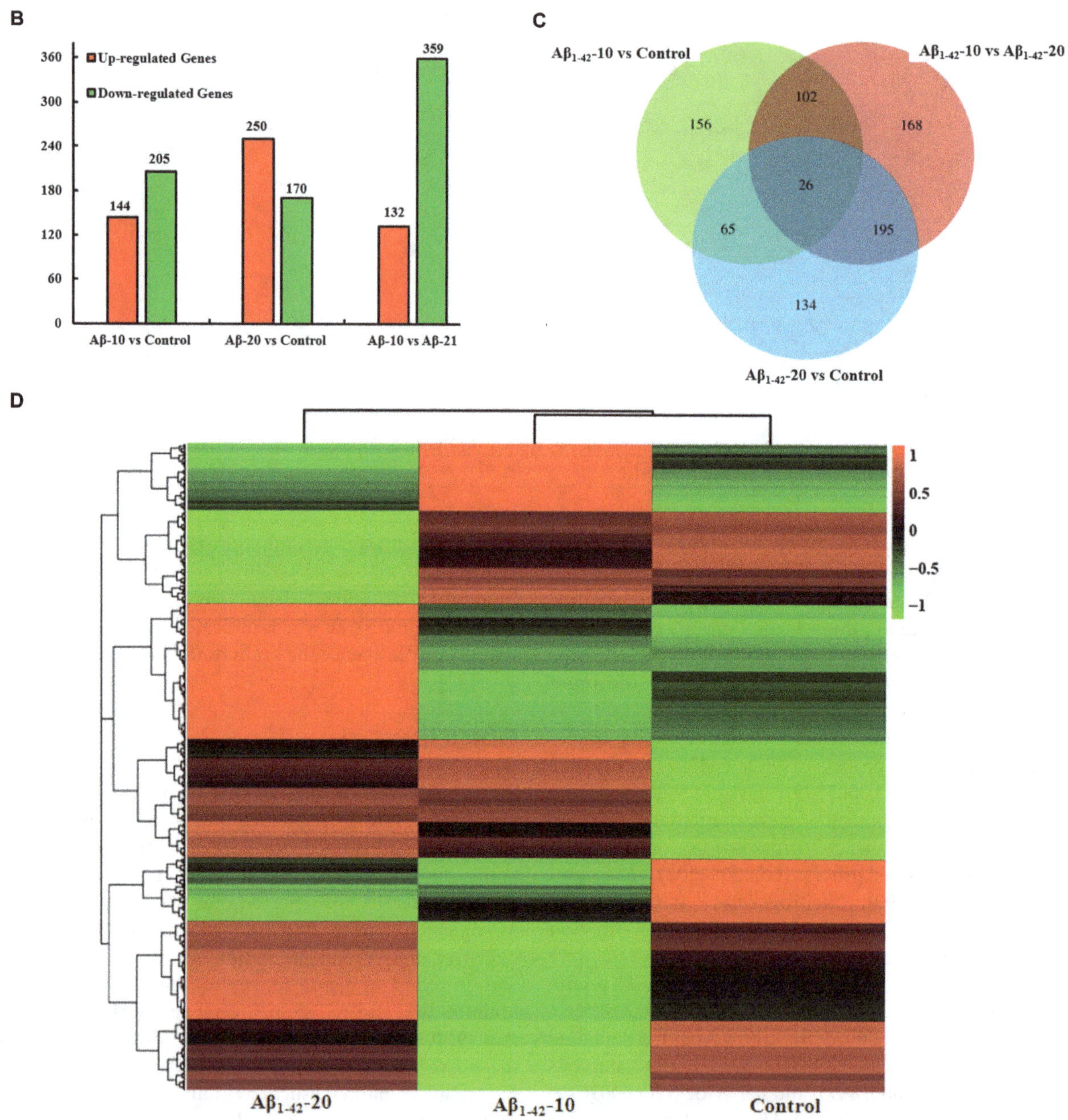

FIGURE 10 | Small intestine transcriptome analysis in the deficit rats by injected $A\beta_{1-42}$. **(A)** The statistics of transcriptome sequences. **(B)** DEGs in the small intestine at different concentrations of $A\beta_{1-42}$. **(C)** Venn diagram of DEGs. **(D)** The heat map of the relative expressions of DEGs in all three groups.

TABLE 1 | Differentially expressed genes (DEGs) in the small intestine of deficient rat injected at different concentration of $A\beta_{1-42}$.

Genes	FoldChange		log2FoldChange		Up–down	*p*-value	
	Normal/Aβ-10	Normal/Aβ-20	Normal/Aβ-10	Normal/Aβ-20		Normal/Aβ-10	Normal/Aβ-20
Slc5a4b	0.09	0.27	−3.47	−1.86	Down	0.000000	0.000494
Nts	0.41	4.57	−1.27	2.19	Down	0.002207	0.000056
Fkbp5	0.27	2.81	−1.90	1.49	Down	0.000004	0.000132
Cubn	0.40	2.81	−1.33	1.49	Down	0.000323	0.000132
Defa8	0.03	0.08	−5.11	−3.66	Down	0.000000	0.000000
AABR07000398.1	0.45	3.21	−1.17	1.68	Down	0.000995	0.000002
LOC257642	0.45	4.12	−1.15	2.04	Down	0.032226	0.012780
Hpse	5.37	0.39	2.43	−1.36	Up	0.000050	0.002196
Nop10	2.12	10.70	1.09	3.42	Down	0.032836	0.000000
Arhgdib	2.22	0.49	1.15	−1.03	Up	0.006915	0.007868
AABR07065789.1	2.13	7.85	1.09	2.97	Down	0.026618	0.000001
Reg3g	2.72	0.35	1.44	−1.52	Up	0.000232	0.000032
Rps24	4.88	66.16	2.29	6.05	Down	0.000000	0.000000
Pou2af1	2.14	0.36	1.10	−1.47	Up	0.048293	0.001217
Adh6	2.32	0.14	1.21	−2.88	Up	0.004548	0.000000
RGD1311933	2.24	5.12	1.16	2.36	Down	0.006467	0.000000
Rps27	2.08	19.07	1.05	4.25	Down	0.003563	0.000000
Wfdc21	2.46	0.45	1.30	−1.15	Up	0.002445	0.002823
Rps27a-ps1	3.22	6.84	1.69	2.77	Down	0.000020	0.000000
Ccl21	3.20	0.30	1.68	−1.73	Up	0.001820	0.000047
Pdx1	3.20	0.49	1.68	−1.03	Up	0.007298	0.037669
AABR07051670.1	7.56	0.36	2.92	−1.49	Up	0.000008	0.000992
Igkv5-48	30.08	0.32	4.91	−1.65	Up	0.000000	0.000302
AABR07051684.1	23.10	0.27	4.53	−1.91	Up	0.001867	0.003488
AABR07065768.3	23.64	0.11	4.56	−3.25	Up	0.032367	0.000002
Akp3	13.94	0.13	3.80	−2.93	Up	0.000000	0.000000

microbiota can lead to changes in brain function, thereby affecting the host behavior (Vuong et al., 2017). Recent studies showed a significant correlation between the changes in gut microbiota and cognitive behavior (Dinan and Cryan, 2017). The modulation of gut microbiota by germ-free animals, probiotics or antibiotics intervention, and fecal microbiota transplantation (FMT) can influence the cognitive behavior of the host (Hu et al., 2016). Our data were in agreement with previous studies, showing that the gut microbiota in two AD-like model rats was altered as compared to the normal rats, as the abundance of *Clostridia* and *Clostridiales* in $A\beta_{1-42}$-induced groups increased significantly ($p < 0.05$), while the groups administered OMO can reverse those changes, especially the probiotic *Lactobacillus* and *Akkermansia* increased distinctly ($p < 0.05$).

The probiotic administration had a marked effect on the cognitive behavior. The prototype probiotic bacterium has been found to up-regulate the hormone oxytocin and systemic immune responses in order to achieve a broad range of health benefits involving wound healing, mental health, metabolism, and myoskeletal maintenance (Servin, 2004; Erdman and Poutahidis, 2016). Studies showed that *Lactobacillus pentosus* var. plantarum C29 from kimchi, a traditional food manufactured by fermenting vegetables (Park et al., 2014), was beneficial to health. It can also protect the memory deficits by inducing the expressions of BDNF and p-CREB in scopolamine-induced memory-deficient mice (Jung et al., 2012), anti-inflammatory amelioration of age-dependent memory impairment in Fischer 344 rats (Jeong et al., 2015), and ameliorate memory impairment and inflammation in D-galactose-induced accelerated aging mouse (Woo et al., 2014). Another study also showed that *L. plantarum* could attenuate anxiety-related behavior and protect against stress-induced dysbiosis in adult zebrafish (Davis et al., 2016). *Lactobacilli* and *Bifidobacteria* exhibited antagonistic activities against microbial pathogens (Servin, 2004). Our data were in agreement with previous studies showing that *Lactobacillus* can ameliorate memory deficiencies (**Figure 4H**); the relative abundance of $A\beta_{1-42}$-induced *Lactobacillus* was reduced starkly, especially in the high-dose group. As a result of OMO administration, the relative abundance of *Lactobacillus* was increased significantly; also, the MWM tests showed that the learning and memory abilities were improved (**Figure 3B**). These results suggested that OMO can promote the abundance of *Lactobacillus* and ameliorate the memory deficiencies.

Fructo-oligosaccharides (FOS) are commonly regarded as a type of prebiotics, favorably stimulating the growth of *Bifidobacteria* and *Lactobacilli*. FOS from *Stevia rebaudiana* roots

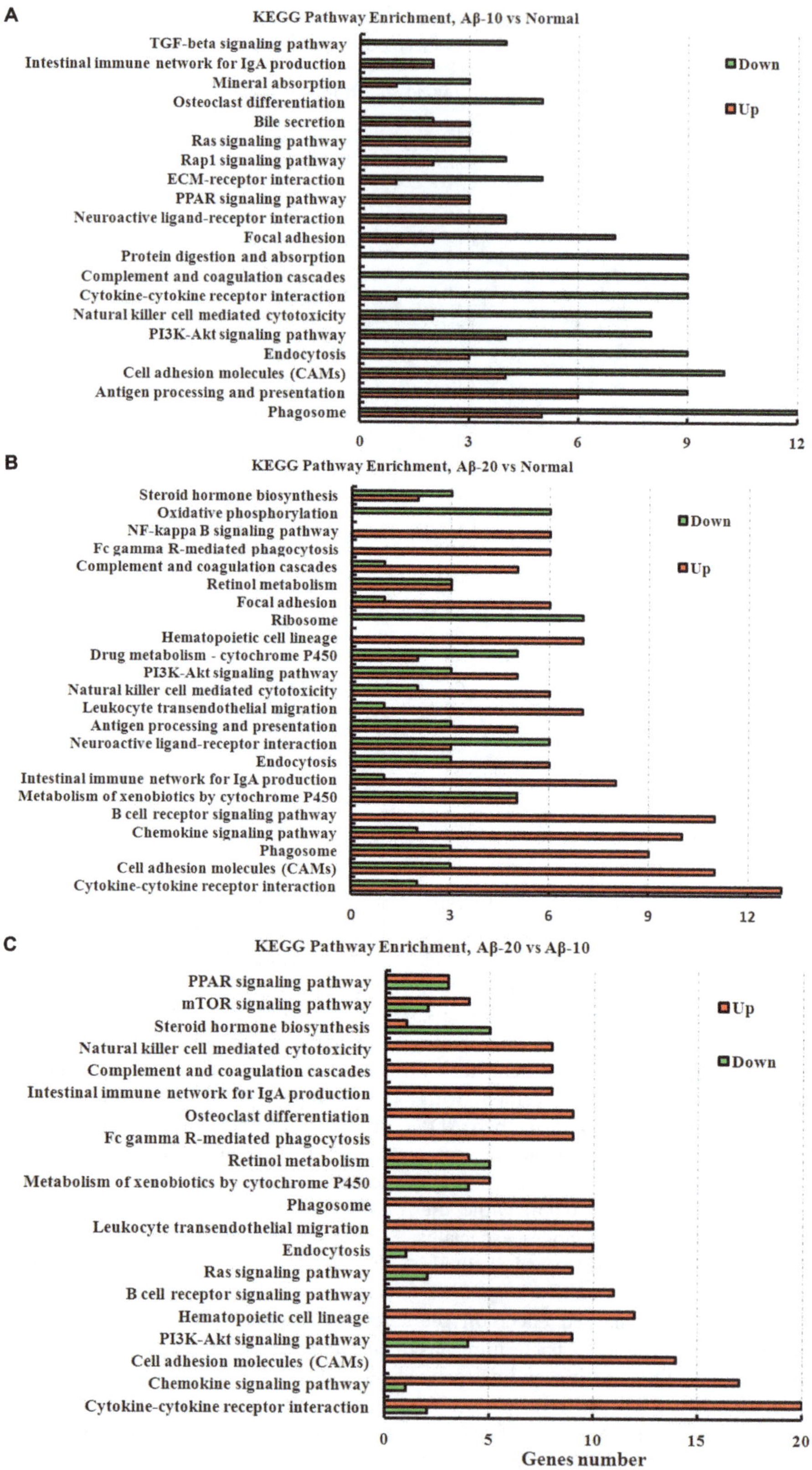

FIGURE 11 | The KEGG pathway enrichment of DEGs in the small intestine transcriptome in deficient rats induced by $A\beta_{1-42}$. **(A)** The group of Aβ-10 vs. the Normal; **(B)** the group of Aβ-20 vs. the Normal; **(C)** the group of Aβ-20 vs. the Aβ-10.

A

A-a. Statistics of Aβ_{1-42}-induced deficits rat brain RNA sequences mapped

Sample	Useful reads	Map event	Map reads	Map reads/%	Multiple reads	Multiple reads/%	Unique reads	Unique reads/%
Aβ_{1-42}-10	142490562	411476820	129291217	90.74	60113374	46.49	69177843	53.51
Aβ_{1-42}-20	143270656	444440717	131174213	91.56	63112535	48.11	68061678	51.89
Control	144332070	413610803	131924767	91.40	61196946	46.39	70727821	53.61

A-b. Statistics of Aβ_{1-42}-induced deficits rat brain RNA sequences mapped events

Sample	Map events count	Mapped to gene	Mapped to gene/%	Mapped to inter gene	Mapped to inter gene/%	Mapped to exon	Mapped to exon/%
Aβ_{1-42}-10	411476820	397038221	96.49	14438599	3.51	387464643	94.16
Aβ_{1-42}-20	444440717	431078830	96.99	13361887	3.01	418683541	94.20
Control	413610803	398932568	96.45	14678235	3.55	388408941	93.91

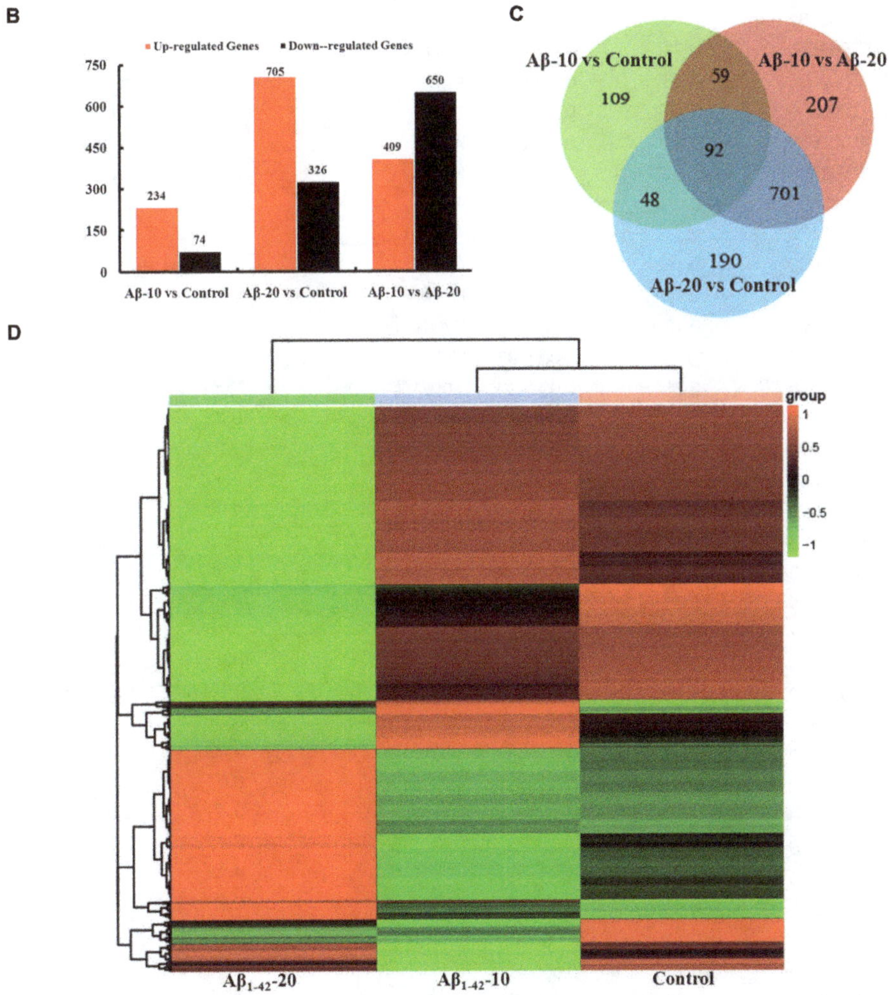

FIGURE 12 | Brain transcriptome analysis in the deficit rats by injected Aβ_{1-42}. **(A)** Statistics of the transcriptome sequences. **(B)** The differentially expressed genes in the brain at different concentration of Aβ_{1-42}. **(C)** Venn diagram of DEGs. **(D)** The heat map of the relative expressions of DEGs in all the three groups.

enhanced the growth of specific strains of both *Bifidobacteria* and *Lactobacilli*, especially, with respect to their fermentation ability (Sanches Lopes et al., 2016). FOS are reserve carbohydrates with important positive health effects and technological applications in the food industry. Another previous study indicated that short-chain fructooligosaccharides could be used optimally in combination with *Bifidobacterium animalis* or *B. longum* strains for the development of synbiotic foods or dietary supplements (Valdés-Varela et al., 2017). Our results showed that FOS from *M. officinalis* also enhances the growth

TABLE 2 | Differentially expressed genes in the brain of the deficient rats injected at different concentrations of $A\beta_{1-42}$.

Genes	Aβ-10		Aβ-20	
	Foldchange (Normal/Aβ-10)	*p*-value	Foldchange (Normal/Aβ-20)	*p*-value
Cbln1	10.94	0.000000	0.13	0.000105
Grm4	2.39	0.000030	0.21	0.002146
Pcp2	60.50	0.000000	0.09	0.000007
Uncx	36.00	0.000034	0.09	0.000041
Adora2a	2.31	0.000004	15.53	0.000001
Wdr66	3.13	0.000018	0.19	0.001367
Lhx5	Infinity	0.000034	0.20	0.007717
Barhl2	3.13	0.036893	0.09	0.000025
Lhx1	30.79	0.000182	0.10	0.000055
Slc6a4	10.61	0.004566	0.23	0.015495
Gabra6	107.05	0.000000	0.06	0.000000
Rgs9	2.88	0.000000	10.66	0.000012
Tph2	4.79	0.007662	0.21	0.006924
Arhgap6	2.00	0.001638	8.30	0.000186
Btg1	2.16	0.000475	0.34	0.034729
Rxrg	2.33	0.000179	15.69	0.000004
Neurod1	3.51	0.000000	0.11	0.000025
Car8	3.90	0.000000	0.12	0.000060
St14	2.78	0.017265	0.13	0.000206
Trim54	0.36	0.000003	11.11	0.000192
Grid2	2.34	0.000518	0.21	0.002420
Slc30a3	0.46	0.000006	5.77	0.000880
En2	191.37	0.000000	0.10	0.000026
Arhgef33	9.12	0.000000	0.11	0.000050
Tac1	4.23	0.000000	31.52	0.000000
Slc1a6	2.00	0.016579	0.11	0.000032
Crtam	2.24	0.000013	0.28	0.010983
Crtam	Infinity	0.000115	0.08	0.000020
Drd2	2.73	0.000002	10.76	0.000026
Cga	22.26	0.002718	0.08	0.000031
Kcnh5	0.37	0.000000	4.25	0.007422
Nyx	3.68	0.036361	0.13	0.000541
Fibcd1	2.76	0.000000	24.48	0.000000
Satb2	0.47	0.000200	43.65	0.000000
Hes3	7.22	0.008186	0.07	0.000006
Irx3	15.47	0.004015	0.14	0.001121
Adamts18	3.02	0.045565	0.11	0.000091
Il16	3.40	0.000000	0.10	0.000019
Tfap2b	3.39	0.022277	0.19	0.003907
Ppp1r17	17.05	0.000000	0.12	0.000083
Impg1	Infinity	0.009945	0.08	0.000060
Fat2	33.50	0.000000	0.10	0.000009
Irx2	9.63	0.003845	0.11	0.000157
Rgl3	3.76	0.000002	0.11	0.000045
Barhl1	21.79	0.003154	0.20	0.011641
Cdhr1	2.16	0.001501	18.13	0.000003
Glra1	3.33	0.005627	0.22	0.005136
Cbln2	0.43	0.000035	0.21	0.042611
Pax3	Infinity	0.035388	6.15	0.008361
Kcns1	0.12	0.000000	0.10	0.000187
Skor1	35.05	0.005526	0.16	0.000376
Zic1	3.08	0.000000	0.35	0.049800
Zic4	2.01	0.047534	14.65	0.000001
Cpne7	2.09	0.000020	77.78	0.000000
Emx1	0.46	0.001804	0.35	0.038103
Kcng4	2.18	0.000235	0.30	0.023002
Zfp521	3.24	0.000000	0.20	0.001811
Calb2	3.89	0.000000	0.17	0.000482
LOC688778	0.46	0.000054	51.87	0.000000
Atp2a3	4.19	0.000000	0.13	0.000074
Ptpn22	Infinity	0.035388	0.07	0.000080
Gng7	2.88	0.000000	24.88	0.000000
Asic4	2.15	0.000048	11.89	0.000008
Npas4	2.04	0.000529	13.37	0.000006
Cbln3	108.68	0.000000	0.08	0.000002
Adra1d	0.49	0.000370	4.54	0.006404
Ctxn3	3.24	0.006074	0.16	0.000811
Drd1	2.50	0.000005	35.19	0.000000
Syndig1l	3.07	0.000000	17.72	0.000001
Cdh15	2.20	0.000772	0.20	0.001638
Cnpy1	36.47	0.000030	0.11	0.000160
Robo3	0.22	0.000001	26.35	0.001324
Cyp11b2	0.23	0.000000	6.98	0.004899
Lrrc10b	2.40	0.000035	34.15	0.000000
Mab21l2	4.00	0.000280	0.17	0.000872
Slc6a5	4.53	0.003476	0.08	0.000009
Myom3	6.95	0.000135	0.33	0.049080
Svep1	2.27	0.000253	0.13	0.000107
Tll1	2.15	0.034882	0.20	0.003254
Irx1	5.63	0.001444	0.23	0.009492
Eomes	10.74	0.030867	0.07	0.000011
Tmem215	0.34	0.000002	10.90	0.000267
Spp1	3.32	0.000003	0.15	0.000348
Comp	6.67	0.000051	0.29	0.024367
Shisa8	3.49	0.000142	0.13	0.000128
Gpr6	2.45	0.000035	72.86	0.000000
Gdf10	4.42	0.001245	0.16	0.000964
Zic2	2.20	0.001201	0.21	0.002489
Dao	11.94	0.000011	0.12	0.000114
Lrp2	3.58	0.000003	0.28	0.013024
AABR07010944.1	Infinity	0.006930	0.12	0.001066
Sdc1	4.80	0.000003	0.11	0.000046

of some probiotics similar to that of *Bifidobacteria* and *Lactobacilli*.

The microbiota can modulate the changes in the gut barrier as well as metabolic and inflammatory responses. Gut barrier function is a key to maintaining a balanced response between the host and its microbiome. This highly complex system involves numerous microbiota-derived factors. *Akkermansia muciniphila* is positively correlated with a lean phenotype, reduced body weight gain, amelioration of metabolic responses, and restoration of gut barrier function is effectuated by the modulation of mucus layer thickness (Bland, 2016; Derrien et al., 2016; Greer et al., 2016; Henning et al., 2017; Van Herreweghen et al., 2017). Our data in D-galactose-induced deficient rats showed that the *Akkermansia* were increased ($p < 0.05$, **Figure 2D**), and the intestinal pathological tissue changes (**Figure 1E**) were improved after administration of OMO, thereby indicating that OMO administration can improve the gut barrier function via targeting the abundance of *Akkermansia*, but need more studies.

Increased gut permeability (leaky gut) and alterations in gut microbiota are now widely accepted as an important link with the etiology, course, and treatment of several neuropsychiatric disorders (Anderson et al., 2016). Gut microbiota-released LPS contributes to chronic inflammation and oxidative stress (Le Sage et al., 2017). Moreover, inflammation was first implicated in AD pathology and development, with the neuropathological findings of activated inflammatory cells (microglia and astrocytes) and inflammatory proteins (for example, cytokines and complement), surrounding the amyloid plaques and the nerve fiber tangles (Alkasir et al., 2017). Our study showed that OMO administration could reduce the levels of LPS in TNBS-induced IBD mice and some pro-inflammatory cytokines in both $A\beta_{1-42}$ induced deficit rats (**Figure 3C**) and TNBS-induced IBD mice (**Figures 5C, 6**). On the other hand, it can increase the levels of some anti-inflammatory cytokines, which suggested that the administration of OMO (prebiotics) can improve the host inflammatory immune response. The data also showed that OMO administration could enhance the oxidative stress, similar to elevated SOD, MDA, CAT, and inhibiting the MDA production in the D-galactose-induced deficit rats (**Figure 1D**). The gut microbiota is known to play a vital role in those responses (Vanegas et al., 2017), although not fully understood. Taken together, we can summarize that OMO administration influences the host inflammatory immune response and oxidative stress by regulating the gut microbiota.

Preliminary data suggested that FOS increases fecal *Bifidobacteria*, induce immunoregulatory dendritic cell (DC) responses, and reduce the disease activity in patients with Crohn's disease (Benjamin et al., 2011). Moreover, *Bifidobacteria* are predominant bacterial species in the human gut microbiota and have been considered to exert a beneficial effect on human health by maintaining the equilibrium of the resident organisms. *B. longum* with FOS reduces TNF-α, CRP, serum AST levels, HOMA-IR, serum endotoxin, steatosis, and the non-alcoholic steatohepatitis activity index significantly (Malaguarnera et al., 2012). Human milk contains *B. breve*, *Streptococcus thermophilus*, and short-chain galactooligosaccharides/long-chain fructooligosaccharides with pectin-derived acidic oligosaccharides conferring a protective role against gastrointestinal infections: ameliorating the AD symptoms, modulating the immune response, binding the viral particles, and protecting against rotavirus infection (Rigo-Adrover et al., 2017). The combination of fermented formula with short-chain galactooligosaccharides and long-chain fructooligosaccharides was well-tolerated showing a low overall crying time, low incidence of infantile colic infection, and a stool-softening effect in healthy term infants (Vandenplas et al., 2017). After a broad spectrum antibiotics treatment, the IBD mice model showed that FOS from *M. officinalis* also increases fecal *Bifidobacteria*, ameliorates the symptoms of IBD, and modulates the immune response; the $A\beta_{1-42}$ induced deficient rats showed a similar effect.

The gut microbiota can regulate the activity in the peripheral and central nervous system by various means of communication including vagal nerve and adrenergic nerve activation as well as producing several molecular candidates such as neurotransmitters, neuropeptides, endocrine hormones, and immunomodulators. Host stress hormones, such as noradrenaline, might affect the bacterial activities or signal between bacteria may change the microbial diversity and actions of the gut microbiota. However, these bacteria are capable of synthesizing and releasing several neurotransmitters and neuromodulators or eliciting the synthesis and release of neuropeptides from enteroendocrine cells. Previous studies showed that *Lactobacillus* and *Bifidobacterium* species could produce short-chain fatty acids; *Escherichia*, *Bacillus*, and *Saccharomyces* spp. can produce norepinephrine; spore-forming microbes can produce 5-HT; *Bacillus* can produce dopamine, and *Lactobacillus* can produce acetylcholine (Wall et al., 2014; Potgieter et al., 2015; Yano et al., 2015; Alkasir et al., 2017). In this study, the monoamine neurotransmitter (NE, DA, 5-HT, and 5-HIAA) levels in the brain tissue were reduced in $A\beta_{1-42}$ induced deficient rats, and the OMO administration can reverse this decreasing tendency. Thus, we can conclude that OMO influences some bacteria that affect the synthesis and release of some neurotransmitters and neuromodulators. Similar effects were observed in mice subjected to chronic stress, where the observed behavioral, neurochemical, genetic, and neuroendocrine changes after prebiotic (fructooligosaccharides and galactooligosaccharides) administration could be mediated partially by short chain fatty acids (SCFAs) (Burokas et al., 2017); the increased levels of acetate, propionate, and n-butyrate correlated with behavior and gene expression.

We also observed novel changes in microbiota composition, especially the increase in *Bifidobacterium*, immunological enhancement (**Figures 5, 6**), and gut barrier impairment (**Figure 5**) in TNBS-induced IBD mice. Previous reports showed that *Bifidobacterium* combined with *L. acidophilus*, *L. casei*, and *L. fermentum* for 12 weeks can affect the cognitive function and some metabolic statuses in AD patients (Akbari et al., 2016), and *B. longum* 1714 reduced the stress and improved the memory in healthy volunteers (Allen et al., 2016). The abundance of *Bacteroides* was also increased with OMO administration in the two AD-like animal models (**Figures 3, 5**). *Bacteroides* are strict anaerobes critical since the initiation of life (Arboleya et al., 2015), and some strains have been used as probiotics. Previous studies have shown that *Bacteroides fragilis* could reverse the autism-like behavior in mice (Hsiao et al., 2013).

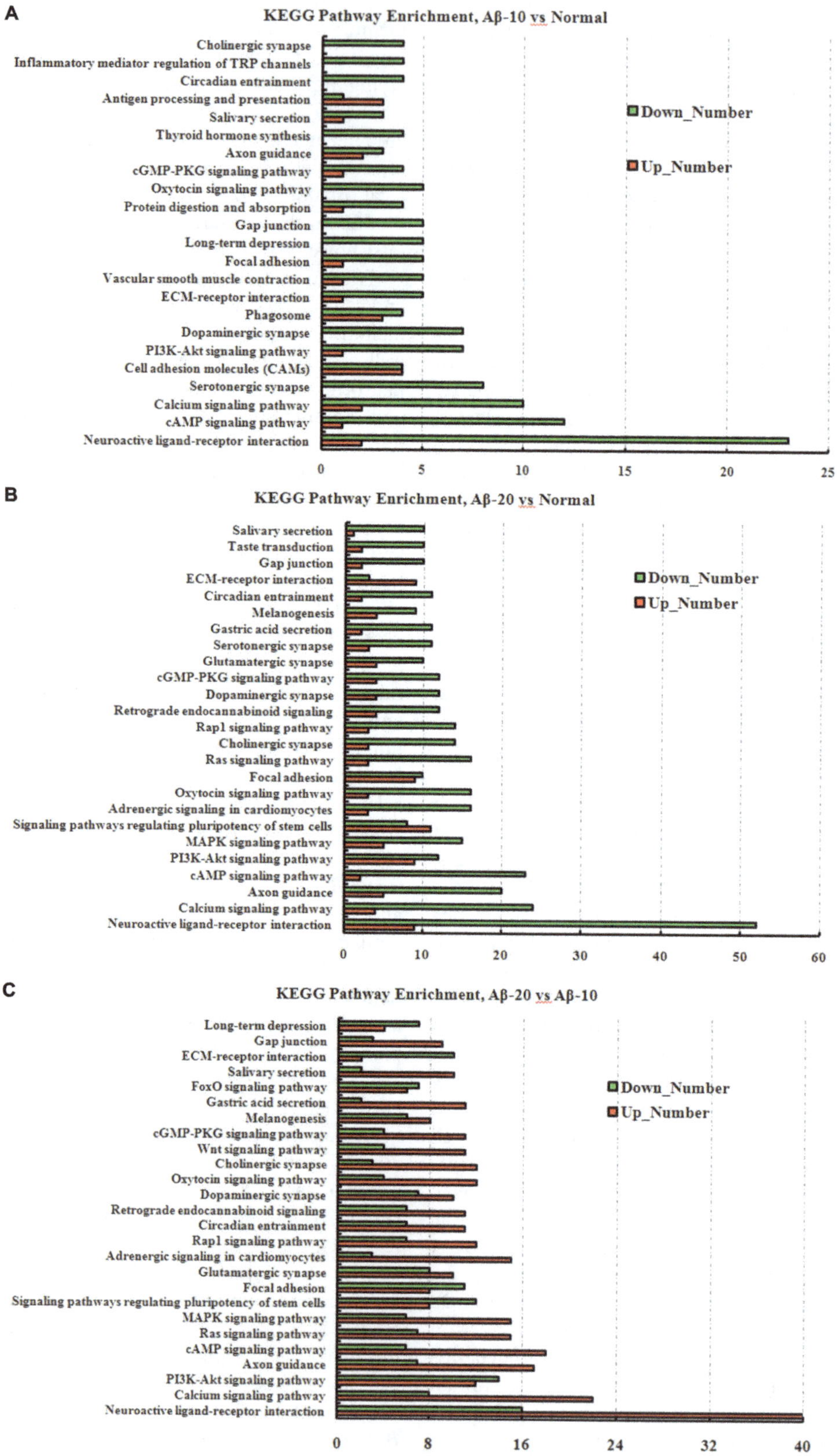

FIGURE 13 | The KEGG pathway enrichment of DEGs in brain transcriptome in the deficit rats induced by Aβ$_{1-42}$. **(A)** The group of Aβ-10 vs. the Normal; **(B)** the group of Aβ-20 vs. the Normal; **(C)** the group of Aβ-20 vs. the Aβ-10.

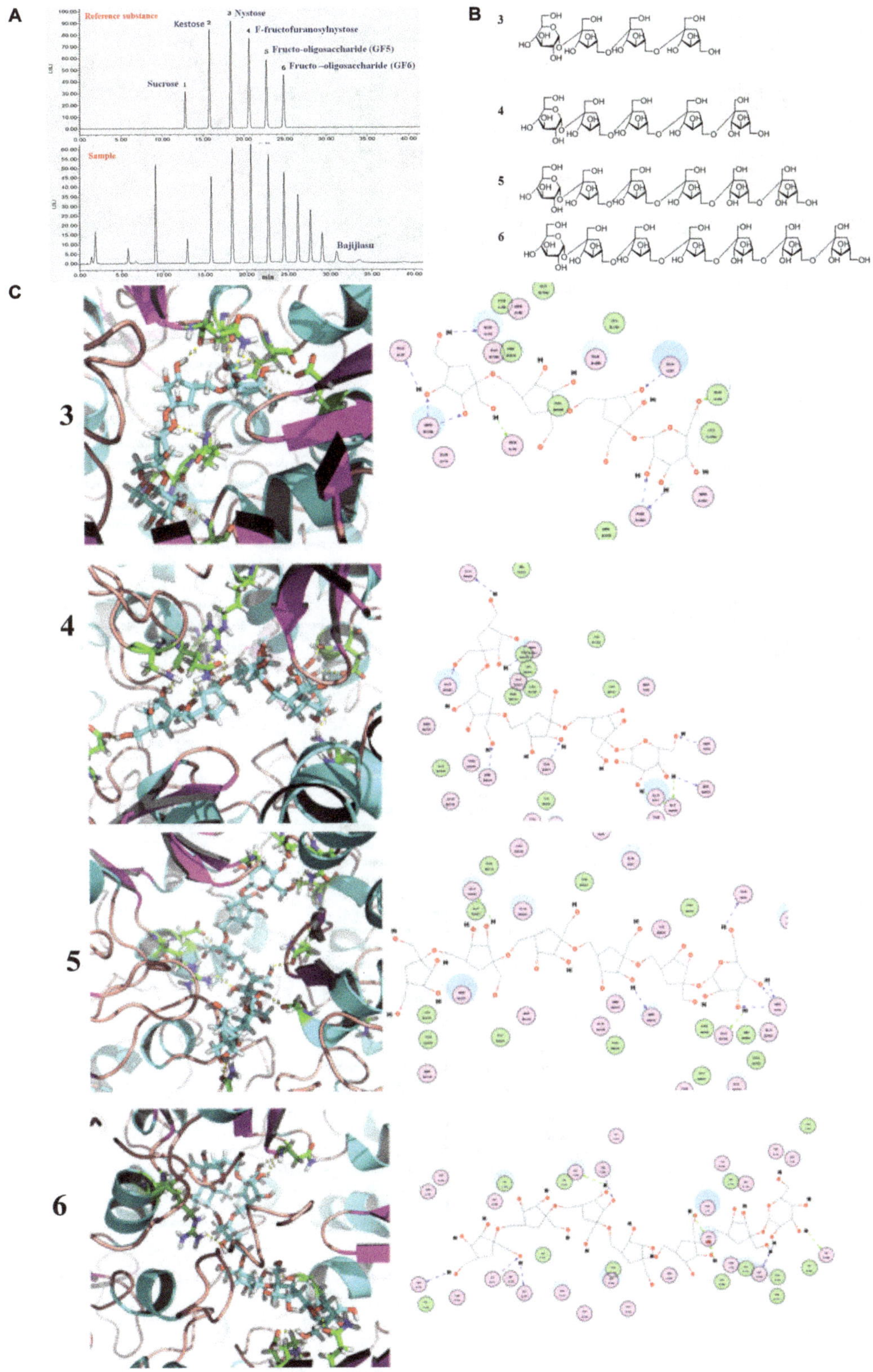

FIGURE 14 | Binding pattern of fructooligosaccharides from *Morinda officinalis*: **(A)** HPLC-ELSD analysis of fructooligosaccharides from *M. officinalis*. **(B)** The chemical structure of nystose (3), *F*-fructofuranose nystose (4), fructooligosaccharide (GF5, 5), fructooligosaccharide (GF6, 6); **(C)** The docked poses were ranked by CDOCKER- ENERGY and the top 10 poses with the co-crystal ligand for SusCD were retained. The data revealed compounds 3, 4, 5, and 6 with CDOCKER-ENERGY of −52.0244180, −75.5881, −101.88, and −110.387, respectively.

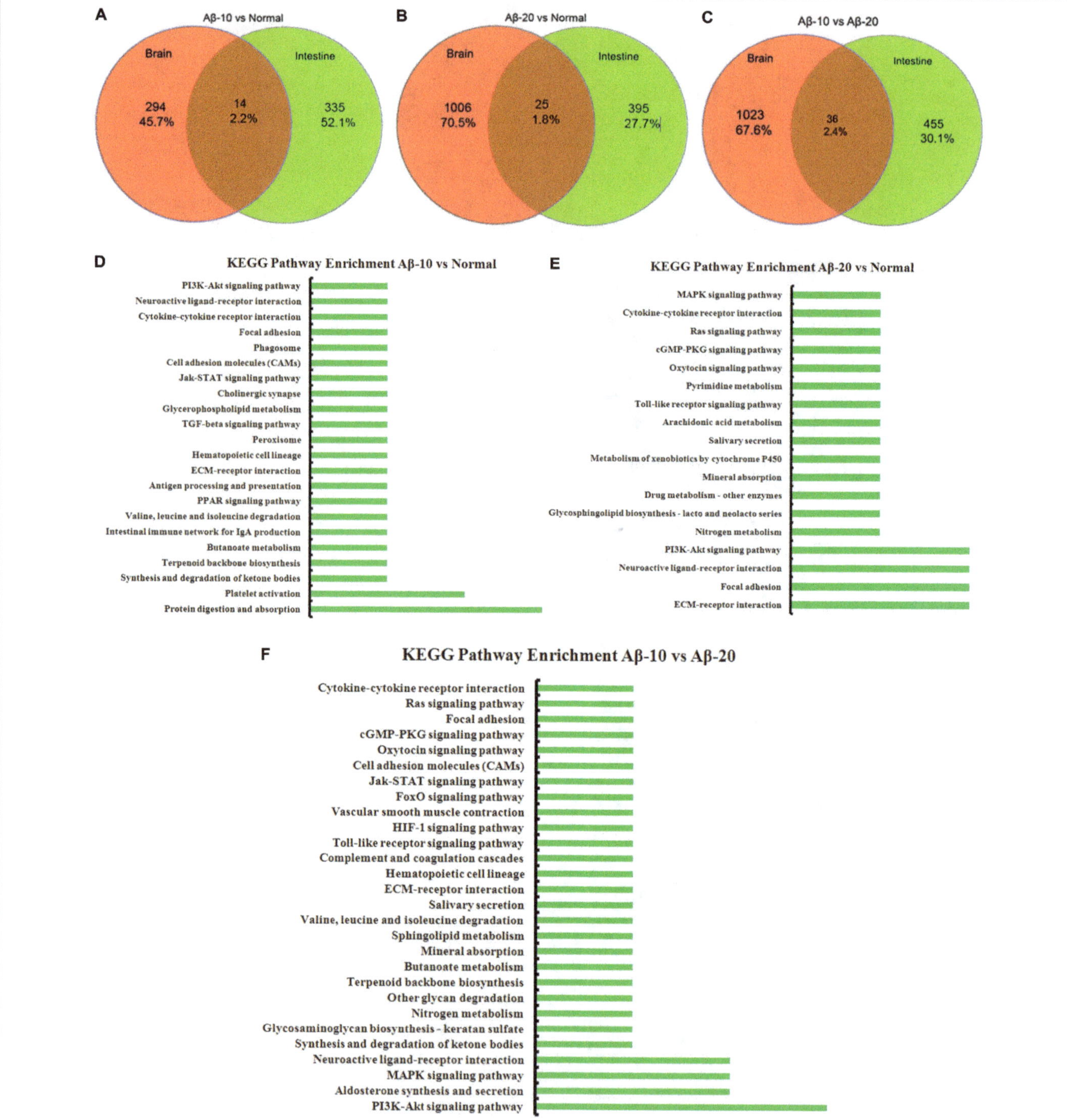

FIGURE 15 | The interactive information analysis of DEGs in brain and intestine in deficient rats by injected $A\beta_{1-42}$. **(A–C)** Wayne chart of DEGs in the brain and intestine transcriptome. **(D–F)** KEGG pathway enrichment of DEGs in the brain and intestine transcriptome.

The gut microbiota contains highly diverse microbial communities that play a critical role in the metabolic, immunological, and protective functions in health. This phenomenon is influenced by several factors including genetics, host physiology (age of the host, disease, and stress) and environmental factors such as living conditions and use of medications. Increasingly, diet has been recognized as a key environmental factor that mediates the composition and metabolic function of the gut microbiota. Furthermore, the consumption of specific dietary ingredients, such as oil, fibers, and prebiotics, is an avenue that modulates the microbiota. Studies on pigs also suggests that the combination with fructooligosaccharides might represent a valuable symbiotic strategy to increase the probiotic levels of bacteria and survival in the gastrointestinal tracts for feed and food applications (Tanner et al., 2015). The administration of such oligosaccharides is attributable to high interindividual variation of the communities in fecal bacteria from pet cats and dogs (Garcia-Mazcorro et al., 2017). In this study, the fructooligosaccharides were extracted from *M. officinalis*, which was widely used in soup, wine, and sweetmeats in South China. Fructo-oligosaccharides are soluble fiber extensively used as prebiotics that is conventionally associated with the stimulation of beneficial bacteria such as *Bifidobacteria* and *Lactobacilli*, among other gut members. However, the mechanisms underlying the fructooligosaccharides stimulation of the beneficial bacteria are yet unknown. A previous study showed that the obtained nutrients process of bacteria require cell membrane protein machines called SusCD complexes (extracellular substrate binding proteins and SusC transporter) (Glenwright et al., 2017), in order to detect the binding capacities between SusCD and nutrients (as starch and other dietary polysaccharides) can evaluate the activity of prebiotics of nutritional ingredients. In this study, the molecular docking analysis was carried out for the evaluation of the binding capacities between SusCD and fructooligosaccharides from *M. officinalis*. The molecular docking study was conducted using the CDOCKER protocol for the four polysaccharides from *M. officinalis* using the Discovery Studio 2.5 (DS2.5) Provisional software. A total of four components (**Figures 14A,B**) from *M. officinalis* were assimilated by literature search, and 1048 poses were generated for all the compounds investigated. The docked poses were ranked by the CDOCKER-ENERGY, and the top 10 poses with the co-crystal ligand for SusCD were retained (**Figure 14**). The data revealed 4 hits namely, compounds 3 (Nystose), 4 (*F*-fructofuranosylnystose), 5 (fructooligosaccharide, GF5), and 6 (fructooligosaccharide, GF6) with CDOCKER-ENERGY -52.0244180, -75.5881, -101.88, and -110.387, respectively (**Figure 14C**). This indicated that the 4 polysaccharides might exert a potent binding activity on SusCD. The interaction between the SusCD protein and the four compounds was further analyzed using the receptor-ligand interaction module in DS. The analysis between SusCD and compound 3 revealed that 9 hydrogen bond interactions appeared in the docked pose. The analysis between SusCD and compound 5 revealed that 9 hydrogen bond interactions appeared in the docked pose. The analysis between SusCD and compound 5 revealed that 7 hydrogen bond interactions appeared in the docked pose. The analysis between SusCD and compound 6 revealed that 9 hydrogen bond interactions appeared in the docked pose. These results suggested that the fructooligosaccharides from *M. officinalis* could be absorbed sufficiently by bacteria with the help of SusCD, serving as optimal nutritional ingredients or prebiotics for bacteria.

The changes in behavior and gut microbiota, as a result of different concentrations of $A\beta_{1-42}$, coincided with the alterations in gene expression in critical brain and intestinal regions. The transcriptome analysis of intestine and brain tissues at the 5th week induced by $A\beta_{1-42}$ showed that the expression of some genes changed significantly (**Figures 10, 12**). Furthermore, to understand the genetic pathways of the gut-brain axis, the significant DEGs both in the brain and intestine were analyzed to identify the gene elements by an interactive information using the Wayne chart (**Figures 15A–C**), which revealed that the interactive genes were increased by the $A\beta_{1-42}$ levels (14 for Aβ-10 vs. normal, while 25 for Aβ-20 vs. normal, $p < 0.05$). The KEGG pathway enrichment analysis showed that the DEGs were primarily enriched in protein digestion and absorption and platelet activation for Aβ-10 induced group (**Figure 15D**). This phenomenon might be attributed to the colonic bacteria that might not be able to run well or are lost, the non-digestible peptides and proteins (collagen) could not be fermented, and some short-chain fatty acids such as butyrate, propionate, and acetate are deficient, which resulted in platelet activation. Thus, the expressions of Col1a1, Col3a1, and Col14a1 mRNA were changed. With the altered mRNA expression of Lamc2, Sstr3, Nts, Spp1, Il6r, Vip, Kcnk3, and Nr4a1, the PI3K-Akt signaling pathway, neuroactive ligand-receptor interaction, focal adhesion, and ECM-receptor interaction were activated in the Aβ-20-induced group (**Figure 15E**). With the increased levels of $A\beta_{1-42}$ levels, the mRNA expressions of Igsf8, Kcnk3, and Mef2c were changed, and the KEGG pathway enrichment analysis showed that the aldosterone synthesis and secretion and MAPK signaling pathway were influenced (**Figure 15F**). Together with the changes in the gut microbiota community diversity shown in **Figure 8**, and the transcriptome analysis data of intestine and brain, we concluded that the $A\beta_{1-42}$ levels in hippocampus interact the gut and microbiota, although further studies are essential for substantiation.

Antibiotics intervention in APPSWE/PS1ΔE9 mouse model suggests that the diversity of the gut microbiota community can regulate the host innate immunity mechanisms that impact Aβ amyloidosis (Minter et al., 2016). The fecal microbiota transplantation implemented from Aβ precursor protein (APP) transgenic mice to non-transgenic wild-type mice showed a drastically increased level of cerebral Aβ levels, thereby indicating a microbial involvement in the development of Aβ pathology, and microbiota contributes to the development of neurodegenerative diseases (Harach et al., 2017; Liu et al., 2017). We also observed that the diversity in the gut microbiota community altered with the levels of Aβ and the induced time (**Figure 8**). Although the complex networks of communication between the gut microbiota and the brain are not yet fully elucidates, it is clear that prebiotics strongly modulates the ecology of the microbiota. However, the role of the microbial composition and the vast quantity, diversity, and functional capabilities of all these gut microorganisms on the brain and behavior are yet to be determined.

CONCLUSION

Taken together, these data provide further evidence for a beneficial role of fructooligosaccharides (prebiotics) from *M. officinalis* and the effects on microbiota-brain-gut axis in

AD, but need more studies. This study characterized OMO as a promising naturally occurring chemical constituent and suggested microbiota-brain-gut axis as a putative new therapeutic target for the treatment of various neurological diseases by using *M. officinalis* in conventional medicine.

ETHICS STATEMENT

The animal protocols used in this work were approved by the Institutional Animal Care and Use committee of the Center of Laboratory Animals of the Guangdong Institute of Microbiology (GT-IACUC20160426).

AUTHOR CONTRIBUTIONS

DC designed the study, carried out the computational analyses and wrote the manuscript. JY and GL collected animal physiological data and fecal samples and extracted ruminal DNA. XY and XT collected animal physiological data and brain samples. DC, TY, and OS collected data regarding the microbial metabolic networks and transcriptome analysis. YX and QW helped to design the study and to develop the metagenomic analysis tools and wrote the manuscript. GZ helped with computational tool development and statistical analyses (PCA). All authors read and approved the final manuscript.

FUNDING

The present work was supported by the financial support from the Guangdong Science and Technology Plan Projects (2015A020211021; 2016A050502032), the Guangzhou Science and Technology Plan Projects (201504281708257; 201604020009), the High-level Leading Talent Introduction Program of GDAS (2016GDASRC-0102), and the Nanyue Microbial Talents Cultivation Fund of Guangdong Institute of Microbiology and the Guangzhou Medical University Research Projects (2016C28).

ACKNOWLEDGMENTS

The authors would like to thank Zhang Heming, Burton B. Yang for helpful discussions in the preparation of this manuscript. Sequencing service was provided by Personal Biotechnology Co., Ltd., Shanghai, China.

REFERENCES

Abbott, A. (2011). Dementia: a problem for our age. *Nature* 475, S2–S4. doi: 10.1038/475S2a

Akbari, E., Asemi, Z., Daneshvar Kakhaki, R., Bahmani, F., Kouchaki, E., Tamtaji, O. R., et al. (2016). Effect of probiotic supplementation on cognitive function and metabolic status in Alzheimer's disease: a randomized, double-blind and controlled trial. *Front. Aging Neurosci.* 8:256. doi: 10.3389/fnagi.2016.00256

Alkasir, R., Li, J., Li, X., Jin, M., and Zhu, B. (2017). Human gut microbiota: the links with dementia development. *Protein Cell.* 8, 90–102. doi: 10.1007/s13238-016-0338-6

Allen, A. P., Hutch, W., Borre, Y. E., Kennedy, P. J., Temko, A., Boylan, G., et al. (2016). *Bifidobacterium longum* 1714 as a translational psychobiotic: modulation of stress, electrophysiology and neurocognition in healthy volunteers. *Transl. Psychiatry* 6:e939. doi: 10.1038/tp.2016.191

Anderson, G., Seo, M., Berk, M., Carvalho, A. F., and Maes, M. (2016). Gut permeability and microbiota in Parkinson's disease: role of depression, tryptophan catabolites, oxidative and nitrosative stress and melatonergic pathways. *Curr. Pharm. Des.* 22, 6142–6151. doi: 10.2174/1381612822666160906161513

Arboleya, S., Sanchez, B., Milani, C., Duranti, S., Solis, G., Fernandez, N., et al. (2015). Intestinal microbiota development in preterm neonates and effect of perinatal antibiotics. *J. Pediatr.* 166, 538–544. doi: 10.1016/j.jpeds.2014.09.041

Benjamin, J. L., Hedin, C. R., Koutsoumpas, A., Ng, S. C., McCarthy, N. E., Hart, A. L., et al. (2011). Randomised, double-blind, placebo-controlled trial of fructo-oligosaccharides in active Crohn's disease. *Gut* 60, 923–929. doi: 10.1136/gut.2010.232025

Bland, J. (2016). Intestinal microbiome, *Akkermansia muciniphila*, and medical nutrition therapy. *Integr. Med.* 15, 14–16.

Burokas, A., Arboleya, S., Moloney, R. D., Peterson, V. L., Murphy, K., Clarke, G., et al. (2017). Targeting the microbiota-gut-brain axis: prebiotics have anxiolytic and antidepressant-like effects and reverse the impact of chronic stress in mice. *Biol. Psychiatry* 82, 472–487. doi: 10.1016/j.biopsych.2016.12.031

Cabili, M. N., Trapnell, C., Goff, L., Koziol, M., Tazon-Vega, B., Regev, A., et al. (2011). Integrative annotation of human large intergenic noncoding RNAs reveals global properties and specific subclasses. *Genes Dev.* 25, 1915–1927. doi: 10.1101/gad.17446611

Cai, B., Cui, C. B., Chen, Y. H., Luo, Z. P., Yang, M., and Yao, Z. W. (1996). Antidepressant effect of inulin- type oligosaccharides from *Morinda officinalis* How in mice. *Chin. J. Pharmacol. Toxicol.* 10, 109–112.

Chen, D. L., Li, N., Lin, L., Long, H. M., Lin, H., Chen, J., et al. (2014a). Confocal mirco-Raman spectroscopic analysis of the antioxidant protection mechanism of the oligosaccharides extracted from *Morinda officinalis* on human sperm DNA. *J. Ethnopharmacol.* 153, 119–124. doi: 10.1016/j.jep.2014.01.021

Chen, D. L., Yong, T. Q., Yang, J., Zheng, C. Q., Shuai, O., and Xie, Y. Z. (2017). Docking studies and biological evaluation of a potential β-secretase inhibitor of 3-hydroxyhericenone F from *Hericium erinaceus*. *Front. Pharmacol.* 8:219. doi: 10.3389/fphar.2017.00219

Chen, D. L., Zhang, P., Lin, L., Shuai, O., Zhang, H. M., Liu, S. H., et al. (2013). Protective effect of Bajijiasu against β-amyloid-induced neurotoxicity in PC12 cells. *Cell Mol. Neurobiol.* 33, 837–850. doi: 10.1007/s10571-013-9950-7

Chen, D. L., Zhang, P., Lin, L., Zhang, H. M., Deng, S. D., Wu, Z. Q., et al. (2014b). Protective effects of bajijiasu in a rat model of Aβ25-35-induced neurotoxicity. *J. Ethnopharmacol.* 154, 206–217. doi: 10.1016/j.jep.2014.04.004

Choi, Y. J., Yang, H. S., Jo, J. H., Lee, S. C., Park, T. Y., Choi, B. S., et al. (2015). Anti-amnesic effect of fermented Ganoderma lucidum water extracts by lactic acid bacteria on scopolamine-induced memory impairment in rats. *Prev. Nutr. Food Sci.* 20, 126–132. doi: 10.3746/pnf.2015.20.2.126

Davis, D. J., Doerr, H. M., Grzelak, A. K., Busi, S. B., Jasarevic, E., Ericsson, A. C., et al. (2016). *Lactobacillus plantarum* attenuates anxiety-related behavior and protects against stress-induced dysbiosis in adult zebrafish. *Sci. Rep.* 6:33726. doi: 10.1038/srep33726

Derrien, M., Belzer, C., and de Vos, W. M. (2016). *Akkermansia muciniphila* and its role in regulating host functions. *Microb. Pathog.* 106, 171–181. doi: 10.1016/j.micpath.2016.02.005

Dinan, T. G., and Cryan, J. F. (2017). The microbiome-gut-brain axis in health and disease. *Gastroenterol. Clin. North Am.* 46, 77–89. doi: 10.1016/j.gtc.2016.09.007

Erdman, S. E., and Poutahidis, T. (2016). Microbes and oxytocin: benefits for host physiology and behavior. *Int. Rev. Neurobiol.* 131, 91–126. doi: 10.1016/bs.irn.2016.07.004

Gao, J., Zhou, R., You, X., Luo, F., He, H., Chang, X., et al. (2016). Salidroside suppresses inflammation in a D-galactose-induced rat model of Alzheimer's disease via SIRT1/NF-κB pathway. *Metab. Brain Dis.* 31, 771–778. doi: 10.1007/s11011-016-9813-2

Garcia-Mazcorro, J. F., Barcenas-Walls, J. R., Suchodolski, J. S., and Steiner, J. M. (2017). Molecular assessment of the fecal microbiota in healthy cats and dogs before and during supplementation with fructo-oligosaccharides (FOS) and inulin using high-throughput 454-pyrosequencing. *PeerJ* 5:e3184. doi: 10.7717/peerj.3184

Gareau, M. G. (2014). Microbiota-gut-brain axis and cognitive function. *Adv. Exp. Med. Biol.* 817, 357–371. doi: 10.1007/978-1-4939-0897-4_16

Glenwright, A. J., Pothula, K. R., Bhamidimarri, S. P., Chorev, D. S., Baslé, A., Firbank, S. J., et al. (2017). Structural basis for nutrient acquisition by dominant members of the human gut microbiota. *Nature* 541, 407–411. doi: 10.1038/nature20828

Greer, R. L., Dong, X., Moraes, A. C., Zielke, R. A., Fernandes, G. R., Peremyslova, E., et al. (2016). *Akkermansia muciniphila* mediates negative effects of IFNγ on glucose metabolism. *Nat. Commun.* 7:13329. doi: 10.1038/ncomms13329

Harach, T., Marungruang, N., Duthilleul, N., Cheatham, V., Mc Coy, K. D., Frisoni, G., et al. (2017). Reduction of Abeta amyloid pathology in APP/PS1 transgenic mice in the absence of gut microbiota. *Sci. Rep.* 7:41802. doi: 10.1038/srep41802

Henning, S. M., Summanen, P. H., Lee, R. P., Yang, J., Finegold, S. M., Heber, D., et al. (2017). Pomegranate ellagitannins stimulate the growth of *Akkermansia muciniphila* in vivo. *Anaerobe* 43, 56–60. doi: 10.1016/j.anaerobe.2016.12.003

Hsiao, E. Y., McBride, S. W., Hsien, S., Sharon, G., Hyde, E. R., McCue, T., et al. (2013). Microbiota modulate behavioral and physiological abnormalities associated with neurodevelopmental disorders. *Cell* 155, 1451–1463. doi: 10.1016/j.cell.2013.11.024

Hu, X., Wang, T., and Jin, F. (2016). Alzheimer's disease and gut microbiota. *Sci. China Life Sci.* 59, 1006–1023. doi: 10.1007/s11427-016-5083-9

Huang, H. C., Zheng, B. W., Guo, Y., Zhao, J., Zhao, J. Y., Ma, X. W., et al. (2016). Antioxidative and neuroprotective effects of curcumin in an Alzheimer's disease rat model co-treated with intracerebroventricular streptozotocin and subcutaneous D-galactose. *J. Alzheimers Dis.* 52, 899–911. doi: 10.3233/JAD-150872

Jeong, J. J., Woo, J. Y., Kim, K. A., Han, M. J., and Kim, D. H. (2015). *Lactobacillus pentosus* var. *plantarum* C29 ameliorates age-dependent memory impairment in Fischer 344 rats. *Lett. Appl. Microbiol.* 60, 307–314. doi: 10.1111/lam.12393

Jiang, C., Li, G., Huang, P., Liu, Z., and Zhao, B. (2017). The gut microbiota and Alzheimer's disease. *J. Alzheimers Dis.* 58, 1–15. doi: 10.3233/JAD-161141

Jung, I. H., Jung, M. A., Kim, E. J., Han, M. J., and Kim, D. H. (2012). *Lactobacillus pentosus* var. *plantarum* C29 protects scopolamine-induced memory deficit in mice. *J. Appl. Microbiol.* 113, 1498–1506. doi: 10.1111/j.1365-2672.2012.05437.x

Le Sage, F., Meilhac, O., and Gonthier, M. P. (2017). *Porphyromonas gingivalis* lipopolysaccharide induces pro-inflammatory adipokine secretion and oxidative stress by regulating Toll-like receptor-mediated signaling pathways and redox enzymes in adipocytes. *Mol. Cell. Endocrinol.* 446, 102–110. doi: 10.1016/j.mce.2017.02.022

Leung, K., and Thuret, S. (2015). Gut microbiota: a modulator of brain plasticity and cognitive function in ageing. *Healthcare* 3, 898–916. doi: 10.3390/healthcare3040898

Li, X., Lu, F., Li, W., Xu, J., Sun, X. J., Qin, L. Z., et al. (2016). Minocycline ameliorates D-galactose- induced memory deficits and loss of Arc/Arg3.1 expression. *Mol. Biol. Rep.* 43, 1157–1163. doi: 10.1007/s11033-016-4051-6

Li, Y. F., Liu, Y. Q., Yang, M., Wang, H. L., Huang, W. C., Zhao, Y. M., et al. (2004). The cytoprotective effect of inulin-type hexasaccharide extracted from *Morinda officinalis* on PC12 cells against the lesion induced by corticosterone. *Life Sci.* 75, 1531–1538. doi: 10.1016/j.lfs.2004.02.029

Li, Y. F., Yuan, L., Xu, Y. K., Yang, M., Zhao, Y. M., and Luo, Z. P. (2001). Antistress effect of oligosaccharides extracted from *Morinda officinalis* in mice and rats. *Acta Pharmacol. Sin.* 22, 1084–1088.

Liang, C. Y., Liang, Y. M., Liu, H. Z., Zhu, D. M., Hou, S. Z., Wu, Y. Y., et al. (2017). Effect of *Dendrobium officinale* on D-galactose-induced aging mice. *Chin. J. Integr. Med.* doi: 10.1007/s11655-016-2631-x [Epub ahead of print].

Ling, Z. X., Xia, L., Jia, X. Y., Cheng, Y. W., Luo, Y. Q., Li, Y., et al. (2014). Impacts of infection with different toxigenic *Clostridium difficile* strains on faecal microbiota in children. *Sci. Rep.* 4:7485. doi: 10.1038/srep07485

Liu, K. L., He, Y. G., Yu, L. X., Chen, Y., and He, R. (2017). Elevated formaldehyde in the cecum of APP/PS1 mouse. *Microbiol. China* 44, 1761–1766.

Malaguarnera, M., Vacante, M., Antic, T., Giordano, M., Chisari, G., Acquaviva, R., et al. (2012). *Bifidobacterium longum* with fructo-oligosaccharides in patients with non alcoholic steatohepatitis. *Dig. Dis. Sci.* 57, 545–553. doi: 10.1007/s10620-011-1887-4

Mayer, E. A., Knight, R., Mazmanian, S. K., Cryan, J. F., and Tillisch, K. (2014). Gut microbes and the brain: paradigm shift in neuroscience. *J. Neurosci.* 34, 15490–15496. doi: 10.1523/JNEUROSCI.3299-14.2014

Minter, M. R., Zhang, C., Leone, V., Ringus, D. L., Zhang, X., Oyler-Castrillo, P., et al. (2016). Antibiotic-induced perturbations in gut microbial diversity influences neuro-inflammation and amyloidosis in a murine model of Alzheimer's disease. *Sci. Rep.* 6:30028. doi: 10.1038/srep30028

Park, K. Y., Jeong, J. K., Lee, Y. E., and Daily, J. W. III (2014). Health benefits of kimchi (Korean fermented vegetables) as a probiotic food. *J. Med. Food* 17, 6–20. doi: 10.1089/jmf.2013.3083

Petra, A. I., Panagiotidou, S., Hatziagelaki, E., Stewart, J. M., Conti, P., and Theoharides, T. C. (2015). Gut-microbiota-brain axis and its effect on neuropsychiatric disorders with suspected immune dysregulation. *Clin. Ther.* 37, 984–995. doi: 10.1016/j.clinthera.2015.04.002

Pistollato, F., Sumalla Cano, S., Elio, I., Masias Vergara, M., Giampieri, F., and Battino, M. (2016). Role of gut microbiota and nutrients in amyloid formation and pathogenesis of Alzheimer disease. *Nutr. Rev.* 74, 624–634. doi: 10.1093/nutrit/nuw023

Potgieter, M., Bester, J., Kell, D. B., and Pretorius, E. (2015). The dormant blood microbiome in chronic, inflammatory diseases. *FEMS Microbiol. Rev.* 39, 567–591. doi: 10.1093/femsre/fuv013

Rhee, S. H., Pothoulakis, C., and Mayer, E. A. (2009). Principles and clinical implications of the brain-gut-enteric microbiota axis. *Nat. Rev. Gastroenterol. Hepatol.* 6, 306–314. doi: 10.1038/nrgastro.2009.35

Rieder, R., Wisniewski, P. J., Alderman, B. L., and Campbell, S. C. (2017). Microbes and mental health: a review. *Brain Behav. Immun.* 66, 9–17. doi: 10.1016/j.bbi.2017.01.016

Rigo-Adrover, M., Pérez-Berezo, T., Ramos-Romero, S., van Limpt, K., Knipping, K., Garssen, J., et al. (2017). A fermented milk concentrate and a combination of short-chain galacto-oligosaccharides/long-chain fructo-oligosaccharides/pectin-derived acidic oligosaccharides protect suckling rats from rotavirus gastroenteritis. *Br. J. Nutr.* 117, 209–217. doi: 10.1017/S0007114516004566

Russo, R., Cristiano, C., Avagliano, C., De Caro, C., La Rana, G., Raso, G. M., et al. (2017). Gut-brain axis: role of lipids in the regulation of inflammation, pain and CNS diseases. *Curr. Med. Chem.* doi: 10.2174/0929867324666170216113756 [Epub ahead of print].

Sanches Lopes, S. M., Francisco, M. G., Higashi, B., de Almeida, R. T., Krausová, G., Pilau, E. J., et al. (2016). Chemical characterization and prebiotic activity of fructo-oligosaccharides from *Stevia rebaudiana* (Bertoni) roots and in vitro adventitious root cultures. *Carbohydr. Polym.* 152, 718–725. doi: 10.1016/j.carbpol.2016.07.043

Scott, K. A., Ida, M., Peterson, V. L., Prenderville, J. A., Moloney, G. M., Izumo, T., et al. (2017). Revisiting Metchnikoff: age-related alterations in microbiota-gut-brain axis in the mouse. *Brain Behav Immun.* 65, 20–32. doi: 10.1016/j.bbi.2017.02.004

Servin, A. L. (2004). Antagonistic activities of lactobacilli and bifidobacteria against microbial pathogens. *FEMS Microbiol. Rev.* 28, 405–440. doi: 10.1016/j.femsre.2004.01.003

Sun, L., Luo, H., Bu, D., Zhao, G., Yu, K., Zhang, C., et al. (2013). Utilizing sequence intrinsic composition to classify protein-coding and long non-coding transcripts. *Nucleic Acids Res.* 41:e166. doi: 10.1093/nar/gkt646

Tan, B. X., Chen, C. F., Chen, J. W., Su, W., Li, X. Y., Lin, R. S., et al. (2000a). Mechanism of BA-JI-SU in invigorating kidney to anti-aging. *J. New Chin. Med.* 32, 36–38.

Tan, B. X., Su, W., Chen, J. W., Chen, C. F., Wang, Y., and Li, X. Y. (2000b). improvement effect of bajiasu on spatial learning and memory ability of rats. *Tradit. Chin. Drugs Res. Clin. Pharmacol.* 11, 95–97.

Tanner, S. A., Lacroix, C., Del'Homme, C., Jans, C., Zihler Berner, A., Bernalier-Donadille, A., et al. (2015). Effect of *Bifidobacterium thermophilum* RBL67 and fructo-oligosaccharides on the gut microbiota in Göttingen minipigs. *Br. J. Nutr.* 114, 746–755. doi: 10.1017/S0007114515002263

Trapnell, C., Hendrickson, D. G., Sauvageau, M., Goff, L., Rinn, J. L., and Pachter, L. (2013). Differential analysis of gene regulation at transcript resolution with RNA-seq. *Nat. Biotechnol.* 31, 46–53. doi: 10.1038/nbt.2450

Valdés-Varela, L., Ruas-Madiedo, P., and Gueimonde, M. (2017). *In vitro* fermentation of different fructo-oligosaccharides by *Bifidobacterium* strains for the selection of synbiotic combinations. *Int. J. Food Microbiol.* 242, 19–23. doi: 10.1016/j.ijfoodmicro.2016.11.011

Van Herreweghen, F., Van den Abbeele, P., De Mulder, T., De Weirdt, R., Geirnaert, A., Hernandez-Sanabria, E., et al. (2017). In vitro colonisation of the distal colon by *Akkermansia muciniphila* is largely mucin and pH dependent. *Benef. Microbes* 8, 81–96. doi: 10.3920/BM2016.0013

Vandenplas, Y., Ludwig, T., Bouritius, H., Alliet, P., Forde, D., Peeters, S., et al. (2017). Randomised controlled trial demonstrates that fermented infant formula with short-chain galacto-oligosaccharides and long-chain fructo-oligosaccharides reduces the incidence of infantile colic. *Acta Paediatr.* 106, 1150–1158. doi: 10.1111/apa.13844

Vanegas, S. M., Meydani, M., Barnett, J. B., Goldin, B., Kane, A., Rasmussen, H., et al. (2017). Substituting whole grains for refined grains in a 6-wk randomized trial has a modest effect on gut microbiota and immune and inflammatory markers of healthy adults. *Am. J. Clin. Nutr.* 105, 635–650. doi: 10.3945/ajcn.116.146928

Vuong, H. E., Yano, J. M., Fung, T. C., and Hsiao, E. Y. (2017). The microbiome and host behavior. *Annu. Rev. Neurosci.* 40, 21–49. doi: 10.1146/annurev-neuro-072116-031347

Wall, R., Cryan, J. F., Ross, R. P., Fitzgerald, G. F., Dinan, T. G., and Stanton, C. (2014). Bacterial neuroactive compounds produced by psychobiotics. *Adv. Exp. Med. Biol.* 817, 221–239. doi: 10.1007/978-1-4939-0897-4_10

Wang, L., Feng, Z., Wang, X., Wang, X., and Zhang, X. (2010). DEGseq: an R package for identifying differentially expressed genes from RNA-seq data. *Bioinformatics* 26, 136–138. doi: 10.1093/bioinformatics/btp612

Wang, X., Li, G. J., Hu, H. X., Ma, C., Ma, D. H., Liu, X. L., et al. (2016). Cerebral mTOR signal and pro-inflammatory cytokines in Alzheimer's disease rats. *Transl. Neurosci.* 7, 151–157. doi: 10.1515/tnsci-2016-0022

Wei, Y., Lu, C., Chen, J., Cui, G., Wang, L., Yu, T., et al. (2017). High salt diet stimulates gut Th17 response and exacerbates TNBS-induced colitis in mice. *Oncotarget* 8, 70–82. doi: 10.18632/oncotarget.13783

Woo, J. Y., Gu, W., Kim, K. A., Jang, S. E., Han, M. J., and Kim, D. H. (2014). *Lactobacillus pentosus* var. *plantarum* C29 ameliorates memory impairment and inflammaging in a D-galactose-induced accelerated aging mouse model. *Anaerobe* 27, 22–26. doi: 10.1016/j.anaerobe.2014.03.003

Yano, J. M., Yu, K., Donaldson, G. P., Shastri, G. G., Ann, P., Ma, L., et al. (2015). Indigenous bacteria from the gut microbiota regulate host serotonin biosynthesis. *Cell* 161, 264–276. doi: 10.1016/j.cell.2015.02.047

Zeng, G. F., Zhang, Z. Y., Lu, L., Xiao, D. Q., Zong, S. H., and He, J. M. (2013). Protective effects of ginger root extract on Alzheimer disease-induced behavioral dysfunction in rats. *Rejuvenation Res.* 16, 124–133. doi: 10.1089/rej.2012.1389

Zhan, P. Y., Peng, C. X., and Zhang, L. H. (2014). Berberine rescues D-galactose-induced synaptic/memory impairment by regulating the levels of Arc. *Pharmacol. Biochem. Behav.* 117, 47–51. doi: 10.1016/j.pbb.2013.12.006

Zhong, L., Huang, F., Shi, H., Wu, H., Zhang, B., Wu, X., et al. (2016). Qing'E formula alleviates the aging process in D-galactose-induced aging mice. *Biomed. Rep.* 5, 101–106. doi: 10.3892/br.2016.667

2

Differential Roles of Environmental Enrichment in Alzheimer's Type of Neurodegeneration and Physiological Aging

*Vladimir V. Salmin[1], Yulia K. Komleva[2,3], Natalia V. Kuvacheva[2,3], Andrey V. Morgun[4], Elena D. Khilazheva[2,3], Olga L. Lopatina[2,3], Elena A. Pozhilenkova[2,3], Konstantin A. Shapovalov[1], Yulia A. Uspenskaya[3] and Alla B. Salmina[2,3]**

[1] Department of Medical and Biological Physics, Krasnoyarsk State Medical University named after Prof. V.F. Voino-Yasenetsky, Krasnoyarsk, Russia, [2] Department of Biochemistry, Medical, Pharmaceutical and Toxicological Chemistry, Krasnoyarsk State Medical University named after Prof. V.F. Voino-Yasenetsky, Krasnoyarsk, Russia, [3] Research Institute of Molecular Medicine and Pathobiochemistry, Krasnoyarsk State Medical University named after Prof. V.F. Voino-Yasenetsky, Krasnoyarsk, Russia, [4] Department of Pediatrics, Krasnoyarsk State Medical University named after Prof. V.F. Voino-Yasenetsky, Krasnoyarsk, Russia

Correspondence:
Alla B. Salmina
allasalmina@mail.ru

Impairment of hippocampal adult neurogenesis in aging or degenerating brain is a well-known phenomenon caused by the shortage of brain stem cell pool, alterations in the local microenvironment within the neurogenic niches, or deregulation of stem cell development. Environmental enrichment (EE) has been proposed as a potent tool to restore brain functions, to prevent aging-associated neurodegeneration, and to cure neuronal deficits seen in neurodevelopmental and neurodegenerative disorders. Here, we report our data on the effects of environmental enrichment on hippocampal neurogenesis *in vivo* and neurosphere-forming capacity of hippocampal stem/progenitor cells *in vitro*. Two models – Alzheimer's type of neurodegeneration and physiological brain aging – were chosen for the comparative analysis of EE effects. We found that environmental enrichment greatly affects the expression of markers specific for stem cells, progenitor cells and differentiated neurons (Pax6, Ngn2, NeuroD1, NeuN) in the hippocampus of young adult rats or rats with Alzheimer's disease (AD) model but less efficiently in aged animals. Application of time-lag mathematical model for the analysis of impedance traces obtained in real-time monitoring of cell proliferation *in vitro* revealed that EE could restore neurosphere-forming capacity of hippocampal stem/progenitor cells more efficiently in young adult animals (fourfold greater in the control group comparing to the AD model group) but not in the aged rats (no positive effect of environmental enrichment at all). In accordance with the results obtained *in vivo*, EE was almost ineffective in the recovery of hippocampal neurogenic reserve *in vitro* in aged, but not in amyloid-treated or young adult, rats. Therefore, EE-based neuroprotective strategies effective in Aβ-affected brain could not be directly extrapolated to aged brain.

Keywords: environmental enrichment, neurogenesis, neurosphere, Alzheimer's disease, aging, time-lag model

INTRODUCTION

Environmental enrichment (EE) is considered as an environment with numerous sensorimotor, cognitive, and social stimulations able to affect brain plasticity, to restore brain functional reserves, and to facilitate establishment of novel connections actual for preventive or rehabilitation strategies. Modeling EE is currently widely used in experiments aimed to study synaptogenesis, neurogenesis, and brain connectivity (Komleva Iu et al., 2013). EE stimulates neurogenesis and synapse turnover, integration of newly-formed cells into neuronal ensembles, modifies epigenetic mechanisms controlling resistance to oxidative stress, modulates production of neurotransmitters and molecules with neurotrophic activity, prevents apoptosis, suppresses neuroinflammation, affects neuron-glia interactions, thereby enhancing cognition, learning, and social communications in animals or humans with or without brain pathology (Herring et al., 2011; Cotel et al., 2012; Komleva Iu et al., 2013; Leger et al., 2015; Grinan-Ferre et al., 2016; Stuart et al., 2017). These effects well-correspond to those observed in people practicing so-called cognitive training because of their professional duties or personal habits and demonstrating good preservation of cognitive functions even at the eldest period of life (Mora, 2013). However, action of EE depends on experimental conditions, duration of exposure, severity of brain injury, age, gender etc., thereby, the observed effects of EE on neuroplasticity might be different and even unexpected (Ming and Song, 2011; Valero-Aracama et al., 2015).

Growing number of experimental and clinical findings suggest that EE might serve as an effective strategy to restore the functional capacity of damaged brain, i.e., in Alzheimer's disease (AD), in neurodevelopmental disorders, after stroke, etc. (Janssen et al., 2014; Polito et al., 2014; Cioni et al., 2016; Rosbergen et al., 2016). Particularly, prevention or treatment of Alzheimer-type neurodegeneration is one of the most challenging questions in the modern neuroscience which is directly linked to the controlled modulation of hippocampal plasticity (Balietti et al., 2012) In such context, EE provides a lot of premises for its effective application: prevention of hippocampal astroglial dysfunction in the AD transgenic mice (Rodriguez et al., 2013), up-regulation of brain-derived growth factor expression in the hippocampus of senescence-accelerated prone mice (Yuan et al., 2012), prevention of amyloid β (Aβ) deposition and memory impairment in AD model mice (Maesako et al., 2012), modulation of hippocampal synaptic proteins expression (Barak et al., 2013).

In contrast, EE action in aging brain is not deciphered in detail, even aging itself is the certain risk for AD development (Avila et al., 2010). Moreover, precise molecular mechanisms of EE effects on neuroplasticity in aged or AD brain remain to be unclear or even contradictory (Herring et al., 2011; Cotel et al., 2012; Bezzina et al., 2015; Huttenrauch et al., 2016). Impairment of hippocampal adult neurogenesis in aging is a well-known phenomenon caused by the shortage of brain stem cell pool, alterations in the local microenvironment within the neurogenic niches, or deregulation of stem cell development (Ali et al., 2015; Moraga et al., 2015). It is well-known that there is an obvious contrast between Alzheimer-type neurodegeneration and physiological aging, however, both of them are associated with progressive cognitive deficits and impairment of brain plasticity. Healthy aging brain is characterized by moderate decline in neurogenesis affecting the structure and function of the entorhinal-hippocampal circuit which is in the focus of neurodegeneration seen in AD due to the toxic action of Aβ, oxidative stress, excitotoxicity, and neuroinflammation (Hollands et al., 2016). In physiologically aging brain, no significant changes in the number of neural stem cells (NSCs) residing within the hippocampal neurogenic niche have been detected (Hattiangady and Shetty, 2008). In contrast, gradual decrease of NSCs and neural progenitor cells (NPCs) number has been reported in the experimental APP/PS1/nestin-GFP triple transgenic mouse model of AD (Zeng et al., 2016). Thus, the earliest stages of adult neurogenesis (stem cell maintenance, self-renewal, and proliferation) are significantly affected in AD neurodegeneration but not in healthy aging. Since enhancing neurogenesis was proposed as a therapeutic approach in neurodegeneration (Hollands et al., 2016), one may assume that EE could produce different effects on aging-associated and AD-compromised hippocampal neurogenesis. Despite several experimental and clinical observations on EE action in elderly subjects with or without AD, little information is available on the comparative efficacy of EE in AD and healthy aging.

So, whether EE-induced changes are equally beneficial in aging brain and in AD? The subject has received increased attention with the deciphering the biological mechanisms of late-life brain alterations: reduced neurogenesis and synapse turnover (Mostany et al., 2013), suppressed release of neuropeptides and neurotrophic factors (Forlenza et al., 2015), appearance of white matter lesions and pathological blood–brain barrier permeability (Marin-Padilla and Knopman, 2011; Firbank et al., 2012). Several studies suggest that EE affects epigenetic mechanisms controlling neuroplasticity, promotes remyelination, or reduces glia-supported neuroinflammation in the neurogenic niches in the aged brain (Williamson et al., 2012; Yang et al., 2012; Neidl et al., 2016). However, alterations in neurogenesis and the capacity of so-called "neurogenic reserve" may have different patterns and degree of progression in normal aging and in AD (Esiri and Chance, 2012).

Assessment of neurogenesis represents an appropriate system to analyze the activity of factors with presumptive neuroprotective properties. *In vivo*, neurogenesis can be studied with the approach based on the detection of markers expression in cells at different stages of development within the neurogenic niches or along their migratory paths in the brain (Roybon et al., 2009). Apart from this, some neurogenesis-associated events are easily reproduced *in vitro* due to ability of neurogenic non-differentiated cells to produce non-adherent spherical clusters of cells known as neurospheres (NS). NS-forming capacity is a parameter which is widely used for the assessment of neurogenic potential of neural stem/progenitor cells as well as the action of regulatory molecules, neurotoxic substances, or drug candidates (Pacey et al., 2006). Positive effects of EE on neurogenesis *in vivo* have been shown (Monteiro et al., 2014; Clemenson et al., 2015), however, there are very limited data on NS development *in vitro* in AD or aging (Heo et al., 2007; Diaz-Moreno et al., 2013).

Recently, we have demonstrated EE-mediated enhancement of neurosphere-forming capacity of NSCs obtained from the brains of AD rat model (Kuvacheva et al., 2015). It should be mentioned that analysis of data obtained with NS culture systems is hampered by the relative shortage of tools for adequate interpretation within the context of cell cycle- and proliferation-related events. Modeling the cell growth kinetics has been in the focus of researchers for a long time (Baker et al., 1998), but mathematic analysis of kinetic features of stem cells behavior in several subsequent NS generations *in vitro* was undertaken in few studies only (Ma et al., 2007). Development of correct mathematical models of NS establishment in the short-term experimental conditions (when reduction of cell population due to cell death might be contingently neglected) would provide new opportunities for rapid and effective analysis of endogenous and exogenous stimuli targeting neurogenesis. Moreover, current achievements in the application of NS cultures for AD modeling *in vitro* (Choi et al., 2013; Ghate et al., 2014) or novel attempts to restore brain functions with NSCs transplantation therapy (Waldau and Shetty, 2008) determine the needs in the appropriate mathematical modeling of NS-generation *in vitro* to clarify mechanisms underlying neurogenesis modulation in a given microenvironment.

Thus, we may entertain the hypothesis that: (i) effects of EE on neurogenesis are different in healthy brain aging and in brain affected by Alzheimer's type of neurodegeneration; (ii) combination of *in vivo* and *in vitro* approaches to the assessment of neurogenesis with the mathematical modeling of neurogenic reserve could help us to identify the neurogenesis stage which is a main "target" for the action of EE in normal and damaged brain. Therefore, the goal of this study was to compare the effects of *in vivo* EE in the Alzheimer's type of neurodegeneration and physiological brain aging with the special focus on hippocampal neurogenesis *in vivo* and NS-forming capacity of hippocampal stem/progenitor cells *in vitro*.

Experimental Procedures

Modeling Environmental Enrichment *In Vivo*

Wistar male rats ($n = 64$) were maintained in standard cages with water and standard diet with free access to food and water. The following groups of animals were included in the experiment: (i) young adult rats, 7–9 months old ($n = 40$) kept under standard conditions (SC, $n = 20$) or in the environmental enrichment (EE, $n = 20$); (ii) elderly rats, 23–25 months old ($n = 24$) kept under SC or in the EE. In SC, rats were housing in the cages sized 50 cm × 30 cm × 18 cm (five animals in one cage). In EE, rats were housing for 60 days in cages sized 78 cm × 48 cm × 39 cm (10 animals in one cage) equipped with various devices to provide extensive physical and explanatory activity (tunnels, houses, hammocks, stairs, boxes, wheels) (Jankowsky et al., 2003).

Modeling Alzheimer-Type Neurodegeneration

In the group of young adult rats, 10 animals kept under SC and 10 animals kept in EE have been used for modeling AD with intracerebral bilateral stereotaxic-guided (Narishige Scientific Instrument Lab) injections of 5 μl (2 μg/μl) aggregated Aβ1-42 (Sigma-Aldrich) into CA1 zones of hippocampus at the day 60 of SC or EE housing according to the protocol described (Li et al., 2011). For this procedure, anesthesia with chloral hydrate (0.35 g/kg) has been applied, and the following stereotaxic coordinates have been chosen: A/P = 3.0 mm, M/L = ± 2.2 mm, D/V = 2.8 mm. Establishment of AD model (Aβ deposition and cognitive impairment) has been confirmed with Thioflavin S staining of brain tissue and neurobehavioral phenotyping of animals (data not shown).

Assessment of Hippocampal Neurogenesis

Expression of markers in NSCs, progenitor cells and differentiated neurons (Pax6, Neurogenin 2, NeuroD1, NeuN) was assessed in the hippocampus of animals in all experimental groups according to the standard protocol of immunohistochemistry with antigen unmasking (proteinase K) procedure. Briefly, 2 μm hippocampal slices were obtained after transcardial perfusion of anesthesized rats with 0.1 M PBS (pH 7.4) and 4% PFA followed by hippocampus fixation in 10% buffered PFA for 24 h. The following primary antibodies have been used: Pax-6 (Abcam, ab78545, mouse monoclonal), 1:100, Neurogenin2 (Abcam, ab26190, rabbit polyclonal), 1:50, NeuroD1 (Abcam, ab60704, mouse monoclonal), 1:100, NeuN (Millipore, ABN78, rabbit polyclonal), 1:500. Alexa-conjugated secondary antibodies were used in 1:500 dilution: Alexa Fluor 488 chicken anti-mouse (for Pax6 detection), Alexa Fluor 488 donkey anti-rabbit (for Neurogenin2 detection), NeuN (rabbit polyclonal) – Alexa Fluor 488 donkey anti-rabbit (for NeuroD1 detection), and Alexa Fluor 488 chicken anti-rabbit (for NeuN detection) on slices. Images were visualized with Olympus CX41 microscope and analyzed with Image J software. Corrected total cell fluorescence (CTCF) was calculated for all the images.

Isolation of Adult Hippocampal Cells with the NS-Forming Capacity

At the day 70 of housing (10 days after AD modeling in the corresponding group of animals), isolation of hippocampus was performed in anesthesized rats according to the standard protocol described (Kuvacheva et al., 2015). After brain tissue dissociation and isolation of hippocampal cells, counting of the cells for further adjusting the viable cell concentrations was done with the Scepter CellCounter (Millipore). Assessment of proliferation of obtained hippocampal cells *in vitro* has been performed by culturing them in NeuroCult®NS-A Proliferation Medium with bFGF and EGF (Stemcell). On the next day after cell plating, development of neurospheres as transparent free-floating cell aggregates with surface microspikes was assessed with phase-contrast microscopy. At the day 3 of NS culture, cells were carefully harvested from the flasks, centrifuged, and suspended in the fresh NeuroCult®NS-A Proliferation Medium.

Real-Time Analysis of Cell Proliferation *In Vitro*

Further real-time analysis of cell proliferation kinetics was done using xCElligence system (Roche) with the gold microelectrode-covered microtiter plates. This method allows electrical impedance monitoring in the real-time manner. For this,

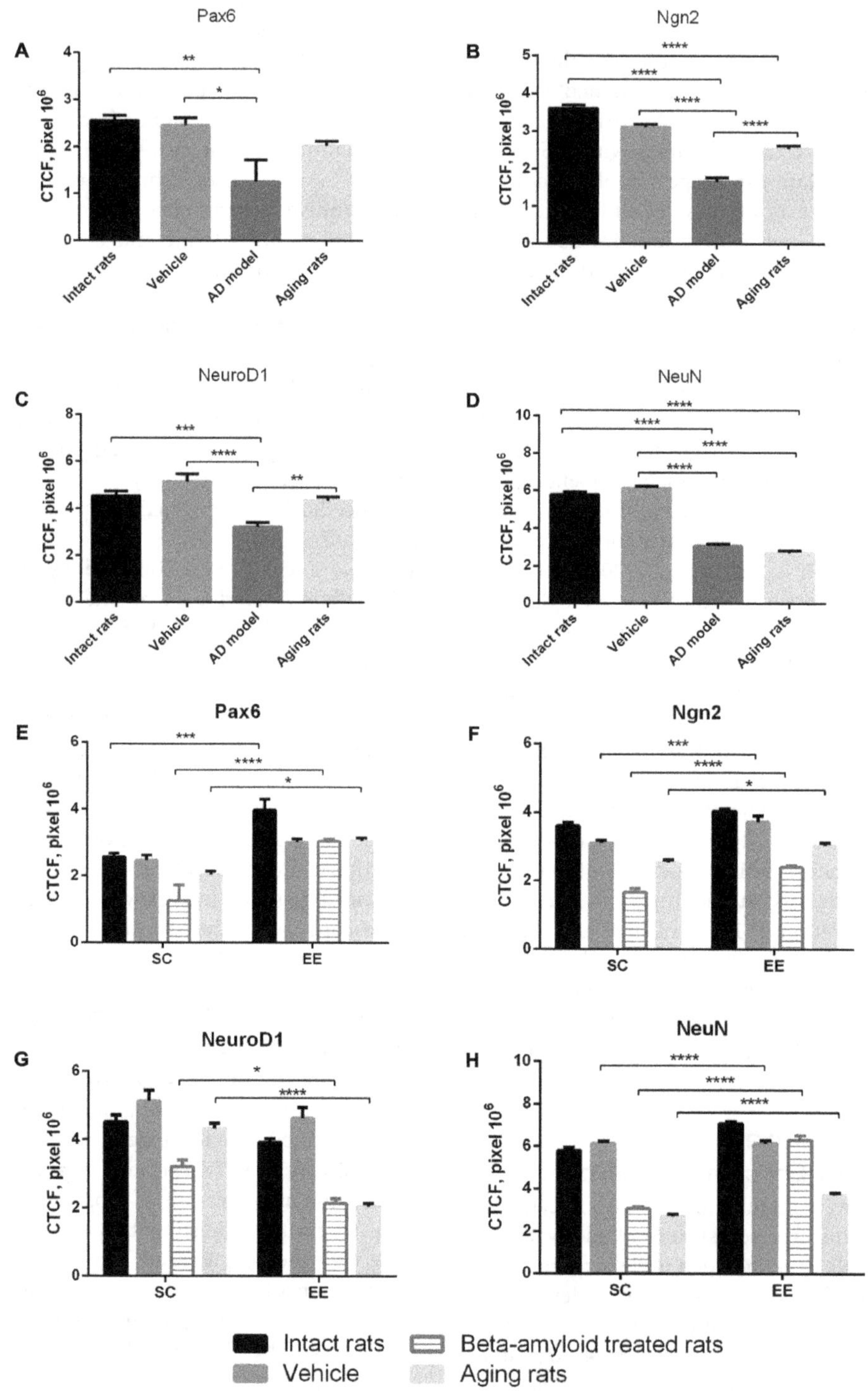

FIGURE 1 | Neurogenesis in the subgranular and granular layers of the dentate gyrus in experimental groups (intact rats, vehicle – sham-operated rats, AD model – Aβ-treated rats, aging rats, SC – standard conditions, EE – environmental enrichment). **(A–D)** Measurement of the CTCF index of different neurogenesis markers between groups under standards conditions (N = 10/per group, one-way ANOVA; Turkey's multiple comparisons test was run between groups). **(A)** Pax6 CTCF index ($p < 0.01$; one-way ANOVA). **(B)** Ngn2 CTCF index ($p < 0.0001$; one-way ANOVA). **(C)** NeuroD1 CTCF index ($p < 0.0001$; one-way ANOVA). **(D)** NeuN CTCF index ($p < 0.0001$; one-way ANOVA). Asterisks indicate statistical differences between groups. *$p < 0.05$; **$p < 0.01$; ***$p < 0.001$; ****$p < 0.0001$. **(E–H)** Measurement of the CTCF index of different neurogenesis markers between groups under standards conditions compared to environmental enrichment (N = 10/per group, statistical significance was determined by two-way ANOVA with a Sidak's test multiple comparisons test). **(E)** Pax6 CTCF index [Interaction $p < 0.05$, $F(3,72) = 2.573$, two-way ANOVA]. **(F)** Ngn2 CTCF index [Interaction ns; environmental factor $p < 0.0001$, $F(1,72) = 68.85$, group factor $p < 0.0001$, $F(3,72) = 130.7$, two-way ANOVA]. **(G)** NeuroD1 CTCF index [Interaction $p = 0.0001$, $F(3,72) = 7.91$, two-way ANOVA]. **(H)** NeuN CTCF index [Interaction $p < 0.0001$, $F(3,72) = 47.92$, two-way ANOVA]. Asterisks indicate statistical differences between groups. *$p < 0.05$; ***$p < 0.001$; ****$p < 0.0001$.

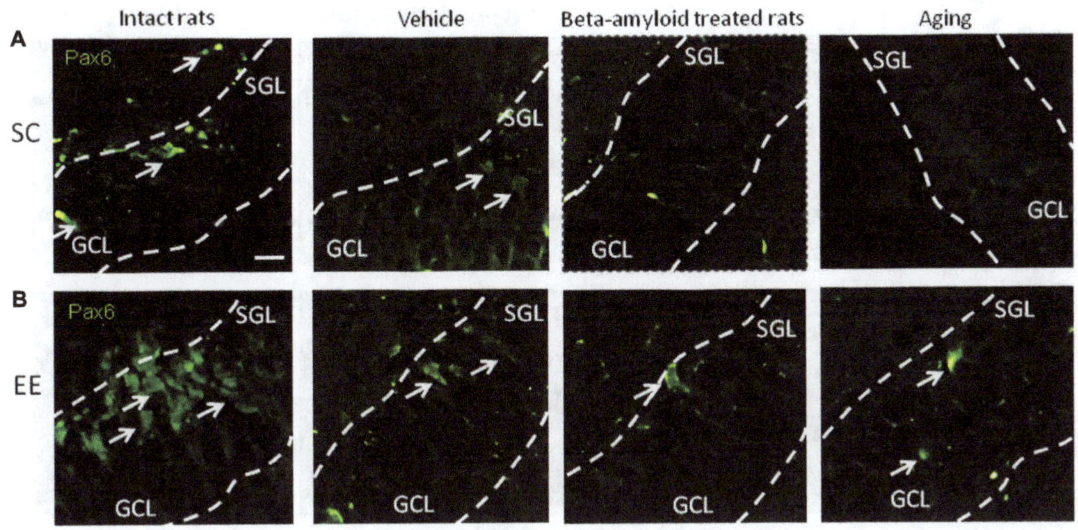

FIGURE 2 | Immunohistochemical (IHC) detection of Pax6 expression in intact, vehicle-, Aβ-treated, and aged rats kept under standard conditions (SC) **(A)** and environmental enrichment (EE) **(B)**. Representative photomicrographs show Pax6 immunostaining in the granular cell layer (GCL) and subgranular layer (SGL) of dentate gyrus. Pax6 was visualized using primary anti-Pax6 monoclonal antibody and secondary chicken anti-mouse IgG conjugated with green fluorescent dye Alexa Fluor 488.

1.2–2.5 × 10^4 cells/ml were cultured in NeuroCult®NS-A Proliferation Medium (100 μl per well, four wells for each series) at +37°C, 5% CO_2 with the measurements intervals of 5 min (from time 0 to 4.5 h) and 15 min (from 4.5 to 24 h).

Statistical Analysis

Non-linear regression analysis was done with the Origin 8.5 software (OriginLab). We applied user-defined function models. All regression models indicate the confidence coefficient χ^2 not worsen than 10^{-4}, and determination coefficient R^2 not less than 0.99. Statistical analysis was performed with the GraphPad Prism 6.0 software. Statistical significance was determined by one-way or two-way ANOVA with a Sidak's test multiple comparisons test. The data are presented as mean and standard deviation.

RESULTS

Immunohistochemical analysis of molecular markers expression in cells at different stages of neurogenesis (Pax6, Neurogenin 2, NeuroD1, NeuN) in the hippocampus revealed that their levels were dramatically affected in Aβ-treated rats and in the group of aging animals (**Figures 1A–D**). Noteworthy, EE did not affect the expression of the markers in the hippocampus of intact or sham-operated rats. EE demonstrated pronounced restorative effect on the impaired neurogenesis in the animals with AD model comparing with the elderly rats (**Figures 1E–H**). Among all the markers, most prominent changes were observed in the expression of NeuroD1 (reduction in all the tested animals subjected to EE).

Expression of Pax6 was efficiently restored by EE in all the groups tested (**Figure 2**). It is well-known that Pax6 is a transcription factor controlling proliferation of multipotent stem/progenitor cells in hippocampus and cortex being predominantly expressed by radial glia. High expression of Pax6 is usually followed by the elevated expression of Neurogenin 2 in amplifying unipotent progenitors, which is later replaced with the expression of NeuroD1 in neuronally committed cells of hippocampus where it is required for their survival (Roybon et al., 2009). At the final stage of neurogenesis, mature neurons in the granule zone of hippocampus are highly enriched in NeuN with the evident elevation in animals kept in EE, particularly in those having AD-type of neurodegeneration (**Figure 3**).

To analyze plausible mechanisms of the observed effect of EE at the initial stage of hippocampal adult neurogenesis, we further used the experimental model suitable for the assessing the kinetic parameters of cell proliferation *in vitro*. Evaluation of NS-forming capacity of hippocampal stem/progenitor cells is rather reliable tool to get the integral pattern of neurogenic cells proliferation and differentiation in the controlled conditions where cell cluster formation and development resemble the events occurring *in vivo* (Malik et al., 2015), particularly at the earliest steps of neurogenesis that were more sensitive to the action of EE *in vivo* (as shown above). We found that being cultured *in vitro*, adult hippocampal stem/progenitor cells produce NS whose appearance could be detected and analyzed with real-time impedance measurements. Recently, we have presented actual impedance traces for NS obtained from the animals with AD model kept under SC or EE (Kuvacheva et al., 2015). For analyzing the kinetic parameters of cell proliferation we applied several assumptions shown below.

Cell index (C) which is the impedance value corresponds to the number of adherent cells, therefore, cell sedimentation leads to the elevation of cell index. If the medium viscosity is not changed, then cell sedimentation to the microplate bottom

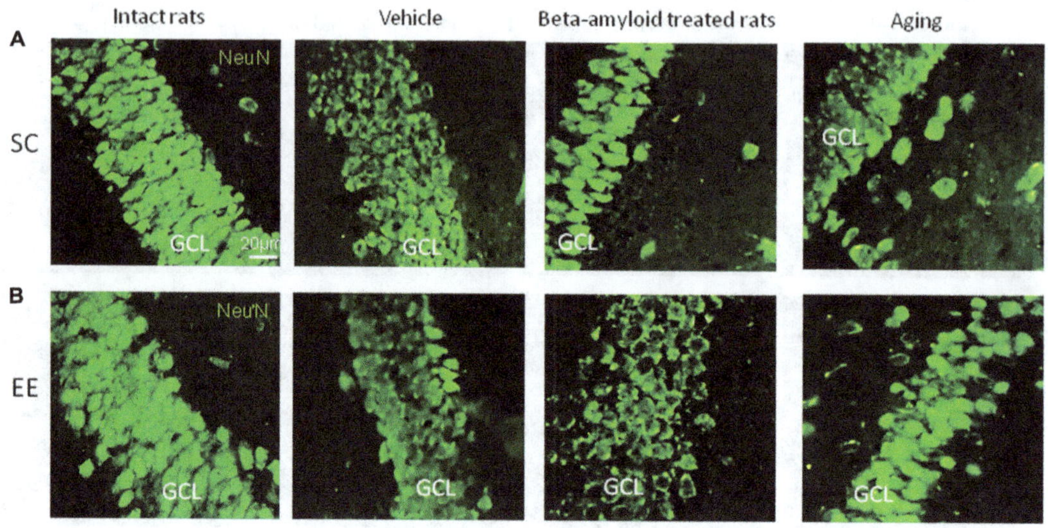

FIGURE 3 | Immunohistochemical (IHC) detection of NeuN expression in intact, vehicle-, Aβ-treated, and aged rats kept under standard conditions (SC) **(A)** and environmental enrichment (EE) **(B)**. Representative photomicrographs show NeuN immunostaining in the granular cell layer (GCL) of dentate gyrus. NeuN was visualized using primary anti-NeuN antibody and secondary donkey anti-rabbit IgG conjugated with green fluorescent dye Alexa Fluor 488.

demonstrates constant velocity, and C is progressively rising at the initial phase of cell culture with the linear dependence on the time:

$$C = \eta t + C_0.$$

Constant parameter η characterizes velocity of cell sedimentation, C_0 is the cell index obtained for the adherent cells at the initial point of measurements. The described process corresponds to the phase A (attachment of cells to the plate). Let assume that cells might be at any phase of cell cycle at this period. Phase I_1 of the impedance trace corresponds to the period after the complete cell adhesion (interphase of the cell cycle) when maximal value of cell index (C_{max}) is not changed. It is well-known that just before mitosis cell adhesion is weakened, and flattened cells acquire round shape (VanHook, 2014), therefore formation of NS leads to decrease of C value. This process corresponds to the mitotic phase M_1. Phase I_2 (interphase) demonstrates stable C value established just before entering mitosis in the 2nd generation of cells. This period is followed by reducing cell adhesion in the 2nd cell generation which corresponds to the mitotic phase M_2 (**Figure 4A**).

Thus, we postulate that in the given experimental conditions: (i) cell proliferation is synchronized; (ii) mitosis-associated loss of cell adhesion leads to C decline; (iii) two generations of cells are present in the system during 24 h of cell culture on microelectrode-covered microplates.

To exclude the impact of cell sedimentation velocity on C kinetics, lets adopt the cell index value as $C = C_{max}$ at the initial phase A. We may use the parameter shown below to take into account all the changes in C caused by the decreasing number of adherent cells:

$$C_N = C_{max} - C$$

Normalization of cell index changes (c_N) allows considering some deviations in cell concentrations in the microplate wells:

$$c_N = \frac{C_N}{C_{N\,max}}$$

Typical curve for c_N kinetics is shown in **Figure 4B**.

In order to analyze the observed changes in c_N, we may apply a lag model developed for explaining the proliferative kinetics of cell population with the synchronized growth (Baker et al., 1998). For this purpose we must use bell-shaped distribution of cells along the different phases of cell cycle. Let's propose that the probability of cell detachment out of microelectrode caused by alterations in adhesion mechanisms would have Boltzmann's distribution of time, whereas normalized changes in c_N value could be covered by the following equation:

$$c_N = c_0 + \frac{A_1}{1 + \exp\left(\frac{t_C - t}{t_M}\right)},$$

where c_0 – value of normalized changes of cell index at the initial point of measurements $t = 0$, A_1 – amplitude of normalized changes of cell index at the point of completing the 1st cycle of proliferation, t_c – duration of cell cycle, t_M – duration of phase M_1 (**Figure 2B**), presumably, corresponding to the duration of mitotic phase in the synchronously proliferating cell population.

The equation given above does not account for any time delay between the cell cycle initiation and beginning of cell index changes. To do this we will introduce another parameter – time-lag t_L, and we will consider a shift from the half-time of mitotic phase duration in the previous cell division (before the

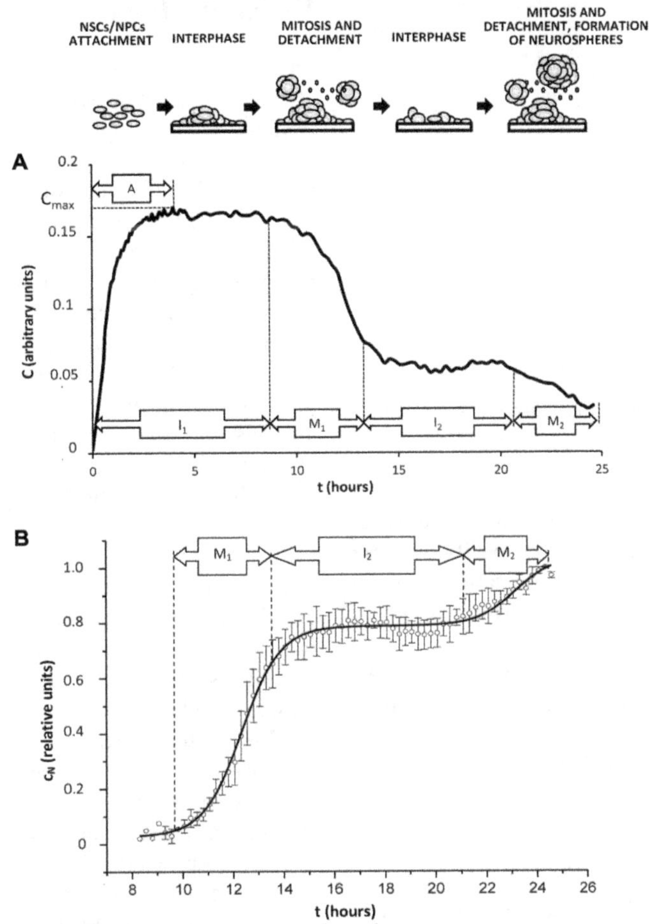

FIGURE 4 | Typical kinetics of cell index in the conditions promoting generation of neurospheres *in vitro*. Cells (NSCs, NPCs) isolated from rat hippocampus were plated in the microelectrode-covered plates of xCELLigence system for impedance measurements as described in Section "Experimental Procedures." Time of incubation is shown as t, hours. **(A)** A representative curve of cell index kinetics (indicated as C, arbitrary units) reflects real impedance trace obtained from the xCELLigence system during 24 h of cell culture. Cell index kinetics corresponds to changes in the number of attached cells during cell cycle progression. A – attachment phase, $I_{1,2}$ – interphase of 1st or 2nd cell cycle (interphasic cells attach to the microelectrode-covered plate), $M_{1,2}$ – mitosis in the 1st or 2nd cell cycle (mitotic cells detach from the microelectrode-covered plate). Corresponding changes in the cell culture are shown schematically at the top of the figure.
(B) Normalized and approximated cell index (indicated as c_n, relative units) was calculated from the real cell index C as shown in Section "Results," and relates to the number of detached cells. Solid curve corresponds to the best regression model.

measurements). Then, the equation covering cell index changes due to 1st mitosis would be as follows:

$$c_N = c_0 + \frac{A_1}{1 + \exp\left(\frac{t_C - t_L - 0.5 t_M - t}{t_M}\right)}$$

Second mitosis will be accounted by introducing the second summand:

$$c_N = c_0 + \frac{A_1}{1 + \exp\left(\frac{t_C - t_L - 0.5 t_M - t}{t_M}\right)} + \frac{A_2}{1 + \exp\left(\frac{2^* t_C - t_L - 0.5 t_M - t}{t_M}\right)}$$

We have used this equation for non-linear regression analysis of experimental data. **Figure 4B** shows regression solid curve corresponding to the applied model for the cells isolated from young adult rats exposed to EE.

At the first round of regression analysis, we determined the mean value of cell cycle duration t_C with kinetic curves for the normalized changes of cell index for the groups of cells with the well-identified phase of 2nd division. This group included data obtained from EE-treated rats as well as from aged rats housed in SC. Then, the obtained value of cell cycle duration for all the cell types was as follows:

$$t_C = 10.8 \pm 2.5 \text{ hr}.$$

At the second round of regression analysis, we fixed the cell cycle duration t_C, and values of t_M have been estimated for all the cell types. The data obtained for the duration of "mitotic phase" t_M are presented in **Table 1**.

Supposing t_M duration as a time of cell cycle "mismatch" in the synchronously proliferating population, we may assume that when the number of cell generations is $N_g = \frac{t_C}{t_M}$ full

TABLE 1 | Parameters of NS-forming capacity of hippocampal progenitors in rats with the Alzheimer-type neurodegeneration (AD) or physiological aging housed in the standard conditions (SC) or in the environmental enrichment (EE).

Experimental group	t_M (hours)	Ng	Nc	K
Young adult rats (SC)	1.23 ± 0.07	9	512	
Young adult rats (EE)	0.77 ± 0.03	14	16,384	32
AD model rats (SC)	2.23 ± 0.07	5	32	
AD model rats (EE)	1.42 ± 0.05	8	256	8
Elderly rats (SC)	1.66 ± 0.06	7	128	
Elderly rats (EE)	1.57 ± 0.08	7	128	1

t_M – duration of mitotic phase M.
N_g – number of cell generations produced before full desynchronization of cell growth.
N_c – maximal cluster size obtained before full desynchronization of cell growth.
K – coefficient of cluster size enlargement due to effect of EE.

desynchronization would happen, thereby affecting cells microenvironment and their proliferative capacity. Under the given experimental conditions, desynchronization is most obvious in the cell culture obtained from the group of elderly rats.

Supposing doubling of cell number in every next cell generation, we may adopt that maximal cluster size (number of cells in an aggregate) which might be formed before full desynchronization of cell cycle in the culture is:

$$N_C = 2^{N_g}$$

Therefore, maximal cluster size Nc should be interpreted as neurosphere-forming capacity. It is clearly shown (**Table 1**) that it is dramatically reduced in the elderly rats and – even more visibly – in the rats with AD-type of neurodegeneration. Since NS-forming ability marks the general neurogenic potential (or neurogenic reserve) of cells involved into adult hippocampal neurogenesis, we may conclude that Aβ treatment of young adult rats produces more prominent suppression of neurogenesis than healthy aging. However, the restorative potential of EE might be easily calculated using coefficient K describing changes in Nc:

$$K = \frac{N_C(EE)}{N_C(SC)}$$

As might be expected from our *in vivo* experiments, EE restored Nc more efficiently in young adult animals (fourfold greater in the control group comparing to the AD model group) but not in the elderly rats (no positive effect of EE at all). Thus, 60 days in the conditions of EE produced no any preventive effect on the aging-associated suppression of hippocampal neurogenesis *in vitro*, being, however, relatively effective in the Alzheimer's type of neurodegeneration. This finding well-corresponds to the number of NeuN+ mature neurons in the dentate gyrus in rats kept in SC or EE (**Figure 1H**) where prominent restoration of mature neurons number was evident in the group of amyloid-treated rats but not in the group of aged animals.

DISCUSSION

Our findings clearly indicate that EE restores neurogenesis affected by the toxic action of Aβ or by aging at the earliest stage of niche cell development (before neuronal fate specification) as was evident both *in vivo* and *in vitro*. In contrast to aging brain, amyloid-affected brain was much more susceptible to the action of EE on the neurogenic capacity of cells. These findings confirm our hypothesis that EE may have different efficacy in AD-type of neurodegeneration and healthy aging brain in the context of neurogenesis improvement.

In accordance to previously published data (Hattiangady and Shetty, 2008) we found that expression of Pax6 within the neurogenic niche was not dramatically decreased in aging animals, but demonstrated prominent decline in AD model. However, the number of NeuN-immunopositive mature neurons was reduced both in healthy aging brain and in AD-affected brain in a similar manner. Therefore, it was not surprising that the earliest stages of neurogenesis both *in vivo* and *in vitro* were more sensitive to the action of EE. Particularly, Pax6 expression was greatly improved by EE exposure *in vivo* in Aβ-treated or aging rats, and the expression pattern of the same marker confirmed the highest neurogenic reserve in young adult rats exposed to long-lasting EE.

Unexpectedly, EE promoted obvious reduction in NeuroD1 expression in the hippocampus in AD group or aged group, whereas in the group of young adult animals no significant changes in NeuroD1 expression have been observed upon action of EE. It is known that NeuroD1 controls survival and maturation of neurons born in the adult brain (Gao et al., 2009) being under the control of Wnt-regulated activity of Sox2 and HDAC1 in NSCs (Chen and Do, 2012). This transcription factor may also direct reprogramming of glial cells into functional neurons *in vivo*, particularly, in AD brain (Guo et al., 2014). NeuroD1 overexpression could reduce functional deficits in newly-formed hippocampal neurons in the experimental model of AD (Richetin et al., 2015). In the aging brain, NeuroD expression declines in the hippocampal neurogenic niche (Uittenbogaard and Chiaramello, 2000). Thus, taking into the consideration the role of NeuroD1 in controlling cell fate and differentiation in hippocampal neurogenesis, one may assume that EE-induced reduction of NeuroD1 expression in Aβ-treated or aged rats could relate to some kind of preservation of neurogenic cells in the non-differentiated state, particularly, in the group of aging rats where elevation of NeuN+ neurons number was less evident than in the group with AD model. Since such effect on NeuroD1 expression was not found in young adult animals, changes in NeuroD1-controled cell differentiation might be considered as a "marker" of EE action in Alzheimer-type neurodegeneration or in healthy brain aging.

It should be noted that EE-mediated decline in NeuroD1 expression is in the contrast to the majority of reports on EE-induced expression of main neurogenesis markers, including NeuroD (Terada et al., 2008). However, similar effect was reported in Manuel et al. (2015) where it was attributed to the inhibition of avoidance behavior in fish subjected to EE. Thus, we may conclude that EE-induced reduction in NeuroD1 hippocampal expression in Aβ-treated or aging rats could reflect some adaptive behavioral reactions needed in further investigation.

We also should point out that housing in standard conditions revealed that NeuroD1 expression in healthy aging brain was well-preserved comparing with Aβ-affected brain. In EE-exposed rats, NeuroD1 expression underwent dramatic decline, particularly in the group of aging animals. Different sensitivity of NeuroD1-expressing cells to the action of EE in aging and AD is consistent with the observed effect of EE on the number of NeuN-immunopositive hippocampal mature neurons: stimulatory action of EE was considerably stronger in Aβ-treated rats.

In sum, EE efficiently improves neurogenesis impaired in the Alzheimer-type neurodegeneration (at least in the AD model used in our study) but produces relatively weak effect on neurogenesis in physiologically aging brain. In both cases, earliest stages of neurogenesis (stimuli-induced proliferation of stem cells and progenitors) *in vivo* represent the periods with higher sensitivity to the action of EE.

The essential question now is whether this effect might be reproduced and quantitatively explained *in vitro*? Analysis of neurogenesis *in vivo* is commonly complemented with *in vitro* studies. Along this way, establishment of NS culture *in vitro* is very useful for assessing proliferative and differentiating properties of stem cells and their progeny, however, quantitative insight into the process of NS development and evolution is highly required (Pacey et al., 2006). Characteristic behavior of NSCs/NPCs in NS culture could not be easy interpreted with simple observations and routine statistics. This problem is further complicated when a number of kinetic data appears in the conditions enabling action of various factors *in vivo* (before cell isolation) or *in vitro* (during cell clusters expansion and development). Therefore, we applied original algorithm to produce comparative analysis of EE effects on the neurogenic reserve of NSCs/NPCs obtained from all the tested groups.

We found that mathematical modeling allowed analyzing the kinetics of cell proliferation *in vitro* with high accuracy and in a good correspondence to the data obtained *in vivo*. Moreover, we were able to get the integral parameter (Nc) reflecting neurogenic reserve of stem/progenitor hippocampal cells affected by different factors (aging, amyloid treatment, EE) *in vivo*. We demonstrated that NS-forming capacity of brain stem and progenitor cells was positively affected by EE in young adult animals, aging animals, but not in elderly rats. The observed difference in the effects of EE on aging- or AD-associated impairment of neurospheres generation *in vitro* might be linked to the very recently reported age-related alterations in the duration of cell cycle (particularly, abnormal extension of G1 phase of the cell cycle not associated with a differentiation commitment) in the hippocampal stem cells resulting in neurogenesis decline (Daynac et al., 2016). A rough analogy might be found with G1-lengthening and alterations in G1/S transition in embryonic stem cells leading to imbalance between self-renewal and differentiation (Coronado et al., 2013). Therefore, the observed prevalence of desynchronization-related changes in the neurosphere-forming capacity in the group of elderly rats is very likely caused by the analogous mechanism of cell cycle impairment. Moreover, such alterations in the cell cycle progression that are evident in neurogenic cells derived from the aged brain might contribute to the relative inefficacy of EE in the context of neurogenesis recovery in aging.

In contrast to physiological aging, Aβ is able to increase NSC activity at the earliest steps of AD pathogenesis followed by later decline (Heo et al., 2007; Diaz-Moreno et al., 2013). Furthermore, EE was reported to increase Aβ accumulation in the transgenic AD model mice due to extensive synaptic activity (Jankowsky et al., 2003). Here, we will note that neurospheres-generating capacity of hippocampal stem/progenitor cells might be enhanced by neuronal excitation due to recruitment of latent stem cells into adult neurogenesis (Walker et al., 2008). That is why Aβ-induced alterations in the adult neurogenesis seem to be more profound but at the same time more sensitive to the restorative capacity of EE-provided neuronal excitation than in the healthy aging brain. Thus, it is reasonable to suggest that long-lasting exposure to EE preceding Aβ neurotoxic action results in excitation-mediated mobilization of latent stem cells and partial restoration of neurosphere-forming capacity *in vitro*. However, this effect is less prominent in Aβ-treated rats than in intact young adult animals. In the group of elderly rats, alterations in the duration of cell cycle diminish EE-induced changes in the stem/progenitor cells pool.

Previously, several attempts have been done to get a mathematical model of neurogenesis (Ashbourn et al., 2012; Ziebell et al., 2014). In this study we propose a mathematical model describing early processes in NSCs/NPCs development *in vitro*. Our time-lag model is based on several assumptions and simplifications but proves our data obtained *in vivo* and provides quantitative parameter (Nc) which is suitable for comparative analysis of effects produced by different factors (i.e., age, housing conditions, neurotoxic stimuli). Thus, combination of *in vivo* and *in vitro* approaches with mathematical modeling reveals some important characteristics of EE action on hippocampal neurogenesis in healthy aging brain or in Alzheimer-type neurodegeneration. It is tempting to speculate that the same approach might be further applied for assessing neurogenesis-targeting activity of drug-candidates in preclinical studies.

There is a growing interest to the restoration of impaired neurogenesis and prevention of neurological deficits in physiological aging (Marr et al., 2010; Mattson, 2015), but differential sensitivity of aging brain and Alzheimer's brain to the conditions of EE should be carefully taken into the consideration. Coming back to our initial hypothesis, we may conclude that: (i) early stages of adult hippocampal neurogenesis are more sensitive to the action of EE in the experimental model of Alzheimer-type neurodegeneration or in aging; (ii) EE differently affects neurogenesis in physiological aging and in experimental AD, particularly, Aβ-affected brain is more susceptible to the action of EE comparing with healthy aging brain; (iii) different outcomes of EE action on NSCs/NPCs in AD or in healthy aging brain can be reliably detected with NS-forming assay *in vitro* and time-lag model of synchronized growth.

Thus, it is clear that EE-based neuroprotective strategies effective in the amyloid-affected brain could not be directly extrapolated to neurodegenerative processes associated with physiological brain aging. Therefore, application of EE strategy aimed to enhance adult neurogenesis should be considered as a personalized and pathogenetically based preventive or therapeutic intervention.

ETHICS STATEMENT

All animal experiments were performed in accordance with the principles of humanity set out in the Directive of the European Community (2010/63/EU). Protocols were reviewed and approved by the Local ethics committee of the Krasnoyarsk State Medical University named after Prof. V.F. Voino-Yasenetsky (35/2011).

AUTHOR CONTRIBUTIONS

VS, YK, and AS conceived and designed the research. All authors performed experiments. VS, YK, NK, AM, EK, and KS analyzed data. VS, YK, OL, and EP prepared figures. VS, YK, YU, EP, and AS prepared the initial draft; VS, YK, OL, and AS revised the manuscript. All authors reviewed the final manuscript and approved its publication.

ACKNOWLEDGMENT

The study is supported by the grant given by the President of Russian Federation for the Leading Scientific Teams (N 10241.2016.7).

REFERENCES

Ali, A. A. H., Schwarz-Herzke, B., Stahr, A., Prozorovski, T., Aktas, O., and von Gall, C. (2015). Premature aging of the hippocampal neurogenic niche in adult Bmal1-deficient mice. *Aging* 7, 435–449. doi: 10.18632/aging.100764

Ashbourn, J. M. A., Miller, J. J., Reumers, V., Baekelandt, V., and Geris, L. (2012). A mathematical model of adult subventricular neurogenesis. *J. R. Soc. Interface* 9, 2414–2423. doi: 10.1098/rsif.2012.0193

Avila, J., Insausti, R., and Del Rio, J. (2010). Memory and neurogenesis in aging and Alzheimer's Disease. *Aging Dis.* 1, 30–36.

Baker, C. T., Bocharov, G. A., Paul, C. A., and Rihan, F. A. (1998). Modelling and analysis of time-lags in some basic patterns of cell proliferation. *J. Math. Biol.* 37, 341–371. doi: 10.1007/s002850050133

Balietti, M., Tamagnini, F., Fattoretti, P., Burattini, C., Casoli, T., Platano, D., et al. (2012). Impairments of synaptic plasticity in aged animals and in animal models of Alzheimer's disease. *Rejuvenation Res.* 15, 235–238. doi: 10.1089/rej.2012.1318

Barak, B., Shvarts-Serebro, I., Modai, S., Gilam, A., Okun, E., Michaelson, D. M., et al. (2013). Opposing actions of environmental enrichment and Alzheimer's disease on the expression of hippocampal microRNAs in mouse models. *Transl. Psychiatry* 3:e304. doi: 10.1038/tp.2013.77

Bezzina, C., Verret, L., Halley, H., Dahan, L., and Rampon, C. (2015). Environmental enrichment does not influence hypersynchronous network activity in the Tg2576 mouse model of Alzheimer's disease. *Front. Aging Neurosci.* 7:178. doi: 10.3389/fnagi.2015.00178

Chen, M., and Do, H. (2012). Wnt Signaling in neurogenesis during aging and physical activity. *Brain Sci.* 2, 745–768. doi: 10.3390/brainsci2040745

Choi, Y. J., Park, J., and Lee, S.-H. (2013). Size-controllable networked neurospheres as a 3D neuronal tissue model for Alzheimer's disease studies. *Biomaterials* 34, 2938–2946. doi: 10.1016/j.biomaterials.2013.01.038

Cioni, G., Inguaggiato, E., and Sgandurra, G. (2016). Early intervention in neurodevelopmental disorders: underlying neural mechanisms. *Dev. Med. Child Neurol.* 58(Suppl. 4), 61–66. doi: 10.1111/dmcn.13050

Clemenson, G. D., Deng, W., and Gage, F. H. (2015). Environmental enrichment and neurogenesis: from mice to humans. *Curr. Opin. Behav. Sci.* 4, 56–62. doi: 10.1016/j.cobeha.2015.02.005

Coronado, D., Godet, M., Bourillot, P.-Y., Tapponnier, Y., Bernat, A., Petit, M., et al. (2013). A short G1 phase is an intrinsic determinant of naïve embryonic stem cell pluripotency. *Stem Cell Res.* 10, 118–131. doi: 10.1016/j.scr.2012.10.004

Cotel, M. C., Jawhar, S., Christensen, D. Z., Bayer, T. A., and Wirths, O. (2012). Environmental enrichment fails to rescue working memory deficits, neuron loss, and neurogenesis in APP/PS1KI mice. *Neurobiol. Aging* 33, 96–107. doi: 10.1016/j.neurobiolaging.2010.02.012

Daynac, M., Morizur, L., Chicheportiche, A., Mouthon, M.-A., and Boussin, F. D. (2016). Age-related neurogenesis decline in the subventricular zone is associated with specific cell cycle regulation changes in activated neural stem cells. *Sci. Rep.* 6:21505. doi: 10.1038/srep21505

Diaz-Moreno, M., Hortiguela, R., Goncalves, A., Garcia-Carpio, I., Manich, G., Garcia-Bermudez, E., et al. (2013). Abeta increases neural stem cell activity in senescence-accelerated SAMP8 mice. *Neurobiol. Aging* 34, 2623–2638. doi: 10.1016/j.neurobiolaging.2013.05.011

Esiri, M. M., and Chance, S. A. (2012). Cognitive reserve, cortical plasticity and resistance to Alzheimer's disease. *Alzheimers Res. Ther.* 4:7. doi: 10.1186/alzrt105

Firbank, M. J., Teodorczuk, A., van der Flier, W. M., Gouw, A. A., Wallin, A., Erkinjuntti, T., et al. (2012). Relationship between progression of brain white matter changes and late-life depression: 3-year results from the LADIS study. *Br. J. Psychiatry* 201, 40–45. doi: 10.1192/bjp.bp.111.098897

Forlenza, O. V., Miranda, A. S., Guimar, I., Talib, L. L., Diniz, B. S., Gattaz, W. F., et al. (2015). Decreased neurotrophic support is associated with cognitive decline in non-demented subjects. *J. Alzheimers. Dis.* 46, 423–429. doi: 10.3233/jad-150172

Gao, Z., Ure, K., Ables, J. L., Lagace, D. C., Nave, K.-A., Goebbels, S., et al. (2009). Neurod1 is essential for the survival and maturation of adult-born neurons. *Nat. Neurosci.* 12, 1090–1092. doi: 10.1038/nn.2385

Ghate, P. S., Sidhar, H., Carlson, G. A., and Giri, R. K. (2014). Development of a novel cellular model of Alzheimer's disease utilizing neurosphere cultures derived from B6C3-Tg(APPswe,PSEN1dE9)85Dbo/J embryonic mouse brain. *Springerplus* 3, 161. doi: 10.1186/2193-1801-3-161

Grinan-Ferre, C., Puigoriol-Illamola, D., Palomera-Avalos, V., Perez-Caceres, D., Companys-Alemany, J., Camins, A., et al. (2016). Environmental enrichment modified epigenetic mechanisms in SAMP8 mouse hippocampus by reducing oxidative stress and inflammaging and achieving neuroprotection. *Front. Aging Neurosci.* 8:241. doi: 10.3389/fnagi.2016.00241

Guo, Z., Zhang, L., Wu, Z., Chen, Y., Wang, F., and Chen, G. (2014). In vivo direct reprogramming of reactive glial cells into functional neurons after brain injury and in an Alzheimer's disease model. *Cell Stem Cell* 14, 188–202. doi: 10.1016/j.stem.2013.12.001

Hattiangady, B., and Shetty, A. K. (2008). Aging does not alter the number or phenotype of putative stem/progenitor cells in the neurogenic region of the hippocampus. *Neurobiol. Aging* 29, 129–147. doi: 10.1016/j.neurobiolaging.2006.09.015

Heo, C., Chang, K. A., Choi, H. S., Kim, H. S., Kim, S., Liew, H., et al. (2007). Effects of the monomeric, oligomeric, and fibrillar Abeta42 peptides on the proliferation and differentiation of adult neural stem cells from subventricular zone. *J. Neurochem.* 102, 493–500. doi: 10.1111/j.1471-4159.2007.04499.x

Herring, A., Lewejohann, L., Panzer, A. L., Donath, A., Kroll, O., Sachser, N., et al. (2011). Preventive and therapeutic types of environmental enrichment counteract beta amyloid pathology by different molecular mechanisms. *Neurobiol. Dis.* 42, 530–538. doi: 10.1016/j.nbd.2011.03.007

Hollands, C., Bartolotti, N., and Lazarov, O. (2016). Alzheimer's Disease and Hippocampal adult neurogenesis; exploring shared mechanisms. *Front. Neurosci.* 10:178. doi: 10.3389/fnins.2016.00178

Huttenrauch, M., Walter, S., Kaufmann, M., Weggen, S., and Wirths, O. (2016). Limited effects of prolonged environmental enrichment on the pathology of

5XFAD Mice. *Mol. Neurobiol.* doi: 10.1007/s12035-016-0167-x [Epub ahead of print].

Jankowsky, J. L., Xu, G., Fromholt, D., Gonzales, V., and Borchelt, D. R. (2003). Environmental enrichment exacerbates amyloid plaque formation in a transgenic mouse model of Alzheimer disease. *J. Neuropathol. Exp. Neurol.* 62, 1220–1227. doi: 10.1093/jnen/62.12.1220

Janssen, H., Ada, L., Bernhardt, J., McElduff, P., Pollack, M., Nilsson, M., et al. (2014). An enriched environment increases activity in stroke patients undergoing rehabilitation in a mixed rehabilitation unit: a pilot non-randomized controlled trial. *Disabil. Rehabil.* 36, 255–262. doi: 10.3109/09638288.2013.788218

Komleva Iu, K., Salmina, A. B., Prokopenko, S. V., Shestakova, L. A., Petrova, M. M., Malinovskaia, N. A., et al. (2013). Changes in structural and functional plasticity of the brain induced by environmental enrichment. *Vestn. Ross. Akad. Med. Nauk.* 39–48.

Kuvacheva, N. V., Morgun, A. V., Komleva, Y. K., Khilazheva, E. D., Gorina, Y. V., Lopatina, O. L., et al. (2015). In Vitro modeling of brain progenitor cell development under the effect of environmental factors. *Bull. Exp. Biol. Med.* 159, 546–549. doi: 10.1007/s10517-015-3012-8

Leger, M., Paizanis, E., Dzahini, K., Quiedeville, A., Bouet, V., Cassel, J. C., et al. (2015). Environmental enrichment duration differentially affects behavior and neuroplasticity in adult mice. *Cereb. Cortex* 25, 4048–4061. doi: 10.1093/cercor/bhu119

Li, X., Yuan, H. F., Quan, Q. K., Wang, J. J., Wang, N. N., and Li, M. (2011). Scavenging effect of Naoerkang on amyloid beta-peptide deposition in the hippocampus in a rat model of Alzheimer's disease. *Chin. J. Integr. Med.* 17, 847–853. doi: 10.1007/s11655-011-0896-7

Ma, B. F., Liu, X. M., Zhang, A. X., Wang, P., Zhang, X. M., Li, S. N., et al. (2007). Mathematical models for the proliferation of neural stem/progenitor cells in clonogenic culture. *Rejuvenation Res.* 10, 205–214. doi: 10.1089/rej.2006.0532

Maesako, M., Uemura, K., Kubota, M., Kuzuya, A., Sasaki, K., Asada, M., et al. (2012). Environmental enrichment ameliorated high-fat diet-induced Abeta deposition and memory deficit in APP transgenic mice. *Neurobiol. Aging* 33, 1011.e11–e23. doi: 10.1016/j.neurobiolaging.2011.10.028

Malik, A., Jamasbi, R. J., Kondratov, R. V., and Geusz, M. E. (2015). Development of circadian oscillators in neurosphere cultures during adult neurogenesis. *PLoS ONE* 10:e0122937. doi: 10.1371/journal.pone.0122937

Manuel, R., Gorissen, M., Stokkermans, M., Zethof, J., Ebbesson, L. O., van de Vis, H., et al. (2015). The effects of environmental enrichment and age-related differences on inhibitory avoidance in zebrafish (Danio rerio Hamilton). *Zebrafish* 12, 152–165. doi: 10.1089/zeb.2014.1045

Marin-Padilla, M., and Knopman, D. S. (2011). Developmental aspects of the intracerebral microvasculature and perivascular spaces: insights into brain response to late-life diseases. *J. Neuropathol. Exp. Neurol.* 70, 1060–1069. doi: 10.1097/NEN.0b013e31823ac627

Marr, R. A., Thomas, R. M., and Peterson, D. A. (2010). Insights into neurogenesis and aging: potential therapy for degenerative disease? *Future Neurol.* 5, 527–541. doi: 10.2217/fnl.10.33

Mattson, M. P. (2015). Lifelong brain health is a lifelong challenge: from evolutionary principles to empirical evidence. *Ageing Res. Rev.* 20, 37–45. doi: 10.1016/j.arr.2014.12.011

Ming, G.-L., and Song, H. (2011). Adult neurogenesis in the mammalian brain: significant answers and significant questions. *Neuron* 70, 687–702. doi: 10.1016/j.neuron.2011.05.001

Monteiro, B. M., Moreira, F. A., Massensini, A. R., Moraes, M. F., and Pereira, G. S. (2014). Enriched environment increases neurogenesis and improves social memory persistence in socially isolated adult mice. *Hippocampus* 24, 239–248. doi: 10.1002/hipo.22218

Mora, F. (2013). Successful brain aging: plasticity, environmental enrichment, and lifestyle. *Dialogues Clin. Neurosci.* 15, 45–52.

Moraga, A., Pradillo, J. M., García-Culebras, A., Palma-Tortosa, S., Ballesteros, I., Hernández-Jiménez, M., et al. (2015). Aging increases microglial proliferation, delays cell migration, and decreases cortical neurogenesis after focal cerebral ischemia. *J. Neuroinflamm.* 12, 87. doi: 10.1186/s12974-015-0314-8

Mostany, R., Anstey, J. E., Crump, K. L., Maco, B., Knott, G., and Portera-Cailliau, C. (2013). Altered synaptic dynamics during normal brain aging. *J. Neurosci.* 33, 4094–4104. doi: 10.1523/jneurosci.4825-12.2013

Neidl, R., Schneider, A., Bousiges, O., Majchrzak, M., Barbelivien, A., de Vasconcelos, A. P., et al. (2016). Late-life environmental enrichment induces acetylation events and nuclear factor kappaB-dependent regulations in the hippocampus of aged rats showing improved plasticity and learning. *J. Neurosci.* 36, 4351–4361. doi: 10.1523/jneurosci.3239-15.2016

Pacey, L., Stead, S., Gleave, J., Tomczyk, K., and Doering, L. (2006). Neural stem cell culture: neurosphere generation, microscopical analysis and cryopreservation. *Protoc. Exch.* doi: 10.1038/nprot.2006.215

Polito, L., Chierchia, A., Tunesi, M., Bouybayoune, I., Kehoe, P. G., Albani, D., et al. (2014). Environmental enrichment lessens cognitive decline in APP23 mice without affecting brain sirtuin expression. *J. Alzheimers. Dis.* 42, 851–864. doi: 10.3233/jad-131430

Richetin, K., Leclerc, C., Toni, N., Gallopin, T., Pech, S., Roybon, L., et al. (2015). Genetic manipulation of adult-born hippocampal neurons rescues memory in a mouse model of Alzheimer's disease. *Brain* 138(Pt 2), 440–455. doi: 10.1093/brain/awu354

Rodriguez, J. J., Terzieva, S., Olabarria, M., Lanza, R. G., and Verkhratsky, A. (2013). Enriched environment and physical activity reverse astrogliodegeneration in the hippocampus of AD transgenic mice. *Cell Death Dis.* 4:e678. doi: 10.1038/cddis.2013.194

Rosbergen, I. C. M., Grimley, R. S., Hayward, K. S., Walker, K. C., Rowley, D., Campbell, A. M., et al. (2016). The effect of an enriched environment on activity levels in people with stroke in an acute stroke unit: protocol for a before-after pilot study. *Pilot Feasibility Stud.* 2:36. doi: 10.1186/s40814-016-0081-z

Roybon, L., Hjalt, T., Stott, S., Guillemot, F., Li, J.-Y., and Brundin, P. (2009). Neurogenin2 directs granule neuroblast production and amplification while NeuroD1 specifies neuronal fate during hippocampal neurogenesis. *PLoS ONE* 4:e4779. doi: 10.1371/journal.pone.0004779

Stuart, K. E., King, A. E., Fernandez-Martos, C. M., Dittmann, J., Summers, M. J., and Vickers, J. C. (2017). Mid-life environmental enrichment increases synaptic density in CA1 in a mouse model of Abeta-associated pathology and positively influences synaptic and cognitive health in healthy ageing. *J. Comp. Neurol.* 525, 1797–1810. doi: 10.1002/cne.24156

Terada, M., Kuzumaki, N., Hareyama, N., Imai, S., Niikura, K., Narita, M., et al. (2008). Suppression of enriched environment-induced neurogenesis in a rodent model of neuropathic pain. *Neurosci. Lett.* 440, 314–318. doi: 10.1016/j.neulet.2008.05.078

Uittenbogaard, M., and Chiaramello, A. (2000). Differential expression patterns of the basic helix-loop-helix transcription factors during aging of the murine brain. *Neurosci. Lett.* 280, 95–98. doi: 10.1016/S0304-3940(00)00761-8

Valero-Aracama, M. J., Sauvage, M. M., and Yoshida, M. (2015). Environmental enrichment modulates intrinsic cellular excitability of hippocampal CA1 pyramidal cells in a housing duration and anatomical location-dependent manner. *Behav. Brain Res.* 292, 209–218. doi: 10.1016/j.bbr.2015.05.032

VanHook, A. M. (2014). De-adhesion for mitotic progression. *Sci. Signal.* 7, ec337. doi: 10.1126/scisignal.aaa3737

Waldau, B., and Shetty, A. K. (2008). Behavior of neural stem cells in the Alzheimer brain. *Cell. Mol. Life Sci.* 65, 2372–2384. doi: 10.1007/s00018-008-8053-y

Walker, T. L., White, A., Black, D. M., Wallace, R. H., Sah, P., and Bartlett, P. F. (2008). Latent stem and progenitor cells in the hippocampus are activated by neural excitation. *J. Neurosci.* 28, 5240–5247. doi: 10.1523/jneurosci.0344-08.2008

Williamson, L. L., Chao, A., and Bilbo, S. D. (2012). Environmental enrichment alters glial antigen expression and neuroimmune function in the adult rat hippocampus. *Brain Behav. Immun.* 26, 500–510. doi: 10.1016/j.bbi.2012.01.003

Yang, S., Lu, W., Zhou, D. S., and Tang, Y. (2012). Enriched environment and white matter in aging brain. *Anat. Rec. (Hoboken)* 295, 1406–1414. doi: 10.1002/ar.22526

Yuan, Z., Wang, M., Yan, B., Gu, P., Jiang, X., Yang, X., et al. (2012). An enriched environment improves cognitive performance in mice from the senescence-accelerated prone mouse 8 strain: role of upregulated neurotrophic factor expression in the hippocampus. *Neural Regen. Res.* 7, 1797–1804. doi: 10.3969/j.issn.1673-5374.2012.23.006

Zeng, Q., Zheng, M., Zhang, T., and He, G. (2016). Hippocampal neurogenesis in the APP/PS1/nestin-GFP triple transgenic mouse model of Alzheimer's disease. *Neuroscience* 314, 64–74. doi: 10.1016/j.neuroscience.2015.11.054

Ziebell, F., Martin-Villalba, A., and Marciniak-Czochra, A. (2014). Mathematical modelling of adult hippocampal neurogenesis: effects of altered stem cell dynamics on cell counts and bromodeoxyuridine-labelled cells. *J. R. Soc. Interface* 11, 20140144. doi: 10.1098/rsif.2014.0144

3

Cognitive Function and Brain Atrophy Predict Non-Pharmacological Efficacy in Dementia: The Mihama-Kiho Scan Project2

Ken-ichi Tabei[1,2], Masayuki Satoh[1]*, Jun-ichi Ogawa[3], Tomoko Tokita[4], Noriko Nakaguchi[5], Koji Nakao[6], Hirotaka Kida[1] and Hidekazu Tomimoto[2]*

[1] Department of Dementia Prevention and Therapeutics, Graduate School of Medicine, Mie University, Tsu, Japan, [2] Department of Neurology, Graduate School of Medicine, Mie University, Tsu, Japan, [3] Yamaha Music Foundation, Tokyo, Japan, [4] Department of Health and Welfare, Mihama Town Hall, Mihama, Japan, [5] Department of Health and Welfare, Kiho Town Hall, Kiho, Japan, [6] Department of Neurosurgery, Kinan Hospital, Mihama, Japan

***Correspondence:**
Ken-ichi Tabei
tabei@clin.medic.mie-u.ac.jp;
kenichi.tabei@gmail.com
Masayuki Satoh
bruckner@clin.medic.mie-u.ac.jp

We aimed to determine whether neuropsychological deficits and brain atrophy could predict the efficacy of non-pharmacological interventions. Forty-six participants with mild-to-moderate dementia were monitored for 6 months; 25 underwent an intervention involving physical exercise with music, and 21 performed cognitive stimulation tasks. Participants were categorized into improvement (IMP) and no-IMP subgroups. In the exercise-with-music group, the no-IMP subgroup performed worse than the IMP subgroup on the Rivermead Behavioural Memory Test at baseline. In the cognitive-stimulation group, the no-IMP subgroup performed worse than the IMP subgroup on Raven's Colored Progressive Matrices and the cognitive functional independence measure at baseline. In the no-IMP subgroup, voxel-based morphometric analysis at baseline revealed more extensive gray matter loss in the anterior cingulate gyrus and left middle frontal gyrus in the exercise-with-music and cognitive-stimulation groups, respectively. Participants with mild-to-moderate dementia with cognitive decline and extensive cortical atrophy are less likely to show improved cognitive function after non-pharmaceutical therapy.

Keywords: dementia, exercise with music, cognitive dysfunction, voxel-based morphometry, atrophy, frontal lobe

INTRODUCTION

The World Alzheimer Report has estimated that there were 46.8 million people with dementia worldwide in 2015, and that this number will reach 131.5 million by 2050 (Prince et al., 2015). However, pharmacological treatments are relatively ineffective in halting the progression of dementia. The lack of pharmacological options (e.g., vaccines or disease-modifying agents) has shifted the focus of researchers toward non-pharmacological treatments for dementia, such as cognitive training, aerobic physical exercise, and music therapy (Gates and Sachdev, 2014; Groot et al., 2016; Zhang et al., 2017).

Abbreviations: AD, Alzheimer's disease; CS, cognitive stimulation; ExM, exercise with music; GM, gray matter; IMP, improvement; LM, logical memory; MMSE, Mini-Mental State Examination; no-IMP, no-improvement; RBMT, Rivermead Behavioural Memory Test; RCPM, Raven's Colored Progressive Matrices; VaD, vascular dementia; WF, word fluency.

Accumulating evidence suggests that non-pharmacological treatment may maintain or decrease the rate of cognitive decline in adults with mild cognitive impairment and early stage dementia (Rodakowski et al., 2015). Additionally, the protective effects of aerobic physical exercise against the development and/or progression of dementia have been well documented (Laurin et al., 2001; Abbott et al., 2004; Ravaglia et al., 2008; Erickson et al., 2011). Additional studies have suggested that physical exercise combined with cognitive training exerts a greater positive impact on cognitive function than physical exercise alone (Fabre et al., 2002; Oswald et al., 2006; Shatil, 2013; Satoh et al., 2014, 2017; Tabei et al., 2017). In older adults, physical ExM induces greater positive effects on visuospatial function and leads to more extensive neuroanatomical changes (Tabei et al., 2017) than exercise alone. In participants with mild-to-moderate dementia, ExM also exerts greater positive effects on cognitive function and activities of daily living than CS using portable game consoles or drills (e.g., easy calculations, mazes, and mistake-searching in pictures) (Satoh et al., 2017).

Despite recent advancements, few studies have focused on predicting outcomes following non-pharmacological treatment. Knowledge of such predictors may allow clinicians to modify factors that are likely to attenuate the effects of the intervention and to provide more targeted treatment (Hsu et al., 2017). Indeed, previous studies have demonstrated that clinical and demographic factors can influence the effect of non-pharmacological activities on cognition and on the behavioral and psychological symptoms of dementia (Särkämö et al., 2016; Hsu et al., 2017). However, the neuropsychological factors influencing non-pharmacological treatment, as well as the neural basis of its efficacy, remain unknown. Furthermore, no randomized controlled trials have compared such effects among different non-pharmacological treatment options.

Therefore, the purpose of the present study was to determine whether neuropsychological factors and regional brain atrophy [as measured via voxel-based morphometry (VBM)] can predict the rate of improvement following non-pharmacological treatment in participants with mild-to-moderate dementia and to compare the effects of different non-pharmacological interventions.

MATERIALS AND METHODS

Participants

The present study included participants with mild-to-moderate dementia who had utilized nursing services, such as day care or group homes, in the towns of Mihama and Kiho, which are situated at the southern end of the Kii peninsula in Japan. This study received approval from the Kinan Hospital Research Ethics Committee, and conformed to the tenets of the Declaration of Helsinki, and all participants provided written informed consent. This study was registered at UMIN-CTR (UMIN000017066) on April 7, 2015. The present study included the same participants as a previous study, which investigated the effect of non-pharmacological interventions in participants with mild-to-moderate dementia (Satoh et al., 2017). The inclusion criteria were as follows: (a) current diagnosis of intractable dementia by neurological specialists, based on ICD-10 diagnostic criteria (World Health Organization, 1993); (b) score between 16 and 26 on the MMSE; (c) stable physical and psychological condition; and (d) preserved hearing, visual acuity, and physical movement sufficient to enable participation in the intervention. Participants were excluded if they met any of the following criteria: (a) presence of chronic debilitating disease, such as malignancy or infection; (b) presence of severe cardiac, respiratory, and/or orthopedic disabilities that would prevent participation in the intervention; (c) presence of paresis or coordination disturbances that would prevent participation in the intervention; and (d) diagnosis of treatable dementia.

Diagnoses of AD were performed in accordance with criteria established by the National Institute of Neurologic Disorders and Stroke/Alzheimer Disease and Related Disorders Association (McKhann et al., 1984). Diagnoses of VaD were performed in accordance with criteria established by the National Institute of Neurological Disorders and Stroke/Association Internationale pour la Recherche et l'Enseignement en Neurosciences (Román et al., 1993).

All participants received treatment with anti-dementia drugs, the most common of which was donepezil hydrochloride. Pharmacological and non-pharmacological activities performed in the nursing-care facilities remained unchanged during the 6-months intervention period. Neuropsychological assessments and brain MRI were performed at baseline and following the intervention.

Procedures

Detailed descriptions of the procedures for each non-pharmacological intervention and neuropsychological assessment can be found in our previous report (Satoh et al., 2017).

Physical Exercise With Music (ExM)

Participants participated in 40-min physical exercise sessions once per week over the 6-months intervention period (total number of sessions: 24). The exercise program was developed by the Yamaha Music Foundation based on a program used in our previous study, which investigated the efficacy of physical exercise combined with music in older adults with normal cognitive function (Satoh et al., 2014; Tabei et al., 2017). The program consisted of muscle training for the upper and lower extremities, hand clapping to music, breath and voice training, and singing. The exercise trainers were professional musicians who also held private licenses as physical trainers with the Yamaha Music Foundation.

Cognitive Stimulation (CS)

Participants trained using a program called "Yawaraka Atama Juku (flexible thinking club)" developed by Nintendo Co., Ltd., using a portable game console (Nintendo DS LL,

Kyoto, Japan) and performed drills consisting of easy calculations (Kawashima, 2003), mazes, and mistake-searching in pictures. Each session was 40 min long and were conducted once per week over the 6-months intervention period (total sessions: 24). Each session was moderated by nurses, certified care workers, or psychiatric social workers employed at the respective nursing facility.

Neuropsychological Assessment

The MMSE (Folstein et al., 1975) and RCPM (Raven, 1947) were used to quantify cognitive function. In addition to an overall score, the RCPM task measures performance time, which reflects the psychomotor speed of the participants. Memory was evaluated using the LM-I/-II subtests of the RBMT (Wilson et al., 1985), which requires immediate and delayed recall of a short story. The RBMT contains four stories of varying difficulty and different word counts. We used different stories for the pre- and post-test periods to avoid the influence of familiarity with story content.

Visuospatial ability was assessed using methods described by Strub and Black (2001). Participants were shown images of cubes and Necker cubes, and were then asked to draw a picture of each. Each drawing was scored by assigning one of four possible grades (0: poor, 1: fair, 2: good, and 3: excellent).

Frontal lobe function was assessed using two tasks: WF and Trail Making Test -A/-B (Partington and Leiter, 1949). The WF test consists of category and letter domains. In the categorical WF task, participants were asked to name as many animals as possible in 1 min. In the letter WF task, participants were asked to name as many objects as possible in 1 min beginning with each of the following four phonemes: ka, sa, ta, and te (Dohi et al., 1992). The average scores for these four phonemes were used for statistical analyses.

The Functional Independence Measure was used to evaluate functional performance regarding activities of daily living. The Functional Independence Measure consists of both motor and cognitive function domains. Motor function is assessed on thirteen items, including eating, dressing, evacuation, urination, and walking. Cognitive function is assessed on five items associated with understanding, expression, and memory. The maximum motor function, cognitive function, and overall Functional Independence Measure scores are 91, 35, and 126, respectively, with higher scores indicating better function. These neuropsychological assessments were administered to participants in both groups before and after the 6-month intervention period.

Improvement and No-Improvement Groups

Participants were dichotomized into an IMP or no-IMP subgroup based on MMSE scores following the intervention. Participants with an increased MMSE score of 2 points or more were included in the IMP subgroup, while the remaining participants were included in the no-IMP subgroup. The cut-off of 2 points was determined based on the findings of previous studies, which had shown that changes in MMSE scores of 2 points are beyond the threshold of chance (Morris et al., 1993; Bowie et al., 1999; Ballard et al., 2003).

MRI Acquisition

T1-weighted gradient echo MR images were obtained using a 1.5-T MR scanner (Echelon Oval, Hitachi Medical Corporation, Tokyo, Japan). Scan parameters were as follows: repetition time = Shortest (Automatic); echo time = 11 ms; flip angle = 90°; field of view = 230 mm × 230 mm; slice thickness = 4 mm; gapless; in-plane resolution = 0.45 mm × 0.45 mm. Scans were obtained both before and after the 6-month intervention period.

MRI Analysis

MRI data were analyzed using SPM12 (Wellcome Trust Centre for Neuroimaging, University College London, London, United Kingdom) implemented in MATLAB R2012a (MathWorks, Natick, MA, United States). In the pre-processing phase, images were set to match the anterior to posterior commissure line using an automated MATLAB script. The images were then visually inspected to check for possible scan issues such as field distortion and movement artifacts. Reoriented images were corrected for intensity inhomogeneity and segmented into GM, white matter, cerebrospinal fluid, and other tissues outside the brain using SPM12 tissue probability maps. The images were registered to the East Asian Brains International Consortium for Brain Mapping space template via affine regularization. We created a population-specific template

TABLE 1 | Characteristics of study participants.

Characteristics	Total IMP	No-IMP	*p*-value	ExM IMP	No-IMP	*p*-value	CS IMP	No-IMP	*p*-value
No. of participants	18	28	0.183	11	14	0.690	7	14	0.189
Sex (F/M)	17/1	27/1	0.174	11/0	14/0	0.690	6/1	13/1	0.167
Dementia type (AD/VaD)	17/1	22/6	0.522	10/1	11/3	1.000	7/0	11/3	0.481
Age, y, mean (*SD*)	89.4 (4.9)	86.4 (5.1)	0.053	89.1 (5.7)	85.6 (5.8)	0.143	89.9 (3.6)	87.1 (4.4)	0.178
Years of education, mean (*SD*)	7.4 (1.9)	8.0 (2.0)	0.135	7.3 (1.6)	7.1 (2.3)	0.609	7.6 (2.4)	8.9 (1.3)	0.287
MMSE, mean (*SD*)	20.5 (2.9)	20.8 (4.0)	0.726	20.1 (2.5)	20.6 (3.7)	0.716	21.1 (3.6)	21.0 (4.3)	0.913
Change in MMSE score at the 6-month follow up, mean (*SD*)	3.8 (1.6)	−1.5 (2.1)	<0.001	4.4 (1.6)	−1.5 (2.1)	<0.001	3.0 (1.4)	−1.4 (2.1)	<0.001

IMP, improvement; no-IMP, no improvement; ExM, exercise plus music intervention; CS, cognitive stimulation intervention; AD, Alzheimer's disease; VaD, vascular dementia; MMSE, Mini Mental State Examination.

TABLE 2 | Baseline neuropsychological performance in the IMP and no-IMP subgroups.

	Total IMP	No-IMP	*p*-value	ExM IMP	No-IMP	*p*-value	CS IMP	No-IMP	*p*-value
MMSE	20.5 (2.9)	20.8 (4.0)	0.726	20.1 (2.5)	20.6 (3.7)	0.716	21.1 (3.6)	21.0 (4.3)	0.913
RCPM (score)	20.7 (5.3)	16.8 (6.4)	0.040	20.2 (6.0)	17.7 (7.3)	0.373	21.4 (4.3)	15.9 (5.6)	0.034
RCPM (time)	755.3 (497.1)	780.7 (782.0)	0.497	747.6 (471.6)	1054.3 (1041.2)	0.709	766.3 (570.1)	507.1 (157.2)	0.172
LM-I	5.4 (2.6)	3.1 (2.6)	0.004	5.2 (1.7)	3.2 (2.5)	0.025	5.9 (3.7)	3.0 (2.7)	0.059
LM-II	2.8 (3.2)	2.0 (2.8)	0.473	2.1 (2.6)	1.9 (2.9)	0.727	3.9 (4.0)	2.1 (2.8)	0.443
Cube	0.7 (0.5)	0.8 (0.5)	0.620	0.6 (0.5)	0.5 (0.5)	0.572	0.7 (0.5)	1.0 (0.4)	0.360
Necker cube	0.3 (0.5)	0.4 (0.5)	0.686	0.3 (0.5)	0.1 (0.4)	0.609	0.4 (0.5)	0.6 (0.5)	0.443
WF (animal)	9.9 (2.2)	8.6 (2.8)	0.099	9.7 (2.2)	8.4 (2.9)	0.209	10.1 (2.4)	8.8 (2.8)	0.172
WF (letter)	5.3 (2.0)	4.8 (2.1)	0.381	5.4 (1.6)	5.0 (1.9)	0.609	5.3 (2.6)	4.6 (2.3)	0.527
TMT-A	350.9 (184.5)	373.5 (182.9)	0.685	381.0 (211.9)	398.2 (158.3)	0.652	303.7 (131.9)	354.1 (203.8)	0.856
FIM (total)	118.6 (8.5)	112.2 (14.4)	0.038	116.9 (10.2)	114.6 (10.7)	0.373	121.3 (4.2)	109.9 (17.4)	0.034
FIM (motor)	85.9 (7.5)	82.4 (11.9)	0.070	85.0 (9.2)	85.5 (10.0)	0.403	87.4 (3.7)	79.2 (13.2)	0.110
FIM (cognition)	32.7 (3.0)	30.6 (4.5)	0.033	31.9 (3.3)	30.5 (4.7)	0.291	33.9 (1.9)	30.6 (4.5)	0.025

IMP, improvement; no-IMP, no improvement; ExM, exercise plus music intervention; CS, cognitive stimulation intervention; MMSE, Mini Mental State Examination; RCPM, Raven's Colored Progressive Matrices; LM, Logical Memory; WF, word fluency; TMT, Trail-Making Test; FIM, Functional Independence Measure.

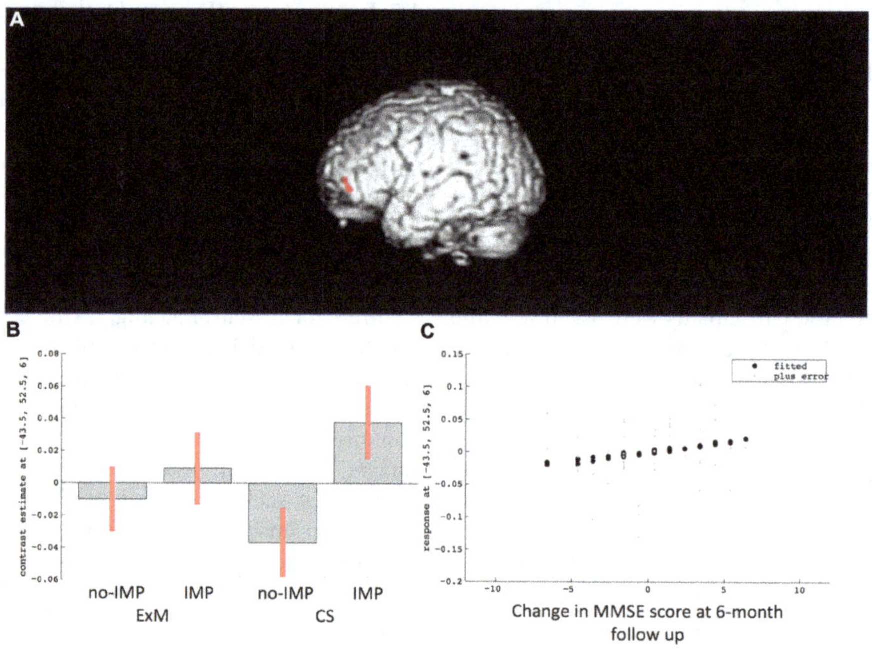

FIGURE 1 | Results of subtraction analysis between the IMP and non-IMP subgroups of the whole cohort **(A,B)**. Correlation between changes in MMSE scores and gray matter (GM) volume **(C)**. IMP, improvement; no-IMP, no-improvement; MMSE, Mini Mental State Examination.

using the SPM12 DARTEL template procedure to directly compare data between the IMP and no-IMP subgroups. We investigated group differences in GM volume, as well as the relationship between neuropsychological assessment results and GM at the whole-brain level. High-dimensional DARTEL was used to create non-linear, modulated-normalized GM and white matter images, which were smoothed using a Gaussian kernel of 8 mm FWHM (full-width at half-maximum). For whole-brain and multiple regression analyses, we assessed the statistical significance at a voxel threshold of $p < 0.005$ (uncorrected), within contiguous clusters of at least 20 voxels. We obtained both MNI and Talairach coordinates to detect the anatomical regions of the clusters. We used a transform from Matthew Brett[1] to convert MNI coordinates to Talairach coordinates, and Talairach Client 2.4.3 (Lancaster et al., 2000) was used to identify the anatomical regions corresponding to Talairach coordinates.

Statistical Analyses

Differences in demographic variables and neuropsychological assessment results between the IMP and no-IMP subgroups were analyzed using independent *t*-tests for continuous data,

[1]http://imaging.mrc-cbu.cam.ac.uk/imaging/MniTalairach

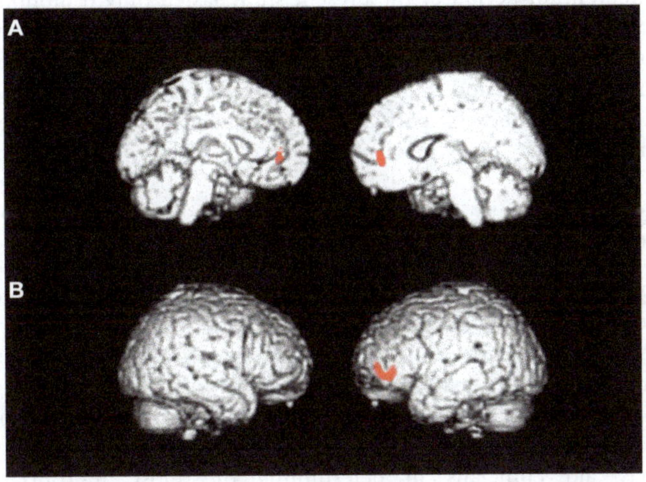

FIGURE 2 | Results of subtraction analysis between the IMP and non-IMP subgroups of the ExM **(A)** and CS groups **(B)**. IMP, improvement; no-IMP, no-improvement; ExM, exercise plus music intervention; CS, cognitive stimulation intervention.

chi-square tests for dichotomous data, and Mann–Whitney *U* tests for non-parametric data. Differences of $p < 0.05$ were considered statistically significant. Statistical analyses were performed using IBM SPSS Statistics software version 20 (IBM Corp., Armonk, NY, United States).

RESULTS

Participant Characteristics

Participants who participated in more than 75% of all sessions (more than 18) and completed the neuropsychological and MRI assessments before and after the intervention were included in the final analysis. Following exclusion of the remaining participants, the ExM and CS groups included 25 and 21 participants, respectively (ExM: AD = 21; VaD = 4; CS: AD = 18, VaD = 3) (**Table 1**). Prior to the intervention, there were no significant differences in sex ratio, dementia type, age, years of education, or MMSE scores between the ExM and CS groups. However, among participants in both ExM and CS groups, MMSE scores were significantly worse in the no-IMP subgroup than in the IMP subgroup at the 6-month follow-up ($p < 0.001$) (**Table 1**).

Neuropsychological Assessments

Baseline cube and Necker cube scores were significantly worse in the ExM group than in the CS group (p = 0.022, 0.01), although no significant differences were observed in the other neuropsychological assessments.

Participants in the no-IMP subgroup had significantly poorer baseline scores on the RCPM, LM-I section of the RBMT, and cognitive functional independence than those in the IMP subgroup (p = 0.04, 0.004, 0.033) (**Table 2**). Furthermore, baseline scores on the LM-I subtest were significantly worse in the no-IMP subgroup than the IMP subgroup (p = 0.025) of the ExM participants. In the CS group, baseline scores on the RCPM test and cognitive functional independence measure were significantly worse in the no-IMP subgroup than in the IMP subgroup (p = 0.034, 0.025, respectively) (**Table 2**).

MRI Assessments

Cube and Necker cube scores were used as covariates. Subtraction analysis revealed more extensive loss of GM in the left middle frontal gyrus in the no-IMP subgroup at baseline, relative to the IMP subgroup (**Figures 1A,B** and **Table 3**). Analysis of MMSE scores at the 6-month follow up revealed that changes in MMSE scores were positively correlated with volume in the left middle frontal gyrus (**Figure 1C** and **Table 3**). Subtraction analysis revealed more extensive GM loss in the anterior cingulate gyrus and left middle frontal gyrus in no-IMP participants in both the ExM (**Figure 2A** and **Table 3**) and CS (**Figure 2B** and **Table 3**) groups at baseline, respectively.

DISCUSSION

The present study aimed to determine whether neuropsychological factors and regional brain atrophy can predict the rate of IMP in participants with mild-to-moderate dementia following non-pharmacological intervention. Among ExM participants, the no-IMP subgroup exhibited poorer baseline performance on the LM-I subtest of the RBMT than participants in the IMP subgroup. Among CS participants, the no-IMP subgroup exhibited poorer baseline RCPM and cognitive functional independence measure scores than participants in the IMP subgroup. Such differences may be associated with differences in cognitive resources required to execute each intervention. Proper execution of the ExM protocol requires the participant to remember the exercise patterns from week to week, while proper execution of the CS protocol requires spatial and

TABLE 3 | Cluster sizes, peak locations, and statistical values for regions showing significant pre-intervention differences between the IMP and no-IMP subgroups.

Contrast	L/R	Area	BA	Talairach coordinates (mm) X	Y	Z	*Z*-value	Cluster size in voxels
IMP > no-IMP (Total)	L	Middle Frontal Gyrus	10	−44	46	−4	2.72	49
IMP > no-IMP (ExM)	R	Anterior Cingulate	32	4	44	−2	2.96	209
IMP > no-IMP (CS)	L	Middle Frontal Gyrus	10	−44	50	3	3.20	433

IMP, improvement; no-IMP, no-improvement; ExM, exercise plus music intervention; CS, cognitive stimulation intervention.

mathematical abilities that allow understanding of geometric designs and missing pieces, as well as expressive abilities and memory function to complete calculations, mazes, and search for mistakes in images. Although previous studies have indicated that exercise and ExM tasks enhance memory in participants with dementia (Radak et al., 2010; Intlekofer and Cotman, 2013; Satoh et al., 2017), our results suggest that execution of the intervention requires a certain amount of memory function reserve. These findings highlight the importance of early intervention, when cognitive function may be somewhat preserved (Dubois et al., 2016).

Voxel-based morphometry analysis revealed more extensive loss of GM in the anterior cingulate gyrus in no-IMP participants of the ExM group, and in the left middle frontal gyrus in the CS group at baseline relative to that observed in the IMP subgroup. These findings may also have been associated with the execution of each intervention. Previous studies have demonstrated that the anterior cingulate gyrus plays a key role in music processing in participants with dementia (Omar et al., 2011; Fletcher et al., 2015; Jacobsen et al., 2015), while the left middle frontal gyrus is associated with calculation (Maurer et al., 2016) and visual search (Weidner et al., 2009) in CS tasks. Therefore, our results indicate that the extent and location of brain atrophy at baseline may represent the neural basis of task execution for each intervention. In addition, these parameters may aid in predicting the efficacy of non-pharmacological treatment.

Previous studies have indicated that characteristic impairments across cognitive domains (Mori et al., 2016), Barthel Index (Formiga et al., 2010), and lower pre-treatment regional cerebral blood flow in the right orbitofrontal cortex (Hongo et al., 2008) can be used to predict better responses to cholinesterase inhibitors treatment in older adults with dementia. Our findings suggest that the efficacy of non-pharmacological treatment can also be predicted based on neural characteristics and the extent of cognitive decline.

The present study has some limitations of note. First, as we did not include healthy controls, further studies are required to investigate differences in neuropsychological factors and regional brain atrophy between healthy individuals and participants with mild-to-moderate dementia. Such findings may allow clinicians to predict the most appropriate non-pharmacological treatment for each participant. Second, the intervention period of the present study lasted only 6 months. Explicit differences in neuropsychological factors and regional brain atrophy may be more evident following a longer intervention period. Future studies should also aim to include a larger number of participants to enhance the accuracy of prediction.

CONCLUSION

Our findings suggest that participants with mild-to-moderate dementia who have experienced cognitive decline, reduced ability to perform activities of daily living, and extensive cortical atrophy are less likely to exhibit IMPs in cognitive function following non-pharmacological treatment. Thus, some characteristics of pre-treatment cognitive dysfunction and regional brain atrophy may aid clinicians in determining the most appropriate non-pharmacological intervention for each participant.

AUTHOR CONTRIBUTIONS

MS: conceived and designed the experiments. TT, NN, and KN: conducted the experiments. KT: analyzed the data. KT and MS: wrote the paper. JO: contributed materials. HK: analyzed and interpreted the data. HT: supervised and interpreted the data. All authors read and approved the final version of the paper.

FUNDING

This study was supported by JSPS KAKENHI Grant-in-Aid for Scientific Research (C) (Grant No: 15K08909) and Grant-in-Aid for Young Scientists (B) (Grant Nos: 25870325 and 17K17811).

ACKNOWLEDGMENTS

We would like to thank Keisuke Okamoto who works in the laboratory, Isamu Nonomura in radiology, and Hideshi Kanai in the community cooperation room at Kinan Hospital, and Takayuki Yotsuji at the Yamaha Music Foundation, for their kind contributions to this study.

REFERENCES

Abbott, R. D., White, L. R., Ross, G. W., Masaki, K. H., Curb, J. D., and Petrovitch, H. (2004). Walking and dementia in physically capable elderly men. *J. Am. Med. Assoc.* 292, 1447–1453. doi: 10.1001/jama.292.12.1447

Ballard, C., Rowan, E., Stephens, S., Kalaria, R., and Kenny, R. A. (2003). Prospective follow-up study between 3 and 15 months after stroke: improvements and decline in cognitive function among dementia-free stroke survivors >75 years of age. *Stroke* 34, 2440–2444. doi: 10.1161/01.STR.0000089923.29724.CE

Bowie, P., Branton, T., and Holmes, J. (1999). Should the mini mental state examination be used to monitor dementia treatments? *Lancet* 354, 1527–1528. doi: 10.1016/S0140-6736(99)03486-8

Dohi, N., Iwaya, T., and Kayamori, R. (1992). *Seishin-kinou Hyouka, the Evaluation of Mental Function.* Tokyo: Ishiyaku Publishers, Inc.

Dubois, B., Hampel, H., Feldman, H. H., Scheltens, P., Aisen, P., Andrieu, S., et al. (2016). Preclinical Alzheimer's disease: definition, natural history, and diagnostic criteria. *Alzheimers Dement.* 12, 292–323. doi: 10.1016/j.jalz.2016.02.002

Erickson, K. I., Voss, M. W., Prakash, R. S., Basak, C., Szabo, A., Chaddock, L., et al. (2011). Exercise training increases size of hippocampus and improves memory. *Proc. Natl. Acad. Sci. U.S.A.* 108, 3017–3022. doi: 10.1073/pnas.1015950108

Fabre, C., Chamari, K., Mucci, P., Masse-Biron, J., and Prefaut, C. (2002). Improvement of cognitive function by mental and/or individualized aerobic training in healthy elderly subjects. *Int. J. Sports Med.* 23, 415–421. doi: 10.1055/s-2002-33735

Fletcher, P. D., Downey, L. E., Golden, H. L., Clark, C. N., Slattery, C. F., Paterson, R. W., et al. (2015). Auditory hedonic phenotypes in dementia: a behavioural and neuroanatomical analysis. *Cortex* 67, 95–105. doi: 10.1016/j.cortex.2015.03.021

Folstein, M. F., Folstein, S. E., and McHugh, P. R. (1975). Mini-mental state: a practical method for grading the cognitive state of patients for the clinician. *J. Psychiatr. Res.* 12, 189–198. doi: 10.1016/0022-3956(75)90026-6

Formiga, F., Fort, I., Robles, M. J., Rodriguez, D., and Regalado, P. (2010). Lower Barthel Index scores predict less prescription of pharmacological therapy in elderly patients with Alzheimer disease. *Dement. Geriatr. Cogn.* 29, 198–203. doi: 10.1159/000278348

Gates, N. J., and Sachdev, P. (2014). Is cognitive training an effective treatment for preclinical and early Alzheimer's disease? *J. Alzheimers Dis.* 42(Suppl. 4), S551–S559. doi: 10.3233/JAD-141302

Groot, C., Hooghiemstra, A. M., Raijmakers, P. G. H. M., van Berckel, B. N. M., Scheltens, P., Scherder, E. J. A., et al. (2016). The effect of physical activity on cognitive function in patients with dementia: a meta-analysis of randomized control trials. *Ageing Res. Rev.* 25, 13–23. doi: 10.1016/j.arr.2015.11.005

Hongo, J., Nakaaki, S., Shinagawa, Y., Murata, Y., Sato, J., Tatsumi, H., et al. (2008). SPECT-identified neuroanatomical predictor of the cognitive effects of donepezil treatment in patients with Alzheimer's disease. *Dement. Geriatr. Cogn.* 26, 556–566. doi: 10.1159/000181148

Hsu, T. J., Tsai, H. T., Hwang, A. C., Chen, L. Y., and Chen, L. K. (2017). Predictors of non-pharmacological intervention effect on cognitive function and behavioral and psychological symptoms of older people with dementia. *Geriatr. Gerontol. Int.* 17(Suppl. 1), 28–35. doi: 10.1111/ggi.13037

Intlekofer, K. A., and Cotman, C. W. (2013). Exercise counteracts declining hippocampal function in aging and Alzheimer's disease. *Neurobiol. Dis.* 57, 47–55. doi: 10.1016/j.nbd.2012.06.011

Jacobsen, J. H., Stelzer, J., Fritz, T. H., Chételat, G., La Joie, R., and Turner, R. (2015). Why musical memory can be preserved in advanced Alzheimer's disease. *Brain* 138, 2438–2450. doi: 10.1093/brain/awv135

Kawashima, R. (2003). *Calculation Drill for Adults Which Improves Brain Function.* Tokyo: Kumon Publication.

Lancaster, J. L., Woldorff, M. G., Parsons, L. M., Liotti, M., Freitas, C. S., Rainey, L., et al. (2000). Automated Talairach atlas labels for functional brain mapping. *Hum. Brain Mapp.* 10, 120–131. doi: 10.1002/1097-0193(200007)10:3<120::AID-HBM30>3.0.CO;2-8

Laurin, D., Verreault, R., Lindsay, J., MacPherson, K., and Rockwood, K. (2001). Physical activity and risk of cognitive impairment and dementia in elderly persons. *Arch. Neurol.* 58, 498–504. doi: 10.1001/archneur.58.3.498

Maurer, S., Tanigawa, N., Sollmann, N., Hauck, T., Ille, S., Boeckh-Behrens, T., et al. (2016). Non-invasive mapping of calculation function by repetitive navigated transcranial magnetic stimulation. *Brain Struct. Funct.* 221, 3927–3947. doi: 10.1007/s00429-015-1136-2

McKhann, G., Drachman, D., Folstein, M., Katzman, R., Price, D., and Stadlan, E. M. (1984). Clinical diagnosis of Alzheimer's disease: report of the NINCDS-ADRDA Work Group under the auspices of Department of Health and Human Services Task Force on Alzheimer's disease. *Neurology* 34, 939–944. doi: 10.1212/WNL.34.7.939

Mori, E., Ikeda, M., Nakagawa, M., Miyagishi, H., and Kosaka, K. (2016). Pretreatment cognitive profile likely to benefit from donepezil treatment in dementia with Lewy bodies: pooled analyses of two randomized controlled trials. *Dement. Geriatr. Cogn.* 42, 58–68. doi: 10.1159/000447586

Morris, J. C., Edland, S., Clark, C., Galasko, D., Koss, E., Mohs, R., et al. (1993). The consortium to establish a registry for Alzheimer's disease (CERAD). Part IV. Rates of cognitive change in the longitudinal assessment of probable Alzheimer's disease. *Neurology* 43, 2457–2465. doi: 10.1212/WNL.43.12.2457

Omar, R., Henley, S. M., Bartlett, J. W., Hailstone, J. C., Gordon, E., Sauter, D. A., et al. (2011). The structural neuroanatomy of music emotion recognition: evidence from frontotemporal lobar degeneration. *Neuroimage* 56, 1814–1821. doi: 10.1016/j.neuroimage.2011.03.002

Oswald, W. D., Gunzelmann, T., Rupprecht, R., and Hagen, B. (2006). Differential effects of single versus combined cognitive and physical training with older adults: the SimA study in a 5-year perspective. *Eur. J. Ageing* 3, 179–192. doi: 10.1007/s10433-006-0035-z

Partington, J. E., and Leiter, R. G. (1949). Partington's pathway test. *Psychol. Serv. Center Bull.* 1, 9–20.

Prince, M., Wimo, A., Guerchet, M., Ali, G. C., Wu, Y. T., and Prina, M. (2015). *World Alzheimer Report 2015 - The Global Impact of Dementia: An Analysis of Prevalence, Incidence, Cost and Trends.* London: Alzheimer's Disease International.

Radak, Z., Hart, N., Sarga, L., Koltai, E., Atalay, M., Ohno, H., et al. (2010). Exercise plays a preventive role against Alzheimer's disease. *J. Alzheimers Dis.* 20, 777–783. doi: 10.3233/JAD-2010-091531

Ravaglia, G., Forti, P., Lucicesare, A., Pisacane, N., Rietti, E., Bianchin, M., et al. (2008). Physical activity and dementia risk in the elderly: findings from a prospective Italian study. *Neurology* 70, 1786–1794. doi: 10.1212/01.wnl.0000296276.50595.86

Raven, J. C. (1947). *Coloured Progressive Matrices Sets A, AB, B. Manual Sections A and 2.* Oxford: Oxford Psychologists Press.

Rodakowski, J., Saghafi, E., Butters, M. A., and Skidmore, E. R. (2015). Non-pharmacological interventions for adults with mild cognitive impairment and early stage dementia: an updated scoping review. *Mol. Aspects Med.* 43, 38–53. doi: 10.1016/j.mam.2015.06.003

Román, G. C., Tatemichi, T. K., Erkinjuntti, T., Cummings, J. L., Masdeu, J. C., Garcia, J. A., et al. (1993). Vascular dementia: diagnostic criteria for research studies. Report of the NINDS-AIREN International Workshop. *Neurology* 43, 250–260. doi: 10.1212/WNL.43.2.250

Särkämö, T., Laitinen, S., Numminen, A., Kurki, M., Johnson, J. K., and Rantanen, P. (2016). Clinical and demographic factors associated with the cognitive and emotional efficacy of regular musical activities in dementia. *J. Alzheimers Dis.* 49, 767–781. doi: 10.3233/JAD-150453

Satoh, M., Ogawa, J. I., Tokita, T., Nakaguchi, N., Nakao, K., Kida, H., et al. (2014). The effects of physical exercise with music on cognitive function of elderly people: Mihama-Kiho project. *PLoS One* 9:e95230. doi: 10.1371/journal.pone.0095230

Satoh, M., Ogawa, J. I., Tokita, T., Nakaguchi, N., Nakao, K., Kida, H., et al. (2017). Physical exercise with music maintains activities of daily living in patients with dementia: Mihama-Kiho project part 21. *J. Alzheimers Dis.* 57, 85–96. doi: 10.3233/JAD-161217

Shatil, E. (2013). Does combined cognitive training and physical activity training enhance cognitive abilities more than either alone? A four-condition randomized controlled trial among healthy older adults. *Front. Aging Neurosci.* 5:8. doi: 10.3389/fnagi.2013.00008

Strub, R. L., and Black, F. W. (2001). *The Mental Status Examination in Neurology*, 4th Edn. Philadelphia, PA: F.A. Davis Company.

Tabei, K. I., Satoh, M., Ogawa, J. I., Tokita, T., Nakaguchi, N., Nakao, K., et al. (2017). Physical exercise with music reduces gray and white matter loss in the frontal cortex of elderly people: the Mihama-Kiho scan project. *Front. Aging Neurosci.* 9:174. doi: 10.3389/fnagi.2017.00174

Weidner, R., Krummenacher, J., Reimann, B., Müller, H. J., and Fink, G. R. (2009). Sources of top-down control in visual search. *J. Cogn. Neurosci.* 21, 2100–2113. doi: 10.1162/jocn.2008.21173

Wilson, B., Cockburn, J., and Baddeley, A. (1985). *The Rivermead Behavioural Memory Test.* Bury St Edmunds: Thames Valley Test Company.

World Health Organization (1993). *International Statistical Classification of Diseases and Related Health Problems*, 10th Rev. Geneva: World Health Organization.

Zhang, Y., Cai, J., An, L., Hui, F., Ren, T., Ma, H., et al. (2017). Does music therapy enhance behavioral and cognitive function in elderly dementia patients? A systematic review and meta-analysis. *Ageing Res. Rev.* 35, 1–11. doi: 10.1016/j.arr.2016.12.003

4

Challenges for Alzheimer's Disease Therapy: Insights from Novel Mechanisms Beyond Memory Defects

Rudimar L. Frozza [1], Mychael V. Lourenco [2,3] and Fernanda G. De Felice [2,4]**

[1] Oswaldo Cruz Institute, Fundação Oswaldo Cruz (FIOCRUZ), Rio de Janeiro, Brazil, [2] Institute of Medical Biochemistry Leopoldo de Meis, Rio de Janeiro, Brazil, [3] Institute of Biophysics Carlos Chagas Filho, Federal University of Rio de Janeiro, Rio de Janeiro, Brazil, [4] Department of Biomedical and Molecular Sciences, Centre for Neuroscience Studies, Queen's University, Kingston, ON, Canada

***Correspondence:**
Rudimar L. Frozza
rudimar.frozza@ioc.fiocruz.br
Fernanda G. De Felice
felice@bioqmed.ufrj.br

Alzheimer's disease (AD), the most common form of dementia in late life, will become even more prevalent by midcentury, constituting a major global health concern with huge implications for individuals and society. Despite scientific breakthroughs during the past decades that have expanded our knowledge on the cellular and molecular bases of AD, therapies that effectively halt disease progression are still lacking, and focused efforts are needed to address this public health challenge. Because AD is classically recognized as a disease of memory, studies have mainly focused on investigating memory-associated brain defects. However, compelling evidence has indicated that additional brain regions, not classically linked to memory, are also affected in the course of disease. In this review, we outline the current understanding of key pathophysiological mechanisms in AD and their clinical manifestation. We also highlight how considering the complex nature of AD pathogenesis, and exploring repurposed drug approaches can pave the road toward the development of novel therapeutics for AD.

Keywords: Alzheimer's disease, inflammation, metabolic derangements, memory defects, preclinical, therapy

INTRODUCTION

Increasing life expectancy has produced a dramatic rise in the number of cases of age-associated diseases, including dementia. Alzheimer's disease (AD) is the most frequent cause of dementia, accounting for 60–80% of all cases (Prince et al., 2016), and epidemiological studies indicate that AD will become even more incident by midcentury, constituting a major personal and societal tragedy. AD is primarily a condition of late life, roughly doubling in prevalence every 5 years after age 65 (Prince et al., 2013), and affects some 47 million people worldwide (Prince et al., 2013). This number is predicted to increase in the next two decades (Prince et al., 2016). The total cost of dementia was estimated around $818 billion in 2010 and has been projected to hit $1 trillion by 2018 worldwide (Prince et al., 2016). This becomes even more dramatic because nearly 60% of people affected by dementia live in low- and middle-income countries.

AD is a complex disorder. While the vast majority of AD cases are sporadic, affecting individuals older than 60 years, genetic mutations cause a rare (<0.5%) familial form of AD, whose symptoms develop earlier, typically between 30 and 50 years of age (Bateman et al., 2010). Further, there is a marked difference in the incidence of AD between women and men. It is estimated that nearly two-thirds of the patients living with AD are women (Alzheimer's Association, 2017), raising the intriguing suggestion that there are biological mechanisms underlying the higher incidence of AD cases in women that still demand to be investigated.

AD is mainly characterized by progressive cognitive impairment. However, as disease progresses, other debilitating non-cognitive symptoms arise, including impaired sleep and appetite, and neuropsychiatric alterations (e.g., depression and apathy) (Ishii and Iadecola, 2015; Lanctôt et al., 2017). In addition, mounting epidemiological studies have supported a link between metabolic disorders and AD (Ott et al., 1996, 1999; Steen et al., 2005; Matsuzaki et al., 2010; Takeda et al., 2010; Crane et al., 2013; De Felice, 2013; De Felice and Lourenco, 2015; Chatterjee et al., 2016). Because AD has been considered a disease of memory, studies on AD pathogenesis have mainly concentrated on how memory and cognitive failure develop, while other symptoms and co-morbidities have remained largely overlooked.

Thus, it is not surprisingly that precise and reliable biomarkers are still lacking for early disease diagnosis. Although conclusive diagnostics has mostly been confirmed through *post-mortem* examination, it is now widely accepted that pathophysiological changes begin to develop decades prior to initial cognitive symptoms, in a preclinical or presymptomatic stage (Sperling et al., 2011a,b). Further, the addition of novel biomarkers to diagnostic criteria has prompted a shift in how AD is considered as pathological entity, increasing the appreciation that it should not be regarded as having discrete and defined clinical stages, but rather as multifaceted process moving along a continuum (Sperling et al., 2011a; van Maurik et al., 2017; **Figure 1**). Relatively accurate diagnosis and timely therapies will likely be achieved when neuropsychological, fluid and imaging biomarkers are used in combination (Viola and Klein, 2015; Dubois et al., 2016; Blennow, 2017).

Although advances in animal and clinical research over the past few decades have improved our knowledge on the pathophysiological course of AD, even drugs with successful preclinical assessment have not been effective in reversing or slowing down AD progression in large clinical trials. These constraints may be due to that clinical trials have predominantly focused on therapies based on anti-amyloid strategies, since the amyloid cascade hypothesis has been placed at the center of therapeutic prospection (Karran et al., 2011; Cummings et al., 2014; Hendrix et al., 2016). Such disappointing outcomes are also suggestive of problems in translating therapies from rodent model species to humans (De Felice and Munoz, 2016). The lack of adequate control for sex differences in animal models adds up to this translational impedance. Therefore, potential therapies that work in a sex of one animal species (usually male rodents) frequently fail to translate to human trials dominated by female participants (often 2:1 female:male in large trials). Furthermore, while neuropathological features of AD are widely recognized, the intricacies of the mechanism involving central and peripheral derangements have not been clearly defined.

Given that AD holds a complex pathology, it has now been believed that more effective treatments could be possible using disease-modifying therapies and drugs targeting multiple molecular pathways (Castellani and Perry, 2012; Cummings et al., 2014; Perry et al., 2014; Stephenson et al., 2014). These should importantly take sex differences into consideration, as recently noticed (Snyder et al., 2016; Zhao et al., 2016). In this review, we discuss recent advances in the AD field, as well as classical and novel mechanisms that might reveal potential new strategies to treat AD.

MOLECULAR PATHOGENESIS OF AD

Tau Phosphorylation, Amyloid Deposition, and Aβ Oligomers

The most distinctive features present in memory-associated brain regions of AD patients are the intracellular neurofibrillary tangles (NFTs) and the extracellular amyloid plaques. The major component of the NFTs is abnormally phosphorylated and aggregated tau protein (Querfurth and LaFerla, 2010; Medeiros et al., 2011; Morris et al., 2011), thereby destabilizing microtubules and compromising axonal transport (Querfurth and LaFerla, 2010; Ittner and Götz, 2011; Medeiros et al., 2011; Morris et al., 2011; Scheltens et al., 2016). It has been recently shown that tangles induce neuronal loss and spatial memory defects (Fu et al., 2017), putatively providing a link between tau pathology and cognitive deficits in early AD. Although pathological alterations of tau were thought to be downstream events of Aβ deposition, it is equally plausible that tau and Aβ act in parallel to enhancing each other's toxic effects and initiate the pathogenic events germane to AD (Small and Duff, 2008; Spires-Jones and Hyman, 2014; Bennett et al., 2017). Fresh evidence has also pointed to soluble, diffusible tau oligomers as important drivers of synaptotoxicity, and possible culprits for the marked progression of tau pathology across the brain (Fá et al., 2016; Carrieri et al., 2017; Piacentini et al., 2017; Puzzo et al., 2017; Reilly et al., 2017).

The amyloid cascade hypothesis suggests that brain accumulation of the amyloid-β peptide (Aβ), produced by sequential cleavage of the amyloid precursor protein (APP) by the β- and γ-secretase enzymes, is a central event in AD (Karran et al., 2011; Selkoe and Hardy, 2016). Soluble Aβ undergoes conformational changes to high β-sheet content, rendering it prone to aggregation into polymeric forms, including soluble oligomers and larger insoluble fibrils. These fibrils ultimately deposit into extracellular amyloid plaques in the AD brains (Stine et al., 2003; Blennow et al., 2006; Finder and Glockshuber, 2007; Lee et al., 2007).

Aβ is physiologically degraded by the peptidases insulin-degrading enzyme, neprilysin, and by endothelin-converting enzyme (Qiu et al., 1998; Iwata et al., 2001; Farris et al., 2003; Leissring et al., 2003). In addition, Aβ can be cleared out by transportation to peripheral circulation across multiple pathways, including the blood-brain barrier, interstitial fluid bulk flow, arachnoid villi, and glymphatic-lymphatic pathways (Tarasoff-Conway et al., 2015). Additionally, Aβ aggregates can be phagocited and degraded by microglia, perivascular macrophages, and astrocytes. Defective clearing systems could thus lead to an imbalance between production and clearance

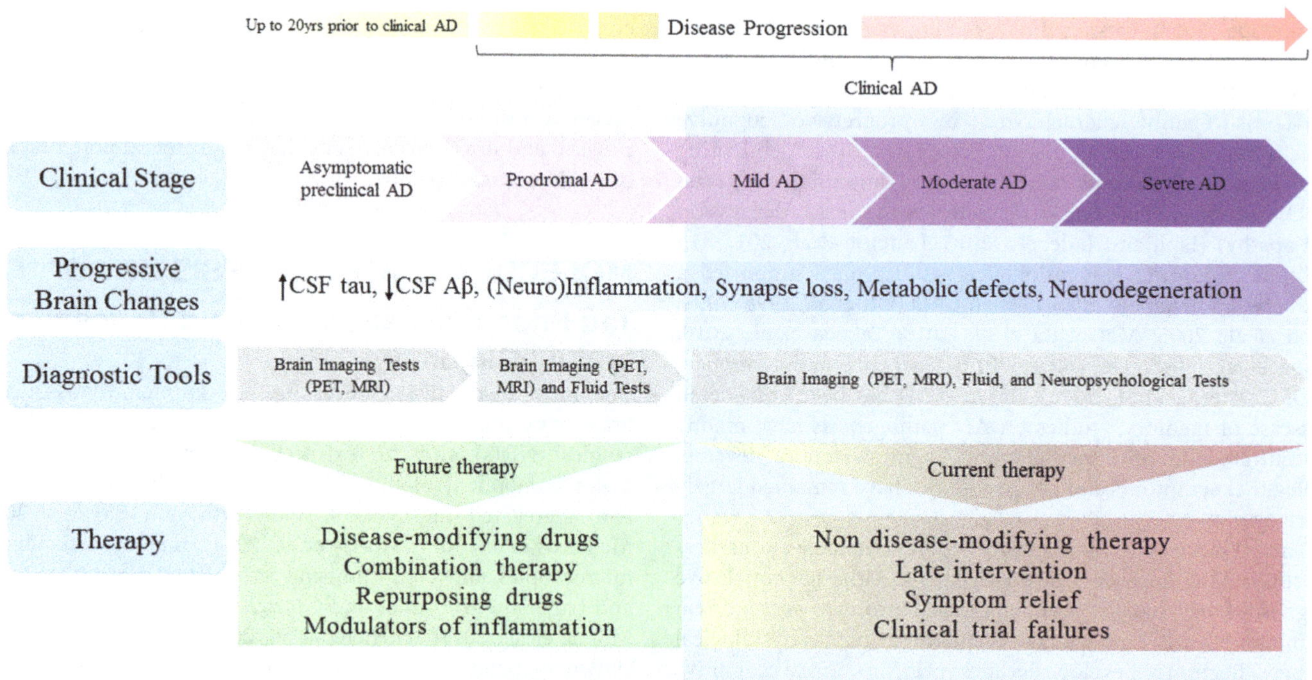

FIGURE 1 | Alzheimer's disease depicted as a continuum: challenges for therapy. Pathophysiological changes in the AD brain begin many years prior to clinical manifestations of disease and move along a continuum, spanning from clinically asymptomatic to severely impaired spectra. Although cognitive symptoms are absent in the preclinical stage, progressive amyloid deposition could drive the patient toward prodromal AD stage, characterized by short-term memory impairment without affecting activity of daily living. As disease progresses, however, many brain areas and their functions become impaired, culminating in severe memory loss and metabolic derangements, both of which affect autonomy. Despite the lack of *bona fide* biomarkers to date, earlier detection will ensure that treatments reach individuals in a timely manner. Given that therapies initially considered promising have disappointed in clinical trials, current AD research pipeline requires a shift toward the use of disease-modifying approaches, combination and/or repurposing therapies, and the search for agents selectively targeting specific modulators of inflammation.

of Aβ in the brain, thereby resulting in subsequent neuronal dysfunction and neurodegeneration (Hardy, 2002).

A growing body of evidence indicates, however, that plaque deposition is not the sole responsible for the impairments observed in AD. On the other hand, the notion that Aβ oligomers (AβOs) are the main toxins responsible for synapse dysfunction and cognitive deficits in AD has attracted considerable attention to improve our understanding of the mechanisms of the disease (Walsh and Selkoe, 2007; Selkoe, 2008; Ferreira and Klein, 2011; Ferreira et al., 2015; Yang et al., 2017). In this context, plaques have been thought to comprise a reservoir from which AβOs diffuse, or may even act sequestering soluble oligomers until they reach a physiological plateau (Selkoe and Hardy, 2016).

A considerable number of studies has reported that AβOs accumulate in the brain and CSF of AD patients (Georganopoulou et al., 2005; Haes et al., 2005; Anker et al., 2009; Xia et al., 2009; Herskovits et al., 2013; Viola et al., 2014; Murakami et al., 2016), and are found in association with synapses in the brains of patients presenting clinical signals of dementia (Koffie et al., 2009; Bjorklund et al., 2012; Perez-Nievas et al., 2013; Bilousova et al., 2016), adding clinical relevance to their role in AD. These studies suggest that synapse-associated AβOs promote detrimental modifications in synapse structure and composition, thereby leading to memory loss. This growing body of evidence props up an early notion that cognitive decline is not only a result of the extracellular accumulation of Aβ and intracellular accumulation of tau but also as a consequence of synapse failure and loss in AD (Terry et al., 1991; Masliah et al., 1992; Selkoe, 2002).

Despite intense research, the exact mechanisms of how AβOs exert their toxicity remains to be fully unveiled. Binding of Aβ aggregates to various receptors may disrupt key neuronal functions. However, the complete identity of receptors to which they bind and the underlying signaling pathways still remain to be fully elucidated (Ferreira et al., 2015).

We now know that AβOs bind to cell surface receptors and trigger multiple aberrant signaling pathways, including calcium signaling (Mattson, 2010; Ferreira et al., 2015), oxidative stress (Smith et al., 1998; Perry et al., 2002; De Felice et al., 2007), derangements in plasticity-related receptors and increased glutamate release from pre-synaptic terminals (Roselli et al., 2005; Shankar et al., 2007; Decker et al., 2010a; Ferreira et al., 2015). In addition, they promote tau hyperphosphorylation (De Felice et al., 2008; Jin et al., 2011), impaired axonal transport (Snyder et al., 2005; Decker et al., 2010b; Miñano-Molina et al., 2011; Bomfim et al., 2012), and drive inhibition of long-term potentiation (LTP) and memory impairment (Rowan et al., 2005; Shankar et al., 2008; Ferreira and Klein, 2011; Ferreira et al., 2015; Yang et al., 2017).

Inflammatory Markers in the Brain

AD pathogenesis appears to include strong interactions with immune mechanisms in the brain. AβOs induce aberrant reactivity of astrocytes and microglia, in the brains of mice and non-human primates (Bomfim et al., 2012; Ledo et al., 2013, 2016; Forny-Germano et al., 2014). Recent studies have further unveiled that disturbances in microglia, as well as interactions with peripheral immune cells, may play key roles in causing synapse loss and neurodegeneration in AD (Browne et al., 2013; Zhang et al., 2013; Baruch et al., 2015, 2016; Guillot-Sestier et al., 2015; Zenaro et al., 2015; Hong et al., 2016a,b). These studies are in line with emerging evidence suggesting that inflammation has a pivotal role in disease pathogenesis, as markers of inflammation, such as TNF-α, IL-1β, IL-6, and other cytokines, have been shown to be increased in the brain, CSF, and plasma of AD patients (Perry et al., 2010; Swardfager et al., 2010; Czirr and Wyss-Coray, 2012; Alcolea et al., 2014; Heneka et al., 2015a; Hong et al., 2016a; Salter and Stevens, 2017).

Increased pro-inflammatory signaling resulting from reactive microglial reduces Aβ clearance, promotes aberrant synaptic pruning (Lee and Landreth, 2010; Mandrekar-Colucci et al., 2012; Heneka et al., 2015a,b; Hong et al., 2016b), prompts Aβ and tau pathologies, and contributes to impaired synapse function (Wang W. Y. et al., 2015). Importantly, TNF-α-dependent mechanisms appear to drive memory defects (Lourenco et al., 2013) and depressive-like behavior in AD mice (Ledo et al., 2016), thereby indicating a causal role of inflammation in deleterious processes linked to AD.

Unfolded Protein Response and Defective Proteostasis

Pro-inflammatory pathways triggered by AβOs, notably via TNF-α, have been reported to induce neuronal stress (Lourenco et al., 2013), likely resulting in defective proteostasis. Furthermore, it has been recently demonstrated that AβOs stimulates eIF2α phosphorylation (Devi and Ohno, 2010, 2013, 2014; Lourenco et al., 2013; Ma et al., 2013; Baleriola et al., 2014). In the brain, eIF2α is a hub that controls protein synthesis-dependent learning and memory and mantain neuronal integrity in health and disease. When phosphorylated, however, eIF2α attenuates the initiation of global protein synthesis (Lourenco et al., 2015).

Aberrant eIF2α phosphorylation and inhibition of protein synthesis have emerged as major molecular pathways driving synapse and memory failure in AD models (Costa-Mattioli et al., 2007; Lourenco et al., 2013, 2015; Ma et al., 2013; Baleriola et al., 2014). In line with this notion, deletion of eIF2α kinases, including PKR, PERK, or GCN2 restores memory and synapse function in mouse models of AD (Lourenco et al., 2013; Ma et al., 2013).

Abnormal accumulation of misfolded proteins in the endoplasmic reticulum triggers the unfolded protein response (UPR), a set of signaling branches aimed at restore cellular homeostasis (Hetz, 2012; Dufey et al., 2014; Hetz and Saxena, 2017). However, when prolonged, UPR signaling might compromise neuronal functions, resulting in neurodegeneration (Lourenco et al., 2015; Freeman and Mallucci, 2016; Hetz and Saxena, 2017). There is now considerable evidence suggesting that AD brain display increased markers of UPR (Hoozemans et al., 2009; Hetz and Saxena, 2017), and that at least the PERK (Ma et al., 2013) and IRE-1a (Lourenco et al., 2013; Duran-Aniotz et al., 2017) branches of UPR are involved in memory defects in AD mice. Further, the chemical chaperone 4-phenylbutyrate alleviates AβO-induced memory defects in mice (Lourenco et al., 2013), thus highlighting the role of UPR in mediating neurotoxicity in AD. The combination of misfolded protein accumulation, activation of brain immune responses and defective proteostasis might thus comprise the very essence of synapse and memory failure in AD.

NOVEL PATHOPHYSIOLOGICAL MECHANISMS IN AD

Scientific breakthroughs during the past decades have expanded our knowledge on cellular and molecular aspects of AD. Nevertheless, AD remains largely idiopathic, and therapies that effectively combat disease progression are still lacking. Given that AD largely associates with memory loss, it is not surprising that the vast majority of studies deal with mechanisms implicated in cognitive deterioration. Hence, much less is known about how brain regions that are not directly linked to memory are affected in AD, as well as about mechanisms underlying its major comorbidities.

Numerous studies have investigated how Aβ impacts the hippocampus and the cortex (Ferreira and Klein, 2011; Musiek and Holtzman, 2015), known to be fundamentally involved in acquisition, consolidation, and recollection of new episodic memories. However, early studies indicated that brain regions not necessarily involved in learning and memory might also be affected in AD. It is noteworthy that AD patients exhibit significant non-cognitive deficits (summarized in the **Table 1**) such as sleep-wake disorders and neuroendocrine alterations attributable to hypothalamic dysfunction (Prinz et al., 1982; White et al., 1996; Csernansky et al., 2006).

Impaired Hypothalamic Function

Disturbances in hypothalamic nuclei have been reported in patients and animal models of AD (Duncan et al., 2012; Lim et al., 2014; Musiek et al., 2015; Musiek and Holtzman, 2016; Stevanovic et al., 2017). Since the hypothalamus is responsible for controlling circadian rhythm, impairments in its function can at least partially account for sleep disturbances. Nonetheless, although initial results have already shed light on how sleep becomes deregulated in AD (Ju et al., 2014; Musiek and Holtzman, 2016; Kincheski et al., 2017), studies investigating whether hypothalamic defects mediate sleep disturbances in AD are still needed.

Derangements in hypothalamic functions play a central role in peripheral metabolism deregulation and its consequences. For instance, hypothalamic inflammation and impaired proteostasis are critical pathogenic events in the establishment of peripheral insulin resistance in metabolic disorders (Zhang et al., 2008; Milanski et al., 2009; Denis et al., 2010; Arruda et al., 2011; Thaler

TABLE 1 | Novel pathophysiological mechanisms in AD.

Feature	Pathophysiological mechanisms	References
Impaired hypothalamic function	– Aβ deposits in hypothalamic nuclei leading to disturbances in circadian rhythm; – Reduced dendrite arborization and neurodegeneration; – Inflammation driving endoplasmic reticulum stress and insulin resistance.	Ogomori et al., 1989; Standaert et al., 1991; Duncan et al., 2012; Lim et al., 2014; Baloyannis et al., 2015; Clarke et al., 2015; Musiek et al., 2015; Musiek and Holtzman, 2016; Kincheski et al., 2017; Stevanovic et al., 2017
Metabolic derangement	– Reduced cerebral glucose metabolism; – Altered peripheral metabolism with hyperglycemia and hyperinsulinemia; – Defective glucose metabolism and insulin signaling induced by Aβ;	Chase et al., 1984; Janson et al., 2004; Rivera et al., 2005; Steen et al., 2005; Lester-Coll et al., 2006; De Felice et al., 2009; de la Monte, 2009; Matsuzaki et al., 2010; Moloney et al., 2010; Bomfim et al., 2012; Talbot et al., 2012; Crane et al., 2013; De Felice, 2013; Lourenco et al., 2013; De Felice and Ferreira, 2014; Clarke et al., 2015
Disturbances in monoamine signaling and mood	– Aβ induces both depressive-like behavior and decreases brain serotonin levels; – Increased microglial activity of IDO might partially explain reduced serotonin levels; – Reduced tryptophan and increased quinolinic acid in plasma might drive depressive-like behavior in AD; – Alterations in the dopaminergic system, including reduced levels of dopamine and its receptors might contribute to hippocampus-dependent memory deficits and reward circuitry dysfunction.	Gibb et al., 1989; Storga et al., 1996; Burns et al., 2005; Bonda et al., 2010; Gulaj et al., 2010; Jürgensen et al., 2011; Ledo et al., 2013, 2016; Romano et al., 2014; Masters et al., 2015; Nobili et al., 2017
Inflammation	– Pro-inflammatory cytokines are elevated in AD brains and mediate neurotoxic signals; – Brain inflammation underlies defective neuronal insulin signaling and peripheral metabolic deregulation; – Inflammation may drive synaptic failure in the monoaminergic systems, thereby linking cognitive and non-cognitive symptoms found in AD patients.	Heneka and O'Banion, 2007; Bonda et al., 2010; Lee and Landreth, 2010; Swardfager et al., 2010; Bomfim et al., 2012; Czirr and Wyss-Coray, 2012; Ledo et al., 2013, 2016; Lourenco et al., 2013; Alcolea et al., 2014; De Felice and Ferreira, 2014; Morales et al., 2014; Clarke et al., 2015; Heneka et al., 2015a,b; Yirmiya et al., 2015; Hong et al., 2016a,a; Santos et al., 2016; Nobili et al., 2017; Salter and Stevens, 2017

Aβ, amyloid-β peptide; AD, Alzheimer's disease; CNS, central nervous system; IDO, indolamine-2,3-dioxygenase; T2D, type 2 diabetes.

et al., 2012; Valdearcos et al., 2015). Nonetheless, very few studies so far investigated hypothalamic dysfunction in AD.

Early *post-mortem* studies identified Aβ deposits in hypothalamic nuclei of AD patients (Ogomori et al., 1989; Standaert et al., 1991), and neurodegeneration with marked retraction of dendrites in early AD (Baloyannis et al., 2015). Further, hypothalamic endoplasmic reticulum stress, inflammation, and insulin resistance were demonstrated in AβO-injected mice and non-human primates (Clarke et al., 2015). Dysfunction triggered by AβOs in the hypothalamus associated with development of persistent peripheral glucose intolerance, which was further demonstrated in several transgenic mouse models of AD (Clarke et al., 2015; Vandal et al., 2015; Stanley et al., 2016), and in human patients (Craft et al., 1992).

Defective Glucose Metabolism and Insulin Signaling

Altered peripheral metabolism with hyperglycemia and hyperinsulinemia, which are cardinal features of type 2 diabetes (T2D), were recently found to positively correlate with development of AD-like brain pathology in humans (Matsuzaki et al., 2010; Crane et al., 2013). Conversely, AD has been associated with increased T2D risk (Janson et al., 2004), suggesting that the connection between AD and T2D may comprise a two-way road. AD progression positively further correlates with reduction of cerebral glucose metabolism in the forebrain, including the posterior parietal lobe and portions of temporal and occipital lobes (Chase et al., 1984).

An important player accounting for impaired glucose metabolism in AD could arise from defects in insulin signaling pathways. AD brains exhibit lower levels of insulin and reduced insulin receptor (IR) expression and sensitivity (Rivera et al., 2005; Steen et al., 2005; Talbot et al., 2012). Further, impairments in insulin signaling downstream machinery have been reported in *post-mortem* brain tissue and in animal models of AD (Steen et al., 2005; Lester-Coll et al., 2006; de la Monte, 2009; Moloney et al., 2010; Bomfim et al., 2012; Craft, 2012; Talbot et al., 2012; Lourenco et al., 2013; Clarke et al., 2015). Recent studies have shown that AβOs are the toxins linked to impaired hippocampal insulin signaling by promoting internalization and cellular redistribution of insulin receptors, blocking downstream hippocampal insulin signaling (De Felice et al., 2009; Ma et al., 2009; Bomfim et al., 2012). Such body of evidence has established novel molecular parallels between AD and T2D.

The precise molecular mechanisms connecting impaired glucose metabolism and insulin signaling to AD pathogenesis remain to be fully determined. Nonetheless, mounting evidence has pointed to inflammation as a critical player linking AD and metabolic diseases, including T2D (De Felice and Ferreira, 2014;

Ferreira et al., 2014; Morales et al., 2014; Heneka et al., 2015b). Overproduction of pro-inflammatory cytokines, notably TNF-α, is a key feature of the pathophysiology of metabolic disorders (Hotamisligil, 2006, 2017). Notably, brain inflammation has recently been proposed to underlie defective neuronal insulin signaling (Bomfim et al., 2012; Lourenco et al., 2013), as well as peripheral metabolic deregulation in AD (Clarke et al., 2015).

Disturbances in Monoamine Signaling and Mood

Mounting evidence supports the notion that microglial activation and brain inflammation could further underlie mood disorders, including depressive behaviors (Yirmiya et al., 2015; Santos et al., 2016). Depression and/or apathy have been reported as frequent comorbidities in AD patients (Lyketsos and Olin, 2002), and have been regarded as risk factors for AD (Green et al., 2003; Ownby et al., 2006; Starkstein and Mizrahi, 2006; Geerlings et al., 2008).

Although clinical and epidemiological studies have revealed a strong connection between AD and depression, the mechanisms connecting these disorders at the molecular and cellular levels have only recently begun to be established. Clues into a mechanistic link between memory and mood disturbances in AD came from recent works showing that AβOs induce both depressive-like behavior and memory deficits in mice and associate with decreased brain serotonin levels (Ledo et al., 2013, 2016) in a similar way to that observed in transgenic mice model of AD (Romano et al., 2014). Reduced serotonin levels may be linked to increased levels and activity of indolamine-2,3-dioxygenase (IDO) follow microglial activation. Interestingly, AD patients were found to have reduced levels of plasma tryptophan and increased quinolinic acid (Gulaj et al., 2010), as well as increased IDO immunoreactivity in microglia (Bonda et al., 2010). Because inflammation plays a significant role in depression, these findings raise the possibility that AβO-induced brain inflammation may constitute a common denominator between cognitive and mood alterations in AD.

Alterations in the dopaminergic system have also been reported in AD patients and experimental models, including reduced levels of dopamine and its receptors (Gibb et al., 1989; Storga et al., 1996; Burns et al., 2005; Jürgensen et al., 2011; Nobili et al., 2017), and are commonly linked to cognitive and non-cognitive symptoms of the disease. It has been recently shown that inflammation and apoptosis take place in the ventral tegmental area, causing selective degeneration of the dopaminergic nuclei before senile plaque deposition, tangles or any sign of neuronal loss in cortical and hippocampal regions in a transgenic mouse model of AD (Nobili et al., 2017).

Given that dopaminergic neurons from ventral tegmental area not only modulate hippocampal synaptic plasticity (Rossato et al., 2009; McNamara et al., 2014; Broussard et al., 2016), but also target the nucleus accumbens and the cerebral cortex (Russo and Nestler, 2013), dopaminergic degeneration in ventral tegmental area might largely contribute to the deficits in hippocampus-dependent memory and reward circuits. These findings may provide an intriguing explanation to recent observations in AD patients indicating that the clinical diagnosis of dementia is associated with early non-cognitive symptoms, such as depression and apathy (Masters et al., 2015). Overall, these recent data suggest that inflammation may drive synaptic failure in the monoaminergic systems, thereby linking the cognitive and non-cognitive symptoms found in AD patients.

CHALLENGES FOR AD THERAPY

Despite intensive investigation of mechanisms of pathogenesis in AD during the past three decades, little has been achieved in terms of effective treatments or approaches to prevent or cure it. Taking into account the dramatic rise in the number of AD cases, huge economic and social hurdle will impact the society if no treatment is developed within the next few years. Additionally, it is noteworthy that advances in therapeutic strategies for AD that lead to even small delays in AD onset or progression would significantly attenuate the global burden of the disease.

Given the conceptual frameshift that occurred in the field in the past few years, AD has not only been viewed with discrete and defined clinical stages, but as a multifaceted process moving along a continuum. Thanks to the evolving biomarker research, it is now recognized that pathophysiological changes begin many years before clinical manifestations of AD. For example, changes in CSF tau levels have been shown to develop ~15 years before the onset of clinical AD, while CSF Aβ42 levels may drop even earlier, up to 20 years before symptom onset (Bateman et al., 2012; Buchhave, 2012; Villemagne et al., 2013; Fagan et al., 2014).

The spectrum of AD spans from clinically asymptomatic to severely impaired (**Figure 1**). However, these boundaries are challenging, given that separation between healthy aging and preclinical AD is not well-defined in our current understanding. This unmet question will likely be addressed in the future, as early detection biomarkers have become a major research focus.

Sex differences should also be taken into account as a biological variable in AD pathogenesis as women constitute the majority of affected people, accounting for nearly two-thirds of AD patients (Alzheimer's Association, 2017). Reasons for the higher frequency of AD among women could be partly explained by the fact that women live longer. However, late-onset AD risk is greater in women even after controlling for their longer lifespan relative to men (Viña and Lloret, 2010). The biological underpinnings of the increased AD risk in women remain largely unknown.

Nonetheless, it is now accepted that the perimenopause to menopause transition disrupts multiple estrogen-regulated systems, thereby affecting multiple domains of cognitive function (Brinton et al., 2015; Christensen and Pike, 2015). Indeed, recent preclinical studies have implicated that a shift in the bioenergetics system of the brain during menopause onset could serve as an early initiating mechanism for increased AD risk in the female brain (Brinton et al., 2015; Mosconi et al., 2017a,b). These biological variables may lead to increased fatty acid catabolism, Aβ deposition, and impaired synaptic plasticity (Liu et al., 2008; Brinton, 2009; Yao and Brinton, 2012), which could serve as a mechanism that triggers AD (Brinton et al., 2015). As a result, it is conceivable that disappointing outcomes in clinical trials may be partially explained by metabolic differences in women and men. Therefore, recommendations to include both female and male animals in preclinical research should be completely embraced by the research community.

While the amyloid cascade hypothesis has dominated research for the past 20 years, the shift toward disease-modifying drug development in the last decade might be imperative to develop approaches that interrupt the underlying disease processes.

Potential benefits for AD therapy can also emerge from combination pharmacotherapy. This strategy has proven effective for several diseases, including tuberculosis, HIV/AIDS, cardiovascular diseases, and cancer (Perry et al., 2014; Hendrix et al., 2016), and holds potential to enhance the efficacy of drugs that are ineffective on their own, but offer synergistic or additive benefits in combination.

Taking into account the well-known high failure rates in drug development targeting the central nervous system, strategies aimed at repurposing already marketed drugs become an interesting option to speed up drug discovery in AD (Appleby and Cummings, 2013). Given that metabolic derangements seem to play a pivotal role in AD, and that a myriad of drugs for metabolic disease have already been labeled for human use, repurposing such compounds may have the potential to accelerate drug development. That is because preclinical toxicology, human safety, tolerability, and pharmacokinetic assessments could move faster. Impaired brain insulin signaling or brain insulin resistance seems play a central role in the molecular pathogenesis of sporadic AD. Thus, targeting brain insulin signaling through the administration of drugs that have already been previously approved for the treatment of diabetes mellitus, such as insulin and drugs that improve insulin sensitivity, could expedite their development for the treatment of AD (Chen et al., 2016). It worthy to note that anti-diabetic compounds, such as insulin, exenatide, and liraglutide, have already been tested in ongoing clinical trials (clinical trial ID NCT01767909, NCT01255163, and NCT01843075, respectively).

Neuroinflammation, especially at the earliest stages, supports a vicious cycle of microglial activation, release of pro-inflammatory factors, and neuronal damage. Additionally, inflammatory mechanisms, such as those driven by TNF-α, may be orchestrated between the brain and the periphery, providing a likely link between AD and peripheral metabolic deregulation (De Felice and Ferreira, 2014; Ferreira et al., 2014; De Felice and Lourenco, 2015). The important role of neuroinflammation in AD is further supported by findings that gene variants for immune receptors, including TREM2, are associated with altered AD risk (Guerreiro et al., 2013; Heneka et al., 2015a).

A considerable body of evidence supports that inflammation could be a therapeutically relevant target in AD. Nevertheless, trials with anti-inflammatory compounds, such as non-steroidal anti-inflammatory drugs (NSAIDs), peroxisome proliferator-activated receptor-γ (PPAR-γ) activators, minocycline, and TNF-α signaling inhibitors have not yet provided exciting outcomes to date (Calsolaro and Edison, 2016), although lifelong use of NSAIDs has been associated with reduced risk of developing AD (Wang J. et al., 2015).

Additional therapeutic approaches with intravenous immunoglobulins and/or monoclonal antibodies are currently under evaluation, and results have not been conclusive yet. These uncertain results could be, to some extent, due to that anti-inflammatory drugs target generic rather than specific neuroinflammatory components in AD. Thus, specific modulators of inflammation at early disease stages will be essential to understand the potential of targeting inflammation in neurodegeneration.

CONCLUDING REMARKS

Although our understanding of AD has considerably increased over recent years, there is a still unmet requirement for effective therapeutics. Properly diagnosing AD is still one of the major hurdles in the field, as reliable biomarkers are lacking. There is fresh and compelling preclinical evidence that brain regions not necessarily involved in learning and memory might also be affected in AD, driving its major comorbidities. As most of therapeutic approaches have had disappointing outcomes so far, it is time to revisit the science underlining our current AD canons, and move toward the search for additional disease mechanisms and keys to treatment. Inflammation plays a critical role in the pathogenesis of AD and seems to drive the metabolic derangements that have been found to positively correlate with disease onset, leading to the emergence of cognitive and non-cognitive symptoms.

A deeper understanding of the complex features underlying major disease symptoms, including behavioral, mood, inflammation, and metabolic disturbances, may contribute to the development of novel and successful therapies. Given the differential prevalence of AD in men and women, sex differences should also be taken into account when studying AD pathophysiology, as they might reveal the need for separate therapeutic approaches. Drugs currently approved for use in AD are not disease-modifying, only confer mild and transient symptomatic management. Intervention at earlier stages using disease-modifying and combination therapy comprised of repourposed drugs and anti-inflammatory agents could pave the road toward successful outcomes in AD therapy.

AUTHOR CONTRIBUTIONS

RF, ML, and FD: planned, researched and wrote the manuscript.

ACKNOWLEDGMENTS

Work in the authors' laboratories has been supported by grants from National Institute for Translational Neuroscience (INNT/Brazil), Conselho Nacional de Desenvolvimento Científico e Tecnológico (CNPq/Brazil), Fundação Carlos Chagas Filho de Amparo à Pesquisa do Estado do Rio de Janeiro (FAPERJ), Alzheimer Society Canada and the International Society for Neurochemistry (ISN).

REFERENCES

Alcolea, D., Carmona-Iragui, M., Suárez-Calvet, M., Sánchez-Saudinós, M. B., Sala, I., Antón-Aguirre, S., et al. (2014). Relationship between β-secretase, inflammation and core cerebrospinal fluid biomarkers for Alzheimer's disease. *J. Alzheimer's Dis.* 42, 157–167. doi: 10.3233/JAD-140240

Alzheimer's Association (2017). 2017 Alzheimer's disease facts and figures. *Alzheimer's Dement.* 13, 325–373. doi: 10.1016/j.jalz.2017.02.001

Anker, J. N., Hall, W. P., Lambert, M. P., Velasco, P. T., Mrksich, M., Klein, W. L., et al. (2009). Detection and identification of bioanalytes with high resolution LSPR spectroscopy and MALDI mass spectrometry. *J. Phys. Chem. C* 113, 5891–5894. doi: 10.1021/jp900266k

Appleby, B. S., and Cummings, J. L. (2013). Discovering new treatments for Alzheimer's disease by repurposing approved medications. *Curr. Top. Med. Chem.* 13, 2306–2327. doi: 10.2174/15680266113136660162

Arruda, A. P., Milanski, M., Coope, A., Torsoni, A. S., Ropelle, E., Carvalho, D. P., et al. (2011). Low-grade hypothalamic inflammation leads to defective thermogenesis, insulin resistance, and impaired insulin secretion. *Endocrinology* 152, 1314–1326. doi: 10.1210/en.2010-0659

Baleriola, J., Walker, C. A., Jean, Y. Y., Crary, J. F., Troy, C. M., Nagy, P. L., et al. (2014). Axonally synthesized ATF4 transmits a neurodegenerative signal across brain regions. *Cell* 158, 1159–1172. doi: 10.1016/j.cell.2014.07.001

Baloyannis, S. J., Mavroudis, I., Mitilineos, D., Baloyannis, I. S., and Costa, V. G. (2015). The hypothalamus in alzheimer's disease. *Am. J. Alzheimer's Dis. Other Dementiasr.* 30, 478–487. doi: 10.1177/1533317514556876

Baruch, K., Deczkowska, A., Rosenzweig, N., Tsitsou-Kampeli, A., Sharif, A. M., Matcovitch-Natan, O., et al. (2016). PD-1 immune checkpoint blockade reduces pathology and improves memory in mouse models of Alzheimer's disease. *Nat. Med.* 22, 135–137. doi: 10.1038/nm.4022

Baruch, K., Rosenzweig, N., Kertser, A., Deczkowska, A., Sharif, A. M., Spinrad, A., et al. (2015). Breaking immune tolerance by targeting Foxp3$^+$ regulatory T cells mitigates Alzheimer's disease pathology. *Nat. Commun.* 6, 7967. doi: 10.1038/ncomms8967

Bateman, R. J., Aisen, P. S., De Strooper, B., Fox, N. C., Lemere, C. A., Ringman, J. M., et al. (2010). Autosomal-dominant Alzheimer's disease: a review and proposal for the prevention of Alzheimer's disease. *Alzheimers. Res. Ther.* 3, 1. doi: 10.1186/alzrt59

Bateman, R. J., Xiong, C., Benzinger, T. L. S., Fagan, A. M., Goate, A., Fox, N. C., et al. (2012). Clinical and biomarker changes in dominantly inherited alzheimer's disease. *N. Engl. J. Med.* 367, 795–804. doi: 10.1056/NEJMoa1202753

Bennett, R. E., DeVos, S. L., Dujardin, S., Corjuc, B., Gor, R., Gonzalez, J., et al. (2017). Enhanced tau aggregation in the presence of amyloid β. *Am. J. Pathol.* 187, 1601–1612. doi: 10.1016/j.ajpath.2017.03.011

Bilousova, T., Miller, C. A., Poon, W. W., Vinters, H. V., Corrada, M., Kawas, C., et al. (2016). Synaptic Amyloid-β oligomers precede p-Tau and differentiate high pathology control cases. *Am. J. Pathol.* 186, 185–198. doi: 10.1016/j.ajpath.2015.09.018

Bjorklund, N. L., Reese, L. C., Sadagoparamanujam, V.-M., Ghirardi, V., Woltjer, R. L., and Taglialatela, G. (2012). Absence of amyloid β oligomers at the postsynapse and regulated synaptic Zn2$^+$ in cognitively intact aged individuals with Alzheimer's disease neuropathology. *Mol. Neurodegener.* 7:23. doi: 10.1186/1750-1326-7-23

Blennow, K. (2017). A review of fluid biomarkers for alzheimer's disease: moving from CSF to blood. *Neurol. Ther.* 6(Suppl. 1), 15–24. doi: 10.1007/s40120-017-0073-9

Blennow, K., de Leon, M. J., and Zetterberg, H. (2006). Alzheimer's disease. *Lancet.* 368, 387–403. doi: 10.1016/S0140-6736(06)69113-7

Bomfim, T. R., Forny-Germano, L., Sathler, L. B., Brito-Moreira, J., Houzel, J.-C., Decker, H., et al. (2012). An anti-diabetes agent protects the mouse brain from defective insulin signaling caused by Alzheimer's disease-associated Aβ oligomers. *J. Clin. Invest.* 122, 1339–1353. doi: 10.1172/JCI 57256

Bonda, D., Mailankot, M., Stone, J., Garrett, M., S. M., Castellani, R. J., Siedlak, S. L., et al. (2010). Indoleamine 2,3-dioxygenase and 3-hydroxykynurenine modifications are found in the neuropathology of Alzheimer's disease. *Redox Rep.* 15, 161–168. doi: 10.1179/174329210X126505066 23645

Brinton, R. D. (2009). Estrogen-induced plasticity from cells to circuits: predictions for cognitive function. *Trends Pharmacol. Sci.* 30, 212–222. doi: 10.1016/j.tips.2008.12.006

Brinton, R. D., Yao, J., Yin, F., Mack, W. J., and Cadenas, E. (2015). Perimenopause as a neurological transition state. *Nat. Rev. Endocrinol.* 11, 393–405. doi: 10.1038/nrendo.2015.82

Broussard, J. I., Yang, K., Levine, A. T., Tsetsenis, T., Jenson, D., Cao, F., et al. (2016). Dopamine regulates aversive contextual learning and associated *in vivo* synaptic plasticity in the hippocampus. *Cell Rep.* 14, 1930–1939. doi: 10.1016/j.celrep.2016.01.070

Browne, T. C., McQuillan, K., McManus, R. M., O'Reilly, J.-A., Mills, K. H. G., and Lynch, M. A. (2013). IFN- production by amyloid -specific Th1 cells promotes microglial activation and increases plaque burden in a mouse model of alzheimer's disease. *J. Immunol.* 190, 2241–2251. doi: 10.4049/jimmunol.1200947

Buchhave, P. (2012). Cerebrospinal fluid levels of β-Amyloid 1-42, but Not of Tau, are fully changed already 5 to 10 years before the onset of alzheimer dementia. *Arch. Gen. Psychiatry* 69, 98. doi: 10.1001/archgenpsychiatry.2011.155

Burns, J. M., Galvin, J. E., Roe, C. M., Morris, J. C., and McKeel, D. W. (2005). The pathology of the substantia nigra in Alzheimer disease with extrapyramidal signs. *Neurology* 64, 1397–1403. doi: 10.1212/01.WNL.0000158423.05224.7F

Calsolaro, V., and Edison, P. (2016). Neuroinflammation in Alzheimer's disease: current evidence and future directions. *Alzheimer's Dement.* 12, 719–732. doi: 10.1016/j.jalz.2016.02.010

Carrieri, C., Cimatti, L., Biagioli, M., Beugnet, A., Zucchelli, S., Fedele, S., et al. (2017). Tau reduction prevents neuronal loss and reverses pathological tau deposition and seeding in mice with tauopathy. *Nat. Nanotechnol.* 481, 454–457. doi: 10.1126/scitranslmed.aag0481

Castellani, R. J., and Perry, G. (2012). Pathogenesis and disease-modifying therapy in Alzheimer's disease: the flat line of progress. *Arch. Med. Res.* 43, 694–698. doi: 10.1016/j.arcmed.2012.09.009

Chase, T. N., Foster, N. L., Fedio, P., Brooks, R., Mansi, L., and Di Chiro, G. (1984). Regional cortical dysfunction in Alzheimer's disease as determined by positron emission tomography. *Ann. Neurol.* 15(Suppl.), S170–S174.

Chatterjee, S., Peters, S. A. E., Woodward, M., Arango, S. M., Batty, G. D., Beckett, N., et al. (2016). Type 2diabetes as a risk factor for dementia in women compared with men: a pooled analysis of 2.3 million people comprising more than 100,000 cases of dementia. *Diabetes Care* 39, 300–307. doi: 10.2337/dc15-1588

Chen, Y., Zhang, J., Zhang, B., and Gong, C. X. (2016). Targeting insulin signaling for the treatment of Alzheimer's disease. *Curr. Top. Med. Chem.* 16, 485–492. doi: 10.2174/1568026615666150813142423

Christensen, A., and Pike, C. J. (2015). Menopause, obesity and inflammation: interactive risk factors for Alzheimer's disease. *Front. Aging Neurosci.* 7:130. doi: 10.3389/fnagi.2015.00130

Clarke, J. R., Lyra E Silva, N. M., Figueiredo, C. P., Frozza, R. L., Ledo, J. H., Beckman, D., et al. (2015). Alzheimer-associated Aβ oligomers impact the central nervous system to induce peripheral metabolic deregulation. *EMBO Mol. Med.* 7, 190–210. doi: 10.15252/emmm.201404183

Costa-Mattioli, M., Gobert, D., Stern, E., Gamache, K., Colina, R., Cuello, C., et al. (2007). eIF2α phosphorylation bidirectionally regulates the switch from short- to long-term synaptic plasticity and memory. *Cell* 129, 195–206. doi: 10.1016/j.cell.2007.01.050

Craft, S. (2012). Alzheimer disease: insulin resistance and AD—extending the translational path. *Nat. Rev. Neurol.* 8, 360–362. doi: 10.1038/nrneurol.2012.112

Craft, S., Zallen, G., and Baker, L. D. (1992). Glucose and memory in mild senile dementia of the alzheimer type. *J. Clin. Exp. Neuropsychol.* 14, 253–267. doi: 10.1080/01688639208402827

Crane, P. K., Walker, R., Hubbard, R. A., Li, G., Nathan, D. M., Zheng, H., et al. (2013). Glucose levels and risk of dementia. *N. Engl. J. Med.* 369, 540–548. doi: 10.1056/NEJMoa1215740

Csernansky, J. G., Dong, H., Fagan, A. M., Wang, L., Xiong, C., Holtzman, D. M., et al. (2006). Plasma cortisol and progression of dementia in subjects with Alzheimer-type dementia. *Am. J. Psychiatry* 163, 2164–2169. doi: 10.1176/ajp.2006.163.12.2164

Cummings, J. L., Morstorf, T., and Zhong, K. (2014). Alzheimer's disease drug-development pipeline: few candidates, frequent failures. *Alzheimers. Res. Ther.* 6, 37. doi: 10.1186/alzrt269

Czirr, E., and Wyss-Coray, T. (2012). The immunology of neurodegeneration. *J. Clin. Invest.* 122, 1156–1163. doi: 10.1172/JCI58656

Decker, H., Jürgensen, S., Adrover, M. F., Brito-Moreira, J., Bomfim, T. R., Klein, W. L., et al. (2010a). N-Methyl-d-aspartate receptors are required for synaptic targeting of Alzheimer's toxic amyloid-β peptide oligomers. *J. Neurochem.* 115, 1520–1529. doi: 10.1111/j.1471-4159.2010.07058.x

Decker, H., Lo, K. Y., Unger, S. M., Ferreira, S. T., and Silverman, M. A. (2010b). Amyloid- peptide oligomers disrupt axonal transport through an NMDA receptor-dependent mechanism that is mediated by glycogen synthase kinase 3 in primary cultured hippocampal neurons. *J. Neurosci.* 30, 9166–9171. doi: 10.1523/JNEUROSCI.1074-10.2010

De Felice, F. G. (2013). Alzheimer' s disease and insulin resistance : translating basic science into clinical applications. *J. Clin. Invest.* 123, 531–539. doi: 10.1172/JCI64595

De Felice, F. G., and Ferreira, S. T. (2014). Inflammation, defective insulin signaling, and mitochondrial dysfunction as common molecular denominators connecting type 2 diabetes to alzheimer disease. *Diabetes* 63, 2262–2272. doi: 10.2337/db13-1954

De Felice, F. G., and Lourenco, M. V. (2015). Brain metabolic stress and neuroinflammation at the basis of cognitive impairment in Alzheimer's disease. *Front. Aging Neurosci.* 7:94. doi: 10.3389/fnagi.2015.00094

De Felice, F. G., and Munoz, D. P. (2016). Opportunities and challenges in developing relevant animal models for Alzheimer's disease. *Ageing Res. Rev.* 26, 112–114. doi: 10.1016/j.arr.2016.01.006

De Felice, F. G., Velasco, P. T., Lambert, M. P., Viola, K., Fernandez, S. J., Ferreira, S. T., et al. (2007). Abeta oligomers induce neuronal oxidative stress through an N-methyl-D-aspartate receptor-dependent mechanism that is blocked by the Alzheimer drug memantine. *J. Biol. Chem.* 282, 11590–11601. doi: 10.1074/jbc.M607483200

De Felice, F. G., Vieira, M. N. N., Bomfim, T. R., Decker, H., Velasco, P. T., Lambert, M. P., et al. (2009). Protection of synapses against Alzheimer's-linked toxins: insulin signaling prevents the pathogenic binding of Abeta oligomers. *Proc. Natl. Acad. Sci. U. S. A.* 106, 1971–1976. doi: 10.1073/pnas.08091 58106

De Felice, F. G., Wu, D., Lambert, M. P., Fernandez, S. J., Velasco, P. T., Lacor, P. N., et al. (2008). Alzheimer's disease-type neuronal tau hyperphosphorylation induced by A beta oligomers. *Neurobiol. Aging* 29, 1334–1347. doi: 10.1016/j.neurobiolaging.2007.02.029

de la Monte, S. M. (2009). Insulin resistance and Alzheimer's disease. *BMB Rep.* 42, 475–481. doi: 10.5483/BMBRep.2009.42.8.475

Denis, R. G., Arruda, A. P., Romanatto, T., Milanski, M., Coope, A., Solon, C., et al. (2010). TNF-α transiently induces endoplasmic reticulum stress and an incomplete unfolded protein response in the hypothalamus. *Neuroscience* 170, 1035–1044. doi: 10.1016/j.neuroscience.2010.08.013

Devi, L., and Ohno, M. (2010). Phospho-eIF2α level is important for determining abilities of BACE1 reduction to rescue cholinergic neurodegeneration and memory defects in 5XFAD mice. *PLoS ONE* 5:e12974. doi: 10.1371/journal.pone.0012974

Devi, L., and Ohno, M. (2013). Deletion of the eIF2α kinase GCN2 fails to rescue the memory decline associated with alzheimer's disease. *PLoS ONE* 8:e77335. doi: 10.1371/journal.pone.0077335

Devi, L., and Ohno, M. (2014). PERK mediates eIF2α phosphorylation responsible for BACE1 elevation, CREB dysfunction and neurodegeneration in a mouse model of Alzheimer's disease. *Neurobiol. Aging* 35, 2272–2281. doi: 10.1016/j.neurobiolaging.2014.04.031

Dufey, E., Sepúlveda, D., Rojas-Rivera, D., and Hetz, C. (2014). Cellular mechanisms of endoplasmic reticulum stress signaling in health and disease. 1. An overview. *Am. J. Physiol. Physiol.* 307, C582–C594. doi: 10.1152/ajpcell.00258.2014

Dubois, B., Hampel, H., Feldman, H. H., Scheltens, P., Aisen, P., Andrieu, S., et al. (2016). Preclinical Alzheimer's disease: definition, natural history, and diagnostic criteria. *Alzheimers Dement.* 12, 292–323. doi: 10.1016/j.jalz.2016.02.002

Duncan, M. J., Smith, J. T., Franklin, K. M., Beckett, T. L., Murphy, M. P., St. Clair, D. K., et al. (2012). Effects of aging and genotype on circadian rhythms, sleep, and clock gene expression in APPxPS1 knock-in mice, a model for Alzheimer's disease. *Exp. Neurol.* 236, 249–258. doi: 10.1016/j.expneurol.2012.05.011

Duran-Aniotz, C., Cornejo, V. H., Espinoza, S., Ardiles, Á. O., Medinas, D. B., Salazar, C., et al. (2017). IRE1 signaling exacerbates Alzheimer's disease pathogenesis. *Acta Neuropathol.* 134, 489–506. doi: 10.1007/s00401-017-1694-x

Fagan, A. M., Xiong, C., Jasielec, M. S., Bateman, R. J., Goate, A. M., Benzinger, T. L. S., et al. (2014). Longitudinal change in CSF biomarkers in autosomal-dominant alzheimer's disease. *Sci. Transl. Med.* 6:226ra30. doi: 10.1126/scitranslmed.3007901

Fá, M., Puzzo, D., Piacentini, R., Staniszewski, A., Zhang, H., Baltrons, M. A., et al. (2016). Extracellular tau oligomers produce an immediate impairment of LTP and memory. *Sci. Rep.* 6:19393. doi: 10.1038/srep19393

Farris, W., Mansourian, S., Chang, Y., Lindsley, L., Eckman, E. A., Frosch, M. P., et al. (2003). Insulin-degrading enzyme regulates the levels of insulin, amyloid beta-protein, and the beta-amyloid precursor protein intracellular domain *in vivo*. *Proc. Natl. Acad. Sci. U.S.A.* 100, 4162–4167. doi: 10.1073/pnas.0230450100

Ferreira, S. T., Clarke, J. R., Bomfim, T. R., and De Felice, F. G. (2014). Inflammation, defective insulin signaling, and neuronal dysfunction in Alzheimer's disease. *Alzheimer's Dement.* 10, S76–S83. doi: 10.1016/j.jalz.2013.12.010

Ferreira, S. T., and Klein, W. L. (2011). The Aβ oligomer hypothesis for synapse failure and memory loss in Alzheimer's disease. *Neurobiol. Learn. Mem.* 96, 529–543. doi: 10.1016/j.nlm.2011.08.003

Ferreira, S. T., Lourenco, M. V., Oliveira, M. M., and De Felice, F. G. (2015). Soluble amyloid-β oligomers as synaptotoxins leading to cognitive impairment in Alzheimer's disease. *Front. Cell. Neurosci.* 9:191. doi: 10.3389/fncel.2015.00191

Finder, V. H., and Glockshuber, R. (2007). Amyloid-beta aggregation. *Neurodegener. Dis.* 4, 13–27. doi: 10.1159/000100355

Forny-Germano, L., Lyra e Silva, N. M., Batista, A. F., Brito-Moreira, J., Gralle, M., Boehnke, S. E., et al. (2014). Alzheimer's disease-like pathology induced by amyloid- oligomers in nonhuman primates. *J. Neurosci.* 34, 13629–13643. doi: 10.1523/JNEUROSCI.1353-14.2014

Freeman, O. J., and Mallucci, G. R. (2016). The UPR and synaptic dysfunction in neurodegeneration. *Brain Res.* 1648, 530–537. doi: 10.1016/j.brainres.2016.03.029

Fu, H., Rodriguez, G. A., Herman, M., Emrani, S., Nahmani, E., Barrett, G., et al. (2017). Tau pathology induces excitatory neuron loss, grid cell dysfunction, and spatial memory deficits reminiscent of early alzheimer's disease. *Neuron* 93, 533.e5–541.e5. doi: 10.1016/j.neuron.2016.12.023

Geerlings, M. I., Den Heijer, T., Koudstaal, P. J., Hofman, A., and Breteler, M. M. B. (2008). History of depression, depressive symptoms, and medial temporal lobe atrophy and the risk of Alzheimer disease. *Neurology* 70, 1258–1264. doi: 10.1212/01.wnl.0000308937.30473.d1

Georganopoulou, D. G., Chang, L., Nam, J.-M., Thaxton, C. S., Mufson, E. J., Klein, W. L., et al. (2005). From the cover: nanoparticle-based detection in cerebral spinal fluid of a soluble pathogenic biomarker for Alzheimer's disease. *Proc. Natl. Acad. Sci. U. S. A.* 102, 2273–2276. doi: 10.1073/pnas.0409336102

Gibb, W. R., Mountjoy, C. Q., Mann, D. M., and Lees, A. J. (1989). The substantia nigra and ventral tegmental area in Alzheimer's disease and Down's syndrome. *J. Neurol. Neurosurg. Psychiatry* 52, 193–200.

Green, R. C., Cupples, L. A., Kurz, A., Auerbach, S., Go, R., Sadovnick, D., et al. (2003). Depression as a risk factor for Alzheimer disease: the MIRAGE Study. *Arch. Neurol.* 60, 753–759. doi: 10.1001/archneur.60.5.753

Guerreiro, R., Wojtas, A., Bras, J., Carrasquillo, M., Rogaeva, E., Majounie, E., et al. (2013). TREM2 variants in Alzheimer's Disease. *N. Engl. J. Med.* 368, 117–127. doi: 10.1056/NEJMoa1211851

Guillot-Sestier, M. V., Doty, K. R., Gate, D., Rodriguez, J., Leung, B. P., Rezai-Zadeh, K., et al. (2015). Il10 deficiency rebalances innate immunity to mitigate Alzheimer-like pathology. *Neuron.* 85, 534–548. doi: 10.1016/j.neuron.2014.12.068

Gulaj, E., Pawlak, K., Bien, B., and Pawlak, D. (2010). Kynurenine and its metabolites in Alzheimer's disease patients. *Adv. Med. Sci.* 55, 204–211. doi: 10.2478/v10039-010-0023-6

Haes, A. J., Chang, L., Klein, W. L., and Van Duyne, R. P. (2005). Detection of a biomarker for Alzheimer's disease from synthetic and clinical samples using a nanoscale optical biosensor. *J. Am. Chem. Soc.* 127, 2264–2271. doi: 10.1021/ja044087q

Hardy, J. (2002). The amyloid hypothesis of Alzheimer's disease: progress and problems on the road to therapeutics. *Science* 297, 353–356. doi: 10.1126/science.1072994

Hendrix, J. A., Bateman, R. J., Brashear, H. R., Duggan, C., Carrillo, M. C., Bain, L. J., et al. (2016). Challenges, solutions, and recommendations for Alzheimer's disease combination therapy. *Alzheimer's Dement.* 12, 623–630. doi: 10.1016/j.jalz.2016.02.007

Heneka, M. T., Carson, M. J., Khoury, J., El, Landreth, G. E., Brosseron, F., Feinstein, D. L., et al. (2015a). Neuroinflammation in Alzheimer's disease. *Lancet Neurol.* 14, 388–405. doi: 10.1016/S1474-4422(15)70016-5

Heneka, M. T., and O'Banion, M. K. (2007). Inflammatory processes in Alzheimer's disease. *J. Neuroimmunol.* 184, 69–91. doi: 10.1016/j.jneuroim.2006.11.017

Heneka, M. T., Golenbock, D. T., and Latz, E. (2015b). Innate immunity in Alzheimer's disease. *Nat. Immunol.* 16, 229–236. doi: 10.1038/ni.3102

Herskovits, A. Z., Locascio, J. J., Peskind, E. R., Li, G., and Hyman, B. T. (2013). A luminex assay detects amyloid β oligomers in alzheimer's disease cerebrospinal fluid. *PLoS ONE* 8:e67898. doi: 10.1371/journal.pone.0067898

Hetz, C. (2012). The unfolded protein response: controlling cell fate decisions under ER stress and beyond. *Nat. Rev. Mol. Cell Biol.* 13, 89–102. doi: 10.1038/nrm3270

Hetz, C., and Saxena, S. (2017). ER stress and the unfolded protein response in neurodegeneration. *Nat. Rev. Neurol.* 13, 477–491. doi: 10.1038/nrneurol.2017.99

Hoozemans, J. J. M., van Haastert, E. S., Nijholt, D. A. T., Rozemuller, A. J. M., Eikelenboom, P., and Scheper, W. (2009). The unfolded protein response is activated in pretangle neurons in Alzheimer's disease hippocampus. *Am. J. Pathol.* 174, 1241–1251. doi: 10.2353/ajpath.2009.080814

Hong, S., Beja-Glasser, V. F., Nfonoyim, B. M., Frouin, A., Li, S., Ramakrishnan, S., et al. (2016a). Complement and microglia mediate early synapse loss in Alzheimer mouse models. *Science* 352, 712–716. doi: 10.1126/science.aad8373

Hong, S., Dissing-Olesen, L., and Stevens, B. (2016b). New insights on the role of microglia in synaptic pruning in health and disease. *Curr. Opin. Neurobiol.* 36, 128–134. doi: 10.1016/j.conb.2015.12.004

Hotamisligil, G. S. (2006). Inflammation and metabolic disorders. *Nature* 444, 860–867. doi: 10.1038/nature05485

Hotamisligil, G. S. (2017). Inflammation, metaflammation and immunometabolic disorders. *Nature* 542, 177–185. doi: 10.1038/nature21363

Ishii, M., and Iadecola, C. (2015). Metabolic and non-cognitive manifestations of Alzheimers disease: the hypothalamus as both culprit and target of pathology. *Cell Metab.* 22, 761–776. doi: 10.1016/j.cmet.2015.08.016

Ittner, L. M., and Götz, J. (2011). Amyloid-β and tau — a toxic pas de deux in Alzheimer's disease. *Nat. Rev. Neurosci.* 12, 65–72. doi: 10.1038/nrn2967

Iwata, N., Tsubuki, S., Takaki, Y., Shirotani, K., Lu, B., Gerard, N. P., et al. (2001). Metabolic regulation of brain Abeta by neprilysin. *Science* 292, 1550–1552. doi: 10.1126/science.1059946

Janson, J., Laedtke, T., Parisi, J. E., O'Brien, P., Petersen, R. C., and Butler, P. C. (2004). Increased risk of type 2 diabetes in Alzheimer disease. *Diabetes* 53, 474–481. doi: 10.2337/diabetes.53.2.474

Jin, M., Shepardson, N., Yang, T., Chen, G., Walsh, D., and Selkoe, D. J. (2011). Soluble amyloid -protein dimers isolated from Alzheimer cortex directly induce Tau hyperphosphorylation and neuritic degeneration. *Proc. Natl. Acad. Sci. U.S.A.* 108, 5819–5824. doi: 10.1073/pnas.1017033108

Jürgensen, S., Antonio, L. L., Mussi, G. E. A., Brito-Moreira, J., Bomfim, T. R., De Felice, F. G., et al. (2011). Activation of D1/D5 dopamine receptors protects neurons from synapse dysfunction induced by amyloid-β oligomers. *J. Biol. Chem.* 286, 3270–3276. doi: 10.1074/jbc.M110.177790

Ju, Y.-E. S., Lucey, B. P., and Holtzman, D. M. (2014). Sleep and Alzheimer disease pathology–a bidirectional relationship. *Nat. Rev. Neurol.* 10, 115–119. doi: 10.1038/nrneurol.2013.269

Karran, E., Mercken, M., and Strooper, B., De (2011). The amyloid cascade hypothesis for Alzheimer's disease: an appraisal for the development of therapeutics. *Nat. Rev. Drug Discov.* 10, 698–712. doi: 10.1038/nrd3505

Kincheski, G. C., Valentim, I. S., Clarke, J. R., Cozachenco, D., Castelo-Branco, M. T. L., Ramos-Lobo, A. M., et al. (2017). Chronic sleep restriction promotes brain inflammation and synapse loss, and potentiates memory impairment induced by amyloid-β oligomers in mice. *Brain Behav. Immun.* 64, 140–151. doi: 10.1016/j.bbi.2017.04.007

Koffie, R. M., Meyer-Luehmann, M., Hashimoto, T., Adams, K. W., Mielke, M. L., Garcia-Alloza, M., et al. (2009). Oligomeric amyloid associates with postsynaptic densities and correlates with excitatory synapse loss near senile plaques. *Proc. Natl. Acad. Sci. U.S.A.* 106, 4012–4017. doi: 10.1073/pnas.0811698106

Lanctôt, K. L., Amatniek, J., Ancoli-Israel, S., Arnold, S. E., Ballard, C., Cohen-Mansfield, J., et al. (2017). Neuropsychiatric signs and symptoms of Alzheimer's disease: new treatment paradigms. *Alzheimer's Dement. Transl. Res. Clin. Interv.* 3, 440–449. doi: 10.1016/j.trci.2017.07.001

Ledo, J. H., Azevedo, E. P., Beckman, D., Ribeiro, F. C., Santos, L. E., Razolli, D. S., et al. (2016). Cross talk between brain innate immunity and serotonin signaling underlies depressive-like behavior induced by Alzheimer's amyloid- oligomers in mice. *J. Neurosci.* 36, 12106–12116. doi: 10.1523/JNEUROSCI.1269-16.2016

Ledo, J. H., Azevedo, E. P., Clarke, J. R., Ribeiro, F. C., Figueiredo, C. P., Foguel, D., et al. (2013). Amyloid-β oligomers link depressive-like behavior and cognitive deficits in mice. *Mol. Psychiatry* 18, 1053–1054. doi: 10.1038/mp.2012.168

Lee, C. Y. D., and Landreth, G. E. (2010). The role of microglia in amyloid clearance from the AD brain. *J. Neural Transm.* 117, 949–960. doi: 10.1007/s00702-010-0433-4

Lee, S., Fernandez, E. J., and Good, T. A. (2007). Role of aggregation conditions in structure, stability, and toxicity of intermediates in the Abeta fibril formation pathway. *Protein Sci.* 16, 723–732. doi: 10.1110/ps.062514807

Leissring, M. A., Farris, W., Chang, A. Y., Walsh, D. M., Wu, X., Sun, X., et al. (2003). Enhanced proteolysis of β-amyloid in APP transgenic mice prevents plaque formation, secondary pathology, and premature death. *Neuron* 40, 1087–1093. doi: 10.1016/S0896-6273(03)00787-6

Lester-Coll, N., Rivera, E. J., Soscia, S. J., Doiron, K., Wands, J. R., and de la Monte, S. M. (2006). Intracerebral streptozotocin model of type 3 diabetes: relevance to sporadic Alzheimer's disease. *J. Alzheimers. Dis.* 9, 13–33. doi: 10.3233/JAD-2006-9102

Lim, A. S. P., Ellison, B. A., Wang, J. L., Yu, L., Schneider, J. A., Buchman, A. S., et al. (2014). Sleep is related to neuron numbers in the ventrolateral preoptic/intermediate nucleus in older adults with and without Alzheimer's disease. *Brain* 137, 2847–2861. doi: 10.1093/brain/awu222

Liu, F., Day, M., Muñiz, L. C., Bitran, D., Arias, R., Revilla-Sanchez, R., et al. (2008). Activation of estrogen receptor-β regulates hippocampal synaptic plasticity and improves memory. *Nat. Neurosci.* 11, 334–343. doi: 10.1038/nn2057

Lourenco, M. V., Clarke, J. R., Frozza, R. L., Bomfim, T. R., Forny-Germano, L., Batista, A. F., et al. (2013). TNF-α mediates PKR-dependent memory impairment and brain IRS-1 inhibition induced by Alzheimer's β-amyloid oligomers in mice and monkeys. *Cell Metab.* 18, 831–843. doi: 10.1016/j.cmet.2013.11.002

Lourenco, M. V., Ferreira, S. T., and De Felice, F. G. (2015). Neuronal stress signaling and eIF2α phosphorylation as molecular links between Alzheimer's disease and diabetes. *Prog. Neurobiol.* 129, 37–57. doi: 10.1016/j.pneurobio.2015.03.003

Lyketsos, C. G., and Olin, J. (2002). Depression in Alzheimer's disease: overview and treatment. *Biol. Psychiatry* 52, 243–252. doi: 10.1016/S0006-3223(02)01348-3

Ma, Q.-L., Yang, F., Rosario, E. R., Ubeda, O. J., Beech, W., Gant, D. J., et al. (2009). Beta-amyloid oligomers induce phosphorylation of tau and inactivation of insulin receptor substrate via c-jun n-terminal kinase signaling: suppression by omega-3 fatty acids and curcumin. *J. Neurosci.* 9, 9078–9089. doi: 10.1523/JNEUROSCI.1071-09.2009

Ma, T., Trinh, M. A., Wexler, A. J., Bourbon, C., Gatti, E., Pierre, P., et al. (2013). Suppression of eIF2α kinases alleviates Alzheimer's disease–related plasticity and memory deficits. *Nat. Neurosci.* 16, 1299–1305. doi: 10.1038/nn.3486

Mandrekar-Colucci, S., Karlo, J. C., and Landreth, G. E. (2012). Mechanisms underlying the rapid peroxisome proliferator-activated receptor- -mediated amyloid clearance and reversal of cognitive deficits in a murine model of alzheimer's disease. *J. Neurosci.* 32, 10117–10128. doi: 10.1523/JNEUROSCI.5268-11.2012

Masliah, E., Ellisman, M., Carragher, B., Mallory, M., Young, S., Hansen, L., et al. (1992). Three-dimensional analysis of the relationship between synaptic pathology and neuropil threads in Alzheimer disease. *J. Neuropathol. Exp. Neurol.* 51, 404–414. doi: 10.1097/00005072-199207000-00003

Masters, M. C., Morris, J. C., and Roe, C. M. (2015). "Noncognitive" symptoms of early Alzheimer disease : a longitudinal analysis. *Neurology* 84, 617–622. doi: 10.1212/WNL.0000000000001238

Matsuzaki, T., Sasaki, K., Tanizaki, Y., Hata, J., Fujimi, K., Matsui, Y., et al. (2010). Insulin resistance is associated with the pathology of Alzheimer disease: the Hisayama study. *Neurology* 75, 764–770. doi: 10.1212/WNL.0b013e3181eee25f

Mattson, M. P. (2010). ER calcium and Alzheimer's disease: in a state of flux. *Sci. Signal.* 3:pe10. doi: 10.1126/scisignal.3114pe10

McNamara, C. G., Tejero-Cantero, Á., Trouche, S., Campo-Urriza, N., and Dupret, D. (2014). Dopaminergic neurons promote hippocampal reactivation and spatial memory persistence. *Nat. Neurosci.* 17, 1658–1660. doi: 10.1038/nn.3843

Medeiros, R., Baglietto-Vargas, D., and Laferla, F. M. (2011). The role of Tau in Alzheimer's disease and related disorders. *CNS Neurosci. Ther.* 17, 514–524. doi: 10.1111/j.1755-5949.2010.00177.x

Milanski, M., Degasperi, G., Coope, A., Morari, J., Denis, R., Cintra, D. E., et al. (2009). Saturated fatty acids produce an inflammatory response predominantly through the activation of TLR4 signaling in hypothalamus: implications for the pathogenesis of obesity. *J. Neurosci.* 29, 359–370. doi: 10.1523/JNEUROSCI.2760-08.2009

Miñano-Molina, A. J., España, J., Martín, E., Barneda-Zahonero, B., Fadó, R., Solé, M., et al. (2011). Soluble oligomers of amyloid-β peptide disrupt membrane trafficking of α-amino-3-hydroxy-5-methylisoxazole-4-propionic acid receptor contributing to early synapse dysfunction. *J. Biol. Chem.* 286, 27311–27321. doi: 10.1074/jbc.M111.227504

Moloney, A. M., Griffin, R. J., Timmons, S., O'Connor, R., Ravid, R., and O'Neill, C. (2010). Defects in IGF-1 receptor, insulin receptor and IRS-1/2 in Alzheimer's disease indicate possible resistance to IGF-1 and insulin signalling. *Neurobiol. Aging* 31, 224–243. doi: 10.1016/j.neurobiolaging.2008.04.002

Morales, I., GuzmÃ¡n-MartÃ-nez, L., Cerda-Troncoso, C., FarÃ-as, G. A., and Maccioni, R. B. (2014). Neuroinflammation in the pathogenesis of Alzheimer's disease. A rational framework for the search of novel therapeutic approaches. *Front. Cell. Neurosci.* 8:112. doi: 10.3389/fncel.2014.00112

Morris, M., Maeda, S., Vossel, K., and Mucke, L. (2011). The many faces of Tau. *Neuron* 70, 410–426. doi: 10.1016/j.neuron.2011.04.009

Mosconi, L., Berti, V., Guyara-Quinn, C., McHugh, P., Petrongolo, G., Osorio, R. S., et al. (2017a). Perimenopause and emergence of an Alzheimer's bioenergetic phenotype in brain and periphery. *PLoS ONE* 12:e0185926. doi: 10.1371/journal.pone.0185926

Mosconi, L., Berti, V., Quinn, C., McHugh, P., Petrongolo, G., Varsavsky, I., et al. (2017b). Sex differences in Alzheimer risk. *Neurology* 89, 1382–1390. doi: 10.1212/WNL.0000000000004425

Murakami, K., Tokuda, M., Suzuki, T., Irie, Y., Hanaki, M., Izuo, N., et al. (2016). Monoclonal antibody with conformational specificity for a toxic conformer of amyloid β42 and its application toward the Alzheimer's disease diagnosis. *Sci. Rep.* 6:29038. doi: 10.1038/srep29038

Musiek, E. S., and Holtzman, D. M. (2015). Three dimensions of the amyloid hypothesis: time, space and "wingmen." *Nat. Neurosci.* 18, 800–806. doi: 10.1038/nn.4018

Musiek, E. S., and Holtzman, D. M. (2016). Mechanisms linking circadian clocks, sleep, and neurodegeneration. *Science* 354, 1004–1008. doi: 10.1126/science.aah4968

Musiek, E. S., Xiong, D. D., and Holtzman, D. M. (2015). Sleep, circadian rhythms, and the pathogenesis of Alzheimer Disease. *Exp. Mol. Med.* 47, e148. doi: 10.1038/emm.2014.121

Nobili, A., Latagliata, E. C., Viscomi, M. T., Cavallucci, V., Cutuli, D., Giacovazzo, G., et al. (2017). Dopamine neuronal loss contributes to memory and reward dysfunction in a model of Alzheimer's disease. *Nat. Commun.* 8:14727. doi: 10.1038/ncomms14727

Ogomori, K., Kitamoto, T., Tateishi, J., Sato, Y., Suetsugu, M., and Abe, M. (1989). Beta-protein amyloid is widely distributed in the central nervous system of patients with Alzheimer's disease. *Am. J. Pathol.* 134, 243–251.

Ott, A., Stolk, R. P., Hofman, A., Van Harskamp, F., Grobbee, D. E., and Breteler, M. M. B. (1996). Association of diabetes mellitus and dementia: the Rotterdam Study. *Diabetologia* 39, 1392–1397. doi: 10.1007/s001250050588

Ott, A., Stolk, R. P., van Harskamp, F., Pols, H. A. P., Hofman, A., and Breteler, M. M. B. (1999). Diabetes mellitus and the risk of dementia: the Rotterdam Study. *Neurology* 53, 1937–1937. doi: 10.1212/WNL.53.9.1937

Ownby, R. L., Crocco, E., Acevedo, A., John, V., and Loewenstein, D. (2006). Depression and risk for Alzheimer disease. *Arch. Gen. Psychiatry* 63, 530. doi: 10.1001/archpsyc.63.5.530

Perez-Nievas, B. G., Stein, T. D., Tai, H. C., Dols-Icardo, O., Scotton, T. C., Barroeta-Espar, I., et al. (2013). Dissecting phenotypic traits linked to human resilience to Alzheimer's pathology. *Brain* 136, 2510–2526. doi: 10.1093/brain/awt171

Perry, D., Sperling, R., Katz, R., Berry, D., Dilts, D., Hanna, D., et al. (2014). Building a roadmap for developing combination therapies for Alzheimer's disease. *Expert Rev. Neurother.* 15, 327–333. doi: 10.1586/14737175.2015.996551

Perry, G., Cash, A. D., and Smith, M. A. (2002). Alzheimer disease and oxidative stress. *J. Biomed. Biotechnol.* 23, 120–123. doi: 10.1155/S1110724302203010

Perry, V. H., Nicoll, J. A. R., and Holmes, C. (2010). Microglia in neurodegenerative disease. *Nat. Rev. Neurol.* 6, 193–201. doi: 10.1038/nrneurol.2010.17

Piacentini, R., Li Puma, D. D., Mainardi, M., Lazzarino, G., Tavazzi, B., Arancio, O., et al. (2017). Reduced gliotransmitter release from astrocytes mediates tau-induced synaptic dysfunction in cultured hippocampal neurons. *Glia* 65, 1302–1316. doi: 10.1002/glia.23163

Prince, M., Bryce, R., Albanese, E., Wimo, A., Ribeiro, W., and Ferri, C. P. (2013). The global prevalence of dementia: a systematic review and metaanalysis. *Alzheimer's Dement.* 9, 63–75. doi: 10.1016/j.jalz.2012.11.007

Prince, M., Comas-Herrera, A., Knapp, M., Guerchet, M., and Karagiannidou, M. (2016). *World Alzheimer Report 2016 Improving Healthcare for People Living with Dementia. Coverage, Quality and Costs Now and in the Future.* Available online at: https://www.alz.co.uk/research/world-report-2016

Prinz, P., Vitaliano, P. P., Vitiello, M. V., Bokan, J., Raskind, M., Peskind, E., et al. (1982). Sleep, EEG and mental function changes in senile dementia of the Alzheimer's type. *Neurobiol. Aging* 3, 361–370.

Puzzo, D., Piacentini, R., Fá, M., Gulisano, W., Li Puma, D. D., Staniszewski, A., et al. (2017). LTP and memory impairment caused by extracellular Aβ and tau oligomers is APP- dependent. *Elife* 6:e26991. doi: 10.7554/eLife.26991

Qiu, W. Q., Walsh, D. M., Ye, Z., Vekrellis, K., Zhang, J., Podlisny, M. B., et al. (1998). Insulin-degrading enzyme regulates extracellular levels of amyloid β- protein by degradation. *J. Biol. Chem.* 273, 32730–32738. doi: 10.1074/jbc.273.49.32730

Querfurth, H. W., and LaFerla, F. M. (2010). Alzheimer's disease. *N. Engl. J. Med.* 362, 329–344. doi: 10.1056/NEJMra0909142

Reilly, P., Winston, C. N., Baron, K. R., Trejo, M., Rockenstein, E. M., Akers, J. C., et al. (2017). Novel human neuronal tau model exhibiting neurofibrillary tangles and transcellular propagation. *Neurobiol. Dis.* 106, 222–234. doi: 10.1016/j.nbd.2017.06.005

Rivera, E. J., Goldin, A., Fulmer, N., Tavares, R., Wands, J. R., and de la Monte, S. M. (2005). Insulin and insulin-like growth factor expression and function deteriorate with progression of Alzheimer's disease: link to brain reductions in acetylcholine. *J. Alzheimers Dis.* 8, 247–268. doi: 10.3233/JAD-2005-8304

Romano, A., Pace, L., Tempesta, B., Lavecchia, A. M., Macheda, T., Bedse, G., et al. (2014). Depressive-like behavior is paired to monoaminergic alteration in a murine model of Alzheimer's disease. *Int. J. Neuropsychopharmacol.* 18, 1–12. doi: 10.1093/ijnp/pyu020

Roselli, F., Tirard, M., Lu, J., Hutzler, P., Lamberti, P., Livrea, P., et al. (2005). Soluble β-amyloid 1-40 induces NMDA-dependent degradation of postsynaptic density-95 at glutamatergic synapses. *J. Neurosci.* 25, 11061–11070. doi: 10.1523/JNEUROSCI.3034-05.2005

Rossato, J. I., Bevilaqua, L. R. M., Izquierdo, I., Medina, J. H., and Cammarota, M. (2009). Dopamine controls persistence of long-term memory storage. *Science* 325, 1017–1020. doi: 10.1126/science.1172545

Rowan, M. J., Klyubin, I., Wang, Q., and Anwyl, R. (2005). Synaptic plasticity disruption by amyloid beta protein: modulation by potential Alzheimer's disease modifying therapies. *Biochem. Soc. Trans.* 33, 563–567. doi: 10.1042/BST0330563

Russo, S. J., and Nestler, E. J. (2013). The brain reward circuitry in mood disorders. *Nat. Rev. Neurosci.* 14, 609–625. doi: 10.1038/nrn3381

Salter, M. W., and Stevens, B. (2017). Microglia emerge as central players in brain disease. *Nat. Med.* 23, 1018–1027. doi: 10.1038/nm.4397

Santos, L. E., Beckman, D., and Ferreira, S. T. (2016). Microglial dysfunction connects depression and Alzheimer's disease. *Brain. Behav. Immun.* 55, 151–165. doi: 10.1016/j.bbi.2015.11.011

Scheltens, P., Blennow, K., Breteler, M. M. B., de Strooper, B., Frisoni, G. B., Salloway, S., et al. (2016). Alzheimer's disease. *Lancet* 388, 505–517. doi: 10.1016/S0140-6736(15)01124-1

Selkoe, D. J. (2002). Alzheimer's disease is a synaptic failure. *Science* 298, 789–791. doi: 10.1126/science.1074069

Selkoe, D. J. (2008). Soluble oligomers of the amyloid β-protein impair synaptic plasticity and behavior. *Behav. Brain Res.* 192, 106–113. doi: 10.1007/978-3-540-76330-7_8

Selkoe, D. J., and Hardy, J. (2016). The amyloid hypothesis of Alzheimer's disease at 25 years. *EMBO Mol. Med.* 8, 1–14. doi: 10.15252/emmm.201606210

Shankar, G. M., Bloodgood, B. L., Townsend, M., Walsh, D. M., Selkoe, D. J., and Sabatini, B. L. (2007). Natural oligomers of the alzheimer amyloid- protein induce reversible synapse loss by modulating an NMDA-type glutamate receptor-dependent signaling pathway. *J. Neurosci.* 27, 2866-75. doi: 10.1523/JNEUROSCI.4970-06.2007

Shankar, G. M., Li, S., Mehta, T. H., Garcia-Munoz, A., Shepardson, N. E., Smith, I., et al. (2008). Amyloid-β protein dimers isolated directly from Alzheimer's brains impair synaptic plasticity and memory. *Nat. Med.* 14, 837–842. doi: 10.1038/nm1782

Small, S. A., and Duff, K. (2008). Linking Aβ and Tau in late-onset Alzheimer's disease: a dual pathway hypothesis. *Neuron* 60, 534–542. doi: 10.1016/j.neuron.2008.11.007

Smith, M. A., Hirai, K., Hsiao, K., Pappolla, M. A., Harris, P. L., Siedlak, S. L., et al. (1998). Amyloid-beta deposition in Alzheimer transgenic mice is associated with oxidative stress. *J. Neurochem.* 70, 2212–2215. doi: 10.1046/j.1471-4159.1998.70052212.x

Snyder, E. M., Nong, Y., Almeida, C. G., Paul, S., Moran, T., Choi, E. Y., et al. (2005). Regulation of NMDA receptor trafficking by amyloid-β. *Nat. Neurosci.* 8, 1051–1058. doi: 10.1038/nn1503

Snyder, H. M., Asthana, S., Bain, L., Brinton, R., Craft, S., Dubal, D. B., et al. (2016). Sex biology contributions to vulnerability to Alzheimer's disease: a think tank convened by the Women's Alzheimer's Research Initiative. *Alzheimer's Dement.* 12, 1186–1196. doi: 10.1016/j.jalz.2016.08.004

Sperling, R. A., Aisen, P. S., Beckett, L. A., Bennett, D. A., Craft, S., Fagan, A. M., et al. (2011a). Toward defining the preclinical stages of Alzheimer's disease: recommendations from the National Institute on Aging-Alzheimer's Association workgroups on diagnostic guidelines for Alzheimer's disease. *Alzheimer's Dement.* 7, 280–292. doi: 10.1016/j.jalz.2011.03.003

Sperling, R. A., Jack, C. R., and Aisen, P. S. (2011b). Testing the right target and right drug at the right stage. *Sci. Transl. Med.* 3:111cm33. doi: 10.1126/scitranslmed.3002609

Spires-Jones, T. L., and Hyman, B. T. (2014). The intersection of amyloid beta and tau at synapses in Alzheimer's disease. *Neuron* 82, 756–771. doi: 10.1016/j.neuron.2014.05.004

Standaert, D. G., Lee, V. M., Greenberg, B. D., Lowery, D. E., and Trojanowski, J. Q. (1991). Molecular features of hypothalamic plaques in Alzheimer's disease. *Am. J. Pathol.* 139, 681–691.

Stanley, M., Macauley, S. L., Caesar, E. E., Koscal, L. J., Moritz, W., Robinson, G. O., et al. (2016). The effects of peripheral and central high insulin on brain insulin signaling and amyloid-β in young and old APP/PS1 mice. *J. Neurosci.* 36, 11704–11715. doi: 10.1523/JNEUROSCI.2119-16.2016

Starkstein, S. E., and Mizrahi, R. (2006). Depression in Alzheimer's disease. *Exp. Rev. Neurother.* 6, 887–895. doi: 10.1586/14737175.6.6.887

Steen, E., Terry, B. M., Rivera, E. J., Cannon, J. L., Neely, T. R., Tavares, R., et al. (2005). Impaired insulin and insulin-like growth factor expression and signaling mechanisms in Alzheimer's disease–is this type 3 diabetes? *J. Alzheimers. Dis.* 7, 63–80. doi: 10.3233/JAD-2005-7107

Stephenson, D., Perry, D., Bens, C., Bain, L. J., Berry, D., Krams, M., et al. (2014). Charting a path toward combination therapy for Alzheimer's disease. *Exp. Rev. Neurother.* 15, 1–7. doi: 10.1586/14737175.2015.1002173

Stevanovic, K., Yunus, A., Joly-Amado, A., Gordon, M., Morgan, D., Gulick, D., et al. (2017). Disruption of normal circadian clock function in a mouse model of tauopathy. *Exp. Neurol.* 294, 58–67. doi: 10.1016/j.expneurol.2017.04.015

Stine, W. B., Dahlgren, K. N., Krafft, G. A., and LaDu, M. J. (2003). *In vitro* characterization of conditions for amyloid-β peptide oligomerization and fibrillogenesis. *J. Biol. Chem.* 278, 11612–11622. doi: 10.1074/jbc.M210207200

Storga, D., Vrecko, K., Birkmayer, J. G. D., and Reibnegger, G. (1996). Monoaminergic neurotransmitters, their precursors and metabolites in brains of Alzheimer patients. *Neurosci. Lett.* 203, 29–32. doi: 10.1016/0304-3940(95)12256-7

Swardfager, W., Lanctt, K., Rothenburg, L., Wong, A., Cappell, J., and Herrmann, N. (2010). A meta-analysis of cytokines in Alzheimer's disease. *Biol. Psychiatry* 68, 930–941. doi: 10.1016/j.biopsych.2010.06.012

Takeda, S., Sato, N., Uchio-Yamada, K., Sawada, K., Kunieda, T., Takeuchi, D., et al. (2010). Diabetes-accelerated memory dysfunction via cerebrovascular inflammation and A deposition in an Alzheimer mouse model with diabetes. *Proc. Natl. Acad. Sci. U.S.A.* 107, 7036–7041. doi: 10.1073/pnas.1000645107

Talbot, K., Wang, H. Y., Kazi, H., Han, L. Y., Bakshi, K. P., Stucky, A., et al. (2012). Demonstrated brain insulin resistance in Alzheimer's disease patients is associated with IGF-1 resistance, IRS-1 dysregulation, and cognitive decline. *J. Clin. Invest.* 122, 1316–1338. doi: 10.1172/JCI59903

Tarasoff-Conway, J. M., Carare, R. O., Osorio, R. S., Glodzik, L., Butler, T., Fieremans, E., et al. (2015). Clearance systems in the brain—implications for Alzheimer disease. *Nat. Rev. Neurol.* 11, 457–470. doi: 10.1038/nrneurol.2015.119

Terry, R. D., Masliah, E., Salmon, D. P., Butters, N., DeTeresa, R., Hill, R., et al. (1991). Physical basis of cognitive alterations in alzheimer's disease: synapse loss is the major correlate of cognitive impairment. *Ann. Neurol.* 30, 572–580.

Thaler, J. P., Yi, C. X., Schur, E. A., Guyenet, S. J., Hwang, B. H., Dietrich, M. O., et al. (2012). Obesity is associated with hypothalamic injury in rodents and humans. *J. Clin. Invest.* 122, 153–162. doi: 10.1172/JCI59660

Valdearcos, M., Xu, A. W., and Koliwad, S. K. (2015). Hypothalamic inflammation in the control of metabolic function. *Annu. Rev. Physiol.* 77, 131–160. doi: 10.1146/annurev-physiol-021014-071656

Vandal, M., White, P., Chevrier, G., Tremblay, C., St-Amour, I., Planel, E., et al. (2015). Age-dependent impairment of glucose tolerance in the 3xTg-AD mouse model of Alzheimer's disease. *FASEB J.* 29, 4273–4284. doi: 10.1096/fj.14-268482

van Maurik, I. S., Zwan, M. D., Tijms, B. M., Bouwman, F. H., Teunissen, C. E., Scheltens, P., et al. (2017). Interpreting biomarker results in individual patients with mild cognitive impairment in the Alzheimer's biomarkers in daily Practice (ABIDE) Project. *JAMA Neurol.* 74, 1481–1491. doi: 10.1001/jamaneurol.2017.2712

Villemagne, V. L., Burnham, S., Bourgeat, P., Brown, B., Ellis, K. A., Salvado, O., et al. (2013). Amyloid β deposition, neurodegeneration, and cognitive decline in sporadic Alzheimer's disease: a prospective cohort study. *Lancet Neurol.* 12, 357–367. doi: 10.1016/S1474-4422(13)70044-9

Viña, J., and Lloret, A. (2010). Why women have more Alzheimer's disease than men: gender and mitochondrial toxicity of amyloid-beta peptide. *J. Alzheimers. Dis.* 20(Suppl. 2), S527–S533. doi: 10.3233/JAD-2010-100501

Viola, K. L., and Klein, W. L. (2015). Amyloid β oligomers in Alzheimer's disease pathogenesis, treatment, and diagnosis. *Acta Neuropathol.* 129, 183–206. doi: 10.1007/s00401-015-1386-3

Viola, K. L., Sbarboro, J., Sureka, R., De, M., Bicca, M. A., Wang, J., et al. (2014). Towards non-invasive diagnostic imaging of early-stage Alzheimer's disease. *Nat. Nanotechnol.* 10, 91–98. doi: 10.1038/nnano.2014.254

Walsh, D. M., and Selkoe, D. J. (2007). Aβ oligomers - A decade of discovery. *J. Neurochem.* 101, 1172–1184 doi: 10.1111/j.1471-4159.2006.04426.x

Wang, J., Tan, L., Wang, H.-F., Tan, C.-C., Meng, X.-F., Wang, C., et al. (2015). Anti-inflammatory drugs and risk of Alzheimer's disease: an updated systematic review and meta-analysis. *J. Alzheimers Dis.* 44, 385–396. doi: 10.3233/JAD-141506

Wang, W.-Y., Tan, M.-S., Yu, J.-T., and Tan, L. (2015). Role of pro-inflammatory cytokines released from microglia in Alzheimer's disease. *Ann. Transl. Med.* 3, 136. doi: 10.3978/j.issn.2305-5839.2015.03.49

White, H., Pieper, C., Schmader, K., and Fillenbaum, G. (1996). Weight change in Alzheimer's disease. *J. Am. Geriatr. Soc.* 44, 265–272. doi: 10.1111/j.1532-5415.1996.tb00912.x

Xia, W., Yang, T., Shankar, G., Smith, I. M., Shen, Y., Walsh, D. M., et al. (2009). A specific enzyme-linked immunosorbent assay for measuring β-amyloid protein oligomers in human plasma and brain tissue of patients with alzheimer disease. *Arch. Neurol.* 66, 190–199. doi: 10.1001/archneurol.2008.565

Yang, T., Li, S., Xu, H., Walsh, D. M., and Selkoe, D. J. (2017). Large soluble oligomers of amyloid β-protein from alzheimer brain are far less neuroactive than the smaller oligomers to which they dissociate. *J. Neurosci.* 37, 152–163. doi: 10.1523/JNEUROSCI.1698-16.2016

Yao, J., and Brinton, R. D. (2012). Estrogen regulation of mitochondrial bioenergetics. *Adv. Pharmacol.* 64, 327–371. doi: 10.1016/B978-0-12-39 4816-8.00010-6

Yirmiya, R., Rimmerman, N., and Reshef, R. (2015). Depression as a microglial disease. *Trends Neurosci.* 38, 637–658. doi: 10.1016/j.tins.2015.08.001

Zenaro, E., Pietronigro, E., Della Bianca, V., Piacentino, G., Marongiu, L., Budui, S., et al. (2015). Neutrophils promote Alzheimer's disease-like pathology and cognitive decline via LFA-1 integrin. *Nat. Med.* 21, 880–886. doi: 10.1038/nm.3913

Zhang, J., Ke, K. F., Liu, Z., Qiu, Y. H., and Peng, Y. P. (2013). Th17 Cell-mediated neuroinflammation is involved in neurodegeneration of Aβ1-42-Induced Alzheimer's disease model rats. *PLoS ONE* 8:e75786. doi: 10.1371/journal.pone.0075786

Zhang, X., Zhang, G., Zhang, H., Karin, M., Bai, H., and Cai, D. (2008). Hypothalamic β/NF-κB and ER stress link overnutrition to energy imbalance and obesity. *Cell* 135, 61–73. doi: 10.1016/j.cell.2008.07.043

Zhao, L., Mao, Z., Woody, S. K., and Brinton, R. D. (2016). Sex differences in metabolic aging of the brain: insights into female susceptibility to Alzheimer's disease. *Neurobiol. Aging* 42, 69–79. doi: 10.1016/j.neurobiolaging.2016. 02.011

5

On the Extraction and Analysis of Graphs from Resting-State fMRI to Support a Correct and Robust Diagnostic Tool for Alzheimer's Disease

Claudia Bachmann[1], Heidi I. L. Jacobs[2,3,4], PierGianLuca Porta Mana[5], Kim Dillen[6], Nils Richter[6,7], Boris von Reutern[6,7], Julian Dronse[6,7], Oezguer A. Onur[6,7], Karl-Josef Langen[8], Gereon R. Fink[6,7], Juraj Kukolja[6,7,9] and Abigail Morrison[1,10]*

[1] Institute of Neuroscience and Medicine (INM-6), Institute for Advanced Simulation (IAS-6), JARA BRAIN Institute I, Jülich Research Centre, Jülich, Germany, [2] Faculty of Health, Medicine and Life Science, School for Mental Health and Neuroscience, Alzheimer Centre Limburg, Maastricht University, Maastricht, Netherlands, [3] Division of Nuclear Medicine and Molecular Imaging, Department of Radiology, Harvard Medical School, Massachusetts General Hospital, Boston, MA, United States, [4] Department of Cognitive Neuroscience, Faculty of Psychology and Neuroscience, Maastricht University, Maastricht, Netherlands, [5] Kavli Institute for Systems Neuroscience, Norwegian University of Science and Technology (NTNU), Trondheim, Norway, [6] Cognitive Neuroscience, Institute of Neuroscience and Medicine (INM-3), Jülich Research Centre, Jülich, Germany, [7] Department of Neurology, University Hospital of Cologne, Cologne, Germany, [8] Cognitive Neuroscience, Institute of Neuroscience and Medicine (INM-4), Jülich Research Centre, Jülich, Germany, [9] Department of Neurology, Helios University Hospital Wuppertal, Wuppertal, Germany, [10] Faculty of Psychology, Institute of Cognitive Neuroscience, Ruhr-University Bochum, Bochum, Germany

***Correspondence:**
Claudia Bachmann
c.bachmann@fz-juelich.de

The diagnosis of Alzheimer's disease (AD), especially in the early stage, is still not very reliable and the development of new diagnosis tools is desirable. A diagnosis based on functional magnetic resonance imaging (fMRI) is a suitable candidate, since fMRI is non-invasive, readily available, and indirectly measures synaptic dysfunction, which can be observed even at the earliest stages of AD. However, the results of previous attempts to analyze graph properties of resting state fMRI data are contradictory, presumably caused by methodological differences in graph construction. This comprises two steps: clustering the voxels of the functional image to define the nodes of the graph, and calculating the graph's edge weights based on a functional connectivity measure of the average cluster activities. A variety of methods are available for each step, but the robustness of results to method choice, and the suitability of the methods to support a diagnostic tool, are largely unknown. To address this issue, we employ a range of commonly and rarely used clustering and edge definition methods and analyze their graph theoretic measures (graph weight, shortest path length, clustering coefficient, and weighted degree distribution and modularity) on a small data set of 26 healthy controls, 16 subjects with mild cognitive impairment (MCI) and 14 with Alzheimer's disease. We examine the results with respect to statistical significance of the mean difference in graph properties, the sensitivity of the results to model and parameter choices, and relative diagnostic power based on both a statistical model and support vector machines. We find that different combinations of graph construction techniques yield contradicting, but statistically significant, relations of graph properties between health conditions, explaining the discrepancy across previous studies, but casting doubt on such analyses as a method to gain insight into disease effects. The production of significant differences in mean graph properties turns out not to be a good predictor of future diagnostic capacity. Highest predictive power, expressed by largest negative surprise values, are achieved for both atlas-driven and data-driven clustering (Ward clustering), as long as graphs are small and clusters large, in combination with edge definitions based on correlations and mutual information transfer.

Keywords: Alzheimer's disease, MCI, graph theory, resting-state fMRI, diagnosis, model by sufficiency, negative surprise

1. INTRODUCTION

The two major challenges in Alzheimer's disease (AD) research consist in firstly, finding an effective treatment that at least slows down the disease progress, and secondly, developing diagnostic tools that can not only detect the disease at the earliest stage, during which no symptoms related to cognitive deficits are apparent (Sperling et al., 2011), but also provide information into the progression of the disease. For the latter challenge it is particularly desirable that the tools can be deployed within the existing medical infrastructure (i.e., not requiring specialized machinery or lab procedures), such that it is feasible to scan a wide range of the elderly population. Diagnosis procedures currently in use include psychological tests, detection of abnormal concentrations of disease specific biomarkers (Amyloid-β, tau proteins) in cerebrospinal fluid and analysis of structural magnetic resonance images (MRI).

Although abnormalities of Amyloid-β concentrations are proposed to be the earliest disease indicator, they are not very reliable in disease prognosis. Moreover, the changes in Amyloid-β concentrations show the strongest increase in the preclinical phase, and are thus uninformative with respect to the further progression of the disease. Tau pathology, which probably spreads along functional networks (Hoenig et al., 2018) better predicts cognitive deficits and progression of the disease (Nelson et al., 2012). However, the two methods measuring Amyloid-β and tau concentrations, lumbar puncture and PET are invasive (Schroeter et al., 2009; Sperling et al., 2011).

Possibly, synaptic dysfunction, another disease marker, corresponds to the onset of AD even before Amyloid-β pathology starts. Additionally, as it gradually worsens throughout the course of the disease, it could serve as diagnostic marker for all stages of AD. Dysfunction of synapses can be indirectly measured via invasive FDG-PET and non-invasive functional MRI, which might directly be combined with structural MRI scans (Schroeter et al., 2009; Sperling et al., 2011). However, a diagnostic framework based on functional MRI has yet to be established.

Although many fMRI studies have investigated changes of functional activity in AD (for a review see Dennis and Thompson, 2014), there is no consensus about which information should be used. Such studies typically examine disrupted cortical connectivity, either locally, considering single brain areas (e.g., Dillen et al., 2017) and their embedding in the network, or globally, analyzing the entire constructed brain graph and the statistics of its graph properties (Gits, 2016).

We argue that in order to develop a robust diagnosis tool applicable to all disease stages, it is preferable to consider global graph properties for the following reasons. First, global graph properties seem to be more robust across sessions; consequently, changes in these properties over time are more likely to reflect disease progression than statistical fluctuations (Telesford et al., 2010; Wang et al., 2014). Second, not all disease progressions follow a stereotypical pattern. Whereas structural evidence of AD is typically found predominantly in entorhinal cortex and hippocampus, in atypical cases atrophy occurs primarily in other areas, such as posterior cortex (Johnson et al., 2012). These atypical cases might be better captured by global properties, since they make use of the entire information provided by the brain. Furthermore, analyzing the statistics of graph properties rather than comparing the properties of single nodes allows the use of data-driven brain clustering, which results in different numbers and locations of brain clusters for each individual.

However, it is challenging to investigate the informativeness of global graph properties due to the innumerable methods of graph construction, comprising both the clustering of the voxels to define the graph's nodes, and the definition of functional connectivity to define its edges. Across the range of previous studies investigating graph properties in AD, a wide variety of methodological approaches for graph construction and properties assessment have been applied and are probably a major source of contradictory observations, such as the comparative length of the shortest path in AD subjects with respect to control being reported in two recent studies as both shorter (Zhao et al., 2012) and longer (Sanz-Arigita et al., 2010).

It is a further challenge to identify an appropriate evaluation method that not only enables us to compare the different graph construction methods, but also permits the results to be combined with other information indicating the probability of a particular health condition. This means that pure classifiers, although they achieve high discrimination performance (Khazaee et al., 2015, 2017) do not meet these requirements because they return a group membership ("AD," "MCI," or "control") and not a probability that can be combined with the results of other diagnostic tests (e.g., derived from Amyloid-β concentration measures) or individual patient risk factors (Porta Mana et al., 2018).

In this article, we address these issues by presenting a methodology for determining which combination of techniques to extract and analyze graphs from resting state fMRI data provides the best basis for a diagnosis tool, assuming a given initial data set. Here, we apply our methodology to a small data set consisting of 26 control (C) elderly patients without any indication of any form of dementia or other cognitive problems, 16 mild cognitive impaired (MCI) subjects and 14 patients suffering from Alzheimer disease (AD) (Dillen et al., 2017). We evaluate the combinations of graph construction and analysis methods using a statistical model that partly compensates for the small data set and also yields probabilities rather than classifications, thus permitting the results to be combined with other probabilities, as discussed above. In addition, we evaluate the graph construction techniques with respect to robustness of results to method configuration parameters and similarity of results across different techniques.

Note that our aim here is not to demonstrate superior classification (for which our data set is in any case too small) or to propose a particular combination of techniques as optimal (as this may vary between settings), but primarily to provide a principled way for determining an appropriate combination of techniques for a given data set, and secondarily to highlight the sensitivity of graph theoretical analysis to the details of graph construction.

To understand how different methods for constructing graphs affect the resultant graph properties, and thus the ability to distinguish between patient groups, we evaluate a range of standard and non-standard methods to construct the graphs. The first step in graph construction consists in clustering adjacent voxels, such that the activity of the resulting region can be expressed by the average of time varying signal of the selected voxels (see **Figure 1**). The decision as to which voxels form a cluster is often based on atlases established for a standard brain with predefined brain regions. In order to map this standard atlas to the functional image or vice versa, registration algorithms are used. Problematic in this step, especially for subjects potentially suffering from neurodegenerative diseases, is the inhomogeneous shrinkage of the brain, which hampers a correct registration (Liu et al., 2017). In addition, individual brain regions derived from standard brain templates are likely to execute several cognitive processes in parallel, such that averaging the activity across the voxels of these functional inhomogeneous regions is not justified (Marrelec and Fransson, 2011). We therefore also include activity driven algorithms, namely region growing and selection (Lu et al., 2003) and Ward clustering, into our evaluation.

In the second step in graph construction, functional connectivity values are calculated based on the averaged signal of the regions. In most studies this is carried out based on the Pearson correlation coefficient, restricting the functional connectivity to non-directional connections. Here we cover a broader range of possible measures in the time domain: linear, non-linear model-free and model-based (Wang et al., 2014) that, depending on their exact realization, result in directed or undirected graphs.

We then calculate a variety of graph measures on the single nodes (weighted degree, cluster coefficient, closeness centrality), edges (weights, shortest path) and the entire graph (modularity). As several of these measures are only well-defined for binary graphs, many studies binarize the weighted graphs obtained from the previous steps into binary graphs, by setting weights above an arbitrary threshold $w_{\min}$ to 1, and those below it to 0 (e.g., Supekar et al., 2008). The drawback here is that there is no validation for an optimal threshold, and information that might be relevant in AD may be lost. To investigate this problem, we analyze the dependence of graph theoretic measures on $w_{\min}$, setting the weights below it to 0 but leaving the values above unchanged.

To assess the suitability of combinations of graph construction and analysis methods to inform a diagnosis tool, we set up a statistical analysis based on a training data set of known health conditions (healthy controls, mild cognitive impairment, and Alzheimer's disease), see section 5.6. The diagnostic usefulness of the analysis pipeline is then defined as the performance of the model against a labeled test data set. A model with good

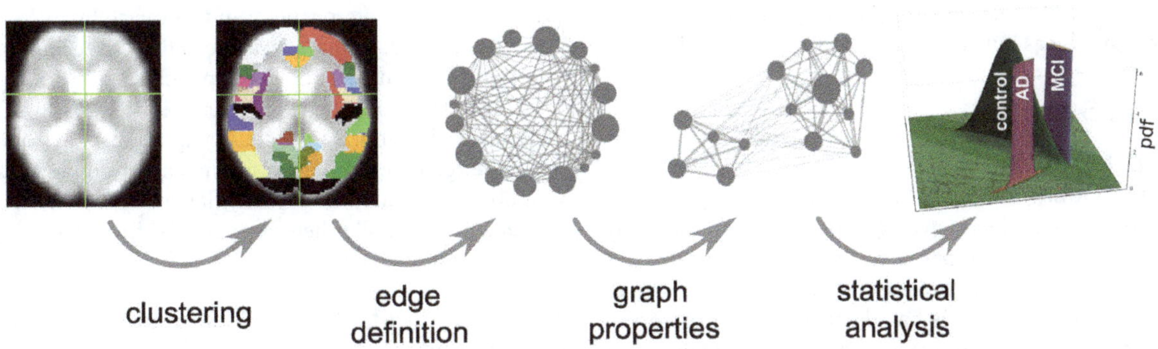

FIGURE 1 | Overview of intermediate steps for graph construction, properties derivation and statistical analysis. Each picture illustrates the result of a processing step starting from the preprocessed functional image (far left), which is clustered into regions, used as the nodes of the graph (second image). The averaged fMRI activity of each region is then used to calculate the edges of the graph (third image) and based on the calculated graph properties (fourth image) of all graphs, the statistical analysis estimates the probability density functions (pdf) of the three health conditions (last image) that are necessary for the evaluation of diagnostic performance based on the negative surprise measure. For the first three steps of the pipeline we investigate a range of different methods, see sections 2.1, 5.3, 5.4, and 5.5 for details.

performance can ultimately be employed in a clinical setting, to assess the probability that a patient has one of the three health conditions. For a more complete discussion of the development and use of the statistical model, see Porta Mana et al. (2018).

In this study we use a statistical model constructed from the following working hypothesis: the empirical means and correlations of graph data from previous patients with a given health condition are sufficient to predict the graph data of a new patient with that same health condition. This is a partially exchangeable model by sufficiency, and the resulting likelihood is a multivariate t distribution (Porta Mana et al., 2018), described in section 5.6. To assess which graph constructions have the greatest predictive power, we calculate their log-probabilities or *negative surprises* (Bartlett, 1952; Good, 1956, 1957a,b, 1983). To validate this approach, we also compare the results of the negative surprise with the classification performance achieved by a support vector machine (SVM).

Our results show that clustering resulting in small graphs with large clusters (Ward and atlas-based clustering) achieve highest negative surprises (and best SVM classification performance). Similarly, amongst the edge definition techniques, model-free methods (linear and non-linear correlations, mutually information transfer) obtain the highest negative surprise values. Conversely, calculating the graph's edge weights according to transfer entropy (model based) achieves limited diagnostic power but the ordering of the individuals based on their average graph properties is very robust toward the applied clustering method and choice of algorithm specific parameters. We further demonstrate that significant differences in the means of graph properties are very sensitive to method choice and to parameterization choices for a given method. Therefore such results, if taken at face value and not validated by alternate methods, may well be artifactual and not provide insight into the effects of a disease. Interestingly, the presence of significant differences in mean values of graph properties is not a reliable predictor of later diagnostic performance. In particular, atlas clustering results in only few significant differences but reaches the highest values for negative surprises and the best classification scores for the SVM. Finally, we show that the effect of setting a threshold on the graphs edge weights has only marginal effect on the negative surprise as long as threshold values are small.

2. RESULTS

2.1. Graph Construction

2.1.1. Vertex Definition by Means of Clustering

A universal property of the clustering algorithms examined here is the existence of a control parameter that regulates how the clusters are formed, and thus preserves a certain feature (or features) of the clusters. In atlas-based clustering, the preserved features are the number of clusters and the number of voxels per cluster. In Ward clustering, the number of resulting clusters is fixed, which we violate to a small extent by deleting very small clusters. In region growing and selection (RGS), the homogeneity of each cluster is preserved. The freedom that each of the algorithms leaves to the non-regulated features can either be considered as a drawback of the algorithm, because it makes graphs less easily comparable, or as an additional feature that might even improve the diagnosis performance.

Figure 2 shows the number of nodes/clusters, the average number of voxels per node and the average heterogeneity of the nodes for two configurations of the RGS algorithm, four configurations of the Ward algorithm, and the atlas algorithm (see section 5.3 and **Table 3**). Most strikingly, the node properties vary far more with respect to the clustering method chosen than with respect to the health condition.

By construction, the number of nodes for atlas clustering are the same for all individuals, and are the smallest over all the clustering methods (top panel). In Ward clustering the number of clusters is a parameter of the algorithm; it is not constant in **Figure 2** because we additionally include a parameter enforcing a minimum cluster size. Thus, the number of nodes for Ward clustering decreases as the minimum number of voxels per cluster p increases from 10 for "ward1" to 25 in "ward4." In RGS clustering we do not have such restrictions and the number of clusters is defined by the voxel dynamics. A consequence of this is that the number of clusters per graph are more widely spread.

The average number of voxels per cluster, shown in the middle panel of **Figure 2**, is unsurprisingly negatively correlated with the number of clusters. For purposes of comparison, the number of voxels for atlas clustering was first calculated for the standard space and then downscaled in proportion to the relation of the total number of voxels present in functional space to those in standard space. An inverse correlation can also be seen in the width of the distributions between the top two panels, for the non-atlas methods. In the case of RGS clustering, this can be explained by the fixation of the heterogeneity to one (see bottom panel of **Figure 2**), leading to quite homogeneous numbers of voxels per cluster, but to a wide range of the number of nodes, namely from 200 to 1200. Since this range is so large, it could be argued that graph properties that depend on this number would not be comparable in a meaningful fashion. In order to take care of such dependencies, we include the number of nodes in our statistical analysis (section 5.6). For Ward clustering we can observe that the numbers of nodes is inversely correlated not only with the average number of nodes and its variability, but also with the average heterogeneity and its variability. We observe the highest degree of heterogeneity for atlas clustering, presumably due to the high number of voxels per cluster.

Comparing node properties between the classes of clustering methods, atlas and ward4 clustering seem to be quite similar, which suggests they might result in similar graph properties and diagnosis performance. In particular, we note that these methods reveal a much smaller heterogeneity for the MCI group than for the control and AD groups.

2.1.2. Edge Definition by Means of Functional Connectivity

The edges of the graphs are constructed in four different ways, described in detail in section 5.4. Linear correlations (*corr*) are based on the Pearson correlation coefficient; non-linear correlations (H_2) result from a non-linear fit of piecewise linear correlations; mutual information transfer (*MIT*) measures the amount of shared information between two time varying signals

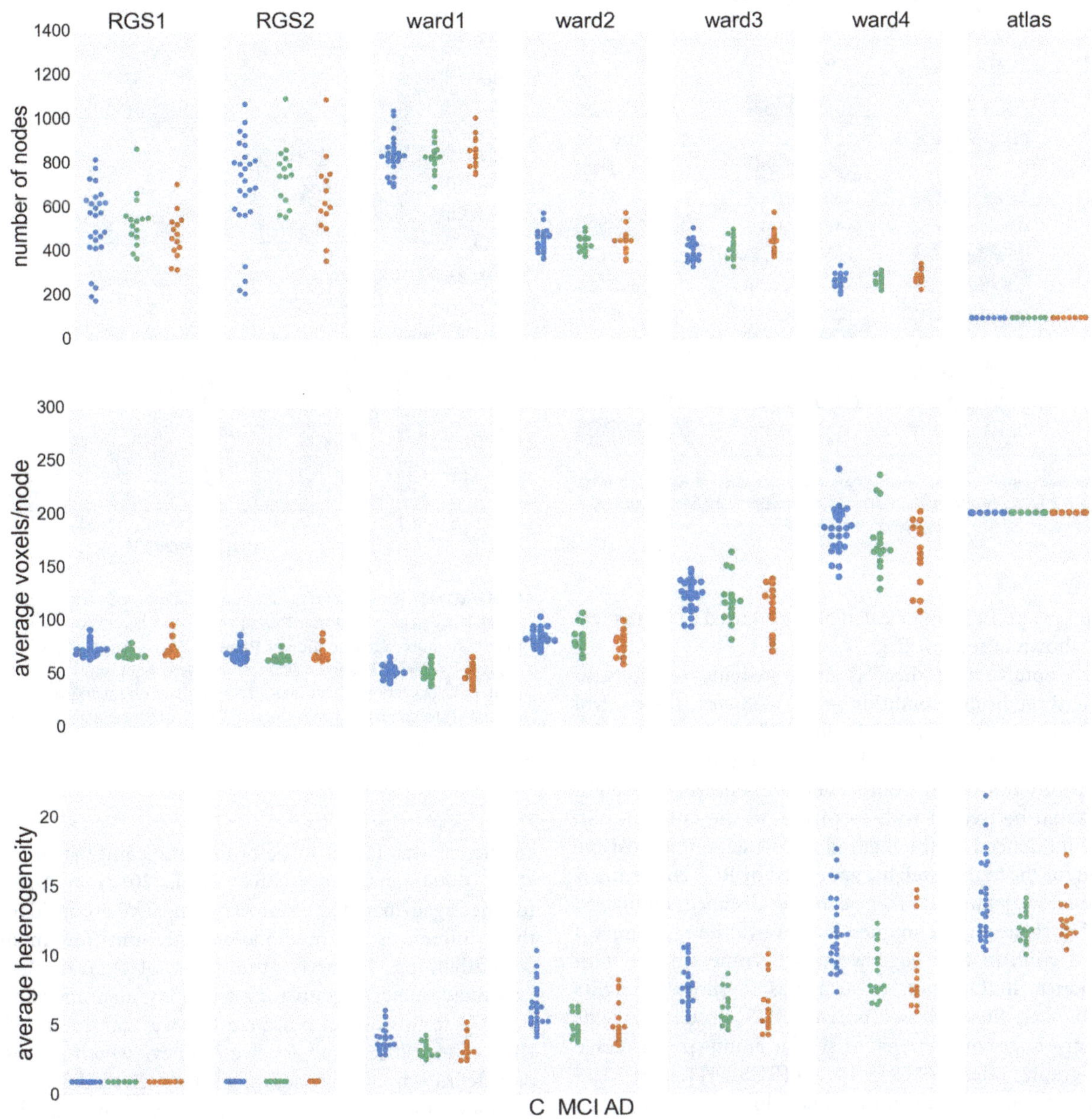

FIGURE 2 | Node properties across different clustering algorithms. For each of the seven clustering methods detailed in section 5.3 and **Table 3**, and each subject categorized in the health conditions: control (C, blue dots), mild cognitive impairment (MCI, green dots), and Alzheimer's disease (AD, orange dots) we calculate the total number of nodes/clusters generated **(Upper Panel)**, the average number of voxels per node **(Middle Panel)**, and the average cluster heterogeneity **(Lower Panel)**.

and transfer entropy (*TE*) describes in how far the future uncertainty is reduced by the preceding activity of the considered pair of nodes. As with the clustering algorithms described in the previous section, we defined differently parameterized variants of these four classes of technique (e.g., generating directed *D* or undirected *U* graphs) which are listed in **Table 4**.

For each combination of vertex (RGS, Ward or atlas) and edge definition technique (*corr*, H_2, *MIT*, *TE*), we averaged over the weights generated in each health condition for each variant of both techniques. For example, for the combination of region growing and transfer entropy (RGS *TE*) we averaged over all combinations of clustering implementation (RGS1 and RGS2) and edge detection (*BTEU*1, *BTEU*2, *BTED*1, *BTED*2). The results are shown in **Table 1** and exhibit a high variability in the mean connection weights. For instance, the combination RGS *TE* yields a maximal mean weight of 0.158 for controls, which is three times lower than the maximum mean weight of 0.493 obtained by the RGS H_2 combination. In particular, RGS clustering yields higher values compared with Ward and atlas clustering for model-free edge definitions (*corr*, H_2, *MIT*). The smallest values are obtained for *TE*. As a consequence, even small thresholds e.g., $w_{\min} = 0.3$ already cause *TE* graphs to disintegrate. Accordingly,

TABLE 1 | Mean and standard deviation of edge weight across different edge definitions.

Combination	$\hat{w}_C$	$\hat{w}_{MCI}$	$\hat{w}_{AD}$
Ward *corr*	0.328 ± 0.021	0.337 ± 0.04	0.315 ± 0.023
RGS *corr*	0.405 ± 0.076	0.363 ± 0.049	0.397 ± 0.113
atlas *corr*	0.319 ± 0.02	0.334 ± 0.054	0.307 ± 0.022
Ward H_2	0.443 ± 0.18	0.398 ± 0.081	0.414 ± 0.057
RGS H_2	0.452 ± 0.1	0.471 ± 0.126	0.493 ± 0.179
atlas H_2	0.36 ± 0.057	0.352 ± 0.039	0.355 ± 0.042
Ward *MIT*	0.201 ± 0.004	0.2 ± 0.007	0.197 ± 0.004
RGS *MIT*	0.221 ± 0.026	0.204 ± 0.011	0.218 ± 0.037
atlas *MIT*	0.196 ± 0.003	0.197 ± 0.008	0.193 ± 0.003
Ward *TE*	0.163 ± 0.013	0.158 ± 0.015	0.156 ± 0.018
RGS *TE*	0.158 ± 0.026	0.149 ± 0.02	0.152 ± 0.042
atlas *TE*	0.163 ± 0.016	0.17 ± 0.011	0.165 ± 0.011

Means and standard deviations are taken across the average edge weight of every individual graph in a health condition. Highest mean edge weights for each combination across the three health conditions are highlighted in gray.

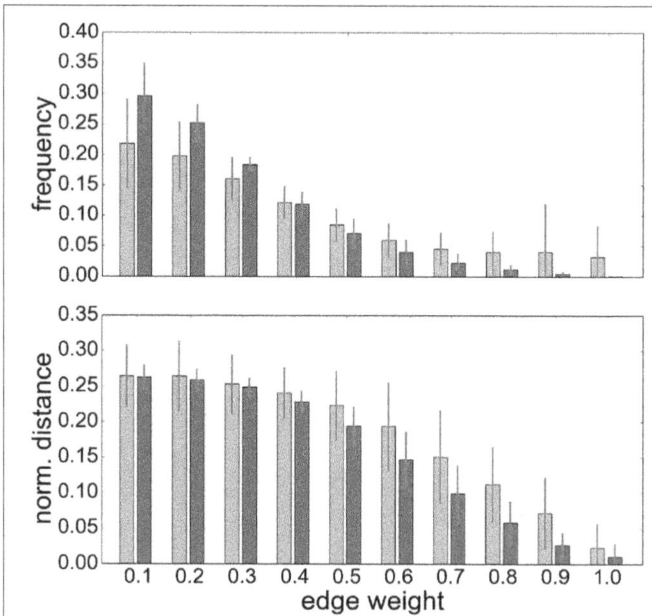

FIGURE 3 | RGS clustering yields stronger long-range connections then Ward clustering. Frequency **(Upper Panel)** and connection distance normalized to maximum graph distance **(Lower Panel)** across a range of graph edge weights calculated based on *BcorrU1* for RGS1 (light gray bars) and ward2 (dark gray) clustering. Mean values and standard deviation (blue vertical lines) are calculated across single histogram values of all subjects independent of health condition.

not all graph properties can be calculated and used for statistical analysis, as shown in section 2.3.

It is also notable that there is no systematic relationship between the three health conditions—for RGS *corr*, the control graphs have the highest mean weight, for RGS H_2, the AD graphs; and for atlas corr, the MCI graphs. These results demonstrate that conclusions drawn on health conditions based on weight statistics should be treated with suspicion, as the outcome can be strongly influenced by the method of calculation. A possible explanation for the higher weights generated by RGS clustering is that it produces a greater number of shorter distances compared with the other clustering techniques. However, although **Figure 3** does indeed confirm that edge weights become smaller with cluster distance, it does not reveal a bias to shorter weights for RGS. In fact, the converse is true: RGS clustering yields stronger long-range connections for similar graph sizes [average number of graph nodes: 379.69 ± 147.99 (RGS), 311.43 ± 33.59 (Ward); average edge weights for distances longer than 0.8: 0.25 (RGS), 0.18 (Ward)]. Therefore we conclude that connecting homogeneous clusters allows stronger long-range connections to be extracted. However, the statistics of the RGS connections has a much larger variance then the ones derived from Ward clustering. This is only partly due to the variance in the number of nodes, since even if we choose three healthy subjects with similar graph size (RGS: 297 ± 2.16, Ward: 297.33 ± 6.6), we still get a higher standard derivation for RGS clustering in the weight distribution ($\sigma_{\text{RGS}}/\sigma_{\text{ward}} = 1.6$).

In the following we will treat the distribution of edge weights as a graph property since it contains information about graph structure.

2.2. Graph Properties

A recent survey by Gits (2016) of studies investigating graph properties in AD reveals no clear and systematic differences between heath conditions. For example, the mean clustering coefficient was found to be both significantly smaller (Supekar et al., 2008) and larger (Zhao et al., 2012) in AD compared to the aged-matched control group. We consider it likely that differences in methodology account for many of the contradictions. However, the stage of AD reached by the examined subject group may also play an important role. To investigate this aspect more closely, we examine the finding by Kim et al. (2015) that local efficiency, which corresponds to our definition of closeness centrality divided by the number of nodes in the network minus one, is increased for MCI, decreased for initial stages of AD and increased for severe AD stages with respect to the control group. The results of applying similar methods (atlas-based clustering combined with *BMITU*) are shown in **Figure 4**. The top panel shows the relationship between the health conditions when closeness centrality is calculated on the full, non-thresholded graph, which reproduces the findings of Kim et al. (2015), at least for initial stages of AD. However, if the measure is calculated on the graphs' rich club, i.e., the sub-graphs consisting of the nodes in the top 10% for degree, a different picture emerges, as shown in the middle panel of **Figure 4**. Here, AD has an increased closeness centrality with respect to both the control and mild cognitive impairment groups, which is in line with advanced AD stages in Kim et al. (2015).

More evidence that the outcome of a graph theoretical analysis can be highly sensitive toward the exact methodological implementation is given by considering the difference between

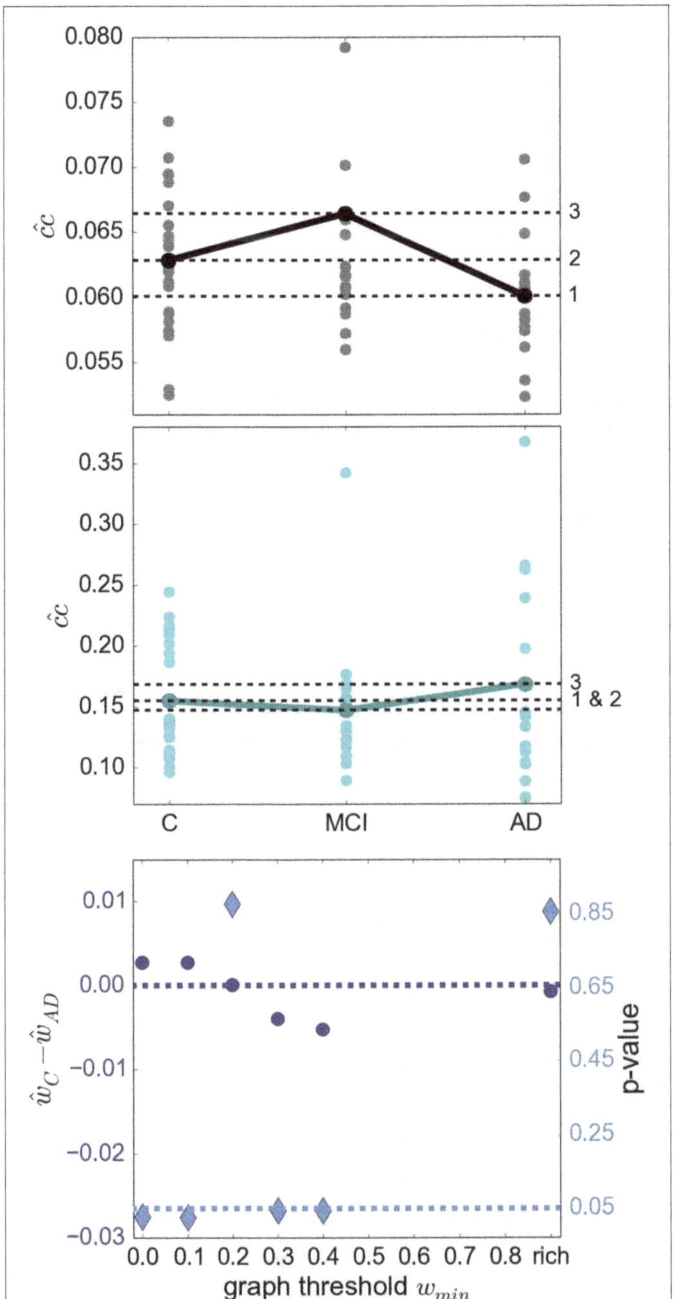

FIGURE 4 | Relationship of sub-graph properties across heath conditions is dependent on graph size. **(Upper Panel)** Average closeness centrality $\hat{cc}$ across graph nodes for complete graphs constructed with atlas *BMITU1* for the different health conditions C (left), MCI (middle) and AD (right). Each dot corresponds to the graph of an individual (connected dots indicate the mean values). **(Middle Panel)** As in top panel, but on the basis of the rich club graphs. **(Lower Panel)** Difference of the averaged ward1 *BMTID2* graph weights of the control group $\hat{w}_C$ and the AD group $\hat{w}_{AD}$ (left vertical axis, blue discs) and significance of this difference (right vertical axis, turquoise diamonds) as functions of the graph thresholding value w_{min}. All $\hat{w}$ are positive and are only calculated as long as graphs are connected (which is the case for $w_{min} < 0.5$). Average is taken across the weights of individual graphs. The dashed dark blue line indicates $\hat{w}_C - \hat{w}_{AD} = 0$; the dashed turquoise line indicates a significance level of 0.05.

the mean weights in the control and the AD conditions, and its significance (section 5.7.1), in dependence on the thresholding weight used to convert weighted graphs into simple graphs. This is illustrated in the bottom panel of **Figure 4**. Here, depending on where we set the threshold for considering an edge to be relevant, results having a significance level of $p < 0.05$ can be observed for both $\hat{w}_C > \hat{w}_{AD}$ ($w_{min} \in \{0.0, 0.1\}$) and $\hat{w}_C < \hat{w}_{AD}$ ($w_{min} \in \{0.3, 0.4\}$).

Extending this analysis, we find that contradictory significant results can be obtained for a variety of graph metrics across (and sometimes within) clustering methods. **Figure 5** shows the percentage of significant results obtained for health condition relationships in average edge weight, weighted degree, shortest path and clustering coefficient. Most strikingly, for most examined relationships, if significant differences are found at all, they are found in both directions, e.g., both for $\hat{d}_C > \hat{d}_{MCI}$ and for $\hat{d}_C < \hat{d}_{MCI}$ (weighted degree). Often a clustering algorithm favors a particular comparison direction, e.g., for the clustering coefficient, RGS clustering yields $\hat{clc}_{MCI} > \hat{clc}_{AD}$ whereas Ward and atlas clustering yields $\hat{clc}_{MCI} < \hat{clc}_{AD}$. However, we also find cases where significant differences are found in both directions with approximately equal frequency, such as $\hat{sp}_C > \hat{sp}_{AD}$ and $\hat{sp}_C < \hat{sp}_{AD}$ for Ward clustering. In addition, we find some clustering algorithms show a systematic behavior across metrics, e.g., for RGS $\hat{x}_C > \hat{x}_{MCI}$ with $x \in \{w, d, sp, clc\}$.

The largest number of significant differences is found for the comparison of controls with MCI, followed by the comparison of controls with AD. Only few significant differences of the means are found for AD and MCI. This relation among the groups is in line with the observed differences in heterogeneity observed for Ward and atlas clustering, for which MCI showed much lower heterogeneity and AD slightly lower values compared to controls (bottom panel of **Figure 2**).

Focusing on the clustering methods that bring about the most significant differences comparing the entire graph properties distributions results, we find the highest fraction for RGS, followed by Ward clustering. Atlas-based clustering yields only a few significant results. **Figure 6** shows the breakdown of the proportion of significant results for each clustering method on the edge definition technique (shown in collated form in **Figure 4**). Notably, transfer entropy (*TE*) only rarely produces significant differences. All other edge definition methods show a similar fraction of significant comparisons. The highest number of significant comparisons across the different graph properties is generated by RGS clustering combined with *MIT*.

To what extent a greater proportion of significant relationships is likely to make this graph construction method a good basis for a diagnostic tool depends on two aspects. First, the significance test is performed only on mean values, but ideally the overall distributions should overlap as little as possible. Second, the correlation between graph properties should be small in order to avoid redundant information.

In this section we considered only the first moments (means) of the graph properties taken from an individual brain. However,

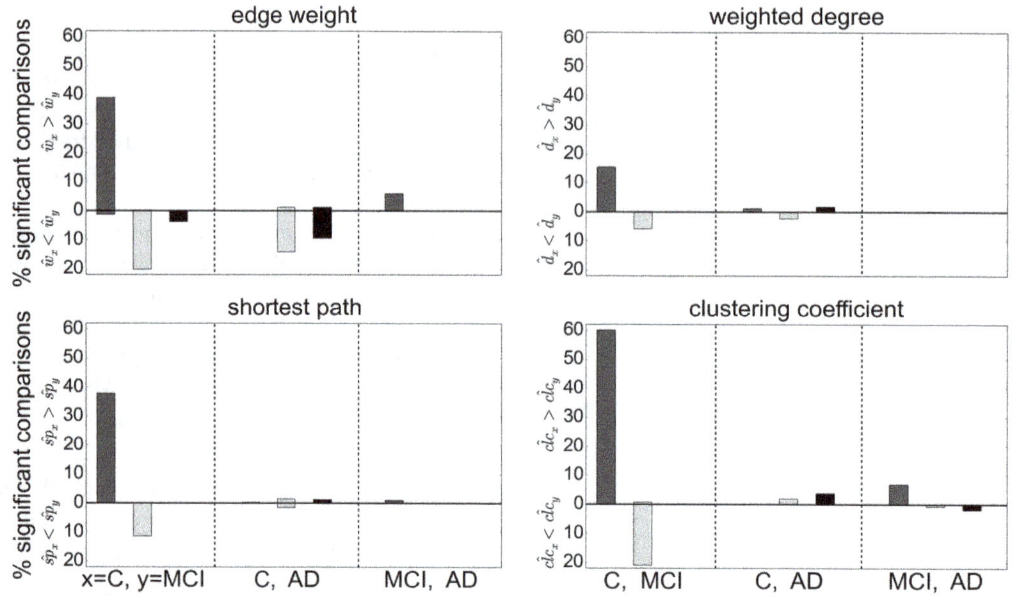

FIGURE 5 | Significant relationships in graph metrics between health conditions dependent on clustering methods. Percentage of significant differences for each clustering method RGS (dark gray), Ward (light gray), and atlas (black) for different averaged graph properties: edge weight **(Upper Left)**, weighted degree **(Upper Right)**, shortest path **(Lower Left)** and clustering coefficient **(Lower Right)**. Fraction of significant differences are calculated for each health condition over all graphs constructed with the corresponding clustering including all variants in parameters, edge definition techniques, thresholds and rich club sub-graphs. The abscissa labels show which pairs of health conditions are compared (C-MCI, C-AD, MCI-AD) and the ordinate labels the direction of the significant differences ("<," ">"). Significance is calculated as in the lower panel of **Figure 4**.

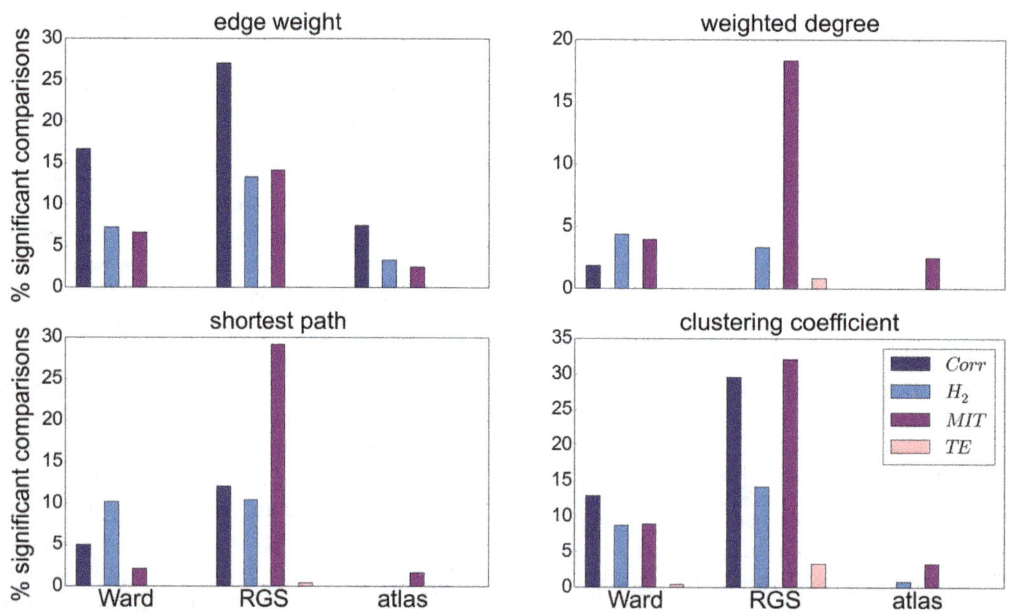

FIGURE 6 | Significant relationships in graph metrics between heath conditions dependent on edge definition methods. Percentage of significant differences for each clustering technique [Ward (left), RGS (middle), atlas (right)] for each class of edge definition method clustering method [*corr* (dark blue) , H_2 (light blue), *MIT* (purple), *TE* (pink)] for averaged graph properties: edge weight **(Upper Left)**, weighted degree **(Upper Right)**, shortest path **(Lower Left)** and clustering coefficient **(Lower Right)**. Fraction of significant differences are calculated for each health condition over all graphs constructed with the corresponding clustering and edge techniques including all variants in parameters, thresholds and rich-club sub-graphs. Significance is calculated as in the lower panel of **Figure 4**.

as explained in section 5.5, we use the first four moments of the individual distributions for our statistical analysis. Since the p-value of the other moments is not calculated, its influence on the statistical analysis cannot be considered.

In order to evaluate the methods based on robustness due to methodical variation, we investigate how the order of subjects (all subjects independent of their health conditions are ordered according to their average value of a certain graph property) is affected by the exact realization of the graph construction methods. Graphs constructed by methods based on similar underlying features of the data will tend to show a systematic ordering of subjects, regardless of the absolute values of the calculated graph metrics. **Figure 7** shows the commonalities and differences, which are illustrated with a dendrogram (see section 5.7.2) calculated on the Euclidean distance between the resulting ordered arrays of average graph weights. The continuous pink area show that graphs constructed using transfer entropy are most robust to the choice of clustering technique. Moreover, linear and non-linear correlations (dark and light blue) occupy contiguous blocks and so are most similar to each other. The leaves denoting atlas clustering (black) are rather spread out, indicating a high sensitivity of this method to the choice of edge definition.

In this section we have shown that the relationship of graph properties between health conditions strongly depends on the methods used for graph construction. For our data we find more significant mean differences for control-AD and control-MCI then for MCI-AD. With respect to clustering and edge definition methods, the largest number of significant differences are found for RGS and Ward clustering, and for model-free edge definitions. These results show that conclusions on how graph properties change due to AD have to be drawn carefully, and ideally validated by other methods, as they can be highly sensitive to the methods used for graph construction.

2.3. Evaluation of Graph Construction Methods Based on Negative Surprise

Having examined the consequences of particular choices for clustering and edge definition techniques in the previous sections, we now evaluate their combinations by considering their ability to help a clinician to discriminate among patient groups. This discrimination is achieved by using the graph data within a statistical model, which specifies the likelihood of the graph data. The model is described in section 5.6; the likelihood is a distribution which depends on a set of parameters. In general, the kind of graph data—i.e., their construction method—and the statistical model with its parameters are interdependent: they cannot be freely varied separately. Therefore our evaluations of the predictive power of the various graph construction methods have to be understood with a caveat: they depend on our specific choice of statistical model.

To quantify the discriminating power for each graph construction combination, we use a metric based on the final probabilities for the correct health conditions known as the log-probability, or *negative surprise* (Bartlett, 1952; Good, 1956, 1957a,b, 1983): a sure event, i.e., with unit probability, has surprise equal to zero; whereas an impossible event, i.e., with zero probability, has surprise equal to infinity, reflecting the fact that its occurrence would be contrary to all our expectations. A high surprise (in absolute value) therefore signals a low predictive power of the data we are using. The expectation or average of the surprises is the Shannon entropy (Shannon, 1948; Bartlett, 1952; McCarthy, 1956; Bernardo, 1979; Jaynes, 2003: section 11.3).

Another possibility, of a more decision-theoretical character, is to consider a metric based on the average utilities obtained with each particular graph-construction method. Given several possible courses of action (e.g., treat or dismiss) and their utilities or costs with respect to each health condition (e.g., treating an Alzheimer patient, dismissing a healthy patient, dismissing an Alzheimer patient, or treating a healthy one), the clinician

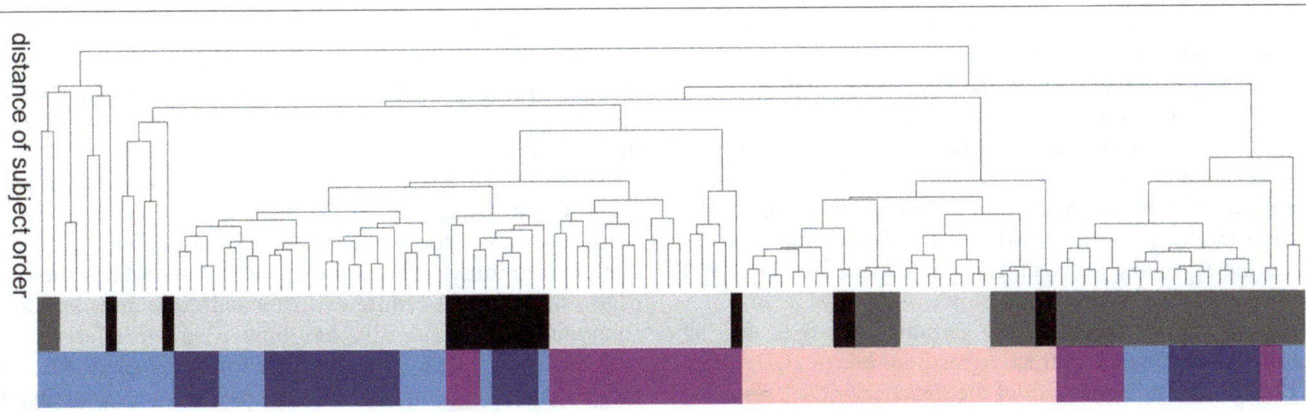

FIGURE 7 | Sensitivity of subject order to clustering and edge detection techniques. The dendrogram shows the distance of subject order, calculated by ordering all subjects according to their average graph edge weights and calculating the Euclidean distance between the resulting rank arrays. For better legibility, instead of naming the dendritic leaves, of which every leaf corresponds to a particular combination of clustering and edge definition techniques, e.g., ward2 *BTED2*, the top row of colors code for the class of clustering method: Ward (light gray), RGS (dark gray) and atlas (black); and the bottom row codes for the class of edge definition method: *corr* (dark blue), H_2 (light blue), *MIT* (purple) and *TE* (pink).

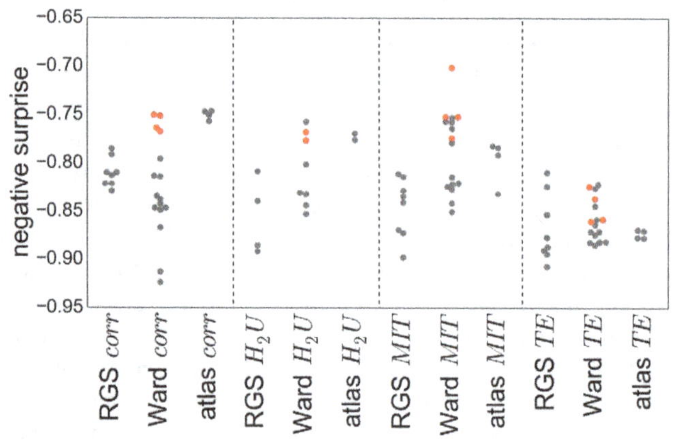

FIGURE 8 | Negative surprise of the different graph construction methods. Each dot represents a specific node clustering (e.g., RGS1) and edge definition (e.g., *BcorrU*1). Dots are grouped together according to their main class (e.g., RGS *corr*). Red dots highlight the results of ward4 clustering. Negative surprise expected by chance is −1.1.

should choose the action that maximizes the expected utility, the expectation being calculated from the final probabilities for the possible health conditions (Sox et al., 2013). This kind of metric therefore requires not only the final probabilities—which depend on the graph-construction method—but also a table of utilities.

Numerical tests show that the two kinds of metric yield similar results, at least for utility tables close to the identity (treating an ill patient and dismissing a healthy one have unit utility; the remaining combinations have zero utility). We therefore choose a metric based on the negative surprise, which is simpler and more intuitive than a utility metric.

In order to have an approximate idea of the relative predictive powers of the graph-construction methods we would like to use a statistical method that can be kept the same, as much as possible, across different methods. For this reason we choose a model based on the working hypothesis of sufficiency of mean and correlations of past data, as explained in the Introduction. This model ignores any restricted range of variability of graph quantities (e.g., positive or bounded). As explained in Porta Mana et al. (2018), this choice is non-standard but does not entail contradictions. The model has some free parameters; their values reflect the fact that the units of measure for the graph quantities make the latter of order unity. This choice of a generic, common statistical model allows us to sidestep the demanding problem of tailoring it for the different graph quantities from our 850 graph-construction methods.

Figure 8 shows the obtained negative surprises for all combinations of graph construction methods except H_2D, which is left out due to an inadequacy of the statistical model, resulting in unrealistic values between −1.26 and −0.66 with a mean and standard deviation of -0.94 ± 0.19.

The differences in negative surprise between the different graph construction method are in general small. The best results are obtained for ward4 clustering combined with mutual information (*MIT*) based edge definition. Across edge definition methods, linear correlation (*corr*) and mutual information give the best results and transfer entropy (*TE*) the worst. The rather poor performance of *TE* edge definition is in line with the small number of significant differences found for this method (compare **Figure 6**). Comparing the different clustering methods, atlas and ward4 clustering give the best results, as long as the edge definition is not *TE*. These two clustering methods have in common a very small number of graph nodes and (correspondingly) the highest number of voxels per cluster (compare **Figure 2**).

As explained above, the comparison of graph-construction methods can be affected by the statistical model and its parameters, especially for small datasets. As a complementary analysis we compare the negative surprises with the classification performances of a support vector machine (SVM, section 5.7.1) based on the same graph constructions. In a clinical setting, a misclassification between control and AD has more severe consequences than between MCI and AD. To avoid introducing an asymmetric misclassification penalty, we perform the classification between pairs of classes only (control-AD, C-MCI, MCI-AD).

Figure 9 shows the relationship between the SVM performance (measured as proportion of correct classifications) against the negative surprise. As long as *TE* edge definition is excluded, the two performance measures are positively correlated. In particular RGS clustering achieves low performance in both negative surprise and SVM classification. Furthermore, atlas clustering achieves a high classification performance across all edge definitions. The exact SVM classification results for each realization of graph construction method are depicted in **Figure S2** (see Supplemental Material).

Figure 10 demonstrates that thresholding graphs has only a minor effect on the negative surprise for small thresholds up to 0.2. No systematic relationship can be observed for the effect of larger thresholds; for example, increasing the threshold to 0.4 causes a decrease in negative surprise for RGS clustering with linear correlations or mutual information, but an increase for atlas clustering with transfer entropy edge detection. Likewise, the creation of highly connected and rich club sub-graphs typically decreases the negative surprise, but in some cases increases it (e.g., RGS H_2U). Overall the highest negative surprise (−0.66) is obtained for ward4 clustering combined with *BMITU*1 thresholded at $w_{\min} = 0.1$.

These results suggest that the best combination of graph construction techniques to use for this data set is the atlas-based or ward4 clustering combined with linear correlation methods or mutual information transfer. Thresholding the graph edges, which might reduce experimental noise and does lower computational complexity, has only a minor effect on the predictive power, as long as threshold values are small. Reducing the graphs complexity via larger thresholds or extracting the rich-club of the graph should be done with care, since the results can change in either direction. Although transfer entropy yields lower negative surprises then the model-free functional connectivity measures, we would not conclude that this edge definition performs worse in general, since it achieves high values in SVM classification. It is very likely that our choice of statistical

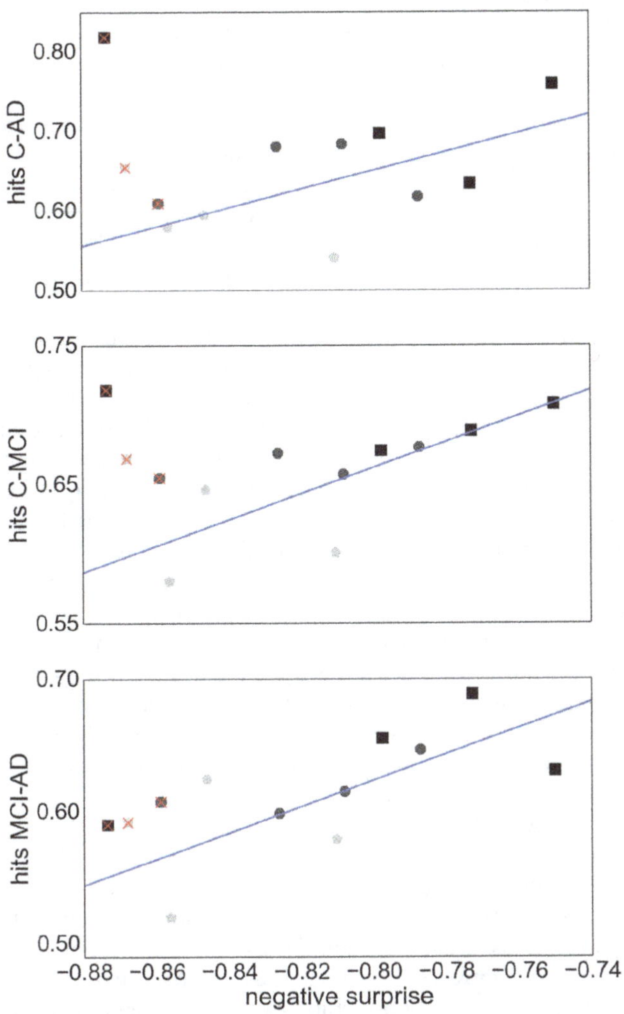

FIGURE 9 | Relationship between SVM classification performance and negative surprise. The average SVM performance achieved by each combination of clustering method and edge definition with respect to each pair of health conditions: control-AD **(Upper Panel)**, control -MCI **(Middle Panel)**, and MCI-AD **(Lower Panel)**, is plotted against the negative surprise calculated for all health conditions. Each marker corresponds to the averaged performance across the parameter space of a specific clustering method [atlas (black squares), Ward (dark gray octagons), RGS (light gray pentagons)] and a specific edge defintion (*corr*, H_2, *MIT*, *TE*). The regression line is calculated for all points but *TE* (superimposed red crosses). Pearson correlation coefficients r of the datasets are $r = 0.59$ **(Upper Panel)**, $r = 0.77$ **(Middle Panel)**, $r = 0.69$ **(Lower Panel)**.

model is not ideal, and a more tailored choice would improve performance.

3. DISCUSSION

In this article we have compared different techniques for constructing and analyzing graphs. By applying a statistical model, we have demonstrated a principled method for choosing a combination of techniques for a given data set. By examining the varied outcomes of the techniques, we have shown how sensitive the results of graph theoretical analyses, such as significant differences in mean properties, can be to the choice of clustering or edge definition technique.

With regards to the predictive power of the graph construction techniques, measured in terms of negative surprise, we find that Ward and atlas clustering yield the highest performance of the clustering techniques, and region growing and selection clustering (RGS) the lowest. In particular, the variant of Ward clustering that produces large clusters and small numbers of nodes (ward4) achieved the highest performance values. Analogously for the edge detection methods, we find better performance for the model-free methods (linear and non-linear correlations, mutual information transfer) than for the model-based method of transfer entropy. For this particular data set, a combination of ward4 clustering with mutual information derived edges achieves best results. Therefore, we would recommend this combination as the primary target for a more narrowly focussed investigation based on a larger data set.

The performances we obtain are above chance level but still far away from optimal prediction of the three health conditions. One reason for this sub-optimal prediction might lie in our choice of statistical model and its parameters. With our small data set (26 controls, 16 MCI, 14 AD) the model and its parameters have a high influence on the final probabilities, and thus on the performance (Porta Mana et al., 2018). We avoided tailoring the statistical model for the theoretic and practical reasons explained in section 2.3. Even if the model is not tailored, the results are consistent with the classification performance of support vector machines (see **Figure 9** and **Figure S2**), for the model-free edge definition techniques.

It remains unclear why Ward and atlas clustering are more successful than RGS, especially in combination with model-free edge definition. One possibility is that this is related to the large variability in graph sizes generated by RGS (**Figure 2**). In addition, the variance of weight distributions across subjects, and the variance of the cluster distances, are much larger in RGS then in Ward clustering (**Figure 3**). This could be related to the variance in the number of nodes; however, choosing graphs similar in size causes even higher variances (section 2.1). Therefore we assume that the number and connectivity of the small functional units extracted by RGS are highly variable across subjects. This variance might be even higher across subjects within a health condition than across health conditions, such that changes due to AD cannot be detected. This assumption might at first glance seem to contradict the high number of significant comparisons observed (**Figure 5**). However, we only calculate the significance level for the means of the distributions and not their entire shape. In addition, it is likely that some graph properties correlate with the graph size, and thus that apparent significant differences in graph properties are simply reflecting significant differences in numbers of nodes detected, and do not provide further information useful for classification or understanding the nature of the disease. Further investigation is needed on this matter.

The low negative surprise of transfer entropy (*TE*) compared with other model-free functional connectivity measures might

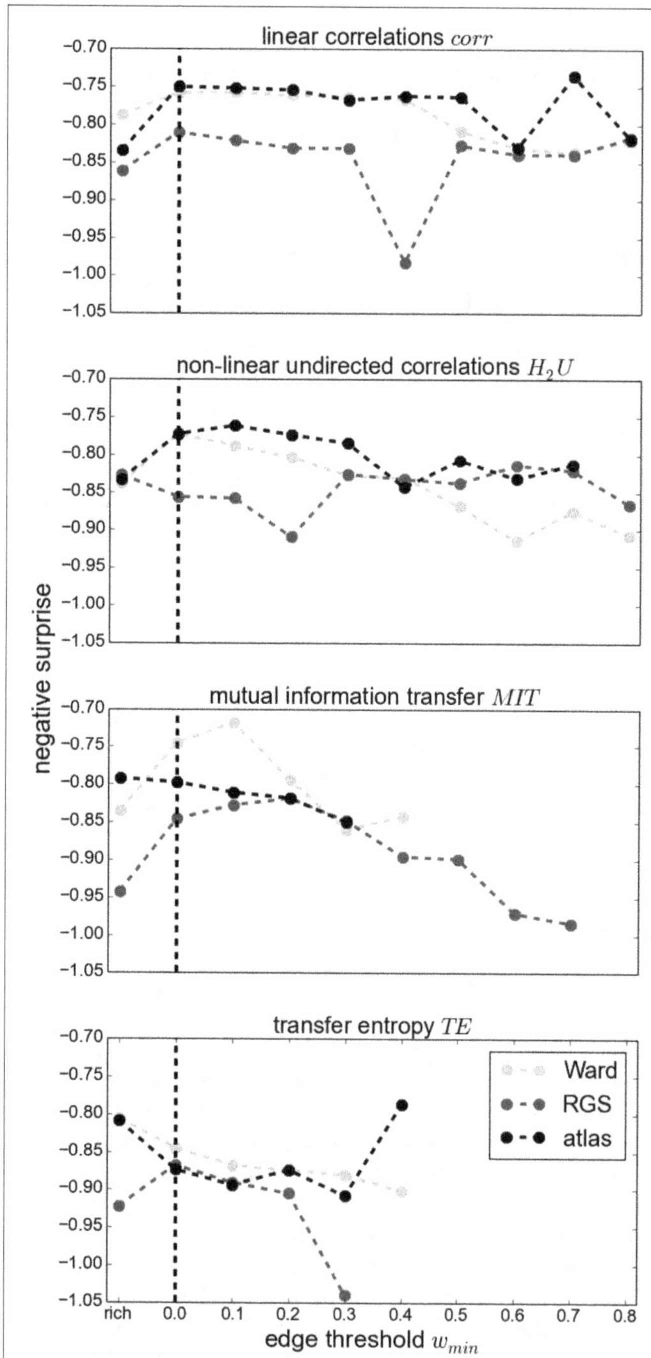

FIGURE 10 | Negative surprise for different graph edge thresholds w_{min} ($w_{min} = 0$ for complete graphs, indicated by a vertical dashed line) and rich club graphs (rich) for different edge definitions: *corr* **(First Panel)**, H_2U **(Second Panel)**, *MIT* **(Third Panel)**, *TE* **(Fourth Panel)** and different clustering methods Ward (light gray), RGS (dark gray) and atlas (black). Each dot is the result of averaging across all possible parameters of a general graph construction method (for $w_{min} = 0$ the average across all points of a swarm in **Figure 8**). Since some methods yield small edge weights, some graphs become unconnected for large w_{min} such that the statistical analysis is not conducted; no values are depicted in this case. Markers are connected for better visual comprehension.

have several reasons. The comparison of the negative surprise with the support vector machine classification suggests that a better choice of a statistical model is possible: the classification results for *TE* are similar to those of the model-free measures. In *TE* the data of a certain time interval in the past is used in order to calculate how much the uncertainty of the future is reduced. Here we use the data of the last 15 s. This time period might be poorly chosen, influencing the overall negative surprise. In addition *TE* is more sensitive to short recording periods than other methods, which may well also result in a reduced performance (Pereda et al., 2005).

With regards to the robustness of the graph theoretical outcomes, we discovered that relationships between mean graph properties, such as closeness centrality, edge weight or clustering coefficient (**Figures 4–6**) were sensitive to choice of clustering and edge definition techniques, to parameter choices for a given technique, and to the manner in which sub-graphs were defined (thresholding value and rich club). For most relationships between graph properties X, we could find significant ($p < 0.05$) differences in both directions, i.e., both $X_{AD} > X_C$ and $X_{AD} < X_C$, for specific choices of clustering and edge definition technique. This strongly suggests that a degree of suspicion should be applied to studies reporting such significant differences, especially if these results are argued to give insight into how a disease affects brain properties, unless the significance level is much more compelling or the reported differences can be validated with alternate methods.

We also investigated the sensitivity to method choice of the ordering of subjects according to a graph theoretic metric (**Figure 7**). In this analysis, transfer entropy was the most consistent. Nevertheless, the distributions of the negative surprises is as broad for transfer entropy as for other edge definitions (**Figure 8**). In general, the exact parameter selection within an edge definition method causes only slight changes in the negative surprise, more crucial is the exact realization of the clustering method: ward4 clustering generally achieves a better performance then ward3 clustering. These two variants differ only in the number of predefined clusters (see Supplemental Material **Figure S1**). Applying a lower threshold w_{min} on the graph's edge weights has little effect on the negative surprise for all methods, as long as only small weights (up to 0.2) are set to zero. Thresholding higher weights or extracting the graph's rich club has unpredictable effects on the results, and so should be used with caution (**Figure 10**). Atlas clustering was least consistent in the subject ordering analysis, suggesting that although it may provide a good basis for a diagnostic tool, care should be taken in reporting discoveries of particular relationships in graph properties between health conditions, as these may well turn out to be critically dependent on the edge definition method used.

Due to the intense computational requirements of the survey performed in this article, we recognize that it would be advantageous to develop heuristics for choosing between graph construction methods without performing the full calculation for each combination. Our results suggest that properties visible at the clustering stage, such as average heterogeneity, may give some indication of predictive performance: graph constructions that result in different degrees of heterogeneity between the health conditions seem to be more discriminable by the later steps of the calculation. More research is needed in this area, which is outside the scope of the current study. In addition, it is tempting to consider t-test results of the mean graph properties as a heuristic. Our results suggest that this approach is largely inadequate. It holds for edge definition via transfer entropy, which gives very few significant results and the negative surprise is rather small compared with the model-free edge definitions. Conversely, region growing clustering yields most significant differences but a generally poor negative surprise. This may be due to graph properties being highly correlated, and so not providing additional information to the statistical model. In addition we used the first four moments (wherever possible) in our statistical model, rather than just the mean, which may also partially account for this apparent contradiction.

In addition to considering the predictive power and robustness of graph construction techniques, we can also evaluate them according to their practicality, i.e., speed of calculation and the extent to which they are easily available in established medical infrastructure and diagnostics. In general, applying graph theoretic measures to fMRI data for improving AD diagnosis makes sense, since MRI scans are already implemented in AD diagnostics for detecting structural changes such as hippocampal dystrophy caused by AD or AD-unrelated pathology (e.g., brain tumors). Softwares such as SPM (Tzourio-Mazoyer et al., 2002) and FSL (Jenkinson et al., 2012) are frequently used in medical research and mainly support clustering that is atlas and independent component analysis based. Ward clustering, which is the fastest of all these clustering methods, is a standard hierarchical clustering method and implemented in all standard programming softwares such as Python and Matlab. The region growing algorithm is not implemented in established softwares and is also computational very demanding. Given that it does not out-perform atlas or Ward clustering, we therefore do not recommend it. For edge definition and graph properties, several software packages are available based on Matlab (Wang et al., 2014; Kruschwitz et al., 2015) or Python[1], which provide a comprehensive range of edge definition and graph analysis methods.

In general we recommend using statistical models and not pure classifiers such as support vector machines as diagnostic tools, since statistical models calculate a probability of a diagnosis rather than assign a classification, i.e., "Given the fMRI scan, person x has a 80% probability of having Alzheimer's disease," rather than "Given the fMRI scan, person x has Alzheimer's disease." Probabilities can be easily combined with other probabilities of other diagnostic tests (Porta Mana et al., 2018) such as cognitive assessment, amyloid beta and tau protein occurrence in cerebrospinal fluid, blood tests, and structural MRI[2] (Johnson et al., 2012). This allows the medical doctor to conclude, for example: "Given the results of the cognitive test *and* cerebrospinal fluid analysis *and* structural and functional MRI scan, person x has a 95% probability of having Alzheimer's disease." After the estimation of the probability for a disease, she has to decide on a treatment, also taking into consideration such factors as "how harmful would the treatment be for a healthy person," which can be expressed in a utility function (Porta Mana et al., 2018). In addition, the statistical model used in this work allows an estimation of how much the model can be trusted, and therefore evaluate whether the sample size is sufficiently large (Porta Mana et al., 2018).

3.1. Relationship to Previous Studies

Studies focusing on the graph properties extracted from resting-state fMRI in AD and its pre-stages generally have one of two aims. The first aim is to identify significant differences in the graph properties between health conditions, and to use these to gain insight into the effects of AD on the physical brain and its cognitive processes. These studies complement the picture revealed by investigations based on structural MRI and functional changes on the basis of EEG and MEG recordings. Typically a variety of graph properties (e.g., nodal degree, clustering coefficient, averaged shortest path, local efficiency, betweenness centrality, global efficiency, small worldness) are calculated, and used to motivate an account of how disease-related modifications to these properties result in a reduced capacity to transfer and process information.

However, such studies reveal entirely contradictory results. For example, the value of the clustering coefficient in AD with respect to controls has been reported to be increased, unchanged, and decreased, respectively (Supekar et al., 2008; Sanz-Arigita et al., 2010; Zhao et al., 2012). Analogous contradictions have been found for the comparative length of the shortest path (Supekar et al., 2008; Sanz-Arigita et al., 2010; Zhao et al., 2012). These contradictions could be caused by methodological differences or by not separating the different states of AD. Our results show ample evidence that the precise choice of graph construction techniques can easily account for contradictory findings, even for atlas based clustering, in which the number and size of clusters is held constant across all subjects (**Figure 5**). Evidence that the separation of different AD stages is relevant was provided by Kim et al. (2015), who demonstrated a non-monotonic behavior of global efficiency, local efficiency and betweenness centrality across different stages of AD and MCI. In our study, we could reproduce the pattern of increase and decrease of closeness centrality across conditions (**Figure 4**). However, we also demonstrate that the same analysis based on the rich club sub-graph yields a different pattern, and that contradictory (but significant) results can be obtained for the same graph construction techniques with different choices of threshold. We thus conclude that differences in graph properties between health conditions are currently ill-suited to provide an account of disease mechanisms in AD, unless either: (1) a specific method of graph construction can be shown to be more representative of the underlying connectivity than other methods, (2) the differences can be shown to be robust to choice of graph construction, (3) the differences can be validated by another analytical approach, or (4) the significance level is shown to be substantially more persuasive than $p < 0.05$.

[1]https://github.com/dpisner453/PyNets.

[2]https://www.alz.org/research/diagnostic_criteria/.

The second category of studies use graph theoretical information as input for machine learning algorithms to classify the health conditions of the subjects. Note that for this purpose it is irrelevant if a difference between health conditions is not robust to method choice, as the goal is not to understand the effects of the disease but to robustly distinguish between conditions. Recent studies have reached very high performance: 100% accuracy in discriminating AD and control (Khazaee et al., 2015), and 93% for AD, MCI and control classification (Khazaee et al., 2017). In the latter work they extract more than two dozen local and global graph properties, resulting in roughly 3,000 features, since each of the local properties is calculated for all brain areas. Only a small subset of features is then used for classification, e.g., in-degree of the left middle temporal gyrus. They found that the classification power of local graph measures is larger than that of the global ones. Local changes in graph properties that do not propagate to global mean values have also been reported for area specific (frontal cortices, parietal and occipital regions) synchronization levels (Sanz-Arigita et al., 2010).

In this work we do not compare node-specific graph properties, because Ward and RGS clustering do not result in the same spatial location of clusters across subjects. Instead, we consider, wherever possible, the first four moments of the entire distributions of graph properties. This is more information than typically used for global measures, where often only the first moment (the mean) of a graph property distribution is taken into consideration. Nevertheless, it is still possible that considering single nodes, of which some may be more damaged by AD than others, could yield a better diagnostic performance. This requires further study in a survey considering only atlas based clustering. Again, this is out of scope of the current study, but we remark that the statistical model methodology we employ here would be equally applicable to such an investigation. The advantage of taking the entire distribution lies in the possibility of using purely data driven clustering algorithms (e.g., Ward clustering) that can be substantially faster than atlas based clustering, since they do not depend on a time and memory consuming registration of the individual brain image to standard space. In addition, the global distribution is more likely to be more robust against brain morphologic abnormalities such as brain tumors or brain shrinkage, and is more stable across recording sessions (Telesford et al., 2010; Wang et al., 2014). Finally, a short recording time might be expected to have a weaker influence on entire graph property distributions then on single nodes. Thus we conclude that global measures are preferable, if a good diagnostic performance can be reached. Although the goal of this work was not classification, we note that we obtain up to (80–90%) correct classification using an off-the-shelf support vector machine on leave-one-out subsets of our data for pairwise (C-AD, C-MCI, AD-MCI) comparisons. Whether global measures can reach the impressive performance shown by Khazaee et al. (2017) can only be investigated on a sufficiently large data set, ideally with several hundred participants.

3.2. Limitations of This Study

In each step of the graph construction and analysis pipeline (**Figure 1**) we set limits to the endless space of possible methods and their corresponding parameters. Here we will shortly summarize the reasons motivating the selection of the methods examined here and the exclusion of others, given the constraint of limited computational and temporal resources. As a general principle, we aimed to include the most commonly used method(s) and additional methods that we found to be reasonable, even if they are not currently frequently used.

Starting with the fMRI pre-processing, we had to decide whether to include global signal regression. The global signal (the average activity across all brain voxels) is assumed to originate partly from vascular and respiratory processes that do not represent neuronal activity. However, there is also evidence that it contains neuronal-signaling based components, since it is negatively correlated with the EEG signal and strongly correlated with the activity of the largest network in the brain (the default mode network, which plays a major role in rest state activity) when noise levels are low (Murphy and Fox, 2017). Without global signal regression, the Pearson correlation distribution derived from the signal of all voxels, or the average activity of clustered voxels, is biased to the right such that negative values are rare and small. The correction for the global signal centers this distribution, such that negative values are much more prominent. This also changes the properties of the graphs extracted from such data, for example an increase in modularity combined with fewer unconnected nodes has been reported (Schwarz and McGonigle, 2011; Hayasaka, 2013).

Speaking against global signal regression is the finding that correction for white matter, CSF and motions yield the most stable graph properties across sessions compared with additional applied global regression (Schwarz and McGonigle, 2011). In diagnostics it is important to have only small variance in the outcome across different sessions if the health condition of a subject is stable, such that small changes that indicate a worsening of the health condition can be rapidly detected. Moreover, we define the edges of our graphs as the absolute values of the functional connectivity values. As the negative part of the correlation distribution is small without global regression, different possible treatment of negative correlations (taking the absolute values or setting them to zero) should have only a small influence on the resulting graph properties, at least when the underlying functional connectivity are based on correlations. Consequently, we elect not to include global signal regression in our pipeline.

In the clustering step, the most commonly used method is to define clusters based on cortical regions defined by a brain atlas. We supplemented this with two data-driven clustering approaches: Ward clustering and RGS clustering. We selected Ward clustering, as it has been shown to perform better than alternative hierarchical clustering methods with respect to reproducibility and accuracy (Thirion et al., 2014). RGS, a method derived from image processing (Lu et al., 2003), was selected because we could adjust the method to produce functionally homogeneous clusters. In this formulation, the only free parameter of the algorithm is the minimal cluster size.

For both data-driven methods, we selected parameters such that graphs did not exceed a maximal size of 1,500 nodes, due to computational limitations. We excluded clustering based on independent component analysis, because of its laborious implementation and the requirement for domain expertise to distinguish noise from activity-related components. We also excluded all clustering algorithms that do not take functional consistency into account, e.g., dividing the voxels into cuboid patches, as has been proposed for structural data (Amoroso et al., 2017).

With regards to methods for edge definition, we limit our survey to functional connectivity measures that act in the time domain and not in the frequency domain, thus omitting frequency based wavelet analysis (Supekar et al., 2008), synchronization likelihood (Sanz-Arigita et al., 2010) and coherence (Wang et al., 2014). The most commonly used and simplest functional connectivity measure is the Pearson correlation coefficient (e.g., Zhao et al., 2012), which we name *BCorrU* in our work. We also test two additional model-free and one model-based method. A further model-based method based on Granger causality was excluded because it is too computationally expensive for larger graphs (Wang et al., 2014).

A thresholding operation is often applied to graphs extracted from fMRI, setting all values below $w_{\min}$ to zero. The aim of this step is to reduce experimental noise, which mainly manifests in the weaker edges, and to make the computation of graph properties computationally less demanding (Bordier et al., 2017). The threshold $w_{\min}$ can be defined in several ways: it can be set arbitrarily, without satisfying a certain demand, or such that certain properties of the graphs are preserved, e.g., average number of edges per vertex (Sanz-Arigita et al., 2010), node density (Zhao et al., 2012), small world behavior (Bassett et al., 2008) or a fixed cluster coefficient. Alternatively, it can be set such that information on the network's community structure is maximized; see, e.g., Bordier et al. (2017). In a variant of the thresholding approach, it has been proposed to transform the edge weights by applying a power law (Schwarz and McGonigle, 2011). In this study, for the sake of simplicity, we examine graph properties as a function of $w_{\min}$ without targeting any specific value of a graph property. Potentially, our results would reveal a different picture if $w_{\min}$ was optimized for each subject to attain, for example, a specific average nodal degree. However, comparison of these two different thresholding mechanisms resulted in no major difference in the relationships of graph properties between the control and AD groups (Sanz-Arigita et al., 2010).

We do not binarize our graphs (setting all values below $w_{\min}$ to zero and those above it to one) as is frequently done (e.g., Zhao et al., 2012), as this leads to a loss of information, and moreover some distributions of graph properties would become discrete (e.g., only ones and zeros for edge weights distributions), such that higher moments would be uninformative. The disadvantage of using weighted graphs lies in the limitation of possible graph properties. Most graph properties are well-defined for binary graphs and have been partly extended to weighted graphs. Here, we calculate the (normalized) weighted degree, shortest path, closeness centrality, clustering coefficient, and the modularity. We only investigate the most commonly used metrics and do not include more complex methods such as the minimal spanning tree (Çiftçi, 2011).

In addition to the restrictions of scope with regards to the examined techniques, a clear limitation of this study is the small data set. As our aim here is primarily to provide a methodology for evaluating and comparing analysis methods, rather than to draw conclusions on the effect of Alzheimer's disease on the graph properties of the cortex, a small data set is less problematic. Indeed, for the explorative survey carried out here, a large data set would have been prohibitively expensive with respect to computational resources. Moreover, many studies applying graph analysis to fMRI data are based on similarly sized data sets, which highlights the importance of raising awareness about the methodological artifacts we have identified.

The results of our survey indicate which combinations of methods are promising in view of Alzheimer diagnosis and should be investigated further in future studies based on larger data sets. Naturally, such studies could yield some quantitatively different results to those reported here, particularly with regard to the classification performance. Nonetheless, we would like to summarize some conclusions of the work that are unlikely to change with a larger data set. First, our results show that different combinations of methods can lead to contradictory findings with regard to significant differences in mean properties (section 2.2). This effect is unlikely to be resolved by a larger sample size. Second, methods showing good robustness with respect to parameter choice for a small sample size (e.g., *TE* edge definition, see **Figure 7**), are likely to remain robust with increasing sample size. Likewise, there is no reason to assume that methods performing well in all circumstances for the small data set, e.g., Ward clustering combined with *corr* edge definition (section 2.3), would perform worse for larger data sets. Finally, we assert that thresholding the graphs of a large data set with a small $w_{\min}$ (as shown in section 2.3) would similarly not result in a sudden jump in negative surprise.

3.3. Application of Approach to Other Analysis Techniques

We have demonstrated a systematic, quantitative approach for comparing and evaluating sequences of algorithms that result in classification of fMRI data based on the first four moments of simple graph theoretic metrics defined on the whole graph. However, the approach we present is equally well suited for assessing pipelines based on other metrics, as we briefly outline in the following.

One possibility is to consider the graph properties of individual nodes, as these have been shown to be very informative (Xia et al., 2014; Khazaee et al., 2015; Wang et al., 2016; Dillen et al., 2017).

This entails the use of atlas based clustering. We speculate that a global analysis of graph properties would be both faster and more robust to brain abnormalities and short recording times, and so would be the preferable approach if equivalent performance levels can be attained.

A second possibility is to extend our approach to a hierarchical analysis. This could potentially be of great use, as previous studies based on PET imaging have suggested that in Alzheimer's disease, long range connections become weaker but local clustering increases (Pagani et al., 2016, 2017). These alterations would not be observable using the graph analyses so far considered, although we have taken the first step by calculating the modularity, which compares the ideal dissection of the given graph into modules with that of a random graph with similar edge weights.

To capture the graph meta-structures it is necessary to cluster graph nodes into modules, or sub-graphs. Modules can be defined either purely functionally, such that each node (ideally) has the strongest connections to the nodes in its own cluster, and the weakest connections to nodes of other clusters, or based on anatomic structures, such that nodes in a cluster are part of large, anatomo-functionally similar brain areas. Analogous to the variety of methods for spatial clustering and edge definition investigated in this study, there are many techniques used to cluster nodes into modules (e.g., k-clustering, hierarchical clustering and spectral clustering, for a review see Schaeffer, 2007 or anatomo-functional clustering, see Pagani et al., 2016), and likewise multiple options for analysing the characteristics of the resulting modular structure (e.g., module degree or participation coefficient; see Guimerá and Nunes Amaral, 2005). Such a comprehensive study is outside the scope of the current work, but could well provide great insight into health condition related alterations in the global network structure of the brain.

4. CONCLUSIONS

In order to achieve a robust and successful Alzheimer's disease diagnosis based on graphs extracted from fMRI data, we recommend clustering that results in rather small graphs with large clusters. Ward clustering, in which the number of clusters can be predefined, is fast, but requires programming knowledge to implement it. Atlas clustering is well established standard fMRI analysis software applications, but it is slow and might be affected by morphologic abnormalities in the brain, such as atrophy which is a common symptom of AD.

Edge weights should be calculated based on correlations or mutually information transfer, especially if a focus of the study is uncovering significant differences in mean graph properties between health conditions. We emphasize that the existence, magnitude *and direction* of such significant differences can be very sensitive to the methods chosen, and the parameterization of those methods, and so such findings should be reported with care, especially if a biological interpretation of said findings is claimed. Transfer entropy rarely gives significant results, but is more robust toward parameter changes in the algorithm and different clustering algorithms. Finding appropriate statistical models may be an additional challenge for this method.

Weak thresholding may be used for complexity reduction as it has little effect on performance. Applying a higher threshold or extracting the rich club sub-graph (The 10% of nodes with highest degree) causes unsystematic changes in the negative surprise and should therefore be used with caution, and validated against the full graph.

In summary, our quantitative evaluation and comparison of graph construction and analysis methods provides insight into how contradicting results come about in studies of graph properties of fMRI data, and identifies a number of potential methodological artifacts. Moreover, it provides a blueprint for establishing appropriate analysis pipelines, and serves as a well-founded starting point for future research on larger data sets.

5. METHODS

5.1. Data Acquisition

The recruitment and neuropsychological assessment of the study participants is given in Dillen et al. (2017). Demographic information is given in **Table 2**.

Anatomical MRI and resting state fMRI (rfMRI) images were obtained from a 3T MR-Brain-PET scanner (Siemens, Erlangen, Germany) in the Memory Clinic Cologne Juelich. The parameters for the single-shot echo planar imaging sequence of the functional (T2* weighted) image are the following: TR = 3,000 ms, TE = 30 ms, FA = 90°, FOV = 200 × 200 mm^2, matrix = 80 × 80, voxel resolution = 2.5 × 2.5 × 2.8, 50 oblique slices parallel to the infra-supratentorial line, gap = 0.28 mm, interleaved, scan time = 7 min. Parameters of the high-resolution T1-weighted structural image based on a magnetization-prepared rapid gradient echo sequence: TR = 2,250 ms, TE = 3.03 ms, FA = 9°, FOV = 256 × 256 mm^2, matrix = 256 × 256, voxel resolution = 1 mm isotropic, 176 sagittal slices, no gap, interleaved, scan time = 314 s. For more detail see Dillen et al. (2017).

5.2. Preprocessing of fMRI-Data and Extraction of Cortical Data

Image preprocessing is accomplished using FMRIB's Software Library tools (FSL; Woolrich et al., 2009; Jenkinson et al., 2012). We carry out the following steps for the structural T1-weighted image: skull-stripping (Smith, 2002) with bias field correction (Keihaninejad et al., 2010; Leung et al., 2011; Popescu et al., 2012) and for the functional T2-weighted image: discarding the first 10 volumes (out of 140 each taken after 3 sec), motion

TABLE 2 | Demographic information of participants.

	Controls	MCI	AD
Number	26	16	14
Age	62.38 [50, 73]	70 [55, 78]	71 [61, 78]
Sex	10 f, 16 m	7 f, 9 m	7 f, 7 m
Years of education	15.3 [8, 25]	12.75 [8, 21]	12.83 [7, 18]

Average and minimal and maximal values [min, max] are given for age and years of education; female (f), male (m).

correction (Beckmann and Smith, 2004), spatial smoothing using a 4 mm full width at half maximum Gaussian kernel, high-pass temporal filtering at 0.02 Hz and a six-parameter, rigid-body linear transformation procedure in MCFLIRT (Jenkinson et al., 2002). More details can be found in Dillen et al. (2017), where the same preprocessing is applied. In addition we carry out white matter and cerebrospinal fluid regression (FSL regfilt, MELODIC) to the functional image in order to reduce noise.

In order to extract only cortical voxels from the entire brain fMRI image, as needed for the data-driven clustering described in the next section, we first register cortical regions (frontal- , occipital-, temporal-, and insular-cortex) defined in the MNI structural atlas (Collins et al., 1995) to the structural and then to the functional space. For this registration we apply the transformation matrix obtained from registering the entire standard brain first to the individual structural brain (linear registration with FSL/FLIRT; Jenkinson and Smith, 2001; Jenkinson et al., 2002) and then to the functional space (non-linear registration with Advanced Normalization Tools, ANTs; Avants et al., 2011). In order to extract only gray matter tissue, we apply the gray matter image of the structural space (segmentation with FSL-FAST; Zhang et al., 2001) registered to functional space as described above, as a mask to the to the functional image.

5.3. Data-Driven and Atlas Based Clustering of Cortical Voxels

In order to construct graphs we cluster cortical voxels into regions using three different methods. Two of these methods, the Ward clustering and the region growing and selection algorithm (RGS) are data driven, such that only neighboring voxels with similar activity are combined into a single region. For these algorithms the number of regions per brain and the participating voxels in a region can differ for each individual and strongly depend on predefined algorithm-specific parameters. The atlas-based cluster algorithm, in contrast, produces the same number of clusters and a constant number of voxels per region across individuals, because the individual brains are mapped onto a standard brain.

5.3.1. Atlas-Based Clustering

For each subject we linearly register the rfMRI image first to the structural, skull-removed image (image segmentation for skull removing with SPM8, Wellcome Department of Cognitive Neurology, London, UKFSL; linear registration with FSL/FLIRT; Jenkinson and Smith, 2001; Jenkinson et al., 2002) and then, through a non-linear mapping, to the MNI standard brain [non-linear registration with Advanced Normalization Tools (ANTs; Avants et al., 2011); MNI 152 standard brain, non-linear 6th generation (Grabner et al., 2006)]. Regions of interest (ROIs) of the resulting functional image in standard space are extracted such that they match the 94 regions identified by the Oxford lateral cortical atlas (regions have a probability above 50%) (Desikan et al., 2006). A demonstration of how the brain is clustered according to the brain areas is given in the first panel of **Figure 12**.

TABLE 3 | Parameters used for the different clustering algorithms.

Method	Minimal number of voxels per cluster *p*	Number of clusters *k*	Threshold *T* of Pearson correlation coefficient
ward1	10	5,000	–
ward2	25	5,000	–
ward3	10	2,000	–
ward4	25	2,000	–
RGS1	55	–	0.75
RGS2	50	–	0.75
atlas	–	–	–

Ward clustering (ward), region growing and selection (RGS), atlas-based clustering (atlas).

5.3.2. Ward Clustering

Ward clustering (Python: *sklearn.cluster.AgglomerativeClustering*, Pedregosa et al., 2011) is a data-driven clustering algorithm, which is initiated by defining each voxel as a cluster and then, in each iteration step, merging the two neighboring clusters (even of different sizes) that after merging show minimal intra-cluster variance compared with all other possible variations of combining two adjacent clusters. In this way, the number of clusters is reduced by one in each iteration step. In our case the clustering stops after k clusters (**Table 3**) are formed. Afterwards, we discard away all clusters that contain less then p voxels (**Table 3**). An example of the outcome of Ward clustering algorithm is depicted in the second panel of **Figure 12**.

5.3.3. Region Growing and Selection

The region growing and selection algorithm is a modified version of the algorithm described in Lu et al. (2003). Region growing implies that each voxel serves as an initial seed (center) and neighboring voxels are added iteratively if they fulfill a certain growing criteria. (**Figure 11A**) The condition proposed for adding a voxel to a region is based on the Pearson correlation coefficient R between the averaged time-varying signals of the pre-merged region and the signal of the voxel to be tested (Lu et al., 2003). If this correlation is higher then a pre-defined threshold T (**Table 3**), the voxel is merged to the region. We tighten the growth criteria by imposing a second condition that allows the merging of voxels only if, in addition to exceeding the correlation threshold, the resulting cluster is also functionally homogeneous. Here, functional homogeneity means that the time-varying signals of all voxels can be expressed as instances of a single signal with varying levels of noise. The number of independent signals in a cluster can be estimated by the spatial functional heterogeneity h (Marrelec and Fransson, 2011):

$$h = n_0 + \frac{e_{n_0} - b_{n_0}}{(e_{n_0} - e_{n_0+1}) - (b_{n_0} - b_{n_0+1})}, \quad (1)$$

where e_n are the eigenvalues of the *NxN* covariance matrix of all N time varing signals in a cluster that exceed the eigenvalues generated by the broken-stick model b_n, such that $e_n > b_n = \sum_{i=n}^{N} 1/i$. The index n_0 accounts for the smallest eigenvalues that fulfill this inequality equation, such that

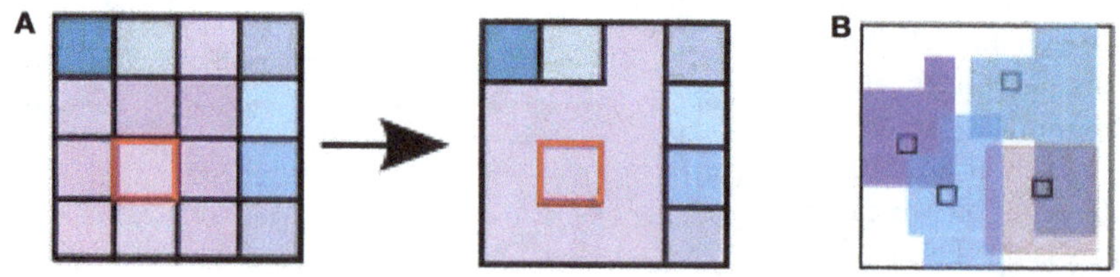

FIGURE 11 | Region growing and selection algorithm. **(A)** Region growing, left: each voxel (colored squares) serves as center for a cluster, right: example of a growing region (purple), only adjacent voxels that fulfill the fusion criteria are added to the growing cluster. **(B)** Region selection. Small regions (pink) with centers overlapping with larger regions (green) get deleted (from left to right) in a iterative manner. Remaining regions can still overlap as long as their centers do not cover other regions. This illustration is in 2D for simplicity, the algorithm used for fMRI data acts in 3D following the same rules.

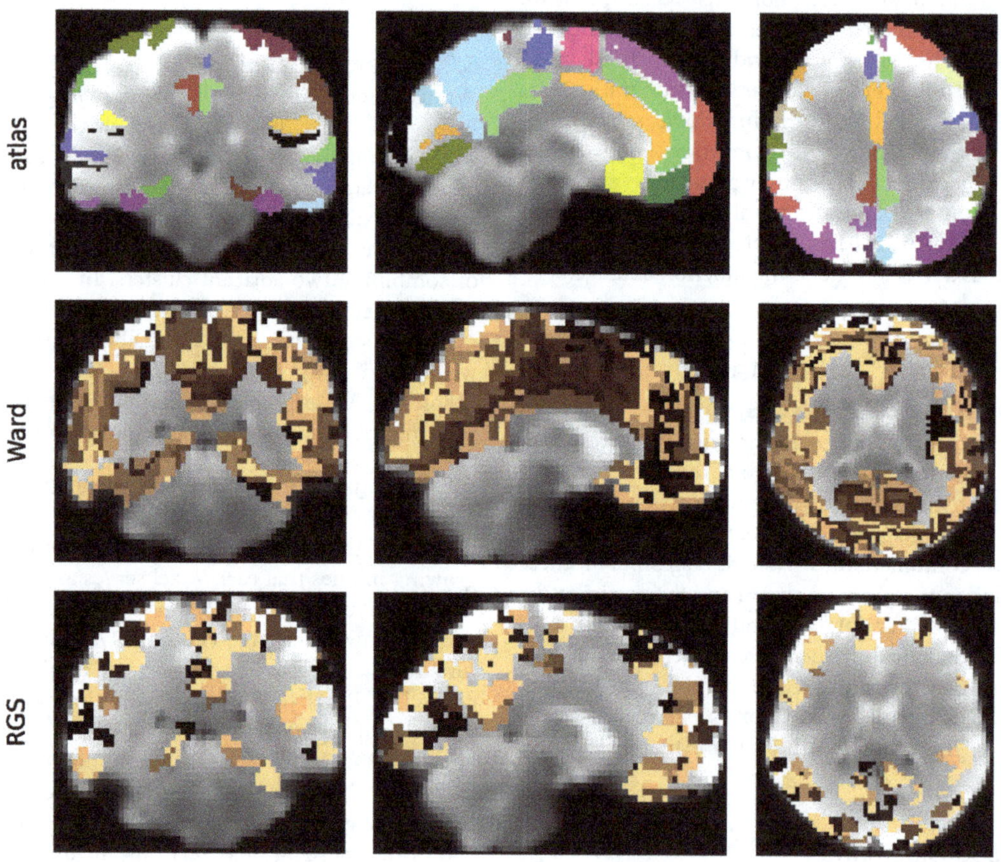

FIGURE 12 | Clustering of the cortical functional image. Illustrated are the clustering outcome of the atlas **(Upper Panel)** and the Ward clustering (ward4, **Middle Panel**) and RGS (RGS1, **Lower Panel**) algorithms for frontal, sagital and horizontal brain sections (from left to right) of a randomly chosen healthy individual. Individual clusters are depicted by a randomly chosen individual color, for clustering parameters see **Table 3**.

$e_{n_0} > b_{n_0}$ and $e_{n_0+1} < b_{n_0+1}$. A value of $h = 1$ indicates a homogeneous cluster.

The region selection algorithm iteratively selects the largest region and deletes all clusters that have their centers in that region, excluding the possibility that centers overlap with other regions. However, clusters can still overlap (**Figure 11B**). Applying this framework does not guarantee that clusters remain spatially connected after deleting regions with overlapping centers. Nevertheless, a check for spatial consistency reveals that only a negligible fraction of the clusters are disrupted in that way. Finally, we took only the clusters that comprised a minimum number of voxels p (**Table 3**). The outcome of RGS is illustrated in the last panel of **Figure 12**.

5.4. Edge Definition

A graph consists of nodes (vertices) that are connected through edges, that might be weighted or binary and directed or undirected. We construct individual brain graphs by defining nodes that represent clusters as described in section 5.3, such that the mean activity of a cluster becomes a node attribute. We presume that all graphs are fully connected and edge weights are defined in terms of functional connectivity. Since functional connectivity can be calculated in several ways, we apply a range of different connectivity measures. In Wang et al. (2014) many such methods are evaluated, taking the structural connectivity of a toy model as reference. As a starting point, for each proposed category of functional connectivity, measured in time, we select the analysis measurement that captures structural connectivity best. We follow this strategy for all proposed measurement categories in Wang et al. (2014), leaving out only Granger causality measures, due to limited computational resources. We thus use linear and non-linear correlation (*corr* and H_2) and mutual information transfer (*MIT*) for the model-free category and transfer entropy (*TE*) for the model-based category. In all groups the bivariate methods perform better then the partial ones. In conclusion we select for each of the families the bivariate implementation that can be both directed and undirected. For consistency we use the same abbreviations for the different methods as in Wang et al. (2014) and the same Matlab toolbox Mulan[3] which they made public. Here we provide only a short description of the applied methods and more details can be inferred from Wang et al. (2014).

Linear correlation (*corr*) are measured based on the Pearson correlation coefficient (Rodgers and Nicewander, 1988) in a pair-wise manner. For directed connectivity (*BCorrD*) delays of up to 5 time steps (**Table 4**) are considered and the largest connectivity value is selected. We do not take into account time lags for undirected correlation (*BCorrU*).

Non-linear correlations (H_2) are based on piece-wise linear correlations of two time signals on which the non-linear curve is fitted (da Silva et al., 1989). Bivariate directed (BH_2D) and bivariate undirected (BH_2U) are defined as above for linear correlations.

Mutual information indicates how much information is shared between two time varying signals by means of Shannon entropy (Grassberger et al., 1991). For *BMITD1* individual histograms of two time series are contrasted to the joint histogram across different time delays. No delays are taken into account in *BMITU*.

Transfer entropy (Schreiber, 2000) describes how far in the past the activity of a node can reduce the uncertainty of the future activity of another node for which the past activity is also considered. Bivariate directed (*BTED*, Chicharro, 2011) and bivariate undirected (*BTEU*) are defined as above for linear correlations.

All methods were tested for a window size that comprises the whole time range (130 time points/6.5 min) and for a sliding window of 50 time points (2.5 min) with an overlap of 10 time points (0.5 min), see **Table 4**. If the methods revealed negative weights, the absolute value was considered. The resulting graphs are directed or undirected weighted graphs with values between zero and one for all methods except non-linear correlations, where values can exceed one.

TABLE 4 | Parameters of the different functional connectivity measures.

Method	Window size	Window overlap	Number of bins	Max. delay
BcorrU1	130	–	–	–
BcorrU2	50	0.2	–	–
BcorrD1	130	–	–	5
BcorrD2	50	0.2	–	5
BH2U1	130	–	10	–
BH2U2	50	0.2	10	–
BH2D1	130	–	10	5
BH2D2	50	0.2	10	5
BMITU1	130	–	5	–
BMITU2	50	0.2	5	–
BMITD1	130	–	5	5
BMITD2	50	0.2	5	5
BTEU1	130	–	–	5
BTEU2	50	0.2	–	5
BTED1	130	–	–	5
BTED2	50	0.2	–	5

Bivariate (B), undirected (U), directed (D), linear correlation (corr), non-linear correlation (H_2U), mutual information entropy (MIT), transfer entropy (TE).

Many studies transfer weighted graphs into binary ones by setting all values below a threshold w_{min} to zero and above to one e.g., Zhao et al. (2012). Following this strategy we also investigate the effect of setting all weights below w_{min} to zero but leaving higher weights unchanged. As far as the remaining graphs are still connected (left panels in **Figure 13**) and single nodes are not disconnected from the network (right panels in **Figure 13**) we study the disease diagnosis capacity for $w_{min} \in \{0.1, 0.2, ...0.7, 0.8\}$. In addition we extract the rich club of the graphs. The rich club is a subgraph that comprises the nodes that are most strongly connected to the network. In this work we define the rich club as the 10% of nodes with highest degree.

5.5. Graph Properties

This section describes the different graph properties that are either characteristics of single nodes (weighted degree, closeness centrality, cluster coefficient), of pairs of nodes (shortest path) or of the entire network (modularity). In the first two cases we get a range of values for each graph. Since we do not know, which are the important features of the resulting distributions, we take the first four moments for our statistical analysis. Because graphs based on data-driven clustering contain different number of nodes and the calculated graph properties might be dependent on the number of nodes, we also include the number of nodes in the subsequent analysis (section 5.6).

5.5.1. Weighted Degree

The weighted degree deg_w describes how strongly a node is connected to all other vertices of the network, obeying the

[3]https://github.com/HuifangWang/MULAN.

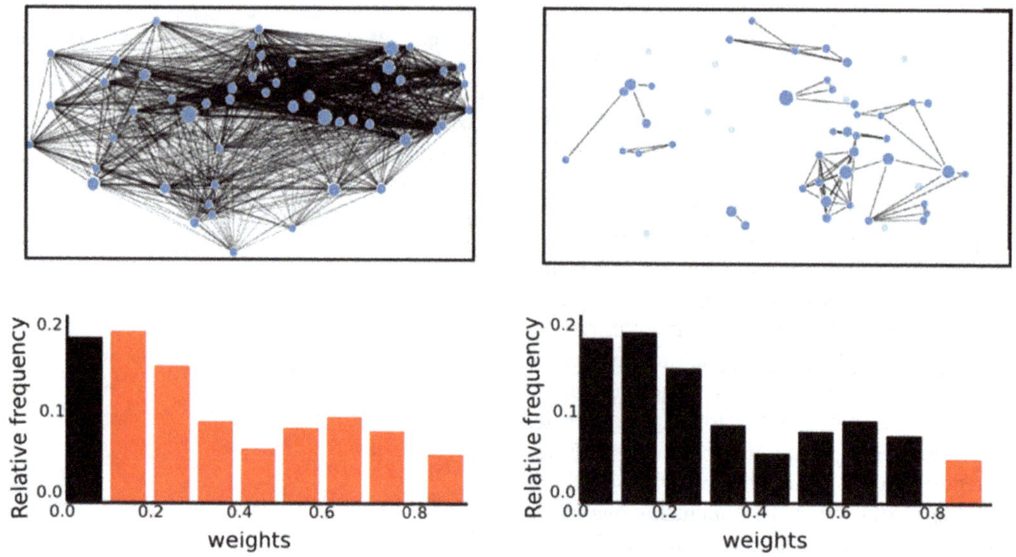

FIGURE 13 | High thresholds on graph edges cause the graphs to dissociate. **(Upper Panel)**, Illustration of graph with edge weights larger then 0.1 ($w_{min} > 0.1$, **Left**) and larger then 0.9 ($w_{min} > 0.9$, **Right**). In the according weight histograms **(Lower Panel)** the red bars correspond to the edges drawn in the upper graph. Edges corresponding to the black bars are not shown.

equation:

$$\deg_w(v) = \sum_{u \in V \setminus \{v\}} w_{uv} \tag{2}$$

where w_{uv} is the weight on the edge between nodes u and v of all nodes V in the graph. This definition implies a high dependency of the weighted degree on the number of nodes in a graph. To address this problem, we normalize the weighted degree

$$\deg_n(v) = \frac{\deg_w(v)}{\deg(v) \cdot w_{\max}} \tag{3}$$

with $w_{\max}$ being the maximal weight of the graph. The resulting values are between 0 and 1.

5.5.2. Shortest Path and Closeness Centrality

The shortest path $\mathrm{dist}_w(u, v)$ between a pair of nodes u and v describes the path that minimizes the sum of the weights of its participating edges. A small shortest path should indicate a strong functional connectivity, therefore we consider the inverse of the graph weights for its calculation. Its computation is carried out using Dijkstra's algorithm (Rivest et al., 2000), which requires the weights to be positive.

Based on the shortest paths of a network we calculate closeness centrality $C_w(v)$ - a measure that indicates how strongly a node v participates in all shortest paths of the graph. It is given by:

$$C_w(v) = \frac{n-1}{\sum_{u \in V \setminus \{v\}} \mathrm{dist}_w(u, v)} \tag{4}$$

Here, n is the number of all nodes V in the graph.

5.5.3. Clustering Coefficient

The clustering coefficient $cc(v)$ describes to what degree the neighbors of a node v are connected among each other and with node v. Since our network is weighted, we use the Zhang-Horvath clustering coefficient (Zhang and Horvath, 2005; Kalna and Higham, 2007), which is an extension to the "standard" algorithm applied to binary graphs:

$$cc(v) = \frac{\sum_{i \neq v} \sum_{j \neq i, j \neq v} \hat{w}_{vi} \hat{w}_{ij} \hat{w}_{jv}}{\left(\sum_{i \neq v} \hat{w}_{vi}\right)\left(\sum_{i \neq v} \hat{w}_{vi}^2\right)} \tag{5}$$

for i, j neighbors of v and $\hat{w}$ denoting the weights normalized by the highest weight in the network, such that $0 \leq \hat{w} \leq 1$.

5.5.4. Modularity

A graph can be partitioned into smaller components. Modularity measures the deviation of the properties of these components as compared to the components of a random graph with the same edge weights. Accordingly, the modularity of a partition p of a network G into communities c is given by Newman (2004):

$$Q(p) = \frac{1}{2m} \sum_{i,j \in V} \left(w_{ij} - \frac{\deg_w(i) \cdot \deg_w(j)}{2m}\right) \delta_{c_i c_j} \tag{6}$$

where $\delta_{c_i c_j}$ is 1, if the community c_i of node i is the same as the community c_j of node j, and 0 otherwise, and $m = \frac{1}{2} \sum_{i,j \in V} w_{ij}$ is the total sum of edge weights in a network. Although there are many different definitions in literature about what a community consists of, we define a community as a group of strongly interconnected nodes that make only weak connections to other communities. In addition, a node can maximally contribute to one community. Hence we want to find the partition that maximizes modularity, which is computationally very demanding, so it is important to use a very effective algorithm. We therefore use the fast algorithm by Blondel et al. (2008), which is implemented in the Python packages community. Unfortunately this implementation is only suitable for undirected graphs, so we investigate modularity only for these type of graphs.

5.6. Statistical Model

The generated graph data is used as input for an exchangeable parametric statistical model. Let us recall that the purpose of the fMRI scan of a patient is to give the clinician a likelihood for the patient's health condition,

$$\mathrm{P}(\text{graph data from fMRI scan} \mid \text{health condition} \wedge \text{prior info}), \tag{7}$$

which she combines with the likelihoods from other tests and her initial probability assignment, to obtain via Bayes's theorem a final probability for the health condition (Sox et al., 2013):

$$\overbrace{\mathrm{P}(\text{health condition} \mid \text{results of all tests} \wedge \text{prior info})}^{\textit{final probability}} \propto$$

$$\textit{likelihoods} \begin{cases} \mathrm{P}(\text{graph data from fMRI scan} \mid \text{health condition} \wedge \text{prior info}) \\ \times \mathrm{P}(\text{results of other tests} \mid \text{health condition} \wedge \text{prior info}) \\ \times \cdots \end{cases}$$

$$\times \underbrace{\mathrm{P}(\text{health condition} \mid \text{prior info})}_{\textit{initial probability}}. \tag{8}$$

The prior information also includes test results from previous patients, so that the prediction becomes more accurate and reliable, the more patients have been previously observed.

The functional dependence of the likelihood on the graph data is determined by the statistical model we use, and may be different for each health condition. The statistical model is determined by additional assumptions or hypotheses. Such hypotheses and the functional form of the likelihood may depend on the particular space of graph data (e.g., real-valued, or positive, or bounded within a finite range, or combinations thereof), and therefore on the graph construction method.

As explained in section 2.3, our purpose is to assess as far as possible the relative predictive power of the different graph construction methods. We therefore would like the functional dependence on the graph data space to be minimal. In the present study we adopt the working hypothesis that only the first and second empirical moments—means and correlations—of the graph data from past patients with the same health condition are relevant to make predictions about a new patient. This hypothesis is adopted for all graph construction methods. We also assume our initial knowledge of the graph data to be approximately invariant under rescalings of their values (Minka, 2001). Finally, we do not take into account the natural range of variability (positive, bounded, etc.) of the graph data; this choice does not seem to impact the predictive power of the model (Porta Mana et al., 2018).

These assumptions almost uniquely determine the statistical model and the likelihood (Porta Mana et al., 2018): it turns out to be a multivariate t distribution (Minka, 2001; Kotz and Nadarajah, 2004; Murphy, 2007). More precisely: select a particular health condition, e.g., Alzheimer's disease. Denote with $\boldsymbol{f}_0$ the d-dimensional vector of graph data obtained from the patient's fMRI scan via a particular graph construction method, and with $(\boldsymbol{f}_i)$ the graph data of n previous patients with the selected health condition. Then the likelihood that the present patient has the selected health condition is

$$\begin{aligned} \mathrm{p}[\boldsymbol{f}_0 \mid (\boldsymbol{f}_i), \kappa_0, \boldsymbol{\delta}_0, \nu_0, \boldsymbol{\Delta}_0, M] &\equiv \mathrm{p}(\boldsymbol{f}_0 \mid \kappa, \boldsymbol{\delta}, \nu, \boldsymbol{\Delta}, M) \\ &= \mathrm{t}\Big[\boldsymbol{f}_0 \Big| \; \nu - d + 1, \boldsymbol{\delta}, \tfrac{\kappa+1}{\kappa(\nu-d+1)} \boldsymbol{\Delta}\Big] \end{aligned} \tag{9}$$

$$\kappa = \kappa_0 + n, \quad \nu = \nu_0 + n,$$

with (10)

$$\boldsymbol{\delta} = \frac{\kappa_0\, \boldsymbol{\delta}_0 + n\overline{\boldsymbol{f}}}{\kappa_0 + n}, \quad \boldsymbol{\Delta} = \boldsymbol{\Delta}_0 + n\,\mathrm{Cov}(\boldsymbol{f}) + \frac{\kappa_0\, n}{\kappa_0 + n} (\overline{\boldsymbol{f}} - \boldsymbol{\delta}_0)(\overline{\boldsymbol{f}} - \boldsymbol{\delta}_0)^{\intercal},$$

where t is a multivariate t distribution with $\nu - d + 1$ degrees of freedom, mean $\boldsymbol{\delta}$, and scale matrix $\frac{\kappa+1}{\kappa(\nu-d+1)} \boldsymbol{\Delta}$, and

$$\overline{\boldsymbol{f}} := \frac{1}{n} \textstyle\sum_i \boldsymbol{f}_i, \qquad \mathrm{Cov}(\boldsymbol{f}) := \frac{1}{n} \sum_i (\boldsymbol{f}_i - \overline{\boldsymbol{f}})(\boldsymbol{f}_i - \overline{\boldsymbol{f}})^{\intercal} \tag{11}$$

are the empirical mean and covariance matrix of the previous graph data.

The parameters κ_0, ν_0, $\boldsymbol{\delta}_0$, $\boldsymbol{\Delta}_0$ should reflect our initial knowledge of the graph parameters. For the reasons explained above and in section 2.3, we fix one set of values identically for all graph construction methods: $\kappa = 1$, $(\boldsymbol{\delta}_0)_a = 0.5$, $\boldsymbol{\Delta}_0 = 2.5\boldsymbol{I}$, where $\boldsymbol{I}$ is the identity matrix. These values yield an initial distribution (before any data from previous patients) centered on positive values of unit order of magnitude, as all the graph data indeed are for each graph construction method.

5.7. Supportive Evaluation Measures of Graph Construction Methods

5.7.1. Significance Test

We measure the significance level of the mean values of a graph property distribution between pairs of the three healthy conditions (control-AD, control-MCI, MCI-AD) based on the Student's t-test, if variances are equal (F-test), and Welch's t-test otherwise. The underlying null hypothesis is that the means of the two data arrays are assumed to be equal, which is rejected for p-values smaller then 0.05.

5.7.2. Dendrograms of Subject Order

Subjects indexed from 1 to 56 (total number of participants) across all health conditions are ordered according to the mean values of a given graph property distribution. The indices of the ordering (the rank) calculated for each graph construction method is then used in order to construct the dendrogram. In the dendrogram, the Euclidean distance between two indices arrays is indicated by the height of the top of the U-link linking the two arrays. In addition, arrays with a small distance are clustered together.

5.7.3. Support Vector Machines

For all complete graphs constructed by all different graph construction methods, we apply a support vector classification (Python: *sklearn.svm.SVC*) on each pair of health conditions (control-AD, control-MCI, MCI-AD). Hereby we choose the graph properties such that the performance of the algorithm maximizes. We use the default parameters and do not optimize performance by varying the kernel coefficient or the penalty parameter of the error term.

ETHICS STATEMENT

This study was part of a larger study, which was approved by the local ethics committee, in accordance with the declaration of Helsinki and performed after informed written consent of each participant. Healthy participants were reimbursed. AD patients were not reimbursed since imaging was part of their diagnostic procedures. We did, however, pay for and organize their traveling costs and lunch.

AUTHOR CONTRIBUTIONS

CB constructed the graphs and calculated and analyzed the graph properties. She also applied the statistical analysis, formulated together with PP, to the data. KD, HJ, NR, BvR, JD, OO, K-JL, GF and JK contributed to the conception of the study design and recruited patients. KD, NR, BvR, and JD organized and performed fMRI scanning. KD and HJ applied primary preprocessing to the fMRI data. The manuscript was written by CB, AM, and PP, with additional editing by HJ and JK.

FUNDING

We acknowledge partial support by the Helmholtz Alliance through the Initiative and Networking Fund of the Helmholtz Association and the Helmholtz Portfolio theme Supercomputing and Modeling for the Human Brain and the German Research Foundation (DFG; grant DI 1721/3-1 [KFO219-TP9]). This work was also supported by a DFG individual grant JA 2336/1-1 (HJ) and by a grant of the Marga and Walter Boll Foundation, Kerpen, Germany, to GF and JK.

ACKNOWLEDGMENTS

PP thanks Mari & Miri for continuous encouragement, affection, and support; the kind staff at Iris; and Buster Keaton and Saitama for filling life with awe and inspiration. We are grateful to Simone Buttler for her important help with regard to the calculation of graph properties, and Fahad Khalid and Andreas Müller of the SimLab Neuroscience at the Jülich Supercomputing Center for their expertise in graph visualization. We also acknowledge the support and expert advice by Alper Yegenoglu, Paulina Dabrowska, and Dr. Jyotika Bahuguna. We would like to thank Dr. Gabriele Stoffels, Dr. Christian Filss, and Nathalie Judov for their assistance and generous support. We also acknowledge the technical support and advice of Prof. Dr. Hans Herzog, Dr. Elena Rota Kops, Lutz Tellmann, and Dr. Daniel Pflugfelder. Finally, we are grateful to Kornelia Frey, Suzanne Schaden, and Silke Frensch for their important help in data acquisition. Thanks are extended to Prof. Dr. Nadim Jon Shah for support with the MRI.

REFERENCES

Amoroso, N., La Rocca, M., Bruno, S., Maggipinto, T., Monaco, A., Bellotti, R., et al. (2017). Brain structural connectivity atrophy in Alzheimer's disease. *arXiv 1709.02369* [preprint].

Avants, B. B., Tustison, N. J., Song, G., Cook, P. A., Klein, A., and Gee, J. C. (2011). A reproducible evaluation of ANTS similarity metric performance in brain image registration. *Neuroimage* 54, 2033–2044. doi: 10.1016/j.neuroimage.2010.09.025

Bartlett, M. S. (1952). The statistical significance of odd bits of information. *Biometrika* 39, 228–237. doi: 10.2307/2334019

Bassett, D. S., Bullmore, E., Verchinski, B. A., Mattay, V. S., Weinberger, D. R., and Meyer-Lindenberg, A. (2008). Hierarchical organization of human cortical networks in health and schizophrenia. *J. Neurosci* 28, 9239–9248. doi: 10.1523/JNEUROSCI.1929-08.2008

Beckmann, C. F., and Smith, S. M. (2004). Probabilistic independent component analysis for functional magnetic resonance imaging. *IEEE Trans. Med. Imaging* 23, 137–152. doi: 10.1109/TMI.2003.822821

Bernardo, J.-M. (1979). Expected information as expected utility. *Ann. Stat.* 7, 686–690.

Blondel, V. D., Guillaume, J.-L., Lambiotte, R., and Lefebvre, E. (2008). Fast unfolding of communities in large networks. *J. Stat. Mech.* 10:P10008. doi: 10.1088/1742-5468/2008/10/P10008

Bordier, C., Nicolini, C., and Bifone, A. (2017). Graph analysis and modularity of brain functional connectivity networks: searching for the optimal threshold. *Front. Neurosci.* 11:441. doi: 10.3389/fnins.2017.00441

Chicharro, D. (2011). On the spectral formulation of Granger causality. *Biol. Cybern.* 105, 331–347. doi: 10.1007/s00422-011-0469-z

Çiftçi, K. (2011). Minimum spanning tree reflects the alterations of the default mode network during Alzheimer's disease. *Ann. Biomed. Eng.* 39, 1493–1504. doi: 10.1007/s10439-011-0258-9

Collins, D. L., Holmes, C. J., Peters, T. M., and Evans, A. C. (1995). Automatic 3-D model-based neuroanatomical segmentation. *Hum. Brain Mapp.* 3, 190–208. doi: 10.1002/hbm.460030304

da Silva, F. L., Pijn, J. P., and Boeijinga, P. (1989). Interdependence of EEG signals: linear vs. nonlinear associations and the significance of time delays and phase shifts. *Brain Topogr.* 2, 9–18.

Dennis, E. L., and Thompson, P. M. (2014). Functional brain connectivity using fMRI in aging and Alzheimer's disease. *Neuropsychol. Rev.* 24, 49–62. doi: 10.1007/s11065-014-9249-6

Desikan, R. S., Ségonne, F., Fischl, B., Quinn, B. T., Dickerson, B. C., Blacker, D., et al. (2006). An automated labeling system for subdividing the human cerebral cortex on MRI scans into gyral based regions of interest. *Neuroimage* 31, 968–980. doi: 10.1016/j.neuroimage.2006.01.021

Dillen, K. N., Jacobs, H. I. L., Kukolja, J., Richter, N., von Reutern, B., Onur, O. A., et al. (2017). Functional disintegration of the default mode network in prodromal Alzheimer's disease. *J. Alzheimer. Dis.* 59, 169–187. doi: 10.3233/JAD-161120

Gits, H. C. (2016). Relating connectivity and graph analysis to cognitive function in Alzheimer's disease. *Michigan J. Med.* 1, 45–65. doi: 10.3998/mjm.13761231.0001.111

Good, I. J. (1956). The surprise index for the multivariate normal distribution. *Ann. Math. Stat.* 27, 1130–1135.

Good, I. J. (1957a). "The appropriate mathematical tools for describing and measuring uncertainty," in *Good Thinking: The Foundations of Probability and Its Applications*, Chap. 16 (Minneapolis, MN: University of Minnesota Press), 173–177. First publ. 1957.

Good, I. J. (1957b). Corrections to "The surprise index for the multivariate normal distribution." *Ann. Math. Stat.* 28:1055.

Good, I. J. (1983). *Good Thinking: The Foundations of Probability and Its Applications*. Minneapolis, MN: University of Minnesota Press.

Grabner, G., Janke, A. L., Budge, M. M., Smith, D., Pruessner, J., and Collins, D. L. (2006). Symmetric atlasing and model based segmentation: an application to the hippocampus in older adults. *Med. Image Comput. Comput. Assist. Interv* 9, 58–66. doi: 10.1007/11866763_8

Grassberger, P., Schreiber, T., and Schaffrath, C. (1991). Nonlinear time sequence analysis. *Int. J. Bifurcation Chaos* 1, 521–547. doi: 10.1142/S0218127491000403

Guimerá, R., and Nunes Amaral, L. A. (2005). Functional cartography of complex metabolic networks. *Nature* 433, 895–900. doi: 10.1038/nature03288

Hayasaka, S. (2013). Functional connectivity networks with and without global signal correction. *Front. Hum. Neurosci.* 7:880. doi: 10.3389/fnhum.2013.00880

Hoenig, M. C., Bischof, G. N., Seemiller, J., Hammes, J., Kukolja, J., Onur, O. A., et al. (2018). Networks of tau distribution in Alzheimer's disease. *Brain* 141, 568–581. doi: 10.1093/brain/awx353

Jaynes, E. T. (2003). *Probability Theory: The Logic of Science*. Cambridge: Cambridge University Press. Available online at: https://archive.org/details/XQUHIUXHIQUHIQXUIHX2, http://www-biba.inrialpes.fr/Jaynes/prob.html

Jenkinson, M., Bannister, P., Brady, M., and Smith, S. (2002). Improved optimization for the robust and accurate linear registration and motion correction of brain images. *Neuroimage* 17, 825–841. doi: 10.1006/nimg.2002.1132

Jenkinson, M., Beckmann, C. F., Behrens, T. E., Woolrich, M. W., and Smith, S. M. (2012). FSL. *Neuroimage* 62, 782–790. doi: 10.1016/j.neuroimage.2011.09.015

Jenkinson, M., and Smith, S. (2001). A global optimisation method for robust affine registration of brain images. *Med. Image Anal.* 5, 143–156. doi: 10.1016/S1361-8415(01)00036-6

Johnson, K. A., Fox, N. C., Sperling, R. A., and Klunk, W. E. (2012). Brain imaging in Alzheimer disease. *Cold Spring Harb. Perspect. Med.* 2:a006213. doi: 10.1101/cshperspect.a006213

Kalna, G., and Higham, D. J. (2007). A clustering coefficient for weighted networks, with application to gene expression data. *AI Commun.* 20, 263–271.

Keihaninejad, S., Heckemann, R. A., Fagiolo, G., Symms, M. R., Hajnal, J. V., and Hammers, A. (2010). A robust method to estimate the intracranial volume across MRI field strengths (1.5T and 3T). *Neuroimage* 50, 1427–1437. doi: 10.1016/j.neuroimage.2010.01.064

Khazaee, A., Ebrahimzadeh, A., and Babajani-Feremi, A. (2015). Identifying patients with Alzheimer's disease using resting-state fMRI and graph theory. *Clin. Neurophysiol.* 126, 2132–2141. doi: 10.1016/j.clinph.2015.02.060

Khazaee, A., Ebrahimzadeh, A., and Babajani-Feremi, A. (2017). Classification of patients with MCI and AD from healthy controls using directed graph measures of resting-state fMRI. *Behav. Brain Res.* 322, 339–350. doi: 10.1016/j.bbr.2016.06.043

Kim, H., Yoo, K., Na, D. L., Seo, S. W., Jeong, J., and Jeong, Y. (2015). Non-monotonic reorganization of brain networks with Alzheimer's disease progression. *Front. Aging Neurosci.* 7:111. doi: 10.3389/fnagi.2015.00111

Kotz, S., and Nadarajah, S. (2004). *Multivariate t Distributions and Their Applications*. Cambridge: Cambridge University Press.

Kruschwitz, J. D., List, D., Waller, L., Rubinov, M., and Walter, H. (2015). GraphVar: a user-friendly toolbox for comprehensive graph analyses of functional brain connectivity. *J. Neurosci. Methods* 245, 107–115. doi: 10.1016/j.jneumeth.2015.02.021

Leung, K. K., Barnes, J., Modat, M., Ridgway, G. R., Bartlett, J. W., Fox, N. C., et al. (2011). Brain MAPS: an automated, accurate and robust brain extraction technique using a template library. *Neuroimage* 55, 1091–1108. doi: 10.1016/j.neuroimage.2010.12.067

Liu, X., Gerraty, R. T., Grinband, J., Parker, D., and Razlighi, Q. R. (2017). Brain atrophy can introduce age-related differences in BOLD response. *Hum. Brain Mapp.* 38, 3402–3414. doi: 10.1002/hbm.23597

Lu, Y., Jiang, T., and Zang, Y. (2003). Region growing method for the analysis of functional MRI data. *Neuroimage* 20, 455–465. doi: 10.1016/S1053-8119(03)00352-5

Marrelec, G., and Fransson, P. (2011). Assessing the influence of different ROI selection strategies on functional connectivity analyses of fMRI data acquired during steady-state conditions. *PLOS ONE* 6:e14788. doi: 10.1371/journal.pone.0014788

McCarthy, J. (1956). Measures of the value of information. *Proc. Natl. Acad. Sci. U.S.A.* 42, 654–655.

Minka, T. (2001). *Inferring a Gaussian Distribution*. Tech. rep., MIT Media Lab, Cambridge, MA. Available online at: http://research.microsoft.com/en-us/um/people/minka/papers/Firstpubl.1998

Murphy, K., and Fox, M. D. (2017). Towards a consensus regarding global signal regression for resting state functional connectivity MRI. *Neuroimage* 154, 169–173. doi: 10.1016/j.neuroimage.2016.11.052

Murphy, K. P. (2007). *Conjugate Bayesian Analysis of the Gaussian Distribution*. Available online at: http://thaines.com/content/misc/gaussian_conjugate_prior_cheat_sheet.pdf

Nelson, P. T., Alafuzoff, I., Bigio, E. H., Bouras, C., Braak, H., Cairns, N. J., et al. (2012). Correlation of Alzheimer disease neuropathologic changes with cognitive status: a review of the literature. *J. Neuropathol. Exp. Neurol.* 71, 362–381. doi: 10.1097/NEN.0b013e31825018f7

Newman, M. E. J. (2004). Analysis of weighted networks. *Phys. Rev. E* 70:056131. doi: 10.1103/PhysRevE.70.056131

Pagani, M., Giuliani, A., Öberg, J., Chincarini, A., Morbelli, S., Brugnolo, A., et al. (2016). Predicting the transition from normal aging to Alzheimer's disease: a statistical mechanistic evaluation of FDG-PET data. *Neuroimage* 141, 282–290. doi: 10.1016/j.neuroimage.2016.07.043

Pagani, M., Giuliani, A., Öberg, J., De Carli, F., Morbelli, S., Girtler, N., et al. (2017). Progressive disintegration of brain networking from normal aging to Alzheimer disease: analysis of independent components of 18F-FDG PET data. *J. Nucl. Med.* 58, 1132–1139. doi: 10.2967/jnumed.116.184309

Pedregosa, F., Varoquaux, G., Gramfort, A., Michel, V., Thirion, B., Grisel, O., et al. (2011). Scikit-learn: machine learning in Python. *J. Mach. Learn. Res.* 12, 2825–2830.

Pereda, E., Quiroga, R. Q., and Bhattacharya, J. (2005). Nonlinear multivariate analysis of neurophysiological signals. *Prog. Neurobiol.* 77, 1–37. doi: 10.1016/j.pneurobio.2005.10.003

Popescu, V., Battaglini, M., Hoogstrate, W. S., Verfaillie, S. C. J., Sluimer, I. C., van Schijndel R. A., et al. (2012). Optimizing parameter choice for FSL-Brain Extraction Tool (BET) on 3D T1 images in multiple sclerosis. *Neuroimage* 61, 1484–1494. doi: 10.1016/j.neuroimage.2012.03.074

Porta Mana, P. G. L., Bachmann, C., and Morrison, A. (2018). Inferring health conditions from fMRI-graph data. *Open Science Framework. arXiv:1803.02626* [preprint]. doi: 10.31219/osf.io/r2huz

Rivest, R. L., Leiserson, C. E., and Cormen, T. H. (2000). *Introduction to Algorithms (MIT Electrical Engineering and Computer Science Series.)* Cambridge, MA: MIT Press.

Rodgers, J. L., and Nicewander, W. A. (1988). Thirteen ways to look at the correlation coefficient. *Am. Stat.* 42, 59–66. doi: 10.1080/00031305.1988.10475524

Sanz-Arigita, E. J., Schoonheim, M. M., Damoiseaux, J. S., Rombouts, S. A., Maris, E., Barkhof, F., et al. (2010). Loss of "small-world" networks in Alzheimer's disease: graph analysis of fMRI resting-state functional connectivity. *PLOS ONE* 5:e13788. doi: 10.1371/journal.pone.0013788

Schaeffer, S. E. (2007). Graph clustering. *Comput. Sci. Rev.* 1, 27–64. doi: 10.1016/j.cosrev.2007.05.001

Schreiber, T. (2000). Measuring information transfer. *Phys. Rev. Lett.* 85, 461–464. doi: 10.1103/PhysRevLett.85.461

Schroeter, M. L., Stein, T., Maslowski, N., and Neumann, J. (2009). Neural correlates of Alzheimer's disease and mild cognitive impairment: a systematic and quantitative meta-analysis involving 1,351 patients. *Neuroimage* 47, 1196–1206. doi: 10.1016/j.neuroimage.2009.05.037

Schwarz, A. J., and McGonigle, J. (2011). Negative edges and soft thresholding in complex network analysis of resting state functional connectivity data. *Neuroimage* 55, 1032–1146. doi: 10.1016/j.neuroimage.2010.12.047

Shannon, C. E. (1948). A mathematical theory of communication. *Bell Syst. Tech. J.* 27, 379–423, 623–656.

Smith, S. M. (2002). Fast robust automated brain extraction. *Hum. Brain Mapp.* 17, 143–155. doi: 10.1002/hbm.10062

Sox, H. C., Higgins, M. C., and Owens, D. K. (2013). *Medical Decision Making, 2nd Edn.* New York, NY: Wiley.

Sperling, R. A., Aisen, P. S., Beckett, L. A., Bennett, D. A., Craft, S., Fagan, A. M., et al. (2011). Toward defining the preclinical stages of Alzheimer's disease: recommendations from the National Institute on Aging-Alzheimer's Association workgroups on diagnostic guidelines for Alzheimer's disease. *Alzheimer. Dement.* 7, 280–292. doi: 10.1016/j.jalz.2011.03.003

Supekar, K., Menon, V., Rubin, D., Musen, M., and Greicius, M. D. (2008). Network analysis of intrinsic functional brain connectivity in Alzheimer's disease. *PLOS Comput. Biol.* 4:e1000100. doi: 10.1371/journal.pcbi.1000100

Telesford, Q. K., Morgan, A. R., Hayasaka, S., Simpson, S. L., Barret, W., Kraft, R. A., et al. (2010). Reproducibility of graph metrics in fMRI networks. *Front. Neuroinformat.* 4:117. doi: 10.3389/fninf.2010.00117

Thirion, B., Varoquaux, G., Dohmatob, E., and Poline, J.-B. (2014). Which fMRI clustering gives good brain parcellations? *Front. Neurosci.* 8:167. doi: 10.3389/fnins.2014.00167

Tzourio-Mazoyer, N., Landeau, B., Papathanassiou, D., Crivello, F., Etard, O., Delcroix, N., et al. (2002). Automated anatomical labeling of activations in SPM using a macroscopic anatomical parcellation of the MNI MRI single-subject brain. *Neuroimage* 15, 273–289. doi: 10.1006/nimg.2001.0978

Wang, H. E., Bénar, C. G., Quilichini, P. P., Friston, K. J., Jirsa, V. K., and Bernard, C. (2014). A systematic framework for functional connectivity measures. *Front. Neurosci.* 8:405. doi: 10.3389/fnins.2014.00405

Wang, Z., Zhang, M., Han, Y., Song, H., Guo, R., and Li, K. (2016). Differentially disrupted functional connectivity of the subregions of the amygdala in Alzheimer's disease. *J. X-Ray Sci. Technol.* 24, 329–342. doi: 10.3233/XST-160556

Woolrich, M. W., Jbabdi, S., Patenaude, B., Chappell, M., Makni, S., Behrens, T., et al. (2009). Bayesian analysis of neuroimaging data in FSL. *Neuroimage* 45, S173–S186. doi: 10.1016/j.neuroimage.2008.10.055

Xia, M., Wang, Z., Dai, Z., Liang, X., Song, H., Shu, N., et al. (2014). Differentially disrupted functional connectivity in posteromedial cortical subregions in Alzheimer's disease. *J. Alzheimers Dis.* 39, 527–543. doi: 10.3233/JAD-131583

Zhang, B., and Horvath, S. (2005). A general framework for weighted gene co-expression network analysis. *Stat. Appl. Genet. Mol. Biol.* 4:Article17. doi: 10.2202/1544-6115.1128

Zhang, Y., Brady, M., and Smith, S. (2001). Segmentation of brain MR images through a hidden Markov random field model and the expectation-maximization algorithm. *IEEE Trans. Med. Imaging* 20, 45–57. doi: 10.1109/42.906424

Zhao, X., Lui, Y., Wang, X., Liu, B., Xi, Q., Guo, Q., et al. (2012). Disrupted small-world brain networks in moderate Alzheimer's disease: a resting-state fMRI study. *PLOS ONE* 7:e33540. doi: 10.1371/journal.pone.0033540

6

Use of Peptides for the Management of Alzheimer's Disease: Diagnosis and Inhibition

*Mohammad H. Baig, Khurshid Ahmad, Gulam Rabbani and Inho Choi**

Department of Medical Biotechnology, Yeungnam University, Gyeongsan, South Korea

***Correspondence:**
Inho Choi
inhochoi@ynu.ac.kr

Alzheimer's disease (AD) is a form of dementia and the most common progressive neurodegenerative disease (ND). The targeting of amyloid-beta (Aβ) aggregation is one of the most widely used strategies to manage AD, and efforts are being made globally to develop peptide-based compounds for the early diagnosis and treatment of AD. Here, we briefly discuss the use of peptide-based compounds for the early diagnosis and treatment of AD and the use of peptide-based inhibitors targeting various Aβ aggregation checkpoints. In addition, we briefly discuss recent applications of peptide-based inhibitors against various AD targets including amyloid beta, β-site amyloid precursor protein cleaving enzyme 1 (BACE1), Glyceraldehyde-3-phosphate dehydrogenase (GAPDH), tyrosine phosphatase (TP) and potassium channel KV1.3.

Keywords: Alzheimer's disease, peptides, amyloid beta, BACE-1, GAPDH, inhibitors, diagnosis

INTRODUCTION

Alzheimer's disease (AD) is the most common fatal neurodegenerative disease (ND), and is characterized by the structural and functional loss of neurons. During the last few decades, AD and its associated risk factors have become major healthcare concerns in most developed countries. Furthermore, it has been reported AD is the fifth-leading cause of death among those aged more than 65 years, and that its incidence exceeds five million cases per year in the United States (Alzheimer's Association, 2017). The World Health Organization (WHO) estimated that the prevalence of AD worldwide will quadruple to reach approximately 114 million by 2050 (Alzheimer's Association, 2017).

Pathological hallmarks of AD include the progressive accretion of plaque outside neurons (extracellular amyloid plaque) and of neurofibrillary tangles inside neurons (hyperphosphorylated tau protein accumulations; VanItallie, 2015). These pathological changes gradually result in neuronal loss and eventual neuron death. Although the etiology and pathogenesis of AD remain imprecise, the amyloid cascade theory is widely accepted and supported by several studies (Drachman, 2014; Herrup, 2015). This hypothesis was further reinforced by the identification of a protective amyloid precursor protein (APP) mutation near the protein's beta-cleavage site, which protects against the development of late onset dementia (Jonsson et al., 2012).

Amyloid-beta (Aβ) is a 39–43 amino acid residue peptide and a key component of extracellular amyloid plaque, and its expression is considered a key event in AD progression (Li et al., 2017). Aβ is the peptide product of the sequential proteolytic cleavages (by β- and γ-secretases) of APP (a type-I transmembrane protein). These proteolytic cleavages result in the generations of two types of Aβ isoforms (Aβ40 and Aβ42), and though Aβ40 is more abundant than Aβ42 in human fluids, Aβ42 aggregates faster and is considered to be the more lethal in terms of neuron survival.

Abbreviations: Aβ, Amyloid-beta; AD, Alzheimer's disease; BACE1, β-site APP cleaving enzyme 1; GAPDH, Glyceraldehyde-3-phosphate dehydrogenase; ND, Neurodegenerative disease; TP, Tyrosine phosphatase.

It has been reported oligomers of diffusible Aβ, such as, protofibrils, prefibrillar aggregates and Aβ-derived diffusible ligands (ADDLs), are the main toxic players during the development and progression of AD (Haass and Selkoe, 2007; Shankar et al., 2008; Funke and Willbold, 2012). Numerous amyloid reduction therapy (ART) clinical trials have failed to provide expected clinical improvements in AD patients, and these failures raise genuine concerns regarding the validity of the amyloid cascade hypothesis and the merits of further research on ART (Extance, 2010; Grundman et al., 2013; Cheng et al., 2017).

Today, due to the extensive efforts of researchers and pharmaceutical companies, peptide-based drugs have emerged as a major class of therapeutics, and as a result, the last decade has witnessed extraordinary scientific and industrial interest in their therapeutic uses (Vlieghe et al., 2010). Such studies are very much on-going and currently, a number of natural and synthetic therapeutic peptides are undergoing clinical trials (Mandal et al., 2014). Generally, these drugs have several advantages over small molecule therapeutics, particularly in terms of their efficacies and fewer side effects (Craik et al., 2013).

Many other fatal NDs, such as, Parkinson's disease (PD), amyotrophic lateral sclerosis (ALS), prion diseases and Huntington's diseases (HD) share the AD characteristic of misfolded protein aggregation. Peptides have proven to be vital tools for ND research, and can be used to study the properties of misfolded proteins and/or peptides. In this review article, we discuss some of the available peptide-based therapeutics used to treat AD, the use of peptide inhibitors to target different aspects of AD, and the use of peptides for the diagnosis and early detection of AD.

THE USE OF PEPTIDES AS DIAGNOSTIC PROBES

Currently, the number of *in vivo* diagnostic techniques available for detection of AD is limited, but early detection of the disease is crucial for effective treatment, because preemptive treatment might control or eliminate early stage disease. Investigations on AD patients have shown amyloid plaque appears several years before cognitive symptoms (Silverman et al., 1997; Thal et al., 2002; Funke and Willbold, 2012). Accordingly, early stage detection and the quantification of amyloid in brain are viewed as important from the prognostic point of view and for evaluating the effects of therapies, and several molecular imaging techniques, including, magnetic resonance imaging (MRI), positron emission tomography (PET) and single-photon emission computed tomography (SPECT) provide means of doing so. These molecular imaging techniques have been reported to be useful for detecting biomarkers of AD (mainly Aβ) and for monitoring the expression of Aβ (Frisoni et al., 2017), and thus, have attracted considerable attention in the AD research field. Furthermore, amyloid ligands have been used as contrast agents to estimate amyloid plaque load, and been shown to stain amyloid plaque specifically in the brain tissues of AD patients, which make these peptides suitable probes for *in vivo* imaging (Kang et al., 2003).

D-enantiomeric peptides (also known as derivatives of ACI-80) are another set of peptides that have been reported to bind Aβ1–42. In one study, ACI-80 also was found to bind Aβ1–42 with high affinity (in the submicromolar range; Funke et al., 2012; Gulyás et al., 2012), and is currently being used as a molecular probe to monitor Aβ1–42 plaque load in the living brain. Findings show when ACI-80 is injected into the brain, it specifically binds to Aβ1–42 and stains dense amyloid deposits in brain but not diffuse plaque (van Groen et al., 2009), which makes it a suitable molecular probe for *in vivo* imaging in AD. In addition, recent studies have described a series of D-enantiomeric peptides that also specifically bind to aggregated Aβ1–42 (Funke et al., 2012), but have greater stabilities and Aβ binding properties than ACI-80. To confirm binding by these peptide derivatives, *ex vivo* immunochemistry was performed using transgenic mouse models of AD, and the ACI-80 derivatives ACI-87-Kφ, ACI-88-Kφ and ACI-89-Kφ were found to bind to aggregated Aβ1–42 with greater affinity than parent ACI-80. These findings suggest these compounds might be useful probes for specific types of Aβ aggregation and plaque *in vivo*.

Larbanoix et al. (2010) used a phage display technique to search for peptide ligands with carrying ability to vectorize an AP-targeting contrast agent, and identified 12 peptide ligands from among 22 sequenced phage clones with high affinity against Aβ42. Two peptides were selected (C-FRHMTEQ-C and C-IPLPFYN-C) as both were found to be present in several copies and to have K_d-values in the picomolar range. For example, C-IPLPFYN-C was found to have a K_d value of 2.2×10^{-10} M, and C-FRHMTEQ-C a K_d value 5.45×10^{-10} M against mouse Aβ42. Both peptides were also tested on human Aβ42, and C-FRHMTEQ-C demonstrated similar affinity against human Aβ42, whereas C-IPLPFYN-C demonstrated greater affinity against human than mouse Aβ42. In addition, a preliminary *in vivo* MRI study on a transgenic mouse model of AD, showed both C-FRHMTEQ-C and C-IPLPFYN-C acted as excellent contrast agents (Larbanoix et al., 2010).

USE OF PEPTIDES AS INHIBITORS AGAINST ALZHEIMER'S DISEASE

Peptide Inhibitors of Amyloid β

Amyloid plaque accumulation and Aβ fibrillation are clinical hallmarks of AD (Hajipour et al., 2017), and thus, the inhibition of amyloid aggregation has been the subject of much research over the last two decades, and the use of peptide-based inhibitors represents a major part of these efforts (Goyal et al., 2017; Folch et al., 2018; **Figure 1**). A large number of these studies have focused on the design of peptide fragments capable of binding to Aβ regions critical for aggregation (Ladner et al., 2004). The peptides designed function by binding to Aβ to either prevent fibril formation or Aβ elongation to

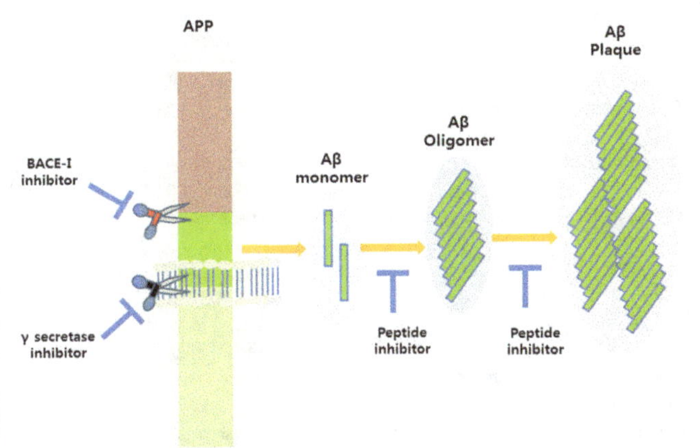

FIGURE 1 | Amyloidogenic amyloid precursor protein (APP) processing and the possible applications of peptide inhibitors to prevent amyloid-beta (Aβ) plaque formation at different disease stages.

prevent the formation of monomers/oligomers. A long list of peptides that specifically target Aβ have been designed (Doig, 2007; Eskici and Gur, 2013), but here, we discuss some of the more recently reported peptides inhibitors of Aβ. **Table 1** shows some of the important peptides described in the literature as inhibitors of AD. Peptide inhibitors that share sequence similar with hydrophobic segments of Aβ are capable of altering Aβ aggregation and reducing the cytotoxicity of Aβ (Wasmer et al., 2008). Austen et al. (2008) described two peptide inhibitors of Aβ, that is, RGKLVFFGR (OR1) and RGKLVFFGR-NH2 (OR2), which were produced by modifying the KLVFF amino acid sequence of Aβ by incorporating RG–/–GR residues at its N- and C-terminals. These inhibitors were both reported to effectively inhibit Aβ fibril formation.

In another study, Wei et al. (2011), reported some new peptide inhibitors based on modifications of the hydrophobic KLVFF amino acid sequence of Aβ, and synthesized a conjugate of the pentapeptide KLVFF and ferrocenoyl (Fc) to improve the lipophilicity and proteolytic stability of peptide inhibitors. In another study, Rangachari et al. (2009) designed two α, β-dehydroalanine (ΔAla) containing peptides based on KLVFF, and found two novel ΔAla-containing peptides (KLVF-ΔA-I-ΔA and KF-ΔA-ΔA-ΔA-F) disrupted Aβ aggregation, though by quite different mechanisms.

Another group of researchers designed and synthesized a decapeptide inhibitor of Aβ1–40 aggregation. This inhibitor (RYYAAFFARR) was designated RR, and unlike other inhibitors was designed to target the extended region of Aβ (Aβ11–23), which consists of a GAG-binding site, a hydrophobic core, and a salt bridge region. RR was found to have high binding affinity for Aβ1–40 (K_d = 1.10 μM), and its binding affinity was markedly greater than that of the known β-sheet breaker peptide iAβ5 (K_d = 156 μM; Liu et al., 2014).

Chalifour et al. (2003) reported results obtained by replacing L-amino acids with D-amino acids with the aims of increase peptide stability and therapeutic potential. The effect of chiral reversal (D-enantiomers) was assessed for five peptides (KKLVFFA, KLVFFA, KIVFFA, KFVFFA and KVVFFA), and it was found they inhibited Aβ aggregation better than L-peptides. In particular, the D-enantiomer of KKLVFFA was found to inhibit the neurotoxic effect of Aβ significantly more than its L counterpart.

Jagota and Rajadas (2013) synthesized three short D-peptides, that is, KKLVFFARRRA, PGKLVYA and KKLVFFA, based on residues of the central hydrophobic core of Aβ (residues 16–20), and examined their effects on Aβ aggregation. Observations suggested these D-peptides effectively inhibited Aβ fibrillogenesis, and two of the three (KKLVFFA and PGKLVYA) were found to improve survival in transgenic *C. elegans*.

β-Site APP Cleaving Enzyme 1 (BACE1)

Beta-site APP cleaving enzyme 1 (BACE1) is a human aspartyl protease, which is believed to play a prime role in the generation of beta amyloid peptides (Aβ) in AD. BACE1 has characteristic bilobal structure and is a membrane-bound aspartyl protease with an open active site, which is less hydrophobic than those of other aspartic proteases and allows up to 11 substrate residues to be accommodated (Hong et al., 2000; Turner et al., 2005). BACE1 levels are elevated in the brain tissues of AD patients and its overexpression in cerebrospinal fluid offers a possible biomarker of early stage disease. When BACE1 is overexpressed it competes with γ-secretase to initiate the cleavage of APP at its β-position. Furthermore, BACE1 inhibition halts Aβ formation at the first step of APP amyloidogenic processing. BACE1 is composed of two signature peptides, that is, DTGS at position 93–96 and DSGT at position 289–292, which come together to form an active site and have the ability to inhibit APP (Yan et al., 2016). Peptides derived from the sequence of BACE1 have also been reported to inhibit APP processing. BACE1 possess a catalytic domain containing a pair of aspartic acid residues at its active site, and Aβ production is blocked by BACE1 inhibition, which reduces Aβ production by depleting C99, acting as a substrate of γ-secretase. The observation that Aβ production was diminished in BACE1 deficient mice supports the view that BACE1 inhibitors reduce Aβ levels (Vassar, 2002).

Glyceraldehyde-3-Phosphate Dehydrogenase (GAPDH)

Glyceraldehyde-3-phosphate dehydrogenase (GAPDH) is a glycolytic enzyme of considerable interest in ND research, especially in AD. Recently, it was revealed that GAPDH interacts with APP, which is known to be involved in AD (Sunaga et al., 1995; Bertram et al., 2007; Butterfield et al., 2010). GAPDH can undergo diverse oxidative modifications that control its structure, function, and activity, and in AD, when exposed to oxidative stress Aβ forms amyloid-like aggregates, which reduce neuron and synapse numbers. Furthermore, insoluble aggregates of GAPDH accelerate Aβ amyloidogenesis and neuronal cell death *in vitro* and *in vivo* (Itakura et al., 2015), and GAPDH aggregation caused by cysteine oxidation and intermolecular disulfide bonding reduces its catalytic

TABLE 1 | List of peptide-based inhibitors reported to be effective against Alzheimer's disease (AD).

Peptides	Description	Reference
RGKLVFFGR (OR1) RGKLVFFGR-NH2 (OR2)	Based on the Aβ (16–20) sequence	Austen et al. (2008)
Fc-KLVFF	Based on the Aβ (16–20) sequence and conjugated with ferrocenoyl (Fc)	Wei et al. (2011)
KLVF-ΔA-I-ΔAKF-ΔA-ΔA-ΔA-F	Based on the Aβ (16–20) sequence and ΔAla	Wei et al. (2011)
RYYAAFFARR	Based on Aβ (11–23)	Liu et al. (2014)
KLVFFA, KKLVFFA, KFVFFA, KIVFFA and KVVFFA	Based on the Aβ (16–20) sequence and replacement of L- with D-amino acids	Chalifour et al. (2003)
PGKLVYA, KKLVFFARRRRA and KKLVFFA	d-peptides of Aβ (16–20)	Jagota and Rajadas (2013)
AuNPs@POMD-pep	Aβ peptide conjugates with gold nanoparticles (AuNPs)	Gao et al. (2015)
IGLMVG-NH2	Based on Aβ (32–37)	Bansal et al. (2016)
HKQLPFFEED	A β-sheet blocker peptide based on the stereochemical structure and characteristic of aggregation of Aβ (1–42)	Lin et al. (2014)
Nonhemolytic 11-residue peptide (NAVRWSLMRPF)	Modified analog of NIVNVSLVK from the E-protein sequence of SARS coronavirus	Ghosh et al. (2017)
AP90	A 23 residue long hairpin peptide (with alternating D- and L-amino acids) reported to inhibit Aβ aggregation.	Kellock et al. (2016)

activity (Nakajima et al., 2007, 2009). Glycyl-L-histidyl-L-lysine-Copper (GHK-Cu) is naturally occurring peptide in human plasma with a stunning array of actions that appear to counter aging-associated diseases and conditions. In plasma the concentration of GHK-Cu is about 200 ng/ml (10^{-7} M^{-1}) at age 20, but decreases to 80 ng/ml at age 60 (Pickart et al., 2015), and interestingly, the enzyme primarily involved in GAPDH gene silencing also belongs to the histone deacetylase (HDACs) protein family. Selective HDAC inhibitors have been shown to possess neuroprotective properties in animal models of brain disease, and have been suggested as potential therapeutics for AD (Fischer et al., 2010). Gly-Pro-Glu (GPE) is present in plasma and brain tissues, and it has been shown to have neuroprotective effects in animal models of NDs, such as, HD, PD and AD (Alexi et al., 1999). Basic structural studies suggest that GPE can interact with single or several Glu receptor types and bind to N-methyl-D-aspartate (NMDA) receptor (Sara et al., 1989). Furthermore, the C-terminal (Glu) GPE is required for NMDA receptor binding and this binding induces the potassium-evoked release of dopamine from nigrostriatal dopaminergic terminals and acetylcholine through an unknown mechanism via NMDA receptor (Sara et al., 1989; Alonso De Diego et al., 2005).

Tyrosine Phosphatase (TP)

STriatal-Enriched tyrosine phosphatase (STEP) is expressed in neurons of the striatum, neocortex, hippocampus and related structures (Pelkey et al., 2002), and targets signaling pathways in the postsynaptic terminals of excitatory glutamatergic synapses (Lombroso et al., 1991; Boulanger et al., 1995). STEP regulates various synaptic actions including glutamate receptor trafficking, which plays critical functions in learning and memory (Karasawa and Lombroso, 2014). Interestingly, it was recently suggested STEP is overactive in AD and schizophrenia (Carty et al., 2012). Endogenous STEP levels also influence the susceptibility of neurons to excitotoxicity and affect the regulation of synaptic proteins by changing synaptic conductivities via the synchronized dephosphorylations of multiple substrates that regulate synaptic plasticity. STEP is an intracellular tyrosine phosphatase (TP) encoded by the *ptpn5* gene, and contains a signature consensus sequence [I/V]HCxAGXXR[S/T]G at its C-terminus that is required for its catalytic activity (Bult et al., 1996), and the active motif (I/V)HCXAGXGR(S/T), also called the P-loop, which houses catalytic Cys for nucleophilic attack is a hallmark of the PTP super-family. Furthermore, a neuroprotective, endogenous tripeptide GPE was reported to protect and rescue cells from Aβ-induced death, and modified analogs of GPE, including modifications at Pro and/or Glu residues, have been synthesized and evaluated (Guan and Gluckman, 2009). Binding of NNZ-2566 (glycyl-L-2-methylprolyl-L-glutamic acid) analogs with Aβ was found to have better neuroprotective effects in infant rats, as compared with GPE (Cacciatore et al., 2012).

Peptide Based Inhibitors Against Potassium Channel KV1.3

Potassium channel KV1.3 was recently identified as a potential target in AD (Rangaraju et al., 2015; Lowinus et al., 2016). Rangaraju et al. (2015) conducted a study on AD and non-AD patients and found Kv1.3 overexpression in the frontal cortices of AD patients, thus suggesting potassium channel KV1.3 to considered a therapeutic target in AD. BmKTX-R11-T28-H33 (ADWX-1), OsK1-K16-D20 and HsTx1 [R14A] are examples of peptides subsequently designed to target Kv1.3 (Norton and Chandy, 2017).

CONCLUSION AND FUTURE PERSPECTIVES

A large amount of research effort has resulted in advancements in the diagnosis and treatment of AD, the etiology of which is considered by most to be explained by the amyloid cascade hypothesis. Furthermore, it is generally considered the early detection of AD is likely to facilitate its treatment using advanced therapeutic approaches, and that the use of peptides for the diagnosis of AD offers an effective means of doing so. Nevertheless, these peptide-based approaches require further development to enable early AD to be efficiently diagnosed and properly treated.

AUTHOR CONTRIBUTIONS

IC and MHB conceived the idea. MHB, KA and GR drafted the review manuscript. IC, MHB, KA and GR critically reviewed the article. IC edited the language and corrected the errors within the manuscript.

REFERENCES

Alexi, T., Hughes, P. E., van Roon-Mom, W. M., Faull, R. L., Williams, C. E., Clark, R. G., et al. (1999). The IGF-I amino-terminal tripeptide glycine-proline-glutamate (GPE) is neuroprotective to striatum in the quinolinic acid lesion animal model of Huntington's disease. *Exp. Neurol.* 159, 84–97. doi: 10.1006/exnr.1999.7168

Alonso De Diego, S. A., Muñoz, P., González-Muñiz, R., Herranz, R., Martín-Martínez, M., Cenarruzabeitia, E., et al. (2005). Analogues of the neuroprotective tripeptide Gly-Pro-Glu (GPE): synthesis and structure-activity relationships. *Bioorg. Med. Chem. Lett.* 15, 2279–2283. doi: 10.1016/j.bmcl.2005.03.015

Alzheimer's Association. (2017). Alzheimer's disease facts and figures. *Alzheimers Dement.* 13, 325–373. doi: 10.1016/j.jalz.2017.02.001

Austen, B. M., Paleologou, K. E., Ali, S. A., Qureshi, M. M., Allsop, D., and El-Agnaf, O. M. (2008). Designing peptide inhibitors for oligomerization and toxicity of Alzheimer's β-amyloid peptide. *Biochemistry* 47, 1984–1992. doi: 10.1021/bi701415b

Bansal, S., Maurya, I. K., Yadav, N., Thota, C. K., Kumar, V., Tikoo, K., et al. (2016). C-terminal fragment, Aβ32–37, analogues protect against aβ aggregation-induced toxicity. *ACS Chem. Neurosci.* 7, 615–623. doi: 10.1021/acschemneuro.6b00006

Bertram, L., McQueen, M. B., Mullin, K., Blacker, D., and Tanzi, R. E. (2007). Systematic meta-analyses of Alzheimer disease genetic association studies: the AlzGene database. *Nat. Genet.* 39, 17–23. doi: 10.1038/ng1934

Boulanger, L. M., Lombroso, P. J., Raghunathan, A., During, M. J., Wahle, P., and Naegele, J. R. (1995). Cellular and molecular characterization of a brain-enriched protein tyrosine phosphatase. *J. Neurosci.* 15, 1532–1544.

Bult, A., Zhao, F., Dirkx, R. Jr., Sharma, E., Lukacsi, E., Solimena, M., et al. (1996). STEP61: a member of a family of brain-enriched PTPs is localized to the endoplasmic reticulum. *J. Neurosci.* 16, 7821–7831.

Butterfield, D. A., Hardas, S. S., and Lange, M. L. (2010). Oxidatively modified glyceraldehyde-3-phosphate dehydrogenase (GAPDH) and Alzheimer's disease: many pathways to neurodegeneration. *J. Alzheimers Dis.* 20, 369–393. doi: 10.3233/JAD-2010-1375

Cacciatore, I., Cornacchia, C., Baldassarre, L., Fornasari, E., Mollica, A., Stefanucci, A., et al. (2012). GPE and GPE analogues as promising neuroprotective agents. *Mini Rev. Med. Chem.* 12, 13–23. doi: 10.2174/138955712798868995

Carty, N. C., Xu, J., Kurup, P., Brouillette, J., Goebel-Goody, S. M., Austin, D. R., et al. (2012). The tyrosine phosphatase STEP: implications in schizophrenia and the molecular mechanism underlying antipsychotic medications. *Transl. Psychiatry* 2:e137. doi: 10.1038/tp.2012.63

Chalifour, R. J., McLaughlin, R. W., Lavoie, L., Morissette, C., Tremblay, N., Boule, M., et al. (2003). Stereoselective interactions of peptide inhibitors with the β-amyloid peptide. *J. Biol. Chem.* 278, 34874–34881. doi: 10.1074/jbc.M212694200

Cheng, Y. S., Chen, Z. T., Liao, T. Y., Lin, C., Shen, H. C., Wang, Y. H., et al. (2017). An intranasally delivered peptide drug ameliorates cognitive decline in Alzheimer transgenic mice. *EMBO Mol. Med.* 9, 703–715. doi: 10.15252/emmm.201606666

Craik, D. J., Fairlie, D. P., Liras, S., and Price, D. (2013). The future of peptide-based drugs. *Chem. Biol. Drug Des.* 81, 136–147. doi: 10.1111/cbdd.12055

Doig, A. J. (2007). Peptide inhibitors of β-amyloid aggregation. *Curr. Opin. Drug Discov. Devel.* 10, 533–539.

Drachman, D. A. (2014). The amyloid hypothesis, time to move on: amyloid is the downstream result, not cause, of Alzheimer's disease. *Alzheimers Dement.* 10, 372–380. doi: 10.1016/j.jalz.2013.11.003

Eskici, G., and Gur, M. (2013). Computational design of new Peptide inhibitors for amyloid β (Aβ) aggregation in Alzheimer's disease: application of a novel methodology. *PLoS One* 8:e66178. doi: 10.1371/journal.pone.0066178

Extance, A. (2010). Alzheimer's failure raises questions about disease-modifying strategies. *Nat. Rev. Drug Discov.* 9, 749–751. doi: 10.1038/nrd3288

Fischer, A., Sananbenesi, F., Mungenast, A., and Tsai, L. H. (2010). Targeting the correct HDAC(s) to treat cognitive disorders. *Trends Pharmacol. Sci.* 31, 605–617. doi: 10.1016/j.tips.2010.09.003

Folch, J., Ettcheto, M., Petrov, D., Abad, S., Pedrós, I., Marin, M., et al. (2018). Review of the advances in treatment for Alzheimer disease: strategies for combating β-amyloid protein. *Neurologia* 33, 47–58. doi: 10.1016/j.nrl.2015.03.012

Frisoni, G. B., Boccardi, M., Barkhof, F., Blennow, K., Cappa, S., Chiotis, K., et al. (2017). Strategic roadmap for an early diagnosis of Alzheimer's disease based on biomarkers. *Lancet Neurol.* 16, 661–676. doi: 10.1016/S1474-4422(17)30159-X

Funke, S. A., Bartnik, D., Glück, J. M., Piorkowska, K., Wiesehan, K., Weber, U., et al. (2012). Development of a small D-enantiomeric Alzheimer's amyloid-β binding peptide ligand for future *in vivo* imaging applications. *PLoS One* 7:e41457. doi: 10.1371/journal.pone.0041457

Funke, S. A., and Willbold, D. (2012). Peptides for therapy and diagnosis of Alzheimer's disease. *Curr. Pharm. Des.* 18, 755–767. doi: 10.2174/138161212799277752

Gao, N., Sun, H., Dong, K., Ren, J., and Qu, X. (2015). Gold-nanoparticle-based multifunctional amyloid-β inhibitor against Alzheimer's disease. *Chemistry* 21, 829–835. doi: 10.1002/chem.201404562

Ghosh, A., Pradhan, N., Bera, S., Datta, A., Krishnamoorthy, J., Jana, N. R., et al. (2017). Inhibition and degradation of amyloid β (Aβ40) fibrillation by designed small peptide: a combined spectroscopy, microscopy, and cell toxicity study. *ACS Chem. Neurosci.* 8, 718–722. doi: 10.1021/acschemneuro.6b00349

Goyal, D., Shuaib, S., Mann, S., and Goyal, B. (2017). Rationally designed peptides and peptidomimetics as inhibitors of amyloid-β (Aβ) aggregation: potential therapeutics of Alzheimer's disease. *ACS Comb. Sci.* 19, 55–80. doi: 10.1021/acscombsci.6b00116

Grundman, M., Dibernardo, A., Raghavan, N., Krams, M., and Yuen, E. (2013). 2012: a watershed year for Alzheimer's disease research. *J. Nutr. Health Aging* 17, 51–53. doi: 10.1007/s12603-013-0002-2

Guan, J., and Gluckman, P. D. (2009). IGF-1 derived small neuropeptides and analogues: a novel strategy for the development of pharmaceuticals for neurological conditions. *Br. J. Pharmacol.* 157, 881–891. doi: 10.1111/j.1476-5381.2009.00256.x

Gulyás, B., Spenger, C., Beliczai, Z., Gulya, K., Kása, P., Jahan, M., et al. (2012). Distribution and binding of ^{18}F-labeled and ^{125}I-labeled analogues of ACI-80, a prospective molecular imaging biomarker of disease: a whole hemisphere post mortem autoradiography study in human brains obtained from Alzheimer's disease patients. *Neurochem. Int.* 60, 153–162. doi: 10.1016/j.neuint.2011.10.010

Haass, C., and Selkoe, D. J. (2007). Soluble protein oligomers in neurodegeneration: lessons from the Alzheimer's amyloid β-peptide. *Nat. Rev. Mol. Cell Biol.* 8, 101–112. doi: 10.1038/nrm2101

Hajipour, M. J., Santoso, M. R., Rezaee, F., Aghaverdi, H., Mahmoudi, M., and Perry, G. (2017). Advances in Alzheimer's diagnosis and therapy: the implications of nanotechnology. *Trends Biotechnol.* 35, 937–953. doi: 10.1016/j.tibtech.2017.06.002

Herrup, K. (2015). The case for rejecting the amyloid cascade hypothesis. *Nat. Neurosci.* 18, 794–799. doi: 10.1038/nn.4017

Hong, L., Koelsch, G., Lin, X., Wu, S., Terzyan, S., Ghosh, A. K., et al. (2000). Structure of the protease domain of memapsin 2 (β-secretase) complexed with inhibitor. *Science* 290, 150–153. doi: 10.1126/science.290.5489.150

Itakura, M., Nakajima, H., Kubo, T., Semi, Y., Kume, S., Higashida, S., et al. (2015). Glyceraldehyde-3-phosphate dehydrogenase aggregates accelerate amyloid-β amyloidogenesis in Alzheimer disease. *J. Biol. Chem.* 290, 26072–26087. doi: 10.1074/jbc.M115.669291

Jagota, S., and Rajadas, J. (2013). Synthesis of D-amino acid peptides and their effect on β-amyloid aggregation and toxicity in transgenic *Caenorhabditis elegans*. *Med. Chem. Res.* 22, 3991–4000. doi: 10.1007/s00044-012-0386-2

Jonsson, T., Atwal, J. K., Steinberg, S., Snaedal, J., Jonsson, P. V., Bjornsson, S., et al. (2012). A mutation in APP protects against Alzheimer's disease and age-related cognitive decline. *Nature* 488, 96–99. doi: 10.1038/nature11283

Kang, C. K., Jayasinha, V., and Martin, P. T. (2003). Identification of peptides that specifically bind $A\beta_{1-40}$ amyloid *in vitro* and amyloid plaques in Alzheimer's disease brain using phage display. *Neurobiol. Dis.* 14, 146–156. doi: 10.1016/s0969-9961(03)00105-0

Karasawa, T., and Lombroso, P. J. (2014). Disruption of striatal-enriched protein tyrosine phosphatase (STEP) function in neuropsychiatric disorders. *Neurosci. Res.* 89, 1–9. doi: 10.1016/j.neures.2014.08.018

Kellock, J., Hopping, G., Caughey, B., and Daggett, V. (2016). Peptides composed of alternating L- and D-amino acids inhibit amyloidogenesis in three distinct amyloid systems independent of sequence. *J. Mol. Biol.* 428, 2317–2328. doi: 10.1016/j.jmb.2016.03.013

Ladner, R. C., Sato, A. K., Gorzelany, J., and de Souza, M. (2004). Phage display-derived peptides as therapeutic alternatives to antibodies. *Drug Discov. Today* 9, 525–529. doi: 10.1016/s1359-6446(04)03104-6

Larbanoix, L., Burtea, C., Laurent, S., Van Leuven, F., Toubeau, G., Vander Elst, L., et al. (2010). Potential amyloid plaque-specific peptides for the diagnosis of Alzheimer's disease. *Neurobiol. Aging* 31, 1679–1689. doi: 10.1016/j.neurobiolaging.2008.09.021

Li, C.-z., Grajales, S., Shuang, S., Dong, C., and Nair, M. (2017). β-amyloid biomarker detection for Alzheimer's disease. *Zhonghua Yi Xue Za Zhi* 1:15. doi: 10.1007/s41664-017-0014-8

Lin, L. X., Bo, X. Y., Tan, Y. Z., Sun, F. X., Song, M., Zhao, J., et al. (2014). Feasibility of β-sheet breaker peptide-H102 treatment for Alzheimer's disease based on β-amyloid hypothesis. *PLoS One* 9:e112052. doi: 10.1371/journal.pone.0112052

Liu, J., Wang, W., Zhang, Q., Zhang, S., and Yuan, Z. (2014). Study on the efficiency and interaction mechanism of a decapeptide inhibitor of β-amyloid aggregation. *Biomacromolecules* 15, 931–939. doi: 10.1021/bm401795e

Lombroso, P. J., Murdoch, G., and Lerner, M. (1991). Molecular characterization of a protein-tyrosine-phosphatase enriched in striatum. *Proc. Natl. Acad. Sci. U S A* 88, 7242–7246. doi: 10.1073/pnas.88.16.7242

Lowinus, T., Bose, T., Busse, S., Busse, M., Reinhold, D., Schraven, B., et al. (2016). Immunomodulation by memantine in therapy of Alzheimer's disease is mediated through inhibition of Kv1.3 channels and T cell responsiveness. *Oncotarget* 7, 53797–53807. doi: 10.18632/oncotarget.10777

Mandal, S. M., Roy, A., Ghosh, A. K., Hazra, T. K., Basak, A., and Franco, O. L. (2014). Challenges and future prospects of antibiotic therapy: from peptides to phages utilization. *Front. Pharmacol.* 5:105. doi: 10.3389/fphar.2014.00105

Nakajima, H., Amano, W., Fujita, A., Fukuhara, A., Azuma, Y. T., Hata, F., et al. (2007). The active site cysteine of the proapoptotic protein glyceraldehyde-3-phosphate dehydrogenase is essential in oxidative stress-induced aggregation and cell death. *J. Biol. Chem.* 282, 26562–26574. doi: 10.1074/jbc.M704199200

Nakajima, H., Amano, W., Kubo, T., Fukuhara, A., Ihara, H., Azuma, Y. T., et al. (2009). Glyceraldehyde-3-phosphate dehydrogenase aggregate formation participates in oxidative stress-induced cell death. *J. Biol. Chem.* 284, 34331–34341. doi: 10.1074/jbc.M109.027698

Norton, R. S., and Chandy, K. G. (2017). Venom-derived peptide inhibitors of voltage-gated potassium channels. *Neuropharmacology* 127, 124–138. doi: 10.1016/j.neuropharm.2017.07.002

Pelkey, K. A., Askalan, R., Paul, S., Kalia, L. V., Nguyen, T. H., Pitcher, G. M., et al. (2002). Tyrosine phosphatase STEP is a tonic brake on induction of long-term potentiation. *Neuron* 34, 127–138. doi: 10.1016/s0896-6273(02)00633-5

Pickart, L., Vasquez-Soltero, J. M., and Margolina, A. (2015). GHK peptide as a natural modulator of multiple cellular pathways in skin regeneration. *Biomed. Res. Int.* 2015:648108. doi: 10.1155/2015/648108

Rangachari, V., Davey, Z. S., Healy, B., Moore, B. D., Sonoda, L. K., Cusack, B., et al. (2009). Rationally designed dehydroalanine ($^{\Delta}$Ala)-containing peptides inhibit amyloid-β (Aβ) peptide aggregation. *Biopolymers* 91, 456–465. doi: 10.1002/bip.21151

Rangaraju, S., Gearing, M., Jin, L. W., and Levey, A. (2015). Potassium channel Kv1.3 is highly expressed by microglia in human Alzheimer's disease. *J. Alzheimers Dis.* 44, 797–808. doi: 10.3233/JAD-141704

Sara, V. R., Carlsson-Skwirut, C., Bergman, T., Jornvall, H., Roberts, P. J., Crawford, M., et al. (1989). Identification of Gly-Pro-Glu (GPE), the aminoterminal tripeptide of insulin-like growth factor 1 which is truncated in brain, as a novel neuroactive peptide. *Biochem. Biophys. Res. Commun.* 165, 766–771. doi: 10.1016/s0006-291x(89)80032-4

Shankar, G. M., Li, S., Mehta, T. H., Garcia-Munoz, A., Shepardson, N. E., Smith, I., et al. (2008). Amyloid-β protein dimers isolated directly from Alzheimer's brains impair synaptic plasticity and memory. *Nat. Med.* 14, 837–842. doi: 10.1038/nm1782

Silverman, W., Wisniewski, H. M., Bobinski, M., and Wegiel, J. (1997). Frequency of stages of Alzheimer-related lesions in different age categories. *Neurobiol. Aging* 18, 377–379; discussion 389–392. doi: 10.1016/s0197-4580(97)00051-1

Sunaga, K., Takahashi, H., Chuang, D. M., and Ishitani, R. (1995). Glyceraldehyde-3-phosphate dehydrogenase is over-expressed during apoptotic death of neuronal cultures and is recognized by a monoclonal antibody against amyloid plaques from Alzheimer's brain. *Neurosci. Lett.* 200, 133–136. doi: 10.1016/0304-3940(95)12098-o

Thal, D. R., Rub, U., Orantes, M., and Braak, H. (2002). Phases of A β-deposition in the human brain and its relevance for the development of AD. *Neurology* 58, 1791–1800. doi: 10.1212/WNL.58.12.1791

Turner, R. T. III., Hong, L., Koelsch, G., Ghosh, A. K., and Tang, J. (2005). Structural locations and functional roles of new subsites S5, S6, and S7 in memapsin 2 (β-secretase). *Biochemistry* 44, 105–112. doi: 10.1021/bi048106k

van Groen, T., Kadish, I., Wiesehan, K., Funke, S. A., and Willbold, D. (2009). *In vitro* and *in vivo* staining characteristics of small, fluorescent, Aβ42-binding D-enantiomeric peptides in transgenic AD mouse models. *ChemMedChem* 4, 276–282. doi: 10.1002/cmdc.200800289

VanItallie, T. B. (2015). Biomarkers, ketone bodies and the prevention of Alzheimer's disease. *Metabolism* 64, S51–S57. doi: 10.1016/j.metabol.2014.10.033

Vassar, R. (2002). β-secretase (BACE) as a drug target for Alzheimer's disease. *Adv. Drug Deliv. Rev.* 54, 1589–1602. doi: 10.1016/S0169-409X(02)00157-6

Vlieghe, P., Lisowski, V., Martinez, J., and Khrestchatisky, M. (2010). Synthetic therapeutic peptides: science and market. *Drug Discov. Today* 15, 40–56. doi: 10.1016/j.drudis.2009.10.009

Wasmer, C., Lange, A., Van Melckebeke, H., Siemer, A. B., Riek, R., and Meier, B. H. (2008). Amyloid fibrils of the HET-s(218–289) prion form a β solenoid with a triangular hydrophobic core. *Science* 319, 1523–1526. doi: 10.1126/science.1151839

Wei, C. W., Peng, Y., Zhang, L., Huang, Q., Cheng, M., Liu, Y. N., et al. (2011). Synthesis and evaluation of ferrocenoyl pentapeptide (Fc-KLVFF) as an inhibitor of Alzheimer's $A\beta_{1-42}$ fibril formation *in vitro*. *Bioorg. Med. Chem. Lett.* 21, 5818–5821. doi: 10.1016/j.bmcl.2011.07.111

Yan, R., Fan, Q., Zhou, J., and Vassar, R. (2016). Inhibiting BACE1 to reverse synaptic dysfunctions in Alzheimer's disease. *Neurosci. Biobehav. Rev.* 65, 326–340. doi: 10.1016/j.neubiorev.2016.03.025

7

Analyzing the Behavior of Neuronal Pathways in Alzheimer's Disease Using Petri Net Modeling Approach

Javaria Ashraf[1], Jamil Ahmad[1], Amjad Ali[2] and Zaheer Ul-Haq[3]*

[1] *Research Center for Modeling and Simulation, National University of Sciences and Technology, Islamabad, Pakistan,*
[2] *Atta-Ur-Rahman School of Applied Biosciences, National University of Sciences and Technology, Islamabad, Pakistan,*
[3] *Dr. Panjwani Center for Molecular Medicine and Drug Research, International Center for Chemical Sciences, University of Karachi, Karachi, Pakistan*

***Correspondence:**
Jamil Ahmad
jamil.ahmad@rcms.nust.edu.pk

Alzheimer's Disease (AD) is the most common neuro-degenerative disorder in the elderly that leads to dementia. The hallmark of AD is senile lesions made by abnormal aggregation of amyloid beta in extracellular space of brain. One of the challenges in AD treatment is to better understand the mechanism of action of key proteins and their related pathways involved in neuronal cell death in order to identify adequate therapeutic targets. This study focuses on the phenomenon of aggregation of amyloid beta into plaques by considering the signal transduction pathways of Calpain-Calpastatin (CAST) regulation system and Amyloid Precursor Protein (APP) processing pathways along with Ca^{2+} channels. These pathways are modeled and analyzed individually as well as collectively through Stochastic Petri Nets for comprehensive analysis and thorough understating of AD. The model predicts that the deregulation of Calpain activity, disruption of Calcium homeostasis, inhibition of CAST and elevation of abnormal APP processing are key cytotoxic events resulting in an early AD onset and progression. Interestingly, the model also reveals that plaques accumulation start early (at the age of 40) in life but symptoms appear late. These results suggest that the process of neuro-degeneration can be slowed down or paused by slowing down the degradation rate of Calpain-CAST Complex. In the light of this study, the suggestive therapeutic strategy might be the prevention of the degradation of Calpain-CAST complexes and the inhibition of Calpain for the treatment of neurodegenerative diseases such as AD.

Keywords: Calpain, CAST, calcium, PKC, APP, Stochastic petri net, Alzheimer disease, Amyloid beta

1. INTRODUCTION

Alzheimer's disease (AD) is a neurodegenerative disorder which has impacted nearly 44 million[1] people around the world and this number is still increasing. AD is the leading cause of dementia in the old age (Ashford, 2004). Unfortunately, it is diagnosed only in one out of four people living with the disease[1]. Clinical characterization of AD includes memory loss and cognitive impairment which further lead to damaged behavioral activities and render a person completely dependent

[1] http://www.alzheimers.net/resources/alzheimers-statistics/

on an external aid (Budson and Price, 2005). AD establishes over time with the appearance of pathological emblems which are senile plaques and neurofibrillary tangles. These lesions comprise of extracellular deposits of Amyloid beta ($A\beta$) (Selkoe, 2000; Golde, 2005; Tam and Pasternak, 2012) and intracellular self-gathered clumps of tau proteins (Lee et al., 2001), respectively. $A\beta$ is a 40–42 amino-acids long peptide which is formed after the proteolytic cleavage of Amyloid Precursor Protein (APP) (Selkoe, 2000; Golde, 2005; Tam and Pasternak, 2012). Previous studies have shown that $A\beta$ monomers are initially non-toxic but their conversion to oligomers makes them toxic (Volles and Lansbury, 2002; Walsh and Selkoe, 2004). Eventually, the abnormal accumulation of oligomers form plaques (Walsh et al., 2002) that deposit into neuronal Endoplasmic Reticulum (ER) (Cuello, 2005) and in extracellular space (Trojanowski and Lee, 2000; Walsh et al., 2000). Aggregation of senile plaques and neurofibrillary tangles cause neuronal cell death and synaptic failure (Tiraboschi et al., 2000; Selkoe, 2002). During the last two decades, several lines of studies have pointed toward the imbalance between $A\beta$ production and its clearance plays a central role in pathogenesis of AD. Since 1992, this hypothesis has earned acquiescence (Hardy and Higgins, 1992) and is known as "***Amyloid cascade hypothesis (ACH)***". It suggests that $A\beta$ and processing of APP are crucial in neuro-degeneration. In AD, aggregation of $A\beta$ is the first step leading toward the formation of senile plaques (Hardy and Selkoe, 2002; Vassar, 2005). APP is a typeI trans-membrane protein produced in ER (Greenfield et al., 1999; Roussel et al., 2013). In neurons, production and metabolism of APP occurs rapidly which makes it a crucial element in neuro-pathogenesis (Lee et al., 2008). The main APP proteolytic processing steps occur at the cell surface and Trans-Golgi networks (TGNs). Proteolysis of APP can occur through the so-called *non-amyloidogenic* and *amyloidogenic Pathways* (**Figure 1**). The first step of non-amyloidogenic pathway is carried out by the enzyme alpha (α)-secretase that breaks down APP into soluble Amyloid precursor protein alpha (sAPPα) and alpha C-terminal fragment (αCTF / CTF83). The catalysis by α-secretase is imperative as it cuts APP within $A\beta$ domain which blocks $A\beta$ formation (Lichtenthaler, 2011). This initial step can also be driven by the beta (β)-secretase / β-site APP-cleaving enzyme (BACE), a transmembrane aspartyl protease (Vassar et al., 1999; Haass, 2004) (**Figure 1**), which constitute amyloidogenic pathway. BACE is a crucial enzyme, that acts as a rate limiting protein in $A\beta$ generation. It breaks down the APP into soluble Amyloid precursor protein beta (sAPPβ) and beta C-terminal fragments (βCTF / CTF99) (Cai et al., 2001). The CTFs are intermediate products of the first step in both pathways which remain attached to the membrane and they are further cleaved by

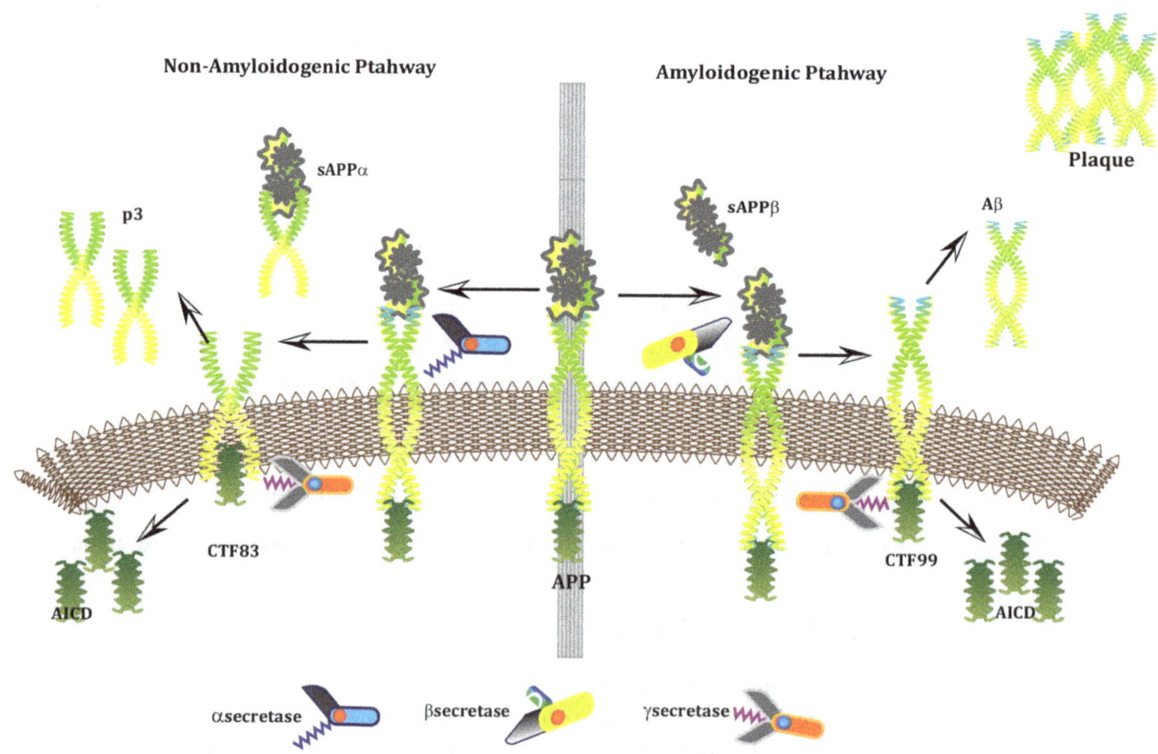

FIGURE 1 | APP and processing products: APP is synthesized in the ER and then transported to the trans-Golgi-network (TGN) where it is cleaved by secretases. In non-amyloidogenic pathway (**left**), cleavage of APP by α-secretase results in the generation of sAPPα and C-terminal fragments CTF83 which is further cleaved by γ-secretase into p3 and AICD. Proteolysis by α-secretase prevents $A\beta$ production as the cleavage site in APP is within the $A\beta$ domain. In amyloidogenic pathway (**right**), APP is cleaved into sAPPβ and CTF99 by β–secretase / BACE activity. Furthermore, CTF99 breaks down into AICD and $A\beta$ by γ-secretase activity. $A\beta$ fragments oligomerize and fibrillize into plaques.

gamma (γ)-secretase (Zhang et al., 2011). In non-amyliodogenic pathway, the fragment α-CTF is cut down by γ-secretase into p38 and the Amyloid Precursor Protein Intracellular Cytoplasmic / C-terminal Domain (AICD). While in amyloidogenic pathway, γ-secretase degrades the βCTF into $A\beta$ and AICD (O'Brien and Wong, 2011) (**Figure 1**).

The Biological Regulatory Networks (BRN) of APP processing, depicted in **Figure 2**, is also built from **Figure 1**. APP processing depends on sequential cleavage by three secretases (α/β-secretase and γ-secretase). In normal conditions, α-secretase residing at the plasma membrane is constitutively active for APP coming to the cell surface and thus favoring non-amyloidogenic pathway (De Strooper and Annaert, 2000). Though there is an interesting fact about APP proteolysis that none of the secretases show special substrate specificity toward APP. There are several transmembrane proteins such as cell surface receptors and ligand, growth factors and cytokines besides APP which undergo ectodomain shedding by enzymes with α-secretase activity (Annaert and Saftig, 2009). In the same manner, BACE shows low affinity toward APP and it is not its exclusive physiological substrate (DeStrooper et al., 2006; Hu et al., 2006). Many observations highlight that in healthy cells APP is frequently processed through non-amyloidogenic pathway to resist amyloid generation while it is altered in pathological conditions (De Strooper and Annaert, 2000). Abnormal processing of APP is stated to be the first and fundamental step in plaques formation in AD pathogenesis (Jonsson et al., 2012). In neuropathological conditions, BACE affinity toward APP increases two folds which leads to enhanced $A\beta$ production (Yang et al., 2003; Li and Südhof, 2004). Recent studies on transgenic mice model have shown that BACE activity is modulated by Calpain activation in AD pathology (Liang et al., 2010). Calpain-Calpastatin system also plays a key role in neurodegeneration. Transgenic mice models have shown that over expression of APP, increased production of $A\beta$, inhibition of Calpastatin (CAST) and activation of Calpain increase neuronal degeneration in AD (Higuchi et al., 2012).

Calpains are protein clan of cysteine/ thiol proteases and their activity depends on Ca^{2+} concentration (Ferreira, 2012). The most studied Calpains, mu(μ)-Calpain (Calpain1) and m-Calpain (Calpain2) are present abundantly in neurons, central nervous system (CNS) and glial cells. Though their distribution differs, Calpain1 is ubiquitous and expressed more in neurons while Calpain2 is present in glial cells (Ono and Sorimachi, 2012; Santos et al., 2012). Calpain1 requires micro-molar concentration of Ca^{2+} (10–50μM), while Calpain2 is activated by mili-molar concentration of Ca^{2+} (250–350μM) *in vitro* (Goll et al., 2003; Ryu and Nakazawa, 2014). Ca^{2+} plays important role in ensuring the cell's vital functions. In addition to calcium, Calpain is tightly regulated in the cell by CAST which is also ubiquitous and solely

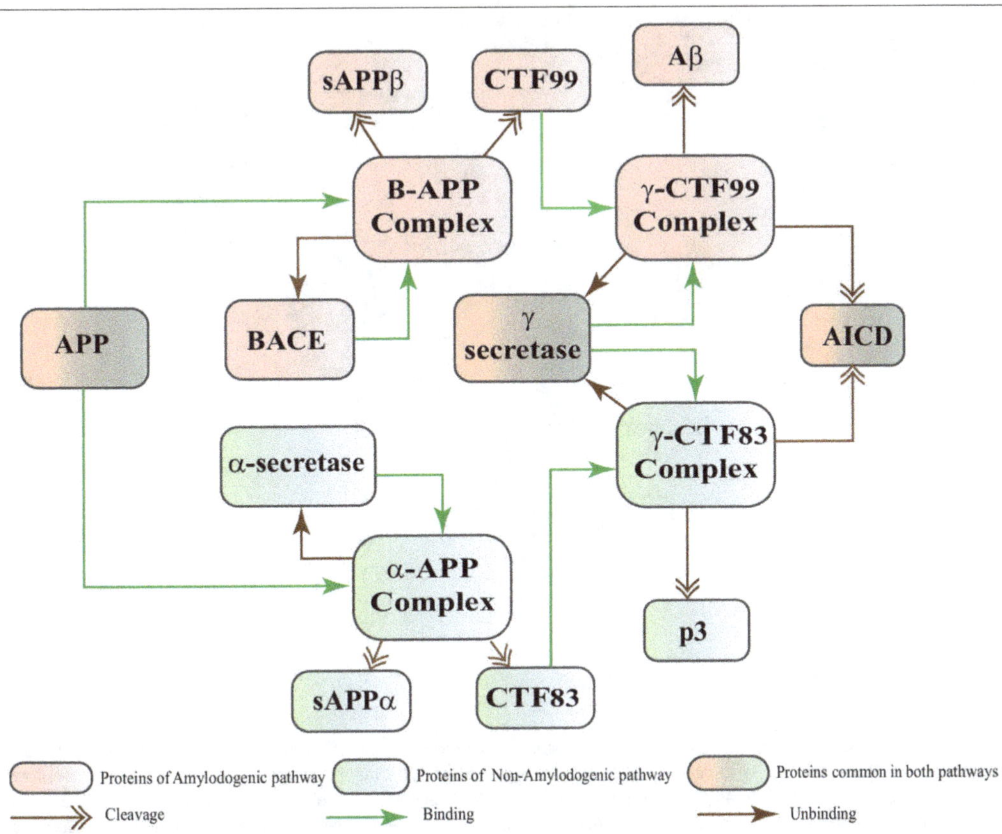

FIGURE 2 | APP processing pathways BRN derived from **Figure 1**.

a specific endogenous inhibitor for both Calpains (Melloni et al., 2006).

CAST is reported as an explicit suicide substrate for Calpain (Yang et al., 2013). The proportion of CAST in a cell is normally larger than Calpain, its ratio with location is crucial in controlling the extent of activation of Calpain within a cell (Todd et al., 2003). CAST interacts with Calpain at different stages i.e., first it constrains Calpain at the membrane where pro-Calpain is attached then it interacts with active Calpain inside cytosol (Hanna et al., 2008). CAST forms a reversible complex with Calpain at both the sites. At membrane, the reversible complex breaks down when Ca^{2+} influx increases to release Calpain. Inside cytosol, Calpain undergoes autolysis to attain active conformation. In response, CAST changes its cellular distribution to make itself widely available in the cytoplasm to counter active Calpain (Todd et al., 2003). Both active Calpain and CAST rejoin in a reversible complex to resist persistent activity of Calpain (De Tullio et al., 1999). Active Calpain modulates CAST by slowly digesting it into small inactive fragments which results in plethora of Calpain in cell leading to pathological condition (Averna et al., 2001b; Tompa et al., 2002) (**Figure 3**). It has been reported that in AD CAST becomes depleted from different regions of the brain as compared to healthy aged brain (Rao et al., 2008). It has also been observed that by controlling Calpain, CAST is indirectly preventing cell membrane damages induced by high Ca^{2+} and $A\beta$ peptide (Vaisid et al., 2008).

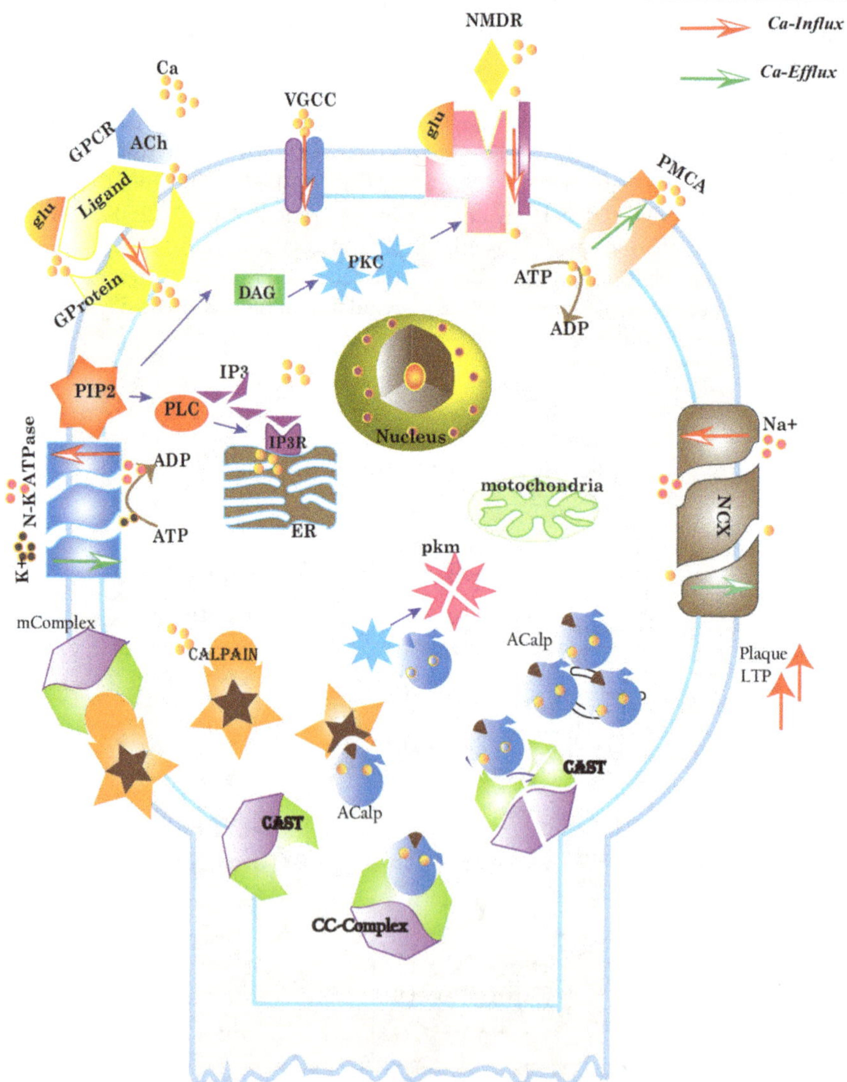

FIGURE 3 | Different calcium channels work in harmony to establish homeostasis in neurons. Calcium influx is controlled by voltage gated (*VGCCs*) or receptor-ligand based (*NMDAR*, *GPCR*) channels. *ER* also release Ca^{2+} into the cytoplasm through inositol-1,4,5-trisphosphate (*IP3R*) and ryanodine receptors. Calcium efflux is carried out by energy (*ATP*) dependent channels such as plasma membrane calcium ATPase (*PMCA*), sodium-potassium ATPase (*NKA*) and sodium-calcium exchanger (*NCX*) channels. Calcium homeostasis influences Calpain-CAST system. At membrane, Calpain is bound to CAST to form *mComplex* at low Ca^{2+} level. At high Ca^{2+} concentration, Calpain is released into cytoplasm and autolysed to active form *ACalp* that again forms complex with CAST (*cComplex*). Gradually the complex breaks down and releases *ACalp* which enhances *Plaque* accumulation and *LTP* events.

CAST pool is regulated by reversible phosphorylation via PKC, which is a Ca^{2+}-activated phospholipid dependent kinase. Moreover, it is de-phosphorylated by protein phosphatases (ppase) (Melloni et al., 2006). Phosphorylation control CAST inhibitory efficiency in brain (Averna et al., 2001a) to regulate its availability for calpain inhibition. Reversible protein phosphorylation regulates many neuronal functions and is important for neuronal signal transduction (Wu and Lynch, 2006). Inactive PKC is converted to Ca^{2+}-bound activated form in the presence of diacylglycerol (DAG) which in turn is activated by receptor based hydrolysis of phosphoinositides 3 (IP3) (Courjaret et al., 2003). The N-terminal region of CAST which is responsible for the function of the protein has a site for phosphorylation by PKC. CAST is phosphorylated by PKC to decrease its inhibitory efficiency toward calpain (Averna et al., 2001a) (**Figure 3**). It has been observed that PKC also regulates APP processing by activating α-secretase (Rossner et al., 2001; Racchi et al., 2003), it promotes non-amylodogenic pathway over β-secretase (Lanni et al., 2004). *In vivo* studies show that in the presence of PKC, secretion of sAPPα increases and $A\beta$ secretion declines (Chen and Fernandez, 2004). Other studies about AD found that PKC has substantial role in AD pathology (Etcheberrigaray et al., 2004; Alkon et al., 2007). Active Calpain also interacts with PKC and converts it into constitutive active enzyme (Yamakawa et al., 2001; Goll et al., 2003). Calpain1 directly starts depletion of PKC from cell by converting it into protein kinase M (PKM) (Yamakawa et al., 2001; Liu et al., 2008). The whole mechanism is also depicted in the form of Calpain-CAST system BRN in **Figure 4**.

The dysregulation of Calcium homeostasis contributes in aging and neurodegeneration (Mattson, 2004; Smith et al., 2005; Stutzmann, 2005). A tremendous deal of work by calcium is tightly regulated in time, space and intensity by intracellular stores, influx and efflux channels (Stutzmann, 2005). At resting stage, extracellular Ca^{2+} concentration ranges from 1.5 to 2.0 mM (Orrenius et al., 2003). While magnitude of Ca^{2+} inside a cell is very low (between 50–100/ 50–300 nM) (LaFerla, 2002; Orrenius et al., 2003) and after activation it can rise to several micromoles. On contrary, inside ER, the level of Ca^{2+} is in the range 100-500μM (LaFerla, 2002) which is approximately 1000 times higher than cytosol concentration at the resting phase. Persistent alteration of Ca^{2+} homeostasis affects production and digestion of pathological proteins such as Calpain, $A\beta$ and tau protein. Dysregulation of cellular Ca^{2+} level is an early and main feature of AD (Mattson et al., 2000; LaFerla, 2002; Small, 2009).

Cytosolic Ca^{2+} is maintained at very low level as compared to extracellular space through several homeostatic mechanisms, working both temporally and spatially (**Figure 3**). These equilibrating apparatuses include voltage-operated channels (VOCs) and receptor operated channels (ROCs) for Ca^{2+} inclusion, Ca^{2+} storage in organelles e.g., ER (Wojda et al., 2008) and Ca^{2+} extrusion to extracellular space. Different ATP-dependent membrane pumps such as plasma membrane calcium ATPase channel (PMCA) and sodium-calcium exchanger (NCX) which are dependent on sodium-potassium ATPase (NKA) (Wojda et al., 2008; Brittain et al., 2012) are used for Ca^{2+} efflux. In different physiological processes, elevation of Ca^{2+} is necessary to switch-on respective proteins. Ca^{2+} inclusion is

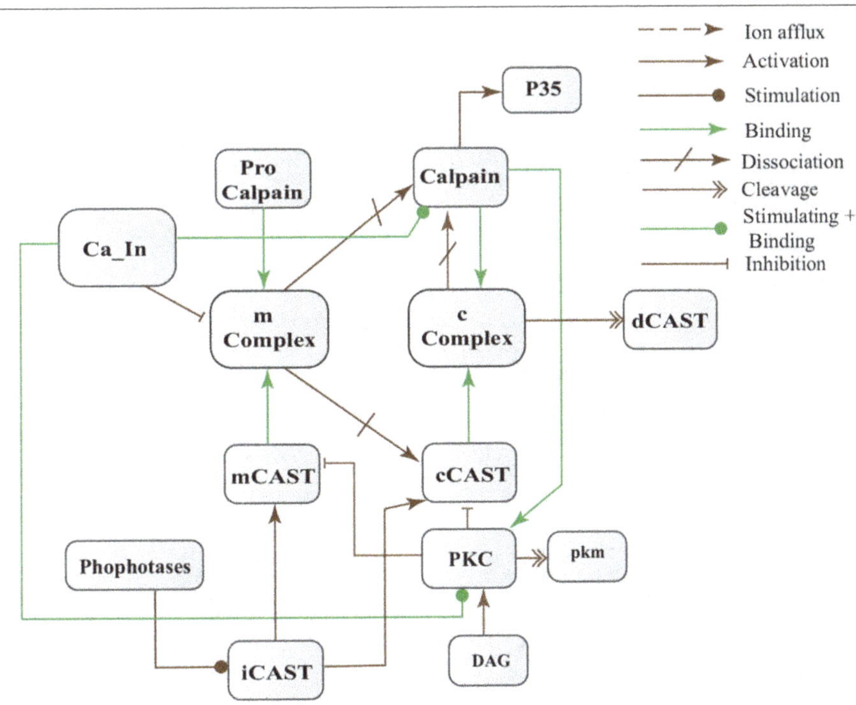

FIGURE 4 | Calpain-CAST system BRN derived from **Figure 3**.

administered by several routes such as N-methyl-D-aspartate receptor (NMDAR), an imperative type of ROCs, which switch into open conformation after binding of endogenous glutamate (glu) as ligand. Another important influx gateway is voltage gated Ca^{2+} channel (VGCC) which is in closed conformation when neuronal membrane is polarized (Schmolesky et al., 2002; Cain and Snutch, 2011). The VGCC adopts open conformation as plasma membrane depolarizes due to Ca^{2+}/ sodium (Na+) influx through ROCs or ion channels (Weber, 2012). Ca^{2+} influx also increases from intracellular stores in ER through store-operated channels. There are two calcium channels in ER which are IP3-sensitive and ryanodine (RyRs)-sensitive Ca^{2+} stores (Berridge, 2009). IP3 driven release of Ca^{2+} starts by binding of G-protein coupled receptor (GPCR) on plasma membrane which induces Phospholipase C (PLC) mediated cleavage of phosphatidylinositol-4,5-bisphosphate (PIP2) on cell membrane into DAG and IP3. IP3 binds to its receptor on ER membrane and stimulate Ca^{2+} release into the cytoplasm (Berridge, 2009; Krebs et al., 2015). Furthermore, depletion of ER stores mediate influx of extracellular Ca^{2+} through store-operated channels (SOCs) (Emptage et al., 2001; Weber, 2012). The mechanism for lowering Ca^{2+} from cell is controlled by PMCA and NCX. Both PMCA and NCX are energy dependent while, NCX is also Na^{+} gradient dependent (Wojda et al., 2008). The BRN of Calcium channels, **Figure 4**, is also helpful in understanding the mechanism underlying the Ca^{2+} homeostasis.

To comprehend the above mentioned neuronal pathways, models are constructed to understand their dynamics. Stochastic

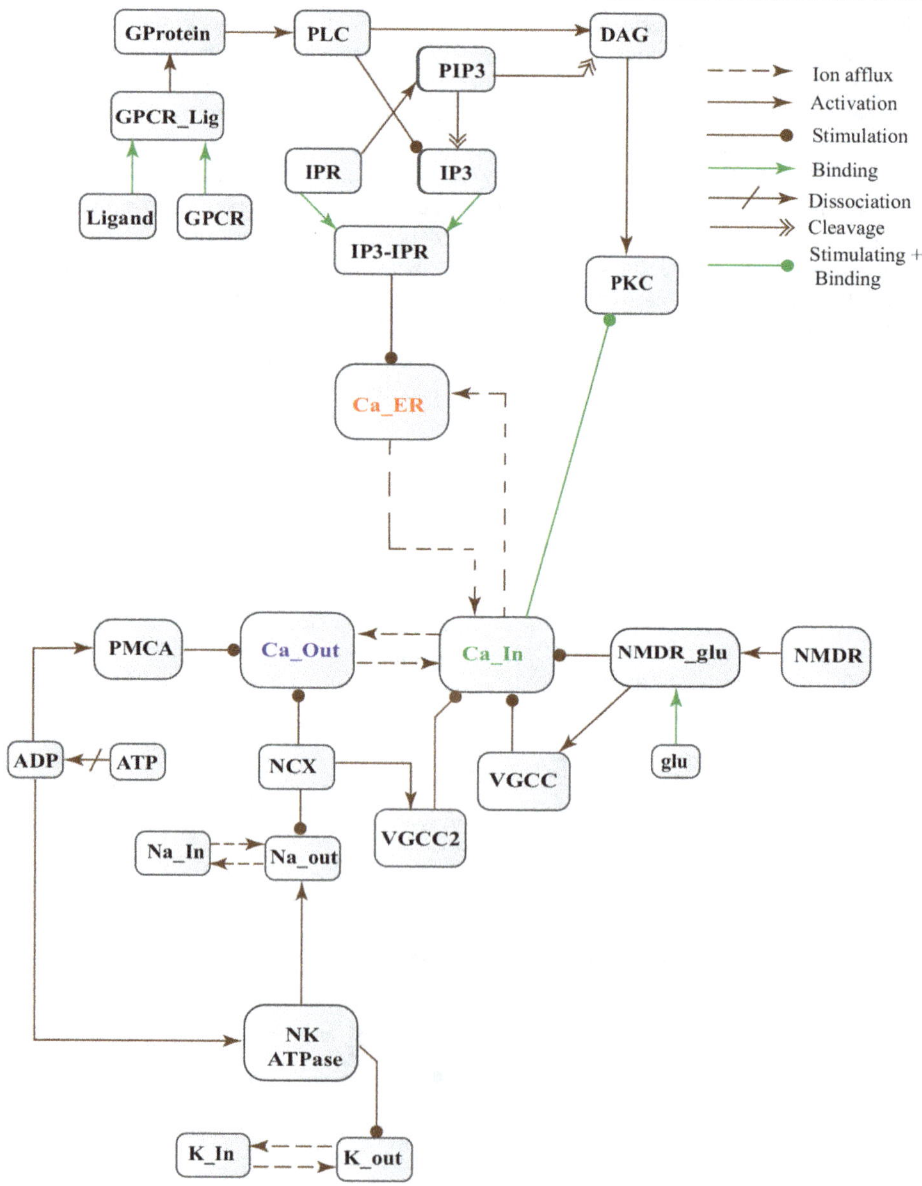

FIGURE 5 | Calcium Influx Efflux BRN derived from **Figure 3**.

approaches describe the randomness of biological system accurately as compared to ordinary differential equations. In BRNs, the activation or inhibition processes take place with random time delays, therefore, stochastic modeling frameworks are more suitable for their modeling. Petri nets provide complementary approach for both qualitative and quantitative modeling and simulation of the dynamical behavior of large systems in an intuitive way (Mounts and Liebman, 1997; Tsavachidou and Liebman, 2002; Tareen and Ahmad, 2015). The study (Tsavachidou and Liebman, 2002) shows that the Petri net models predict the experimental findings which support the soundness of these models. Stochastic petri nets (SPNs) have emerged as a promising tool for modeling and analyzing BRNs in the field of molecular biology (Goss and Peccoud, 1998). The dynamic behaviors of a variety of BRNs have been studied using stochastic simulations (Mura and Csikász-Nagy, 2008; Lamprecht et al., 2011; Castaldi et al., 2012; Marwan et al., 2012).

In this study, we have modeled and analyzed the neuronal physiological system constituting Ca^{2+} channels maintaining homeostasis, CAST regulating Calpain system and APP processing pathways separately and collectively at molecular

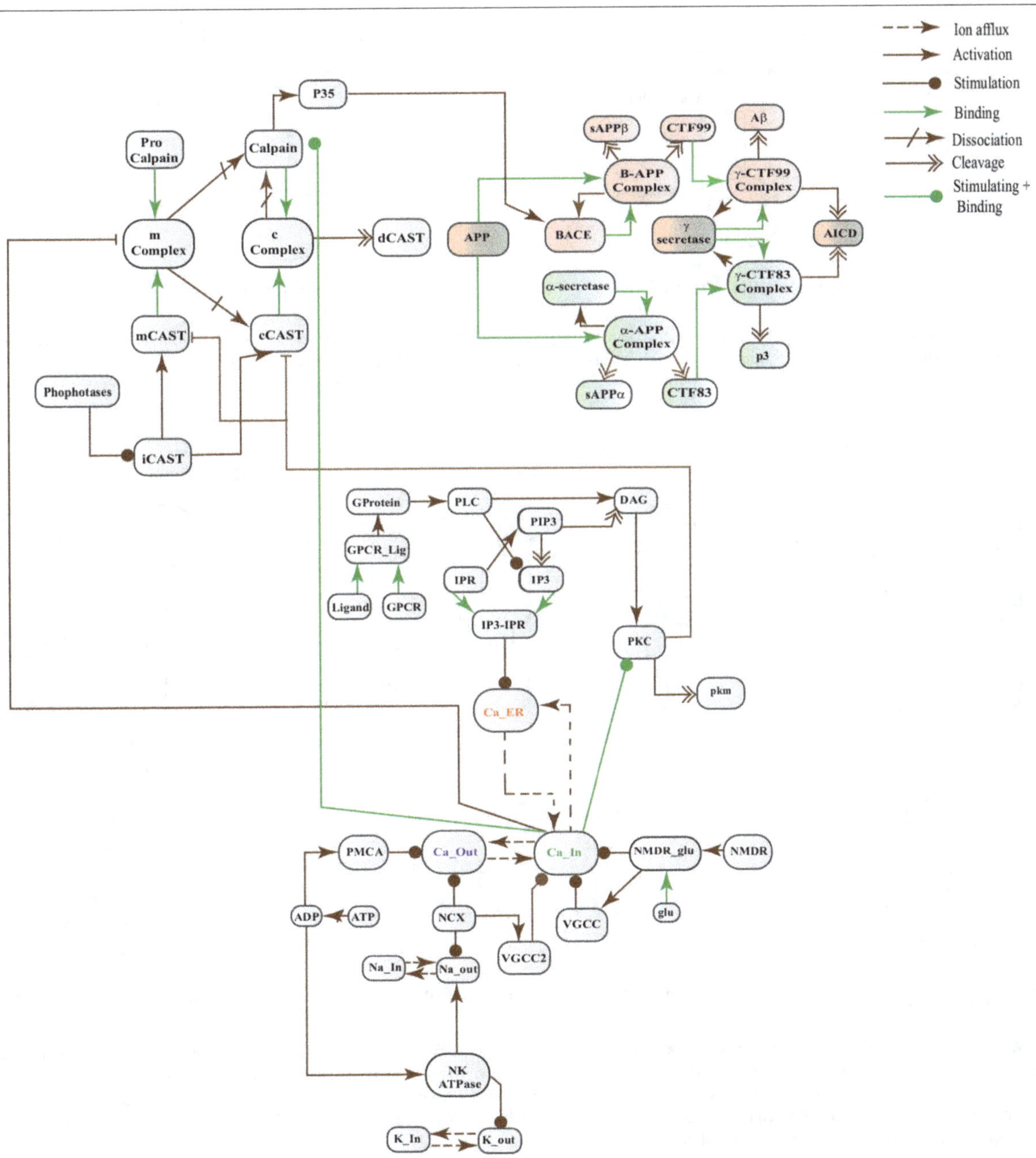

FIGURE 6 | A crosstalk network of three pathways: APP processing pathways, Calcium Channels and Calpain-CAST system.

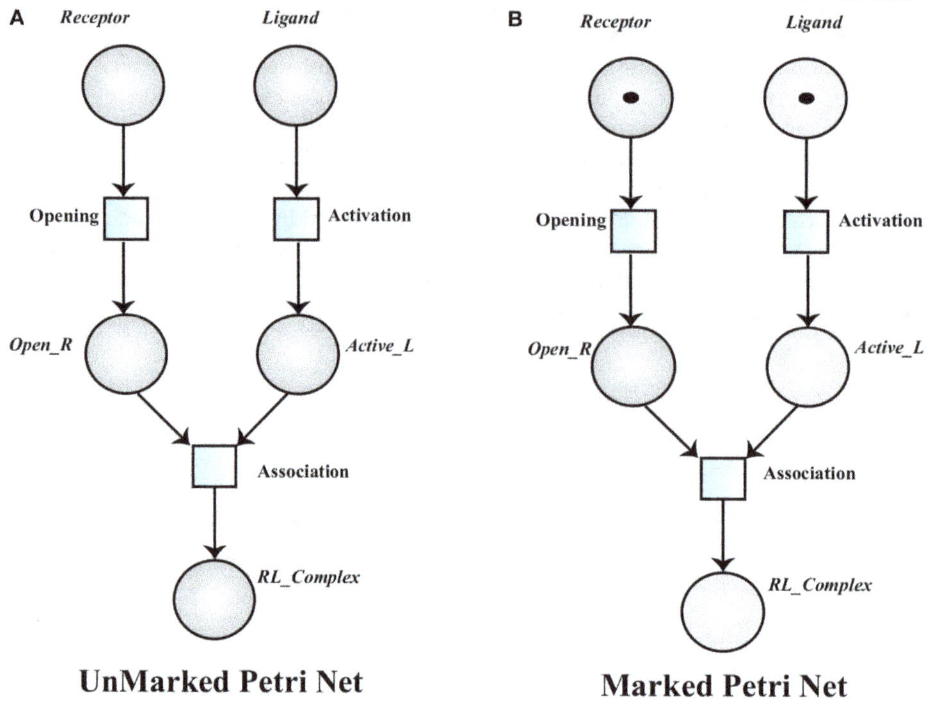

FIGURE 7 | (A) An Unmarked Petri net model of Receptor Ligand binding. *RL_Complex* is formed when *Receptor* is in open conformation (*Open_R*) and *Ligand* is activated into *Active_L*. **(B)**, A marked PN model has tokens which represent initial marking of the Receptor Ligand binding model.

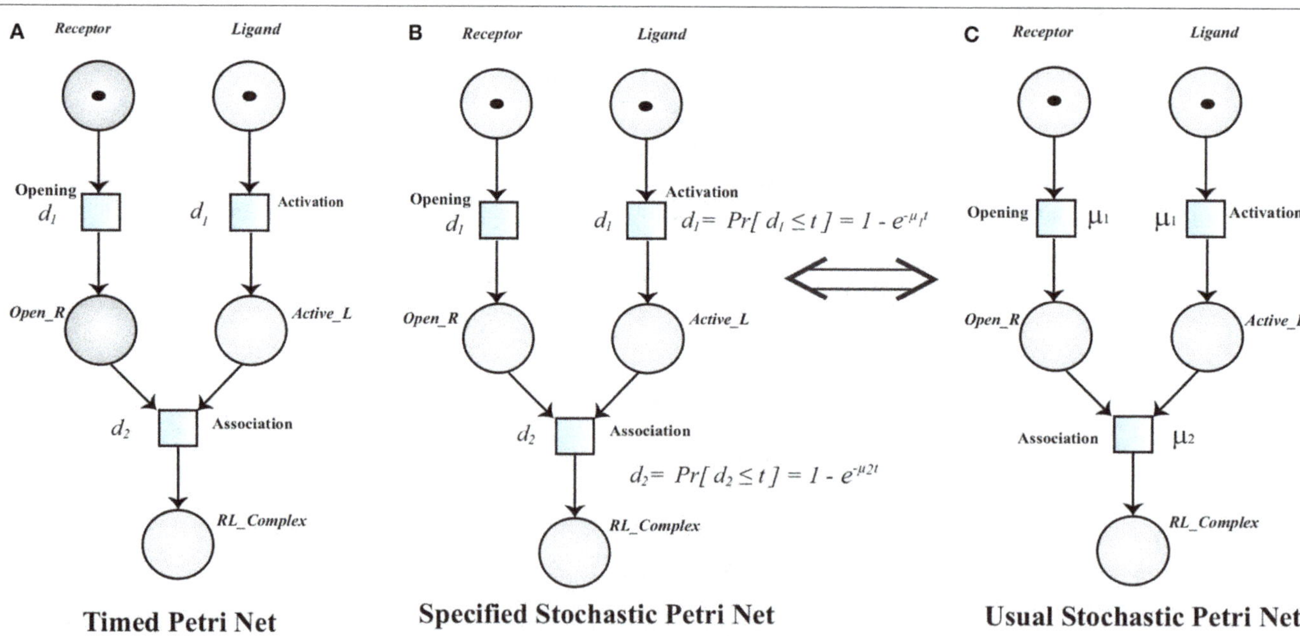

FIGURE 8 | (A) A Timed Petri net model of Receptor Ligand Binding. Initially, the *Receptor* is in close conformation and the *Ligand* is inactive. After enabling of respective transition (*Opening* and *Activation*), *Receptor* adopts open conformation (*Open_R*) and *Ligand* is activated into *Active_L* respectively. The transition *Opening* and *Activation* have an associated time delay d_1. The transitions are fired when the associated time delay is elapsed. *RL_Complex* is formed when *Open_R*, *Active_L* are present and time d_2 is elapsed. **(B,C)** are Specified and Usual Stochastic Petri Nets respectively. The TPN can be converted into SPN when the deterministic firing function d changes into a random variable.

level using SPNs to understand the AD progression mechanism. Particularly, we have analyzed neuronal patho-physiological dynamic behaviors causing the development of hallmark lesions in brain to answer many question e.g., how dysregulation of Ca^{2+} triggers AD? When CAST, the sole inhibitor of Calpain, depletes from the brain cells? how $A\beta$ production increases? and when the accumulation of plaques start? The answers to these questions lie in the modeling of the combined BRN **Figure 6**. The model predicts that Calpain is the main cause of dysregulation, which start with the rise in Ca^{2+} levels in the cytosol. Calpain activates different pathways through which $A\beta$ production and accumulation increases. Plaques start building with time at the age of forty and older. Plaques first enter lag phase and then into rapid growth phase. Calpain slowly degrades CAST which depletes from the cell and eventually neuronal degradation progresses. These results suggest that patho-physiological events such as dysregulation of Ca^{2+} homeostasis, Calpain hyper-activation, CAST degradation and abnormal digestion of APP, all are inter-connected and a cumulative study of these processes through SPN was needed.

2. METHODOLOGY

Petri nets (PNs) have three components namely places, transitions and edges. Place and transition are collectively known as nodes/ vertices of a PN. An arc or edge joins nodes such as a place (*pre-place*) to a transition or a transition to a place (*post-place*) to make a bipartite graph (Petri, 1966). Edges are directed and have weights associated with them. In biological systems, such as BRNs, places (○) represent biological

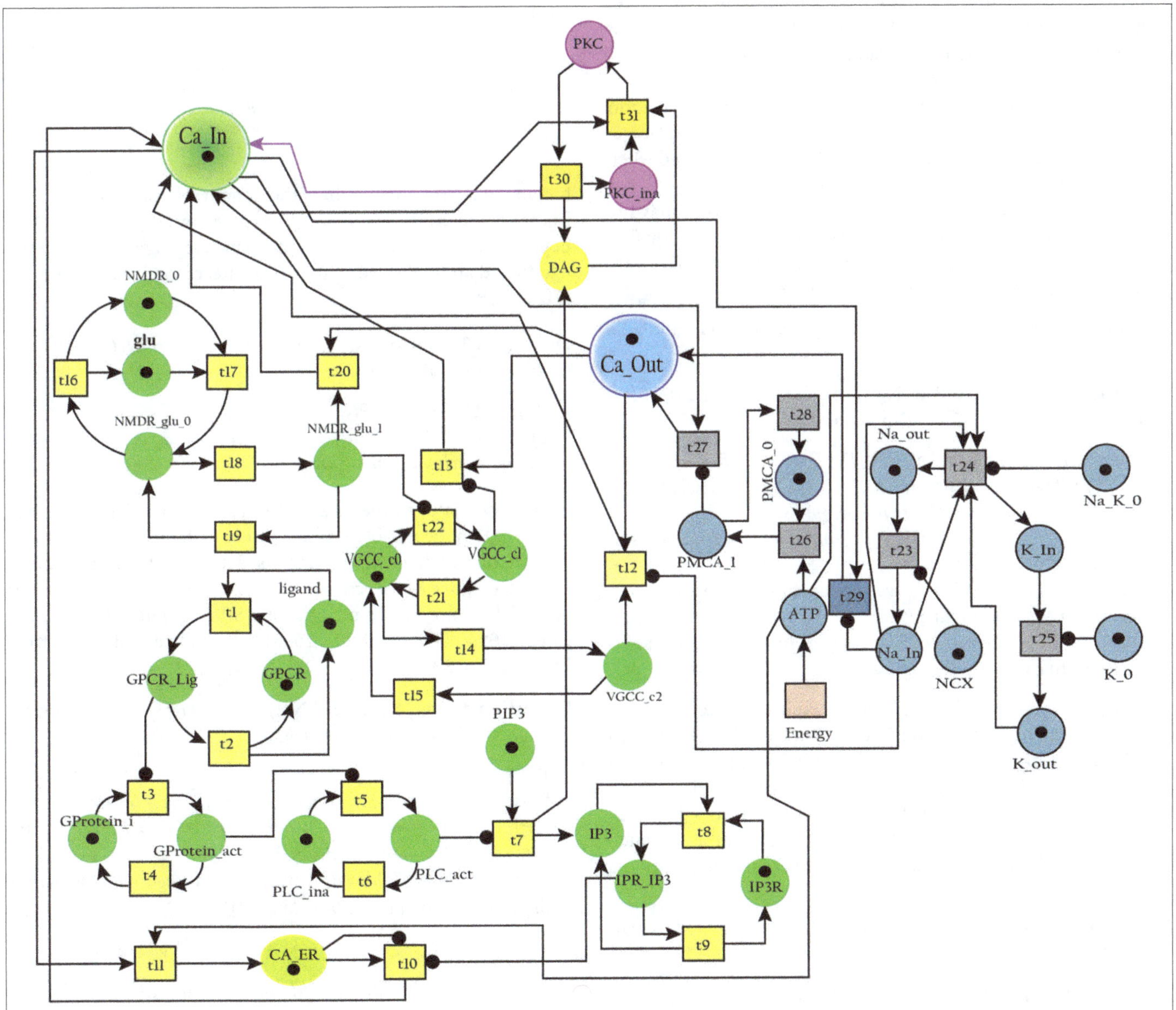

FIGURE 9 | SPN model of the Calcium Channel.

entities e.g., protein or their complexes, gene, mRNA, ions, metabolites and cell or cellular components while transitions (□) represent biochemical reactions e.g., association, activation, decomposition, inhibition, phosphorylation, dephosphorylation and translocation (Tareen and Ahmad, 2015). The weights of edges represent the stoichiometry of reactions. The weight can be one (1) or greater than one (Blätke et al., 2011; Liu et al., 2016). Following are the different types of edges.

- **Standard edge(⟶)** is use to represents a simple biochemical reaction such as synthesis, decomposition, replacement and activation reactions. It is enabled when pre-places have adequate tokens. When the transition is fired, tokens from pre-places are removed and then deposited in post-places according to arc weights.
- **Inhibitor edge(—◦)** connects only a pre-place to a transition. If the corresponding pre-place is not adequately marked i.e., it has less tokens than weight of arc, then, the transition is enabled otherwise, it is un-firable. Tokens are not removed from pre-place in the inhibitor edge.
- **Read edge (—•)** connects only a pre-place to a transition. It enables the transition when the corresponding place is adequately marked. The tokens of a place are not altered when the transition is fired.
- **Equal edge (-•-•)** connects pre-place to transition. It may fire a transition when number of tokens in a pre-place is equal to corresponding arc weight. After firing of transition, tokens are not removed from the respective pre-place.

The following definitions are originally given in David and Alla (2010).

Definition 1 (Unmarked Petri Net). *An unmarked Petri Net (PN) is a five-tuple* $\mathbb{P}= \langle \mathcal{P}, \mathcal{T}, \mathcal{E}, \mathfrak{pre}, \mathfrak{post}\rangle$ *where:*

- $\mathcal{P}$ *is a finite set of places i.e.,* $\mathcal{P} = \{\mathcal{P}_1, \mathcal{P}_2, \mathcal{P}_3 \ldots, \mathcal{P}_n\}$,
- $\mathcal{T}$ *is a finite set of transitions i.e.,* $\mathcal{T} = \{\mathcal{T}_1, \mathcal{T}_2, \mathcal{T}_3, \ldots, \mathcal{T}_n\}$,
- $\mathcal{P} \cap \mathcal{T} = \varnothing$, *both* $\mathcal{P}$ *and* $\mathcal{T}$ *are non-empty sets,*
- $\mathcal{E} \subseteq \mathcal{P} \times \mathcal{T} \cup \mathcal{T} \times \mathcal{P}$, *is a set of input and output edges of transitions.*
- $\mathfrak{pre} : \mathcal{P} \times \mathcal{T} \longrightarrow \mathbb{N}$, *is a weight function that assigns non-negative integers to input edges.*
- $\mathfrak{post} : \mathcal{T} \times \mathcal{P} \longrightarrow \mathbb{N}$, *is a weight function that assigns non-negative integers to output edges.*

A simple unmarked PN is given in **Figure 7A**, to model a receptor-ligand association. A receptor is in closed conformation and ligand is in in-active form. The receptor must undergoes open conformation and then the ligand activates to form an association (*RL_Complex*) with receptor. The places in a PN may have tokens (black dots or positive real numbers) which represent marking of the places. In a marked PN, places are initially assigned tokens.

Definition 2 (Marked Petri Net). *A Marked Petri Net (MPN) is a tuple* $\mathbb{MP}= \langle \mathbb{P}, \check{\mathfrak{m}}_0\rangle$ *where:*

- $\mathbb{P} = \langle \mathcal{P}, \mathcal{T}, \mathcal{E}, \mathfrak{pre}, \mathfrak{post}\rangle$ *is an unmarked PN and*
- $\check{\mathfrak{m}}_0 : \mathcal{P} \longrightarrow \mathbb{Z}_{\geq 0}$, *is an initial marking of the PN.*

The transition associated to a marked place is said to be enabled and it will be fired when the corresponding pre-places have tokens equal or greater than the weight of the associated arc. Receptor opening requires a *Receptor* and ligand activation depends on the presence of an inactive *Ligand.* An active ligand and an opened receptor form a Receptor-Ligand Complex (**Figure 7B**).

TABLE 1 | Transition rates of the SPN model of Calcium Channel.

Tansitions	Rate (μ)	Transitions	Rate (μ)
t1	1	*t17*	1
t2	1	*t18*	1
t3	1	*t19*	1
t4	1	*t20*	1
t5	1	*t21*	1
t6	1	*t22*	1
t7	1	*t23*	1
t8	1	*t24*	1
t9	1	*t25*	1
t10	0.65	*t26*	1
t11	1	*t27*	1
t12	1	*t28*	1
t13	1	*t29*	1
t14	1	*t30*	1
t15	1	*t31*	1
t16	1	*Energy*	1

*The transitions (t) from (**Figure 9**) are listed with their rates. The transitions are adjusted to rates which can reproduce the physiological working of calcium channels.*

Definition 3 (Timed Petri Net). *A Timed Petri Net (TPN) is a tuple* $\mathbb{TP}= \langle \mathbb{MP}, \check{\mathfrak{fn}}\rangle$ *where:*

- $\mathbb{MP}= \langle \mathbb{P}, \check{\mathfrak{m}}\rangle$ *is a MPN.*
- $\check{\mathfrak{fn}} : \mathcal{T} \longrightarrow \mathbb{R}^+$ *is a function that associates a positive real value i.e., time delay to each transition.*

A TPN associates a time delay d_i to a transition $\mathcal{T}_i$. The transition $\mathcal{T}_i$ is said to be enabled when it has sufficient tokens in its pre-places and it is fired when its deterministic delay time is elapsed (**Figure 8**). Stochastic Petri Net (SPN) are used when time delays are random variables. SPN (**Figure 8C**) (Marsan et al., 1994; Heiner et al., 2008) are explicitly derived from TPN (**Figure 8A**).

Definition 4 (Stochastic Petri Net). *A marked stochastic petri net is a pair* $\mathbb{SPN} = \langle \mathbb{MP}, \mathfrak{Rate}\rangle$ *where:*

- $\mathbb{MP} = \langle \mathbb{P}, \check{\mathfrak{m}}_0\rangle$ *is a MPN.*
- $\mathfrak{Rate} : \mathcal{T} \longrightarrow \mathbb{R}^+$, *is a function from the set* $\mathcal{T}$ *of transition to the set of finite positive real numbers.* $\mathfrak{Rate}(\mathcal{T}_i) = \mu_i$, *is the firing rate associated with transition* $\mathcal{T}_i$.
  The random variables d_i *have assigned negative exponential probability distribution function (PDF)* $\check{\mathfrak{fn}}(t)$,

$$\check{\mathfrak{fn}}(t) = Pr[\, d_i \leq t] = 1 - e^{-\mu_i t} \text{ where,}$$

$$Pr[\, d_i \leq t + dt \mid d_i > t] = \mu_i \cdot dt$$

The marking of $\check{\mathfrak{m}}_t$ of SPN is a homogenous Markovanian Chain (HMC) process, which is a class of stochastic processes simply built from the reachability graph of a qualitative PN by

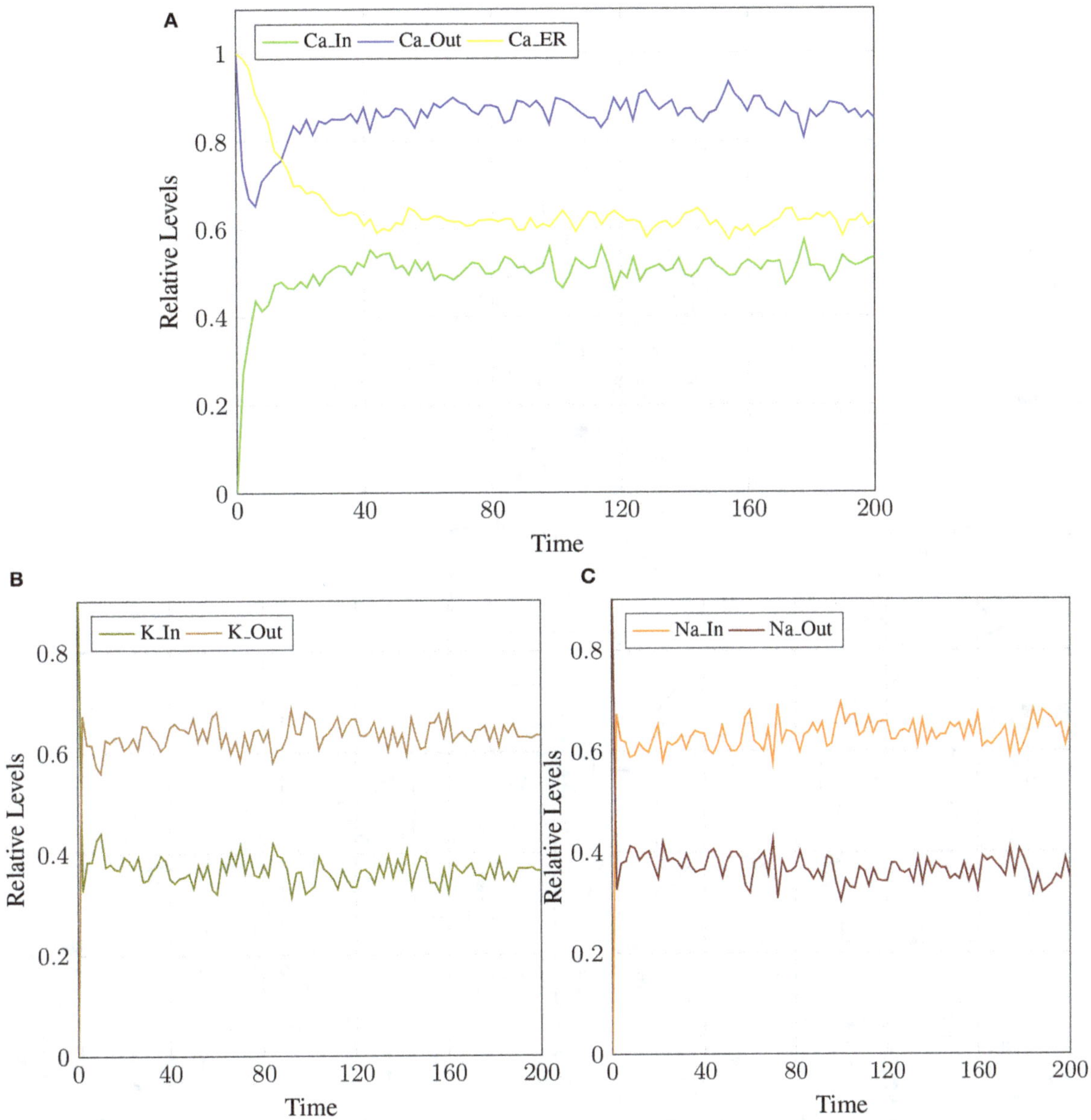

FIGURE 10 | (A) shows Calcium homeostasis which is maintained by influx (***Ca_In***), efflux (***Ca_Out***) and intracellular storage (***Ca_ER***). Calcium efflux is further maintained by coordinated and controlled *in and out* flow of Potassium (***K_In***, ***K_Out***) in **(B)** as well as of the Sodium (***Na_In***, ***Na_out***) ions channels **(C)**.

assigning transition rates to edges between all the states (Heiner et al., 2008). Thus an HMC can be associated with every SPN. Gillespie was the first one who designed special case of Petri nets for reaction networks and called them SPNs (Gillespie, 1976). Snoopy (Marwan et al., 2012) tool is used to design, animate and simulate SPNs of neurodegeneration related BRNs. This tool has been extensively used to model a variety of systems such as software systems, biological systems and production systems. The supplementary file S1 contains a general Enzyme-Substrate BRN that is modeled and simulated through the Petri net modeling tool Snoopy. This file helps to explain the working of the tool (Snoopy).

3. RESULTS

In this study, stochastic modeling and analysis of the neuronal pathways involved in neuro-degradation in AD was carried out. The SPN models of the three main neuronal physiological pathways: Calcium Influx Efflux channels (**Figure 5**), Calpain-CAST regulatory system (**Figure 4**) and APP digesting pathways (**Figure 2**). The SPN model of the crosstalk of these three pathways is also presented.

3.1. SPN of Calcium Influx Efflux Channels

The BRN of Calcium influx efflux channels in **Figure 5** is translated into a SPN model as shown in **Figure 9**. The influx

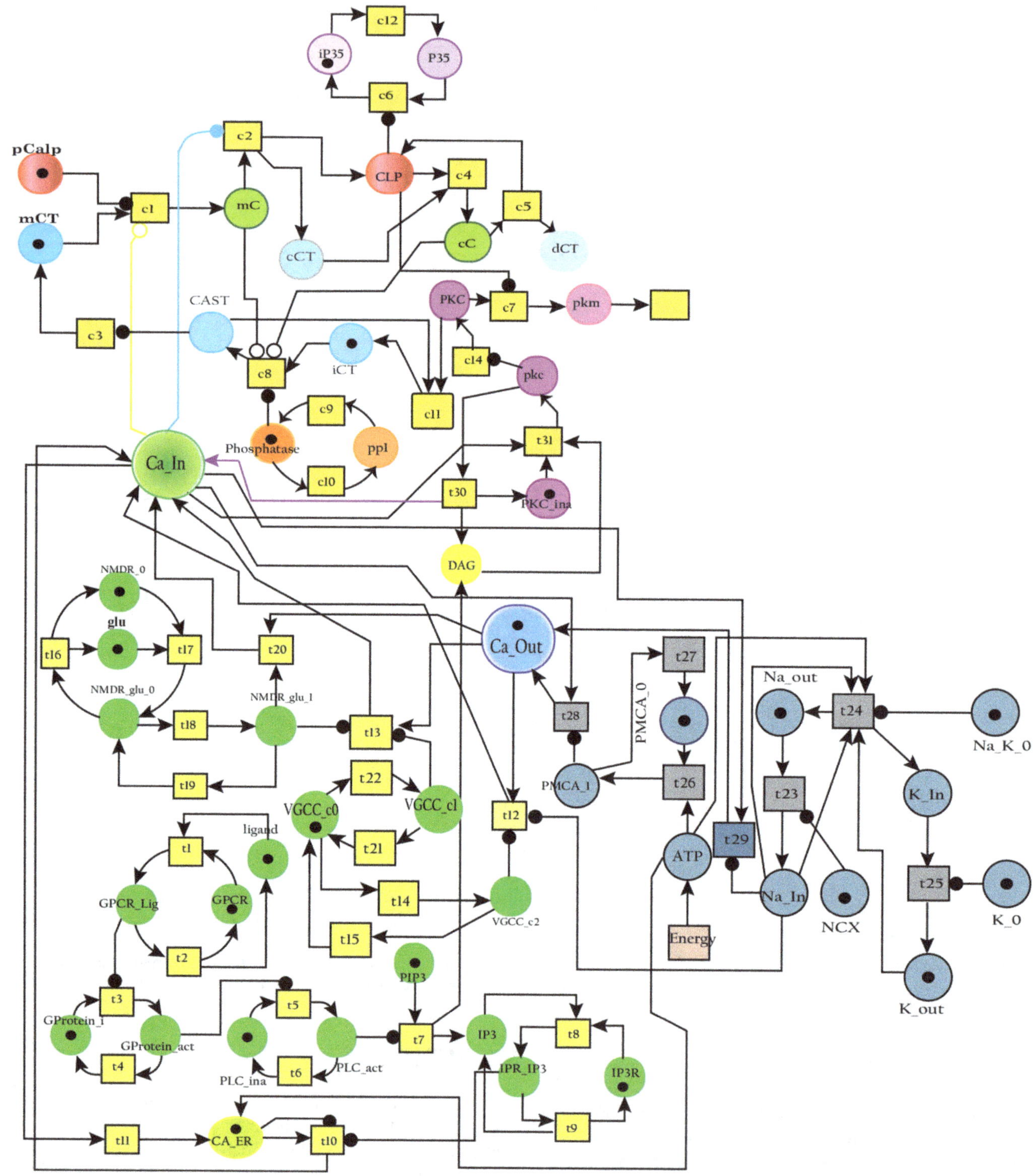

FIGURE 11 | The SPN model of Calpain-CAST system.

channels comprise of receptor based and voltage gated channels (NMDR, VGCC1 / VGCC2). In addition, the GPCR channel regulates intracellular trafficking of Ca^{2+} ions and stimulation of *PKC* signaling pathway. The energy dependent efflux channels (e.g., PMCA and Na-K ATPase) work efficiently in a sync with influx channels to maintain equilibrium between in-out flow of

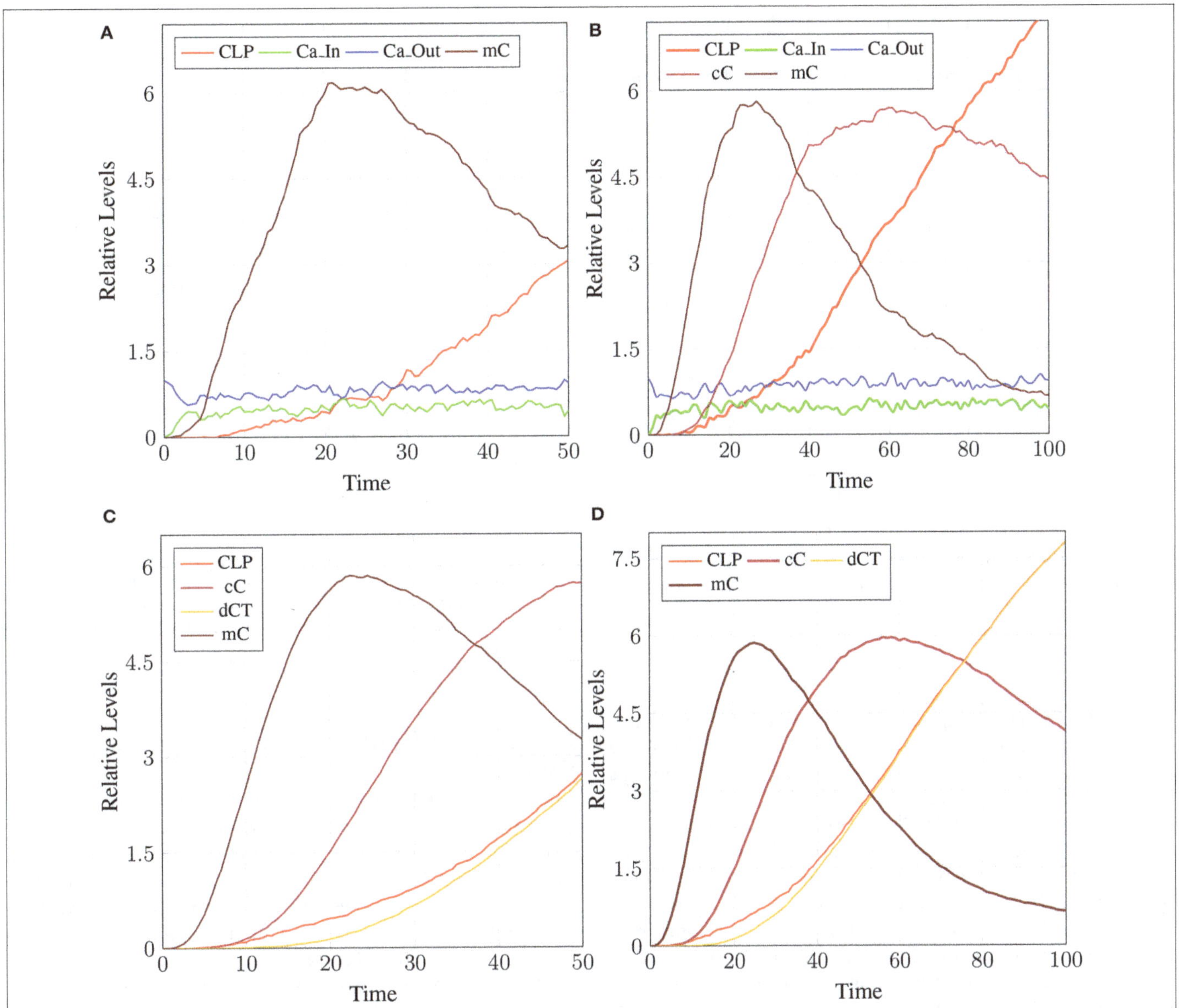

FIGURE 12 | Calpain activation and regulation: In **(A)**, ***CLP*** is bound to CAST in the form of ***mC*** at membrane. As the ***Ca_In*** increases and ***Ca_Out*** decreases the complex ***mC*** breaks down. In an elaborate view **(B)**, ***CLP*** is produced by the break down of the ***mC*** which is again controlled by the formation of ***cC***. In **(C)**, ***mC*** is formed, maintained and eventually degraded into CAST and Calpain. Both Calpain and CAST form complex ***cC*** which decreases the availability of free ***CLP***. *CLP* binding to ***cC*** slowly degrades the CAST which is represented as ***dCT***. **(D)** Both complexes ***mC*** and ***cC*** are formed while ***cC*** is more stable than ***mC***, as rate of degradation of ***mC*** is higher than **(C)**.

Ca^{2+} ions in neurons. Ca^{2+} ions move from ***Ca_In*** place (green) to ***Ca_Out*** place (blue) and vice versa. The places in green colors and transitions (yellow) constitute influx channels. The places in light blue colors and transitions in grey colors make efflux channels. Initially, ***NMDR_0*** place represents that receptor is in close conformation that binds with ***glu*** to form the complex represented by ***NMDR_glu_0*** place. This complex adapts open conformation represented by the place ***NMDR_glu_1*** and then further triggers the opening of VGCC channel represented by the place ***VGCC_c1*** to facilitate Ca^{2+} ions influx. Excess Ca^{2+} ions are deposited into the place ***Ca_ER*** through store-operated channel. The place ***GProtein_i*** represents inactive GPCR, that change into place ***GProtein_act*** by a complex of GPCR and ligand represented by places ***GPCR_Lig*** (complex), ***GPCR*** (receptor) and ***ligand*** respectively. ***GProtein_act*** activates PLC represented by place ***PLC_act***, which mediate cleavage of ***PIP2*** place into ***DAG*** and ***IP3***. The place ***DAG*** activates ***PKC*** by adding Ca^{2+} ion in it. At the surface of ER, IP3 binds with its receptor IP3R, represented by places ***IP3*** and ***IP3R***, which induces Ca^{2+} ions flow into the place ***Ca_ER***. At the same time, Ca outflow is maintained by PMCA, NCX and Na-K ATPase. PMCA channel represented by place ***PMCA_1*** requires ATP (place ***ATP***) to extrude one Ca^{2+} ion into extracellular space. The place ***NCX*** representing NCX pump ensures extrusion of

TABLE 2 | The transition rates of the SPN model of Calpain-CAST regulatory system.

Tansitions	Rate (μ)	Transitions	Rate (μ)	Transitions	Rate (μ)
*t*1	1	*t*17	1	*c*1	0.5
*t*2	1	*t*18	1	*c*2	0.1
*t*3	1	*t*19	1	*c*3	1
*t*4	1	*t*20	1	*c*4	0.02
*t*5	1	*t*21	1	*c*5	0.5
*t*6	1	*t*22	1	*c*6	0.5
*t*7	1	*t*23	1	*c*7	0.3
*t*8	1	*t*24	1	*c*8	0.5
*t*9	1	*t*25	1	*c*9	1
*t*10	0.65	*t*26	1	*c*10	1
*t*11	1	*t*27	1	*c*11	1
*t*12	1	*t*28	1	*c*12	1
*t*13	1	*t*29	1	*c*13	1
*t*14	1	*t*30	1	*c*14	0.5
*t*15	1	*t*31	1		
*t*16	1	*Energy*	1		

*The transitions (t and c) from (**Figure 11**) are listed with their rates. The transitions are adjusted to rates which can reproduce the physiological working of Calpain-CAST regulatory system.*

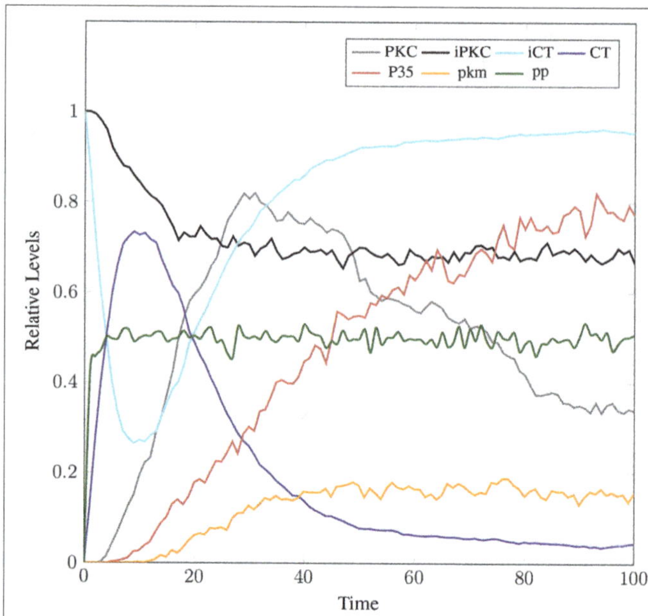

FIGURE 13 | In physiological condition, the helping enzymes (***PKC*** and ***phosphotases***) are periodically activating and deactivating. ***iPKC*** is the dormant form of the cytosol; it activates into ***PKC*** to convert ***mCT*** and ***cCT*** into ***iCT***. Phophotases (***pp***) convert the ***iCT*** into ***CT***. ***PKC*** in the presence of *CLP* is degraded into ***pkm***.

one Ca^{2+} ion by adding three Na ions into the cytoplasm represented by place ***Na_In***. The place ***Na_K_1*** represents active (i.e., depends on ATP) Na-K ATPase pumping that pumps Na out of the neuron (place ***Na_out***) and K into the neuron (place ***K_In***). The place ***VGCC_c2*** representing Ca inflow is also dependent on place ***NCX***, which depolarizes the membrane. The SPN model is simulated after applying and adjusting the rates of transitions in order to reproduce physiological working of the pathway. The transitions are labeled by *t*, transition from ***t1–t22*** are associated with influx channels. ***t1–t10*** are linked to GPCR channel which help in storage of excess Ca^{2+} ions into place ***Ca_ER***. ***t11*** takes Ca^{2+} ions from ***Ca_ER*** into cytoplasm (place ***Ca_In***). Remaining ***t12–t22*** make NMDR and VGCC channels functional. The efflux channels, consisting of NCX, NKA channels and PMCA are connected with transitions ***t23–t29***. The transitions ***t30*** and ***t31*** are involved in activation of PKC which is dependent on calcium. The rates of transitions are shown in parameter in **Table 1**. The simulation results have shown that there is an equilibrium behavior in all channels, which is required to maintain homeostasis in calcium flow. In **Figure 10A**, a stable oscillating behavior can be observed among the places ***Ca_out***, ***Ca_ER*** and ***Ca_In***. Concentration of Ca^{2+} ions in ***Ca_out*** place is higher while it is lower in place ***Ca_In***. Na and K ions, (**Figures 10B,C**) are also oscillating properly, contributing to Ca^{2+} homeostasis and generating nerve impulses through polarization and depolarization. Ca^{2+} homeostasis has pivotal role in cell physiological working. Dysregulation of Ca^{2+} homeostasis will affect the regulation of most of the proteins, enzymes and genes which will have deleterious effects on the physiological processes.

3.2. SPN of Calpain-CAST Regulatory System

The model in **Figure 11** represents Calpain-CAST regulatory system as given in **Figure 4**. In SPN model, due to lower Ca^{2+} level in cytosol, Calpain is in dormant form which is represented by place ***pCalp***. It then attaches to CAST located on membrane (place ***mCT***) to form a reversible complex of CAST and Calpain (place ***mC***). Calpain is activated when cytosolic Ca^{2+} rises to specific concentration (Pal et al., 2001; Ryu and Nakazawa, 2014). Lower level of cytosolic Ca^{2+} represented by place ***Ca_In*** facilitates (place ***mC***), membrane bound inactive reversible Calpain-CAST complex. After the concentration of ***Ca_In*** rises or crosses its threshold, then the short-lived ***mC*** is disintegrated into places ***CLP*** and ***cCT***. The place ***CLP*** shows that Calpain moves to transmembrane and then converts into active form in the presence of Ca^{2+} ions and its autolysis. Now place ***CLP*** shows that Calpain is activated that is free to translocate to cytosol. The place ***cCT*** represents that CAST can again hinder over-activation of ***CLP*** by forming a reversible complex, represented by place ***cC***. The place ***cC***, splits into places ***CLP*** and ***dCT***. In nature, active Calpain breaks down the bounded CAST into small subunits (Rao et al., 2008). The place ***CLP*** shows that it is active and which can be involved in various cellular processes. The place ***CLP*** can cleave place ***P35*** into *p25* which is involved in hyper-activation of cyclin dependent kinase 5 (*cdk5*) (Kusakawa et al., 2000; Lee et al., 2000). The transitions of this system are labeled with *c*. The transition ***c1*** forms complex, place ***mC*** from ***pCalp*** and ***mCT*** at low Ca^{2+} concentration. The ***c2*** breaks complex and activates ***CLP*** when level of Ca^{2+} rises into cytoplasm. The

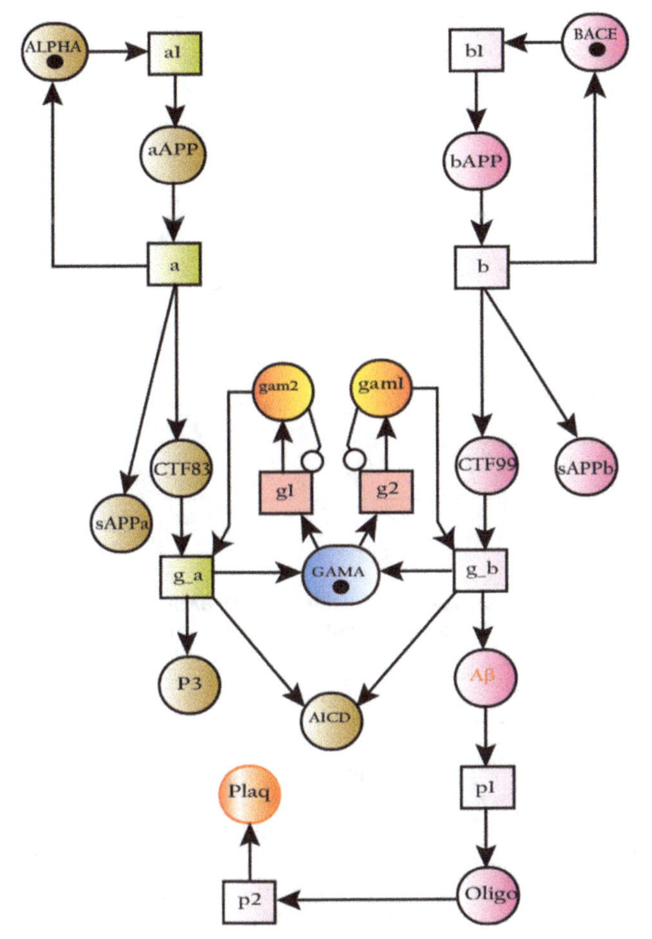

FIGURE 14 | SPN model of non-amyliodogenic (**left**) and amyliodogenic (**right**) of APP processing pathways.

TABLE 3 | The transition rates of the SPN model of APP processing pathways.

Tansitions	Rate (μ)
a	0.5
*a*1	0.5
b	0.3
*b*1	0.3
*g*1	0.5
*g*2	0.5
g_a	0.5
g_b	0.3
*p*1	0.005
*p*2	0.02

*The transitions from **Figure 14** are listed with their rates. The transitions are adjusted to rates which can reproduce the physiological working of amyloidogenic and non-amyloidogenic pathways.*

transition ***c4*** forms complex place ***cC*** by binding ***CT*** and ***CLP*** in cytoplasm and ***c5***, at a very low rate (**Table 2**) slowly degrades the CAST into ***dCT*** and makes the ***CLP*** free. Transitions ***c6***, ***c12*** and ***c13*** are linked to ***CLP*** mediated ***P35*** pathway. ***CLP*** also degrades ***PKC*** into ***pkm*** through ***c7***. Remaining transitions ***c3***, ***c8***, ***c9***, ***c10***, ***c11*** and ***c14*** are associated to CAST regulation through ***PKC*** and phosphotases ***pp***. The **Table 2** lists all reaction rates of associated transitions which are obtained after fine tuning. In **Figure 12A**, the simulation shows that when Ca influx, ***Ca_In***, is lower than its threshold then ***pCalp*** is bounded into complex of Calpain-CAST (***mC***) at membrane. When ***Ca_In*** crosses its threshold, the peak of ***mC*** runs down and ***CLP*** rises representing release and activation of Calpain, (**Figure 12B**). These results are according to experimental findings (De Tullio et al., 1999; Todd et al., 2003) (**Figures 12A,B**). To regulate ***CLP*** activation, ***cC*** appears but gradually the complex peak falls down showing that the ***cC*** is broken down into active ***CLP*** and ***dCT***. The results in **Figures 12C,D** show that as ***CLP*** is rising, both the complexes (***mC*** and ***cC***) are gradually degrading causing depletion of CAST from the cytosol (Averna et al., 2001b; Tompa et al., 2002). In **Figure 13**, regulation of ***PKC***, CAST and phophatases (represented as ***pp***) can be observed. ***iPKC*** converted into ***PKC*** in the presence of Ca^{2+}, which further converts into ***pkm*** by the action of ***CLP***. As shown in the graph of **Figure 13**, ***CT*** is regulating through means of reversible phosphorylation and dephosphorylation expedited by ***PKC*** and ***pp***, respectively.

3.3. APP Processing Pathways

The SPN model of APP processing as shown in **Figure 14** is built by combining both amyliodogenic and non-amyliodogenic pathways (**Figure 2**). APP (place ***aAPP***) is catalyzed by α-secretase (place ***ALPHA***) which produces CTF83 and sAPPα (places ***CTF83*** and ***sAPPa***), whereas digestion of APP (***bAPP***) by β-secretase (place ***BACE***) yields CTF99 and sAPPβ, (represented by places ***CTF99*** and ***sAPPb*** respectively). Further processing is carried out by enzyme γ-secretase (place ***GAMA***) which converts CTF83 into p3 and AICD, while it converts CTF99 into ***Aβ*** and ***AICD***. Aβ accumulate into ***Oligomer*** and finally into ***Plaq***. The transitions ***a***, ***a1*** and ***g_a*** constitute non-amyliodogenic pathway, while transitions ***b***, ***b1*** and ***g_b*** are linked to amyloidogenic pathway. The parameters are set according to **Table 3**, in which the rate of transition of α-secretase (place **ALPHA**) mediated APP processing (***aAPP***) is higher than BACE (***BACE***) driven APP digestion (***bAPP***) (***μ = 0.5, 0.3 respectively)***. The rates of plaques formation and accumulation (transitions: ***p1*** and ***p2***) are also adjusted according to the observations in literature which predict low *Aβ* burden in normal healthy brain (Mawuenyega et al., 2010; Rodrigue et al., 2012).

The simulations in **Figure 15A** shows that all the three enzymes (***ALPHA***, ***BACE***, and ***GAMA***) are available for the proteolysis of APP (in the cell to digest the around-the-clock production of) ***APP***. The **Figure 15B** shows that the product ***sAPPa*** of non-amyloidogenic processing pathway is in higher concentration than the product ***sAPPb*** of amyloidogenic pathway. Production rate of ***sAPPa*** is higher than ***sAPPb***. The graph in **Figure 16A** shows that in the healthy brain plaques are produced and accumulated in a linear fashion. *Aβ* burdens in the form of plaques at elder age i.e., approximately after 60 unit to 100 unit time. In **Figure 16B**, the linear behavior of plaques change to an exponential growth due to the fast accumulation

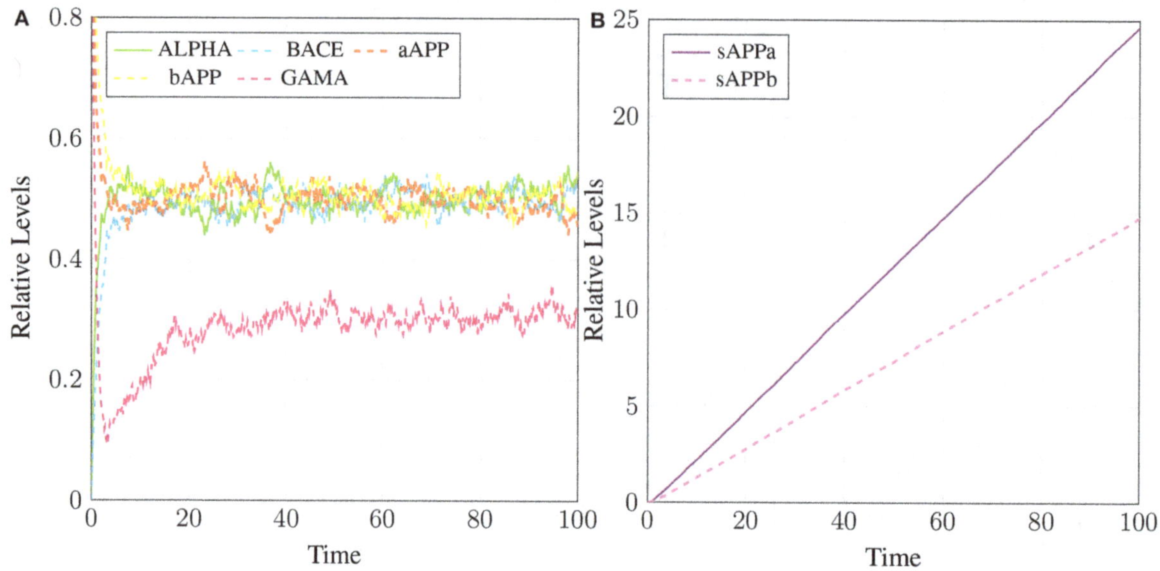

FIGURE 15 | APP processing in physiological conditions: In **(A)**, substrate *aAPP* binds with alpha secretase (***ALPHA***) and ***bAPP*** binds with **BACE**. All the three secretases ***ALPHA*** ,***BACE*** , and ***GAMA*** are oscillating. In **(B)**, concentration of ***sAPPa*** is higher than the concentration of ***sAPPb*** which depicts healthy cell physiology.

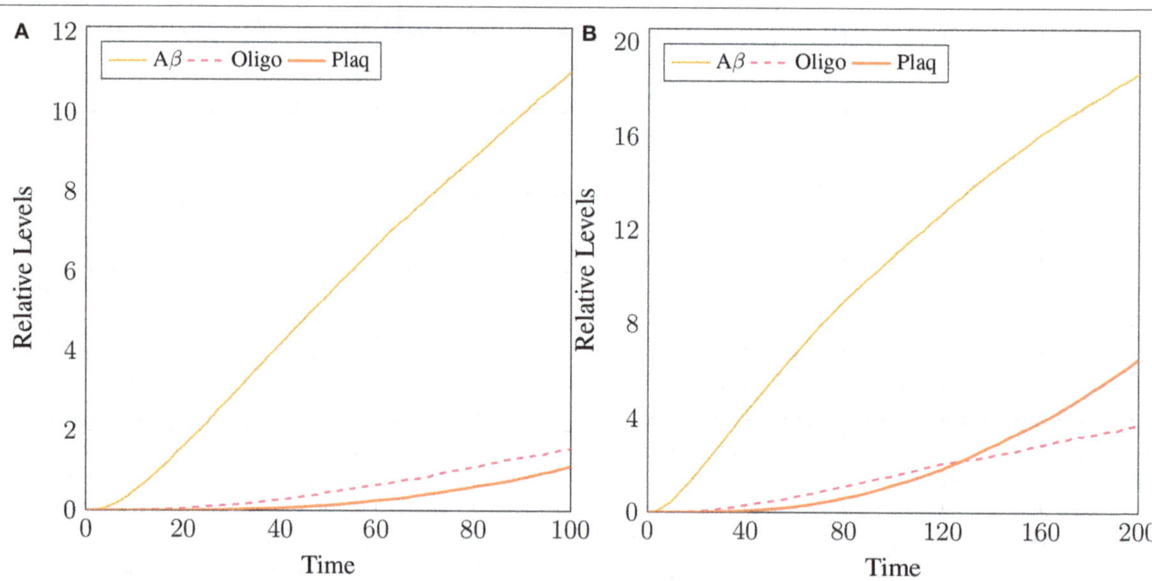

FIGURE 16 | Plaques formation in healthy brain: In **(A,B)** production of plaque is shown over the time period of 100 and 200 unit time, respectively. ***Plaq*** accumulation starts after sixty to eighty unit time. ***Aβ*** and ***Oligo*** show fluctuating behaviors as they start to build-up but degrade with time. First, ***Aβ*** gathers into large quantity to form ***Oligo*** which gradually accumulates into ***Plaq***.

rate with passage of time which depicts the lag phase (no plaques appearance) upto 80 unit time and after it evolves into growth phase (evolution).

3.4. Cross Talk of Calcium Channels, APP and Calpain-CAST Regulatory Pathways

The **Figure 17** represents the SPN model of the crosstalk network in **Figure 6**. The connection that joins the pathways is established through places ***CLP***, ***P35*** and ***BACE***. Active Calpain enhances β-secretase mediated APP cleavage twice than normal (Kusakawa et al., 2000; Liang et al., 2010) which initiates early production and accumulation of plaques (Jack et al., 2010; Braak et al., 2011). As a counter action, PKC ***PKC*** plays its role and enhances the activity of enzyme α-secretase (***ALPHA***) (Skovronsky et al., 2000). In the next connection, Calpain (***CLP***) hinders the functioning of ***PKC*** by degrading it into pkm (place ***pkm***). Aβ

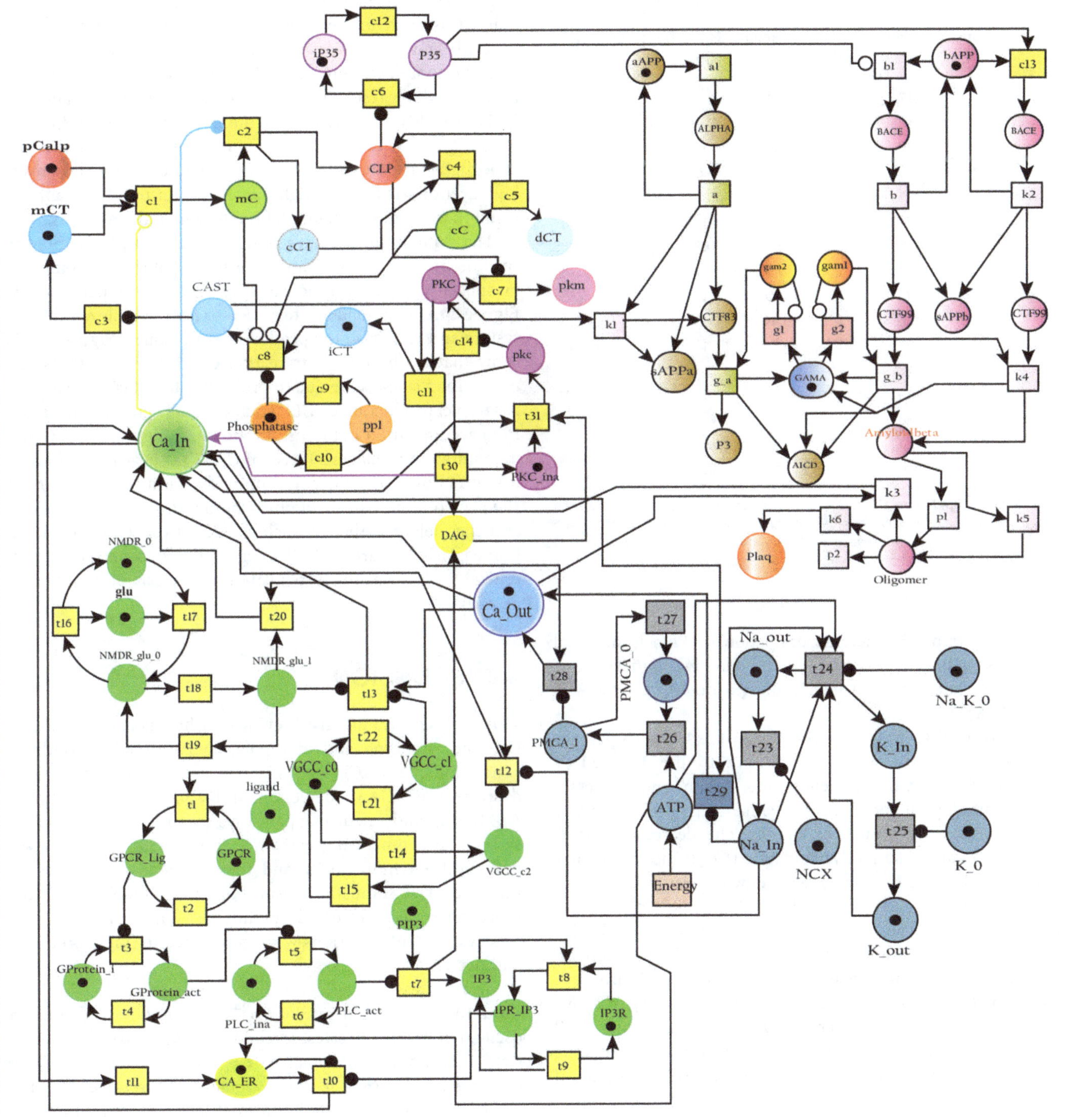

FIGURE 17 | SPN model of the cross talk network of calcium homeostasis, APP processing and Calpain-CAST system Pathways.

oligomers represented by place ***Oligomer*** forms pores into the membrane which instantaneously increases influx of Ca^{2+} ions. The place ***Amyloidbeta*** inhibits the transition **Energy** which indirectly hinders Ca^{2+} extrusion into extracellular space. The new transitions in the crosstalk network are labeled with *k*. The transition ***k1*** connects the place ***PKC*** with ***ALPHA*** while ***P35*** is connected to ***Plaq*** through transitions ***c13***, ***k2***, ***k4***, ***k5***, and ***k6***. The transition ***k3*** joins ***Oligomer*** with ***Ca_In***. The reaction rates of all the transitions are listed in **Table 4**.

The results in **Figure 18** show that ***CLP*** and ***P35*** are accumulating which can directly affect the plaques accumulation process by increase in their deposition rate, as compared to

TABLE 4 | The transitions rates of the SPN model of the crosstalk network.

Tansitions	Rate (μ)	Transitions	Rate (μ)	Transitions	Rate (μ)	Transitions	Rate (μ)
t1	1	*t17*	1	*c1*	0.5	*b*	0.3
t2	1	*t18*	1	*c2*	0.1	*b1*	0.3
t3	1	*t19*	1	*c3*	1	*g1*	0.5
t4	1	*t20*	1	*c4*	0.5	*g2*	0.5
t5	1	*t21*	1	*c5*	0.02	*g_a*	0.5
t6	1	*t22*	1	*c6*	1	*g_b*	0.3
t7	1	*t23*	1	*c7*	0.3	*p1*	0.005
t8	1	*t24*	1	*c8*	0.5	*p2*	0.02
t9	1	*t25*	1	*c9*	1	*k1*	0.5
t10	0.65	*t26*	1	*c10*	1	*k2*	0.6
t11	1	*t27*	1	*c11*	1	*k3*	1
t12	1	*t28*	1	*c12*	0.5	*k4*	0.6
t13	1	*t29*	1	*c13*	1	*k5*	0.01
t14	1	*t30*	1	*c14*	0.5	*k6*	0.04
t15	1	*t31*	1	*a*	0.5		
t16	1	*Energy*	1	*a1*	0.5		

*All the transitions from **Figure 17** are listed with their corresponding rate values. As the SPN is a combination of previous three models, it has only three new connections with transition labeled k. All the transitions are adjusted to rates which can reproduce the patho-physiological condition of the brain.*

results in section 3.3 where accumulation of ***Plaq*** is minimal (**Figure 16A**). It can also be observed that ***mC*** and ***cC*** start declining at later stages which indicates depletion of CAST (**Figure 18A**).

In **Figure 18B**, the concentration of ***sAPPb*** is higher than ***sAPPa*** protein, which is contrary to the **Figure 15B**. Hyper activity of ***CLP*** influences more than one processes in the pathological network by enhancing ***BACE*** activity which increases the growth of ***sAPPb***. The decrease in ***PKC*** concentration and calcium dysregulation (***Ca_In*** rises gradually, ***Ca_Out*** and ***Ca_ER*** both lower down) are also due to over-activation of ***CLP*** (**Figure 18C**). Instability in Calcium equilibrium in neurons appear after 60 unit time which also act as a signal indicating the development of AD. Additionally, degradation of ***PKC*** into ***pkm*** by the action of ***CLP*** also have bidirectional effect on the system. First the availability of active ***CT*** in the cell raises and then ***ALPHA*** secretase driven APP processing slows down (**Figure 18B**). **Figure 18D** represents the translocation and regulation of CAST (***cC*** and***cC***) in the brain cell.

3.5. Therapeutic Intervention

The parameter **Table 5** shows that by changing the rate of reaction of two crucial transitions i.e., ***c2*** and ***c5*** (representing degradation rate of Calpain-CAST complex at membrane and cytosol, respectively) would provide effective strategy to control or stop the development of AD and other related neurological disorders. After applying *in silico* intervention, it can be observed that as the rate of transition ***c2*** is decreased the neurological network move toward stability due to basal or low activity of ***CLP*** (**Figure 19A**). Further, the rate of ***c2*** is set to zero which indicates that ***mC*** is made unbreakable or stable which implies that there would be no production of ***CLP*** (**Figure 19B**). In **Figure 19A**, both the complexes (***mC*** and ***cC***) are maintained for longer time duration which result in low production of ***CLP***, ***Aβ*** and ***Plaq***. In **Figure 19B**, there is neither the production of ***CLP*** nor the formation of ***cC*** due to long life of ***mC*** complex occur and there is negligible production of ***Aβ***. The complex (***mC***) also ensures low level of ***sAPPb*** and high concentration of ***sAPPa*** and as a result there is minor accumulation of ***Plaq*** in the neurons.

The stability of ***mC*** have positive effects in maintaining the calcium homeostasis which regains its equilibrium accompanied by substantial concentration of ***PKC*** and no production of ***P35*** **Figure 20A**. The smaller rate of ***c5*** also favors stable condition of system and can delay the production of plaques. **Figures 19C,D** show that as the rate of transition of *c5* decreases the system maintains a stable state due to prolonged life of ***cC*** which causes basal level production of ***CLP*** and eventually guard against rapid ***Plaq*** accumulation in brains. As shown in **Figure 19D**, ***cC*** helps in maintaining a balanced level of **CAST**, ***sAPPa*** and ***sAPPb*** and it lowers down the concentration and accumulation of ***Aβ*** and ***Plaq***. Also it aids in maintaining homeostasis of other proteins and channels into the cell such as ***PKC***, ***pkm***, ***P35*** and calcium homeostasis (**Figure 20B**). Therefore, these complexes are very critical targets since they regulate homeostasis of many crucial proteins.

4. DISCUSSION

This study contributes in achieving long haul goal of AD research i.e., understanding and manipulating pathological conditions which include BACE and Calpain over-activation, Calcium dysregulation, CAST depletion and abnormal production of Aβ. In this study, neuronal pathways comprising Calpain-CAST system, APP processing pathways and Calcium channels were first modeled individually and then their cross-talk was also modeled. The simulation results of these models predicted a more clearer picture of AD pathogenisis also, on the basis of observations interventions were introduced to linger on the AD pathogenesis.

In a healthy physiological model, rate of Ca^{2+} ions inflow should be lower than rate of Ca^{2+} ions outflow with uniform oscillation within the safest level. Moreover, the concentration of Ca^{2+} ions in intracellular store (***Ca_ER***) is greater than (***Ca_In***) (**Figures 10B,C**) (Korol et al., 2008; Gutierrez-Merino et al., 2014). An equilibrated flow is also observed in other important ions channels such as NCX and NKA, which mediate influx and efflux of Na and K ions. Balance in their flow is obligatory for the adequate efflux of Ca^{2+} ions for maintaining homeostasis (Gutierrez-Merino et al., 2014). Another important physiological pathway, Calpain-CAST regulatory system also depends on Ca^{2+}. The calcium influx and efflux channels are required for the activation and regulation of Calpain.

The simulation results in section 3.2, show that when concentartion of Ca^{2+} is lower inside the cytosol then Calpain is bounded in the complex of Calpain-CAST at membrane.

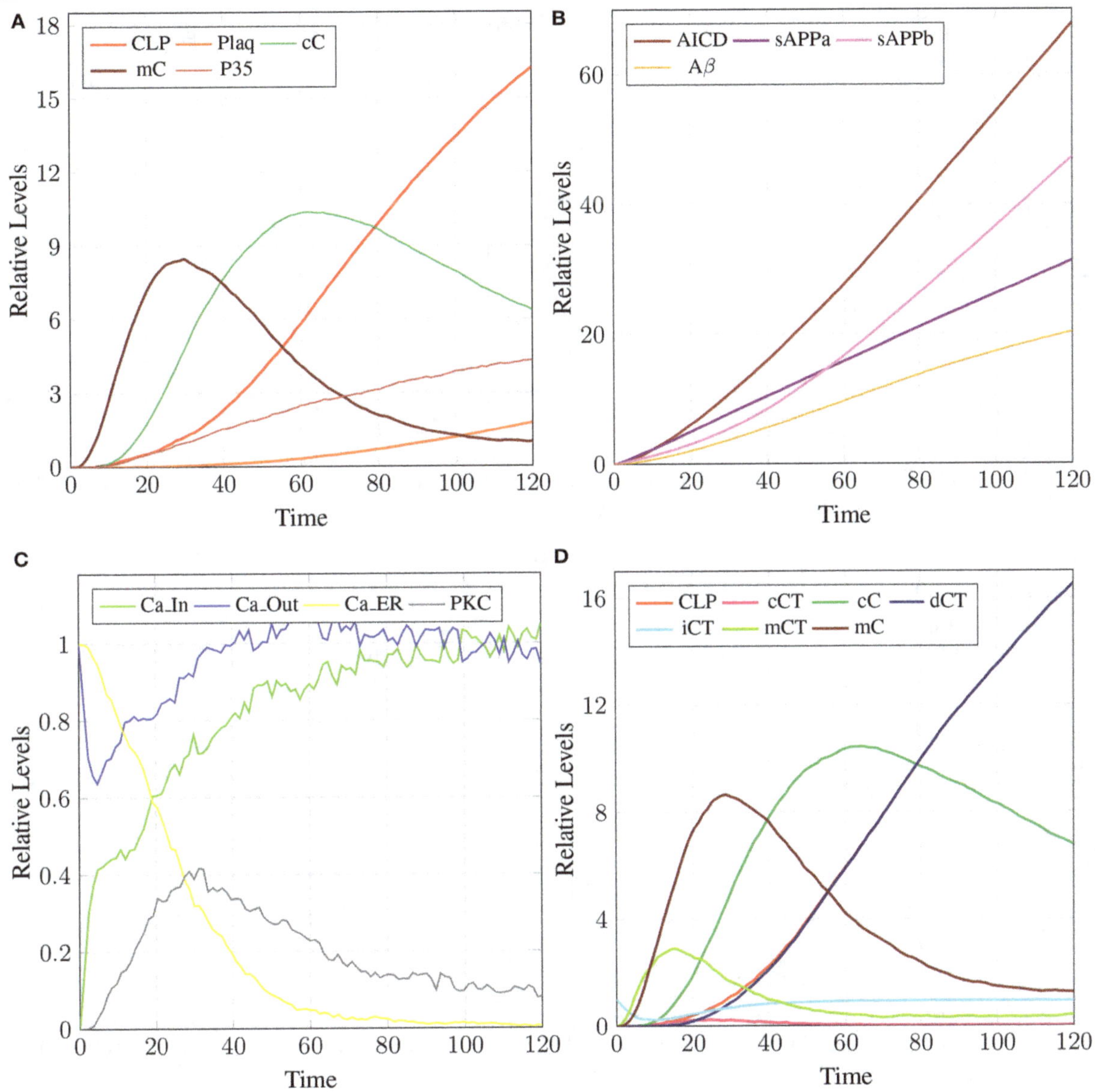

FIGURE 18 | In **(A)**, high concentration of ***CLP*** causes gradual degradation of ***cC*** and further increases the activation of ***P35*** which then activates rapid production of ***Plaq*** leading to the onset of AD. In **(B)**, the production of ***sAPPa*** is lower than the production ***sAPPb*** and ***AICD*** production is higher than both ***sAPPa*** and ***sAPPb***. **(C)** shows slow dysregulation of calcium homeostasis by increase of concentration of ***Ca_In*** from ***Ca_Out*** and ***Ca_ER***. **(D)** shows conversion of ***iCT*** into active form then translocation to membrane ***mCT*** and cytosol ***cCT***. Furthermore, ***cCT*** binds with ***CLP*** to form ***cC***. ***CLP*** gradually degrades CAST into ***dCT***.

TABLE 5 | Transition rate table.

Tansitions	Rate (μ)	Rate (μ)
c2	0.05	0.0
c5	0.005	0.0

Changing the rate of crucial transitions c2 and c5 to study their effects on crosstalk network model ***Figure 17****.*

As concentartion of Ca^{2+} rises, the complex degrades and active Calpain is produced (De Tullio et al., 1999; Todd et al., 2003). To regulate Calpain's activation, CAST appears to form Calpian-CAST complex in cytosol, but gradually its peak falls down which shows release of active Calpain and degradation of CAST. The results in **Figures 12C,D** show that as ***CLP*** rises, both the complexes (***mC*** and ***cC***) gradually degrade which causes depletion of CAST (Averna et al., 2001b; Tompa et al., 2002). PKC also has important role in building a feedback mechanism for Calpain by phosphorylating CAST into inactive form (Averna et al., 2001a). Calpain is also regulating PKC by cleaving it into pkm (Goll et al., 2003) which is persistently active catalytic fragment and quickly disappears (Yamakawa et al., 2001; Liu et al., 2008). PKC also has important roles in the system, it is favoring α-secretase mediated APP cleavage (Rossner et al., 2001; Racchi et al., 2003) and is also involved in inactivation of CAST through phosphorylation

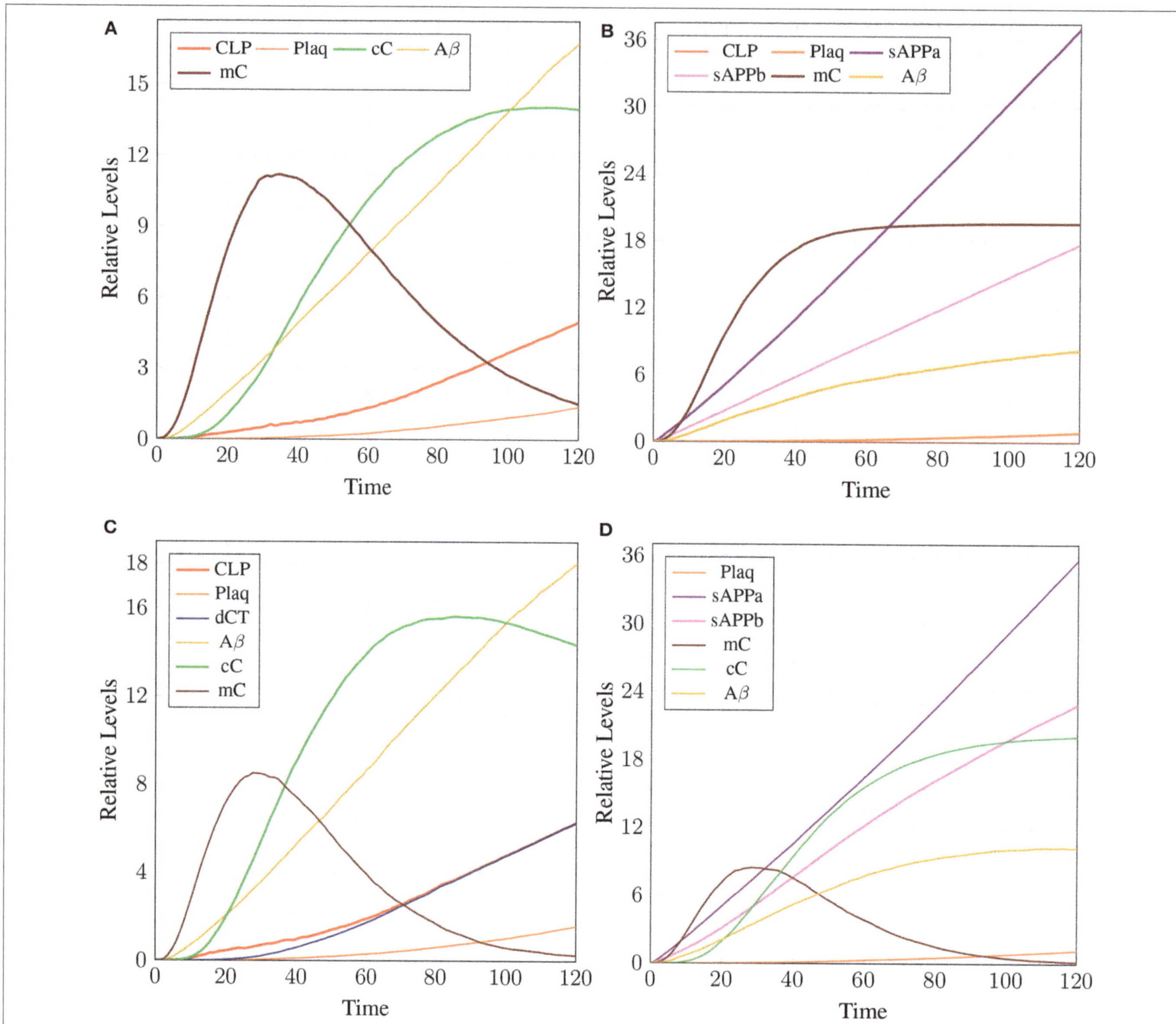

FIGURE 19 | A mild cognitive impairment behavior in **(A,C)**. ***CLP*** is in loosely controlled by ***mC*** and ***cC*** ($c2 = 0.05$ and $c5 = 0.005$). There is low level of ***Plaq*** and significant level of ***Aβ***. By changing the rate of $c2 = 0$ **(B)** there is no conversion of pro-Calpain into ***CLP*** due to long life of ***mC***. Production of ***sAPPb*** and ***Aβ*** are also decreased sufficiently and it lingers on the process of accumulation of ***Plaq***. In **(D)**, *c5* is set to zero which controls level of ***CLP*** after its activation and saves CAST from depletion into ***dCT***. The production of ***sAPPa*** is higher than production of ***sAPPb*** in **(B,D)**.

(Olariu et al., 2002). The inactive CAST regains its active conformation in the presence of phosphatases (Averna et al., 2001a).

Simulation results of the model APP processing pathways show that in a healthy brain all three enzymes of this pathway are available in the cell to digest the around-the-clock production of APP with α-secretase having high affinity as compared to BACE (De Strooper and Annaert, 2000). Consequently, production rate of sAPPα is higher than sAPPβ (**Figure 15B**) which is a depiction of normal physiological behavior (De Strooper and Annaert, 2000; Lichtenthaler, 2011). Studies showed that in healthy brain, plaques produce and accumulate in a linear fashion which is also observed in our studies. Moreover, $A\beta$ burdens in the form of plaques at elder age. This linear behavior of plaques accumulation can adopt exponential growth due to the high accumulation rate with passage of time. In our results the formation of plaques first enter the lag phase (no plaques appearance) upto 80 unit time and then evolve into growth phase (evolution), which is also experimentally reported (Friedrich et al., 2010; Jack et al., 2010; Sperling et al., 2011).

In neuro-pathological model, simulation revealed that the intermediate product sAPPβ of amyloidogenic pathway rises in the AD brain. Higher concentration of sAPPβ can lead to early occurrence of AD (at age of 40 and onward) due

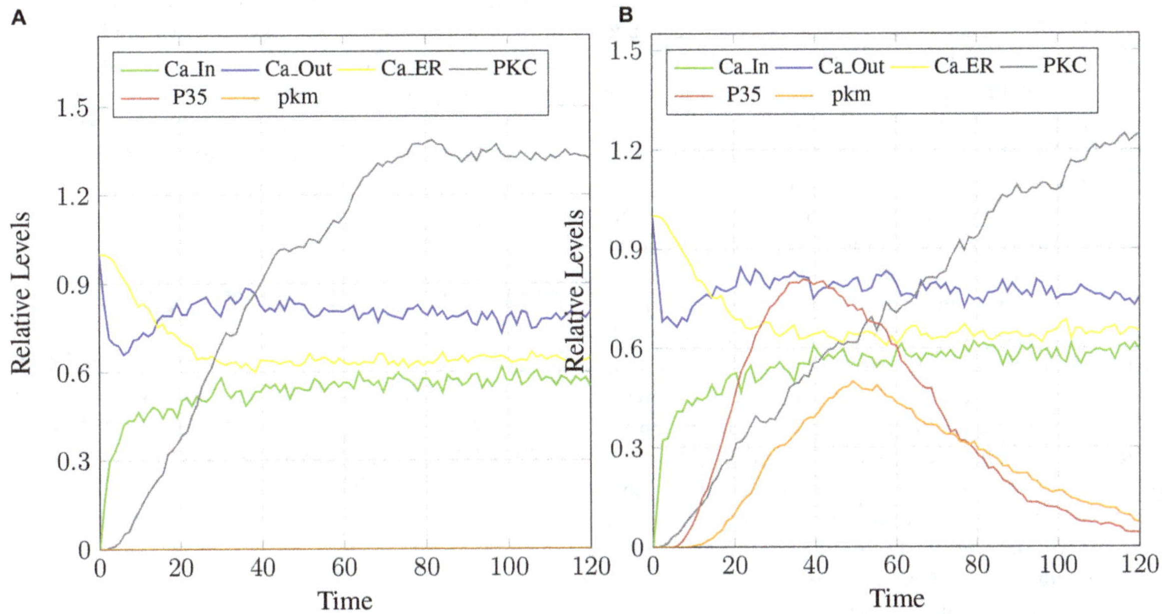

FIGURE 20 | The restoration of Calcium homeostasis. In **(A)**, ***PKC*** is present for longer time and there is no conversion into ***pkm*** also there is no production of ***P35***. In **(B)**, there is less production of ***P35*** and ***pkm***.

to rapid deposition of the plaques in brain of AD patients (Freer et al., 2016). Higher level of sAPPβ also indicate the enhanced activity of BACE which is triggered by over-activation of Calpain. Enhanced activation of Calpain disturbs more than one processes in the pathological network i.e., increased BACE activity, decreased PKC functioning and calcium dysregulation. Initially CAST and its complex with pro-Calpain are in high quantity to control Calpain but with the elevation of calcium influx, the complex starts to degrade. The active Calpain accumulates in cytosol which is then controlled by cytosolic CAST by forming complex with it. After sometime Calpain degrades the CAST in the complex to release itself into the cytosol and eventually CAST and complex deplete from the cell (Higuchi et al., 2012). Depletion of CAST destroys the cell normal functioning and then nervous system deteriorates (Rao et al., 2008, 2014; Kurbatskaya et al., 2016).

After analyzing the neuropathological network, the vague picture of AD development becomes more clear. It provide useful observations such as loss of calcium homeostasis occur after 60 unit time due to intra-neuronal ATP depletion caused by elevation of Calpain (Lipton, 1999; Kurbatskaya et al., 2016) and formation of extracellular ion pores formed by Aβ oligomers (Small et al., 2009). Ca^{2+} disruption increases Calpain concentration in neurons which further elevates the BACE activity toward APP (Liang et al., 2010; Chami and Checler, 2012; Song et al., 2015) via cdk5 dependent pathway as a result of Aβ and sAPPβ levels in neurons built up (Sennvik et al., 2004). In normal healthy brain, the mean burden in the form of plaques are low and it increase in linear fashion from 60 to 90 unit time (Rodrigue et al., 2012; Freer et al., 2016; Kurbatskaya et al., 2016). It is noteworthy that both amyloidogenic and non-amyloidogenic pathways are enabled in an healthy individual but plaques in the brain of AD patient grow rapidly due to increased Calpain mediated cleavage of APP through BACE (Mawuenyega et al., 2010). It can be inferred that all the neuro-pathological events are inter-related where Calpain and its complexes are playing crucial role. Calpain can be called as bone of contention and the complexes are the defenders. This neuropathological network provides valuable knowledge about interventions and offers new therapeutic targets. To stop the Calpain destructive effects, it may be effective strategy to slightly modify the natural process. In the work of Emmaneul and coworkers on cardiovascular remodeling, the Calpain-CAST system has emerged as new effective strategy to prevent angiotension (Letavernier et al., 2008). In our study, Calpain-CAST complexes have also proved to be effective therapeutic targets for delaying the process of neuronal degradation which can save the brains from AD.

5. CONCLUSION

In AD, Aβ has central role as they accumulate into hallmark lesions i.e., plaques. Aβ generates from APP cleavage through amyloidogenic pathway. Progression of the corresponding processing pathway increases due to over-activation of Caplain and depletion of its sole inhibitor CAST. Calpain hyper activation depends on high Calcium concentration in the cytosol. Calpain triggers the production of P35 and the degradation of CAST and PKC. In-Addition, it also triggers the imbalance of calcium homeostasis. All these observations were incorporated into a Stochastic PN models. We gained insight into the mechanism of the AD progression and were able to derive some useful inferences. The first important inference is that under hyper-activation of Calpain, calcium homeostasis dysregulates and CAST starts to degrade gradually. APP processing enzyme

(BACE) increases two folds which starts producing $A\beta$ that slowly accumulates into plaques in AD brains at early age and lesions appear later. The second important inference is about the most crucial protein Calpain that influences many important proteins of neuronal network such as CAST, PKC, P35, and BACE. Furthermore, these proteins together dysregulate calcium homeostasis. Calpain regulation through CAST plays important role in keeping cells safe from neurodegradation. CAST encounters Calpain at two locations in the cell. Initially at membrane, CAST forms complex with inactive Calpain which is short lived and dissociates as the calcium influx increases. In the cytoplasm, active Calpain-CAST complex is long-standing which keeps the Calpain concentration in control but it also degraded slowly by the action of Calpain. From our study, Calpain and Calpain-CAST complexes have emerged as the potential therapeutic targets for the treatment of neurodegenerative pathologies. The pathway modeling of these networks have predicted that we can introduce delays in the production and accumulation of plaques by targeting the Calpain-CAST complexes. The production of Calpain should be kept in safe levels to avoid its hyper activity. It can be achieved implicitly by enhancing activity of Calpain-CAST complexes. The more durable are the complexes, the lesser would be the accumulation of plaques. Another useful strategy can be the designing of inhibitors against the active Calpain using *in silico* methods and *in vitro* experiments. By considering these effective interventions we can increase the chances of healthy life expectancy and can save many lives and families from the adversity of AD.

AUTHOR CONTRIBUTIONS

JAs and JAh conceived research idea, designed and performed the experiments, analyzed the data, wrote the paper, prepared figures and/or tables, reviewed drafts of the paper. AA and ZU-H analyzed the data, prepared tables and/or figures, wrote the paper, reviewed drafts of the paper.

REFERENCES

Alkon, D. L., Sun, M.-K., and Nelson, T. J. (2007). Pkc signaling deficits: a mechanistic hypothesis for the origins of alzheimer's disease. *Trends Pharmacol. Sci.* 28, 51–60. doi: 10.1016/j.tips.2006.12.002

Annaert, W. G., and Saftig, P. (2009). Regulated intramembrane proteolysis—a story about sheddases and I-CliPs. *Semin. Cell Dev. Biol.* 20:125. doi: 10.1016/j.semcdb.2009.03.005

Ashford, J. W. (2004). Apoe genotype effects on Alzheimer's disease onset and epidemiology. *J. Mol. Neurosci.* 23, 157–165. doi: 10.1385/JMN:23:3:157

Averna, M., De Tullio, R., Passalacqua, M., Salamino, F., Pontremoli, S., and Melloni, E. (2001a). Changes in intracellular calpastatin localization are mediated by reversible phosphorylation. *Biochem. J.* 354, 25–30. doi: 10.1042/bj3540025

Averna, M., De Tullio, R., Salamino, F., Minafra, R., Pontremoli, S., and Melloni, E. (2001b). Age-dependent degradation of calpastatin in kidney of hypertensive rats. *J. Biol. Chem.* 276, 38426–38432. doi: 10.1074/jbc.M101936200

Berridge, M. J. (2009). Inositol trisphosphate and calcium signalling mechanisms. *Mol. Cell Res.* 1793, 933–940. doi: 10.1016/j.bbamcr.2008.10.005

Blätke, M. A., Heiner, M., and Marwan, W. (2011). *Petri Nets in Systems Biology.* Technical report, Technical Report, Otto-von-Guericke University Magdeburg.

Braak, H., Thal, D. R., Ghebremedhin, E., and Del Tredici, K. (2011). Stages of the pathologic process in alzheimer disease: age categories from 1 to 100 years. *J. Neuropathol. Exp. Neurol.* 70, 960–969. doi: 10.1097/NEN.0b013e318232a379

Brittain, M. K., Brustovetsky, T., Sheets, P. L., Brittain, J. M., Khanna, R., Cummins, T. R., et al. (2012). Delayed calcium dysregulation in neurons requires both the nmda receptor and the reverse Na+/Ca2+ exchanger. *Neurobiol. Dis.* 46, 109–117. doi: 10.1016/j.nbd.2011.12.051

Budson, A. E., and Price, B. H. (2005). Memory dysfunction. *New Engl. J. Med.* 352, 692–699. doi: 10.1056/NEJMra041071

Cai, H., Wang, Y., McCarthy, D., Wen, H., Borchelt, D. R., Price, D. L., et al. (2001). Bace1 is the major β-secretase for generation of aβ peptides by neurons. *Nat. Neurosci.* 4, 233–234. doi: 10.1038/85064

Cain, S. M., and Snutch, T. P. (2011). Voltage-gated calcium channels and disease. *Biofactors* 37, 197–205. doi: 10.1002/biof.158

Castaldi, D., Maccagnola, D., Mari, D., and Archetti, F. (2012). "Stochastic simulation of the coagulation cascade: a petri net based approach," in *European Conference on Parallel Processing* (Rhodos: Springer).

Chami, L., and Checler, F. (2012). Bace1 is at the crossroad of a toxic vicious cycle involving cellular stress and β-amyloid production in Alzheimer's disease. *Mol. Neurodegenerat.* 7:52. doi: 10.1186/1750-1326-7-52

Chen, M., and Fernandez, H. L. (2004). Stimulation of β-amyloid precursor protein α-processing by phorbol ester involves calcium and calpain activation. *Biochem. Biophys. Res. Commun.* 316, 332–340. doi: 10.1016/j.bbrc.2004.02.052

Courjaret, R., Grolleau, F., and Lapied, B. (2003). Two distinct calcium-sensitive and-insensitive pkc up-and down-regulate an α-bungarotoxin-resistant nachr1 in insect neurosecretory cells (dum neurons). *Eur. J. Neurosci.* 17, 2023–2034. doi: 10.1046/j.1460-9568.2003.02644.x

Cuello, A. C. (2005). Intracellular and extracellular aβ, a tale of two neuropathologies. *Brain Pathol.* 15, 66–71. doi: 10.1111/j.1750-3639.2005.tb00101.x

David, R., and Alla, H. (2010). *Discrete, Continuous, and Hybrid Petri Nets.* Grenoble: Springer Science & Business Media.

De Strooper, B., and Annaert, W. (2000). Proteolytic processing and cell biological functions of the amyloid precursor protein. *J. Cell. Sci.* 113, 1857–1870.

De Tullio, R., Passalacqua, M., Averna, M., Salamino, F., Melloni, E., and Pontremoli, S. (1999). Changes in intracellular localization of calpastatin during calpain activation. *Biochem. J.* 343, 467–472. doi: 10.1042/bj3430467

DeStrooper, B., Saftig, P., Birchmeier, C., and Haass, C. (2006). Control of peripheral nerve myelination by the beta-secretase bace1. *Science* 314, 664–666. doi: 10.1126/science.1132341

Emptage, N. J., Reid, C. A., and Fine, A. (2001). Calcium stores in hippocampal synaptic boutons mediate short-term plasticity, store-operated ca 2+ entry, and spontaneous transmitter release. *Neuron* 29, 197–208. doi: 10.1016/S0896-6273(01)00190-8

Etcheberrigaray, R., Tan, M., Dewachter, I., Kuipéri, C., Van der Auwera, I., Wera, S., et al. (2004). Therapeutic effects of pkc activators in alzheimer's disease transgenic mice. *Proc. Natl. Acad. Sci. U.S.A.* 101, 11141–11146. doi: 10.1073/pnas.0403921101

Ferreira, A. (2012). Calpain dysregulation in Alzheimer's disease. *ISRN Biochem.* 2012:728571. doi: 10.5402/2012/728571

Freer, R., Sormanni, P., Vecchi, G., Ciryam, P., Dobson, C. M., and Vendruscolo, M. (2016). A protein homeostasis signature in healthy brains recapitulates tissue vulnerability to Alzheimer's disease. *Sci. Adv.* 2:e1600947. doi: 10.1126/sciadv.1600947

Friedrich, R. P., Tepper, K., Rönicke, R., Soom, M., Westermann, M., Reymann, K., et al. (2010). Mechanism of amyloid plaque formation suggests an intracellular basis of aβ pathogenicity. *Proc. Natl. Acad. Sci. U.S.A.* 107, 1942–1947. doi: 10.1073/pnas.0904532106

Gillespie, D. T. (1976). A general method for numerically simulating the stochastic time evolution of coupled chemical reactions. *J. Comput. Phys.* 22, 403–434. doi: 10.1016/0021-9991(76)90041-3

Golde, T. E. (2005). The aβ hypothesis: Leading us to rationally-designed therapeutic strategies for the treatment or prevention of alzheimer disease. *Brain Pathol.* 15, 84–87. doi: 10.1111/j.1750-3639.2005.tb00104.x

Goll, D. E., Thompson, V. F., Li, H., Wei, W., and Cong, J. (2003). The calpain system. *Physiol. Rev.* 83, 731–801. doi: 10.1152/physrev.00029.2002

Goss, P. J., and Peccoud, J. (1998). Quantitative modeling of stochastic systems in molecular biology by using stochastic petri nets. *Proc. Natl. Acad. Sci. U.S.A.* 95, 6750–6755. doi: 10.1073/pnas.95.12.6750

Greenfield, J. P., Tsai, J., Gouras, G. K., Hai, B., Thinakaran, G., Checler, F., et al. (1999). Endoplasmic reticulum and trans-golgi network generate distinct populations of Alzheimer β-amyloid peptides. *Proc. Natl. Acad. Sci. U.S.A.* 96, 742–747. doi: 10.1073/pnas.96.2.742

Gutierrez-Merino, C., Marques-da Silva, D., Fortalezas, S., and Samhan-Arias, A. K. (2014). "Cytosolic calcium homeostasis in neurons–control systems, modulation by reactive oxygen and nitrogen species, and space and time fluctuations," in *Neurochemistry*, ed T. Heinbockel (Rijeka: InTech), 59–110.

Haass, C. (2004). Take five–bace and the γ-secretase quartet conduct alzheimer's amyloid β-peptide generation. *EMBO J.* 23, 483–488. doi: 10.1038/sj.emboj.7600061

Hanna, R. A., Campbell, R. L., and Davies, P. L. (2008). Calcium-bound structure of calpain and its mechanism of inhibition by calpastatin. *Nature* 456, 409–412. doi: 10.1038/nature07451

Hardy, J., and Selkoe, D. J. (2002). The amyloid hypothesis of Alzheimer's disease: progress and problems on the road to therapeutics. *Science* 297, 353–356. doi: 10.1126/science.1072994

Hardy, J. A., and Higgins, G. A. (1992). Alzheimer's disease: the amyloid cascade hypothesis. *Science* 256, 184. doi: 10.1126/science.1566067

Heiner, M., Gilbert, D., and Donaldson, R. (2008). "Petri nets for systems and synthetic biology," in *International School on Formal Methods for the Design of Computer, Communication and Software Systems*, eds M. Bernardo, P. Degano, and G. Zavattaro (Bertinoro: Springer), 215–264.

Higuchi, M., Iwata, N., Matsuba, Y., Takano, J., Suemoto, T., Maeda, J., et al. (2012). Mechanistic involvement of the calpain-calpastatin system in alzheimer neuropathology. *FASEB J.* 26, 1204–1217. doi: 10.1096/fj.11-187740

Hu, X., Hicks, C. W., He, W., Wong, P., Macklin, W. B., Trapp, B. D., et al. (2006). Bace1 modulates myelination in the central and peripheral nervous system. *Nat. Neurosci.* 9, 1520–1525. doi: 10.1038/nn1797

Jack, C. R., Knopman, D. S., Jagust, W. J., Shaw, L. M., Aisen, P. S., Weiner, M. W., et al. (2010). Hypothetical model of dynamic biomarkers of the Alzheimer's pathological cascade. *Lancet Neurol.* 9, 119–128. doi: 10.1016/S1474-4422(09)70299-6

Jonsson, T., Atwal, J. K., Steinberg, S., Snaedal, J., Jonsson, P. V., Bjornsson, S., et al. (2012). A mutation in app protects against Alzheimer's disease and age-related cognitive decline. *Nature* 488:96. doi: 10.1038/nature11283

Korol, T. Y., Kostyuk, E., and Kostyuk, P., (2008). Disruption of calcium homeostasis in Alzheimer's disease. *Neurophysiology* 40, 385–392. doi: 10.1007/s11062-009-9064-5

Krebs, J., Agellon, L. B., and Michalak, M. (2015). Ca2+ homeostasis and endoplasmic reticulum (er) stress: an integrated view of calcium signaling. *Biochem. Biophys. Res. Commun.* 460, 114–121. doi: 10.1016/j.bbrc.2015.02.004

Kurbatskaya, K., Phillips, E. C., Croft, C. L., Dentoni, G., Hughes, M. M., Wade, M. A., et al. (2016). Upregulation of calpain activity precedes tau phosphorylation and loss of synaptic proteins in Alzheimer's disease brain. *Acta Neuropathol. Commun.* 4:34. doi: 10.1186/s40478-016-0299-2

Kusakawa, G.-i., Saito, T., Onuki, R., Ishiguro, K., Kishimoto, T., and Hisanaga, S.-i. (2000). Calpain-dependent proteolytic cleavage of the p35 cyclin-dependent kinase 5 activator to p25. *J. Biol. Chem.* 275, 17166–17172. doi: 10.1074/jbc.M907757199

LaFerla, F. M. (2002). Calcium dyshomeostasis and intracellular signalling in Alzheimer's disease. *Nat. Rev. Neurosci.* 3, 862–872. doi: 10.1038/nrn960

Lamprecht, R., Smith, G. D., and Kemper, P. (2011). Stochastic petri net models of ca2+ signaling complexes and their analysis. *Nat. Comput.* 10, 1045–1075. doi: 10.1007/s11047-009-9143-y

Lanni, C., Mazzucchelli, M., Porrello, E., Govoni, S., and Racchi, M. (2004). Differential involvement of protein kinase c alpha and epsilon in the regulated secretion of soluble amyloid precursor protein. *Eur. J. Biochem.* 271, 3068–3075. doi: 10.1111/j.1432-1033.2004.04240.x

Lee, J., Retamal, C., Cuitiño, L., Caruano-Yzermans, A., Shin, J.-E., Van Kerkhof, P., et al. (2008). Adaptor protein sorting nexin 17 regulates amyloid precursor protein trafficking and processing in the early endosomes. *J. Biol. Chem.* 283, 11501–11508. doi: 10.1074/jbc.M800642200

Lee, M.-s., Kwon, Y. T., Li, M., Peng, J., Friedlander, R. M., and Tsai, L.-H. (2000). Neurotoxicity induces cleavage of p35 to p25 by calpain. *Nature* 405, 360–364. doi: 10.1038/35012636

Lee, V. M., Goedert, M., and Trojanowski, J. Q. (2001). Neurodegenerative tauopathies. *Annu. Rev. Neurosci.* 24, 1121–1159. doi: 10.1146/annurev.neuro.24.1.1121

Letavernier, E., Perez, J., Bellocq, A., Mesnard, L., de Castro Keller, A., Haymann, J.-P., et al. (2008). Targeting the calpain/calpastatin system as a new strategy to prevent cardiovascular remodeling in angiotensin ii–induced hypertension. *Circul. Res.* 102, 720–728. doi: 10.1161/CIRCRESAHA.107.160077

Li, Q., and Südhof, T. C. (2004). Cleavage of amyloid-β precursor protein and amyloid-β precursor-like protein by bace 1. *J. Biol. Chem.* 279, 10542–10550. doi: 10.1074/jbc.M310001200

Liang, B., Duan, B.-Y., Zhou, X.-P., Gong, J.-X., and Luo, Z.-G. (2010). Calpain activation promotes bace1 expression, amyloid precursor protein processing, and amyloid plaque formation in a transgenic mouse model of alzheimer disease. *J. Biol. Chem.* 285, 27737–27744. doi: 10.1074/jbc.M110.117960

Lichtenthaler, S. F. (2011). Alpha-secretase in Alzheimer's disease: molecular identity, regulation and therapeutic potential. *J. Neurochem.* 116, 10–21. doi: 10.1111/j.1471-4159.2010.07081.x

Lipton, P. (1999). Ischemic cell death in brain neurons. *Physiol. Rev.* 79, 1431–1568. doi: 10.1152/physrev.1999.79.4.1431

Liu, F., Heiner, M., and Yang, M. (2016). Fuzzy stochastic petri nets for modeling biological systems with uncertain kinetic parameters. *PLoS ONE* 11:e0149674. doi: 10.1371/journal.pone.0149674

Liu, J., Liu, M. C., and Wang, K. K. (2008). Calpain in the cns: from synaptic function to neurotoxicity. *Sci. Signal.* 1, re1. doi: 10.1126/stke.114re1

Marsan, M. A., Balbo, G., Conte, G., Donatelli, S., and Franceschinis, G. (1994). *Modelling With Generalized Stochastic Petri Nets*. New York, NY: John Wiley & Sons, Inc.

Marwan, W., Rohr, C., and Heiner, M. (2012). Petri nets in snoopy: a unifying framework for the graphical display, computational modelling, and simulation of bacterial regulatory networks. *Bact. Mol. Netw. Methods Protocols* 804, 409–437. doi: 10.1007/978-1-61779-361-5_21

Mattson, M. P. (2004). Pathways towards and away from alzheimer's disease. *Nature* 430, 631–639. doi: 10.1038/nature02621

Mattson, M. P., LaFerla, F. M., Chan, S. L., Leissring, M. A., Shepel, P. N., and Geiger, J. D. (2000). Calcium signaling in the er: its role in neuronal plasticity and neurodegenerative disorders. *Trends Neurosci.* 23, 222–229. doi: 10.1016/S0166-2236(00)01548-4

Mawuenyega, K. G., Sigurdson, W., Ovod, V., Munsell, L., Kasten, T., Morris, J. C., et al. (2010). Decreased clearance of cns β-amyloid in Alzheimer's disease. *Science* 330, 1774–1774. doi: 10.1126/science.1197623

Melloni, E., Averna, M., Stifanese, R., De Tullio, R., Defranchi, E., Salamino, F., et al. (2006). Association of calpastatin with inactive calpain a novel mechanism to control the activation of the protease? *J. Biol. Chem.* 281, 24945–24954. doi: 10.1074/jbc.M601449200

Mounts, W. M., and Liebman, M. N. (1997). Application of petri nets and stochastic activity nets to modeling biological pathways and processes. *Int. J. Comput. Simul.* 20, 265–281.

Mura, I., and Csikász-Nagy, A. (2008). Stochastic petri net extension of a yeast cell cycle model. *J. Theor. Biol.* 254, 850–860. doi: 10.1016/j.jtbi.2008.07.019

O'Brien, R. J., and Wong, P. C. (2011). Amyloid precursor protein processing and Alzheimer's disease. *Annu. Rev. Neurosci.* 34, 185–204. doi: 10.1146/annurev-neuro-061010-113613

Olariu, A., Yamada, K., Mamiya, T., Hefco, V., and Nabeshima, T. (2002). Memory impairment induced by chronic intracerebroventricular infusion of beta-amyloid (1–40) involves downregulation of protein kinase c. *Brain Res.* 957, 278–286. doi: 10.1016/S0006-8993(02)03608-9

Ono, Y., and Sorimachi, H. (2012). Calpains–an elaborate proteolytic system. *Biochimica et Biophysica Acta* 1824, 224–236. doi: 10.1016/j.bbapap.2011.08.005

Orrenius, S., Zhivotovsky, B., and Nicotera, P. (2003). Calcium: Regulation of cell death: the calcium–apoptosis link. *Nat. Rev. Mol. Cell Biol.* 4, 552. doi: 10.1038/nrm1150

Pal, G. P., Elce, J. S., and Jia, Z. (2001). Dissociation and aggregation of calpain in the presence of calcium. *J. Biol. Chem.* 276, 47233–47238. doi: 10.1074/jbc.M105149200

Petri, C. (1966). *Kommunikation mit Automaten.* Bonn: Institut für Instrumentelle Mathematik, Schriften Des IIM, No. 3 (1962). English Translation: Communication with Automata, Griffiss Air Force Base. Tech. Rep. RADC-TR-65-377, 1.

Racchi, M., Mazzucchelli, M., Pascale, A., Sironi, M., and Govoni, S. (2003). Role of protein kinase cα in the regulated secretion of the amyloid precursor protein. *Mol. Psychiatry* 8, 209–216. doi: 10.1038/sj.mp.4001204

Rao, M. V., McBrayer, M. K., Campbell, J., Kumar, A., Hashim, A., Sershen, H., et al. (2014). Specific calpain inhibition by calpastatin prevents tauopathy and neurodegeneration and restores normal lifespan in tau p301l mice. *J. Neurosci.* 34, 9222–9234. doi: 10.1523/JNEUROSCI.1132-14.2014

Rao, M. V., Mohan, P. S., Peterhoff, C. M., Yang, D.-S., Schmidt, S. D., Stavrides, P. H., et al. (2008). Marked calpastatin (cast) depletion in Alzheimer's disease accelerates cytoskeleton disruption and neurodegeneration: neuroprotection by cast overexpression. *J. Neurosci.* 28, 12241–12254. doi: 10.1523/JNEUROSCI.4119-08.2008

Rodrigue, K., Kennedy, K., Devous, M., Rieck, J., Hebrank, A., Diaz-Arrastia, R., et al. (2012). β-amyloid burden in healthy aging regional distribution and cognitive consequences. *Neurology* 78, 387–395. doi: 10.1212/WNL.0b013e318245d295

Rossner, S., Mendla, K., Schliebs, R., and Bigl, V. (2001). Protein kinase cα and β1 isoforms are regulators of α-secretory proteolytic processing of amyloid precursor protein *in vivo*. *Eur. J. Neurosci.* 13, 1644–1648. doi: 10.1046/j.0953-816x.2001.01525.x

Roussel, B. D., Kruppa, A. J., Miranda, E., Crowther, D. C., Lomas, D. A., and Marciniak, S. J. (2013). Endoplasmic reticulum dysfunction in neurological disease. *Lancet Neurol.* 12, 105–118. doi: 10.1016/S1474-4422(12)70238-7

Ryu, M., and Nakazawa, T. (2014). "Calcium and calpain activation," in *Neuroprotection and Neuroregeneration for Retinal Diseases*, eds T. Nakazawa, Y. Kitaoka, and T. Harada (Tokyo: Springer), 13–24.

Santos, D. M., Xavier, J. M., Morgado, A. L., Sola, S., and Rodrigues, C. M. (2012). Distinct regulatory functions of calpain 1 and 2 during neural stem cell self-renewal and differentiation. *PLoS ONE* 7:e33468. doi: 10.1371/journal.pone.0033468

Schmolesky, M. T., Weber, J. T., Zeeuw, C. I., and Hansel, C. (2002). The making of a complex spike: ionic composition and plasticity. *Ann. N.Y. Acad. Sci.* 978, 359–390. doi: 10.1111/j.1749-6632.2002.tb07581.x

Selkoe, D. J. (2000). Toward a comprehensive theory for alzheimer's disease. hypothesis: Alzheimer's disease is caused by the cerebral accumulation and cytotoxicity of amyloid β-protein. *Ann. N.Y. Acad. Sci.* 924, 17–25. doi: 10.1111/j.1749-6632.2000.tb05554.x

Selkoe, D. J. (2002). Alzheimer's disease is a synaptic failure. *Science* 298, 789–791. doi: 10.1126/science.1074069

Sennvik, K., Bogdanovic, N., Volkmann, I., Fastbom, J., and Benedikz, E. (2004). β-secretase-cleaved amyloid precursor protein in Alzheimer brain: a morphologic study. *J. Cell. Mol. Med.* 8, 127–134. doi: 10.1111/j.1582-4934.2004.tb00267.x

Skovronsky, D. M., Moore, D. B., Milla, M. E., Doms, R. W., and Lee, V. M.-Y. (2000). Protein kinase c-dependent α-secretase competes with β-secretase for cleavage of amyloid-β precursor protein in the trans-golgi network. *J. Biol. Chem.* 275, 2568–2575. doi: 10.1074/jbc.275.4.2568

Small, D. H. (2009). Dysregulation of calcium homeostasis in Alzheimer's disease. *Neurochem. Res.* 34, 1824–1829. doi: 10.1007/s11064-009-9960-5

Small, D. H., Gasperini, R., Vincent, A. J., Hung, A. C., and Foa, L. (2009). The role of aβ-induced calcium dysregulation in the pathogenesis of Alzheimer's disease. *J. Alzheimer's Dis.* 16, 225–233. doi: 10.3233/JAD-2009-0951

Smith, I. F., Green, K. N., and LaFerla, F. M. (2005). Calcium dysregulation in alzheimer's disease: recent advances gained from genetically modified animals. *Cell Calc.* 38, 427–437. doi: 10.1016/j.ceca.2005.06.021

Song, W.-J., Son, M.-Y., Lee, H.-W., Seo, H., Kim, J. H., and Chung, S.-H. (2015). Enhancement of bace1 activity by p25/cdk5-mediated phosphorylation in Alzheimer's disease. *PLoS ONE* 10:e0136950. doi: 10.1371/journal.pone.0136950

Sperling, R. A., Aisen, P. S., Beckett, L. A., Bennett, D. A., Craft, S., Fagan, A. M., et al. (2011). Toward defining the preclinical stages of Alzheimer's disease: recommendations from the national institute on aging-alzheimer's association workgroups on diagnostic guidelines for Alzheimer's disease. *Alzheimer's Dement.* 7, 280–292. doi: 10.1016/j.jalz.2011.03.003

Stutzmann, G. E. (2005). Calcium dysregulation, ip3 signaling, and Alzheimer's disease. *Neuroscientist* 11, 110–115. doi: 10.1177/1073858404270899

Tam, J. H., and Pasternak, S. H. (2012). Amyloid and alzheimer's disease: inside and out. *Can. J. Neurol. Sci.* 39, 286–298. doi: 10.1017/S0317167100013408

Tareen, S. H. K., and Ahmad, J. (2015). Modelling and analysis of the feeding regimen induced entrainment of hepatocyte circadian oscillators using petri nets. *PLoS ONE* 10:e0117519. doi: 10.1371/journal.pone.0117519

Tiraboschi, P., Hansen, L., Alford, M., Masliah, E., Thal, L., and Corey-Bloom, J. (2000). The decline in synapses and cholinergic activity is asynchronous in Alzheimer's disease. *Neurology* 55, 1278–1283. doi: 10.1212/WNL.55.9.1278

Todd, B., Moore, D., Deivanayagam, C. C., Chattopadhyay, D., Maki, M., Wang, K. K., et al. (2003). A structural model for the inhibition of calpain by calpastatin: crystal structures of the native domain vi of calpain and its complexes with calpastatin peptide and a small molecule inhibitor. *J. Mol. Biol.* 328, 131–146. doi: 10.1016/S0022-2836(03)00274-2

Tompa, P., Mucsi, Z., Orosz, G., and Friedrich, P. (2002). Calpastatin subdomains a and c are activators of calpain. *J. Biol. Chem.* 277, 9022–9026. doi: 10.1074/jbc.C100700200

Trojanowski, J. Q., and Lee, V. M.-Y. (2000). "fatal attractions" of proteins: a comprehensive hypothetical mechanism underlying Alzheimer's disease and other neurodegenerative disorders. *Ann. N.Y. Acad. Sci.* 924, 62–67. doi: 10.1111/j.1749-6632.2000.tb05561.x

Tsavachidou, D., and Liebman, M. N. (2002). Modeling and simulation of pathways in menopause. *J. Am. Med. Inf. Ass.* 9, 461–471. doi: 10.1197/jamia.M1103

Vaisid, T., Barnoy, S., and Kosower, N. (2008). Calpastatin overexpression attenuates amyloid-β-peptide toxicity in differentiated pc12 cells. *Neuroscience* 156, 921–931. doi: 10.1016/j.neuroscience.2008.07.072

Vassar, R. (2005). beta-secretase, app and abeta in Alzheimer's disease. *Subcell Biochem.* 38, 79–103. doi: 10.1007/0-387-23226-5_4

Vassar, R., Bennett, B. D., Babu-Khan, S., Kahn, S., Mendiaz, E. A., Denis, P., et al. (1999). β-secretase cleavage of alzheimer's amyloid precursor protein by the transmembrane aspartic protease bace. *Science* 286, 735–741. doi: 10.1126/science.286.5440.735

Volles, M. J., and Lansbury, P. T. (2002). Vesicle permeabilization by protofibrillar α-synuclein is sensitive to parkinson's disease-linked mutations and occurs by a pore-like mechanism. *Biochemistry* 41, 4595–4602. doi: 10.1021/bi0121353

Walsh, D. M., Klyubin, I., Fadeeva, J. V., Rowan, M. J., and Selkoe, D. J. (2002). Amyloid-beta oligomers: their production, toxicity and therapeutic inhibition. *Biochem. Soc. Trans.* 30, 552–557. doi: 10.1042/bst0300552

Walsh, D. M., and Selkoe, D. J. (2004). Oligomers on the brain: the emerging role of soluble protein aggregates in neurodegeneration. *Protein Pept. Lett.* 11, 213–228. doi: 10.2174/0929866043407174

Walsh, D. M., Tseng, B. P., Rydel, R. E., Podlisny, M. B., and Selkoe, D. J. (2000). The oligomerization of amyloid β-protein begins intracellularly in cells derived from human brain. *Biochemistry* 39, 10831–10839. doi: 10.1021/bi001048s

Weber, J. T. (2012). Altered calcium signaling following traumatic brain injury. *Front. Pharmacol.* 3:60. doi: 10.3389/fphar.2012.00060

Wojda, U., Salinska, E., and Kuznicki, J. (2008). Calcium ions in neuronal degeneration. *IUBMB Life* 60, 575–590. doi: 10.1002/iub.91

Wu, H.-Y., and Lynch, D. R. (2006). Calpain and synaptic function. *Mol. Neurobiol.* 33, 215–236. doi: 10.1385/MN:33:3:215

Yamakawa, H., Banno, Y., Nakashima, S., Yoshimura, S.-i., Sawada, M., Nishimura, Y., et al. (2001). Crucial role of calpain in hypoxic pc12 cell death: calpain, but not caspases, mediates degradation of cytoskeletal proteins and protein kinase c-α and-δ. *Neurol. Res.* 23, 522–530. doi: 10.1179/016164101101198776

Yang, J., Weimer, R. M., Kallop, D., Olsen, O., Wu, Z., Renier, N., et al. (2013). Regulation of axon degeneration after injury and in development by the endogenous calpain inhibitor calpastatin. *Neuron* 80, 1175–1189. doi: 10.1016/j.neuron.2013.08.034

Yang, L.-B., Lindholm, K., Yan, R., Citron, M., Xia, W., Yang, X.-L., et al. (2003). Elevated β-secretase expression and enzymatic activity detected in sporadic Alzheimer disease. *Nat. Med.* 9, 3–4. doi: 10.1038/nm0103-3

Zhang, Y.-w., Thompson, R., Zhang, H., and Xu, H. (2011). App processing in alzheimer's disease. *Mol. Brain* 4:3. doi: 10.1186/1756-6606-4-3

8

The Role of Fluoxetine in Activating Wnt/β-Catenin Signaling and Repressing β-Amyloid Production in an Alzheimer Mouse Model

Min Huang[1†], Yubin Liang[2†], Hongda Chen[3†], Binchu Xu[1], Cuicui Chai[1] and Pengfei Xing[1]*

[1] Department of Neurology, The Seventh Affiliated Hospital, Sun Yat-sen University, Shenzhen, China, [2] Department of Neurology, The First Affiliated Hospital of Jinan University, Guangzhou, China, [3] Department of Traditional Chinese Medicine, The Seventh Affiliated Hospital, Sun Yat-sen University, Shenzhen, China

***Correspondence:**
Min Huang
minhuanghm@163.com

† These authors have contributed equally to this work.

Fluoxetine (FLX) is one of the selective serotonin reuptake inhibitors (SSRIs) antidepressants, which could be used to relieve depression and anxiety among AD patients. This study was designed to search for new mechanisms by which fluoxetine could activate Wnt/β-catenin signaling pathway and reduce amyloidosis in AD brain. Fluoxetine was administered via intragastric injection to APP/tau/PS1 mouse model of Alzheimer's disease (3×Tg-AD) mice for 4 months. In the hippocampus of AD mouse model, there could be observed neuronal apoptosis, as well as an increase in Aβ (amyloid-β) production. Moreover, there is a strong association between down-regulation of Wnt/β-catenin signaling and the alteration of AD pathology. The activity of protein phosphatases of type 2A (PP2A) could be significantly enhanced by the treatment of fluoxetine. The activation of PP2A, caused by fluoxetine, could then play a positive role in raising the level of active β-catenin, and deliver a negative impact in GSK3β activity in the hippocampal tissue. Both the changes mentioned above would lead to the activation of Wnt/β-catenin signaling. Meanwhile, fluoxetine treatment would reduce APP cleavage and Aβ generation. It could also prevent apoptosis in 3×Tg-AD primary neuronal cell, and have protective effects on neuron synapse. These findings imply that Wnt/β-catenin signaling could be a potential target outcome for AD prevention, and fluoxetine has the potential to be a promising drug in both AD prevention and treatment.

Keywords: fluoxetine, Alzheimer's disease, Wnt/β-catenin signaling, protein phosphatases of type 2A (PP2A), amyloid-β

INTRODUCTION

Alzheimer's disease (AD) is a chronic neurodegenerative disease characterized by progressive memory decline and cognitive impairment (Scharre and Chang, 2002). AD has various histopathological hallmarks, including neurofibrillary tangles, cerebral amyloid senile plaques, synaptic and neuronal loss in the brain (Suh and Checler, 2002). Senile plaques, one of the important histopathological hallmarks, consist of a dense core of amyloid-β peptide (Aβ) and the dystrophic neuritis surrounded (Selkoe, 2004). The sequential proteolytic process of β-amyloid precursor protein (APP) through β- and γ-secretases could generate Aβ (Oulès et al., 2012). Previous study shows that Aβ could disrupt synapses and initiate a cascade of toxic events, which might result in neuronal loss (Liu et al., 2014). Another early feature of AD, besides amyloid pathogenesis, is synaptic dysfunction, which might be even prior to Aβ deposition (Miller-Thomas et al., 2016; Zuroff et al., 2017). PP2A plays a core part in dephosphorylation of inactive β-catenin and phosphorylated APP (Seeling et al., 1999; Sontag et al., 2007). Additionally, Aβ generation could also be inhabited simultaneously by drugs that target inactive PP2A (Liu and Wang, 2009; Triaca et al., 2016).

The Wnt/β-catenin signaling pathway has been found to be critical for both neuronal development and maintenance of the nervous system (Patapoutian and Reichardt, 2000). Research shows that Wnt/β-catenin signaling pathway would influence various neuronal processes, such as synaptic differentiation, synaptic function, the function of neuronal circuits, dendrite development, and neuronal plasticity (Rosso and Inestrosa, 2013). Without the activation of the Wnt/β-catenin pathway, β-catenin in the cytoplasm could be phosphorylated by a complex set of proteins, such as glycogen synthase kinase-3β (GSK3β), for ubiquitylation and degradation. However, the GSK3β activity could be inhibited by the activation of the Wnt/β-catenin pathway, which would in term lead to the repression of β-catenin phosphorylation, and, ultimately, result in the degradation of proteasome (Davidson et al., 2005; Zeng et al., 2008). Previous research shows that, in both sporadic and familial AD patients, there could be observed a decreased level of active β-catenin, inactive PP2A, and hyper active GSK3β (Voronkov et al., 2011; Inestrosa and Varela-Nallar, 2014). According to mentioned studies, it could be implied that it would be constructive and therapeutic for AD patients to maintain and rescue Wnt/β-catenin signaling.

Fluoxetine (FLX), as a selective serotonin reuptake inhibitors (SSRIs) antidepressant, could be used to relieve depression and anxiety among AD patients (Modrego, 2010). Moreover, studies suggest another potential application of FLX. For patients with mild cognitive impairment (MCI), which is a prodromal state of AD, Fluoxetine could improve the memory and cognitive function (Mowla et al., 2007). Besides, fluoxetine has been shown to be able to inhibit β-amyloid production, and prevent neuronal degeneration in an APP/PS1 mouse model (Wang et al., 2014; Ma et al., 2017; Sun et al., 2017). Furthermore, Li et al. (2004) have showed that fluoxetine could greatly enhance the phosphorylation of GSK3β. And Pilar-Cuellar et al. (2012) have revealed that fluoxetine could increase the β-catenin level. However, more research would be required to clarify if the neuroprotective effect of fluoxetine is related to the action of Wnt/β-catenin.

The purpose of our research is to explore the role of fluoxetine and its underlying mechanism in alleviating AD symptom. The research would utilize a triple-transgenic mouse model of AD, and measure the AD symptom by PP2A dependent Wnt/β-catenin signaling. Fluoxetine treatment dramatically slowing down the production of Aβ in the hippocampus of AD mouse. Moreover, during the process where fluoxetine positively influences the activation of Wnt/β-catenin signaling, promotion of PP2A activity is found to play a significant role. Ultimately, the mechanisms behind the regulation of fluoxetine in the Wnt/β-catenin signaling pathway were explored.

MATERIALS AND METHODS

Drugs and Reagents

Fluoxetine was manufactured by Sigma-Aldrich (St. Louis, MO, United States). All cell culture reagents were produced from Invitrogen. Penicillin–streptomycin and poly-D-lysine, were manufactured by Sigma-Aldrich (St. Louis, MO, United States). Papain was obtained from Worthington. The Aβ1–42 ELISA kits and Aβ40 ELISA kits were purchased from Nanjing SenBeiJia Biological Technology Co., Ltd. (Nanjing, China). Antibodies information was in the **Table 1**. All other reagents were reagent grade.

Animals and Treatment

This study utilized 3×Tg-AD mice expressing APPswe, PS1M146V, and tauP301L human gene mutants, which were purchased from the Jackson Laboratory (Bar Harbor, ME, United States). In these mice, intracellular Aβ was detected

TABLE 1 | Antibody information.

Antibody	Host	Application	Source	Dilutions
Aβ1–42	Rabbit	WB/IF	Abcam	1:500
APP	Mouse	WB	Abcam	1:3000
CTFβ	Mouse	WB	Santa Cruz	1:500
CTFα	Rabbit	WB	Santa Cruz	1:500
$ADAM_{10}$	Rabbit	WB	Abcam	1:1000
BACE1	Rabbit	WB	Abcam	1:3000
PS1	Mouse	WB	Abcam	1:1000
sAPPα	Mouse	WB	USBiological	1:1000
sAPPβ	Rabbit	WB	Abcam	1:500
C99	Rabbit	WB	Pierce	1:2000
C83	Rabbit	WB	Pierce	1:2000
BDNF	Mouse	WB	Abcam	1:1000
NeuN	Rabbit	IF	Abcam	1:300
Bcl-xL	Rabbit	WB	Abcam	1:1000
Bcl-2	Rabbit	WB	Abcam	1:1000
Cleave-Caspase3	Rabbit	WB	Cell signaling	1:1000
Bax	Rabbit	WB	Abcam	1:1000
PP2Ac	Rabbit	WB	Abcam	1:1000
PP2A pY307	Rabbit	WB	Abcam	1:1000
GSK3β pY216	Rabbit	WB	Abcam	1:1000
GSK3β	Rabbit	WB	Abcam	1:5000
Active β-catenin	Rabbit	WB/IF	Cell signaling	1:2000
Inactive β-catenin	Rabbit	WB	Cell signaling	1:2000
PSD95	Rabbit	WB/IF	Abcam	1:500
Synaptophysin	Rabbit	WB	Abcam	1:1000
GAPDH	Rabbit	WB	Abcam	1:2500

WB, western blot blatting; IF, immunofluorescence.

at ages between 3 and 6 months, and cognitive impairment was detected at the age of 6 months (Oddo et al., 2003a,b; Billings et al., 2005). In the treatment group (Tg + FLX) (n = 12; 6 males and 6 females), fluoxetine was administrated at 10 mg/kg/day, intragastrical injection for 4 months. The fluoxetine administration began at the 4 months of age, just before they developed cognitive impairment and key pathologic features. The dose of fluoxetine was chosen aligning with previous studies (Li et al., 2009), with no gender differences. The rest two groups, the 3×Tg-AD mice group (Tg) (n = 12; 6 males, and 6 females) and male non-transgenic wild-type (WT) mice group (n = 12, 12 males), were treated with drinking water instead. All these three groups were kept under the same standard laboratory conditions with the treatment group, including temperature of 22 ± 2°C, 12-h light/dark cycle, and free access to water and food. Each cage contained 3 or 4 subjects with the same genotype. All experiments were conducted following the *Animal Care and Institutional Ethical Guidelines* in China to minimize animal suffering, for instance, reducing the number of animals used, and utilizing alternatives to *in vivo* techniques, if available. The experiments and procedures utilized in this study were conducted strictly according to the institutional guidelines regarding experimental animal use in Sun Yat-sen University. The protocol was approved by the Animal Ethical and welfare Committee of Sun Yat-sen University (Permit Number: SYXK 2016-0112).

Behavioral Tasks

Morris Water Maze Test

At 8 months of age, all mice were subjected to the Morris water maze task (Mueller et al., 2008) for 5 days (d), as an evaluation of their learning and memory abilities. During the 5-day evaluation, the treatments in both experiment and control groups remained the same. All the apparatus and the test procedure utilized were described before (Vorhees and Williams, 2006). Briefly, the apparatus included a circular white metal pool, whose diameter was 160 cm and height 50 cm, and the pool was filled with 26-cm deep water at constant temperature (22 ± 1°C) throughout the experiment. The water pool was divided into four quadrants by the water maze software, and had a translucent acrylic platform. The translucent acrylic platform was 12 cm in diameter, and 24 cm in height. It was placed in the center of the northwest quadrant, 1~2.0 cm below the water surface.

Spatial Learning Test

The spatial learning task was conducted for five training days with four consecutive trials per day. The location of platform was remained constant with the starting position chosen among four quadrants in sequence at the pool rim every day. At the beginning of each trial, the mice would be gently released into the water with their noses against the wall at each starting point (north, south, east, and west). Every mouse was given a maximum of 60 s to find the hidden platform. If the mouse failed to find the escape platform within 60 s on the training day, it was then manually guided to the platform for 30 s. A camera was mounted in the ceiling directly above the pool to record the escape trace of each mouse. All trials were recorded using an HVS (human visual system) water maze program for subsequent analyses of escape latency (Water Maze 3, Actimetrics, Evanston, IL, United States). All experimental procedures were performed in a blind method, where investigators were blinded to group assignment of each mouse.

Probe Trial

To evaluate short-term and long-term memory consolidation, probe trials were conducted at 24 and 72h, respectively, after the last trial. To perform the memory consolidation evaluation, the platform was removed at first. Then, the mice were placed into the quadrant of the pool opposite to the one pre-placed with the platform. The mice were given 60 s to swim in each probe trial. Both the time spent in the quadrant preplaced with the platform and the time spent across the platform position were recorded to evaluate short-term and long-term memory.

Primary Culture of Hippocampal Neurons

Primary hippocampal neurons were achieved from postnatal (P0–P1) 3×Tg-AD and WT mice pups born within 24 h. After being dissected from the brain, the hippocampi were then digested with 2 mg/mL papain for 30 min at 37°C. Afterwards, the digested tissue was triturated and suspended in DMEM with 10% FBS. Dissociated cells were cultured in the neurobasal medium with 0.5 mM of L-glutamine, 2% B27 supplement, and 50 U/mL of penicillin–streptomycin. All the cultivation process would be conducted in poly-D-lysine-coated 6-well cell culture plates/culture dishes at a density of 0.5 × 10^6 cells/per well. The cells were cultured in a 37°C incubator with 95% O_2 and 5% CO_2. The medium was completely replaced after 4 h, and half of the medium was then replaced every 3 days. On day 13, the neurons were treated with 1 μM fluoxetine (diluted from 20 mM fluoxetine stock solution dissolved in culture medium) for 24 h. Neurons from 3×Tg-AD mice treated with the culture medium were set up as the control group.

ELISA for Aβ1–42 and Aβ40 Levels

Aβ1–42 and Aβ40 levels were assessed by ELISA (enzyme-linked immunosorbent assay). Primary cultured hippocampal neurons and medium from WT, 3×Tg-AD and 3×Tg-AD+fluoxetine groups were collected. The levels of extracellular and intracellular Aβ1–42 and Aβ40 were evaluated through a sandwich ELISA kit, following the manufacturer's instruction.

Western Blot Assay

In the brain tissue-based assay, lysis buffer plus 1 mM PMSF and protease inhibitor cocktail were utilized to homogenize brain tissue samples from different group. In the cell-based assay, the utilized cells were harvested after 24 h of 1 μM of fluoxetine treatment. Then, the harvested cells were lysed with lysis buffer. BCA protein assay kit was utilized to measure protein concentration. And SDS-PAGE was used to extract the same amount of total protein (20 μg per well) from each sample. The extracted protein would then be transferred to polyvinylidene fluoride (PVDF) membranes. After blocking with 5% fat-free milk, corresponding primary antibodies (**Table 1**) were used to probe, which would then be incubated with HRP-conjugated anti-rabbit antibody or HRP-anti-mouse antibody. The blots were developed with ECL detection reagents and visualized with a KODAK Image Station 4000 MM (Carestream Health Inc., New Haven, CT, United States). All band intensities were quantified using Quantity One software.

Immunofluorescence Staining and Histological Analysis

Five-micrometer-thick sagittal paraffin sections of mouse hippocampus were mounted on glass slides. Before incubation, they were pretreated with 0.01 mol/L citrate buffer (pH = 6.0) in hyperthermy for 5 min. 5% goat serum in PBS was used to block the sections for 10 min. After the above pretreatments, there performed two incubations. The first one was performed with primary antibodies at 4°C, overnight. The second incubation was with secondary antibodies (1: 500 in PBS) at 37°C, 1 h. The primary antibodies used were specific to Aβ1–42, NeuN, and β-catenin. The Alexa-Fluor fluorescent dye-conjugated secondary antibodies (anti-mouse and anti-rabbit; Alexa Fluor 488 and 695, Multi Sciences Biotech) were used to detect MAP2 and PSD95. Three equidistant sections including the whole hippocampus were assessed per sample. To analyze and quantify immunoreactive areas, these sections were imaged with fluorescence microscopy (Olympus, Japan) and analyzed with Image-Pro Plus 6.0 software (Media Cybernetics).

TdT-Mediated dUTP Nick-End Labeling

Neurons were washed three times with 0.01 MPBS, 5 min each time. 4% paraformaldehyde was used to fix the neurons for 30 min, and 0.1% Triton X-100 in 0.1% sodium citrate was used to permeate them. The TdT-mediated dUTP nick-end labeling (TUNEL) was conducted via In Situ Cell Death Detection Kit, Fluorescein (Roche), following the manufacturer's protocols. Hoechst 33342 was used to counter stain the neuronal nuclei. Fluorescence images were obtained with an Olympus fluorescent microscope (Olympus), and TUNEL-positive cells were counted under a 20× objective.

Quantitative RT-PCR Analysis (qRT-PCR)

TRIzol reagent (Invitrogen, Carlsbad, CA, United States) was utilized to exact the total RNA from the cells. And a qSYBR-green-containing PCR kit (Qiagen, Germantown, MD, United States) was utilized to conduct reverse transcription and qRT-PCR reactions. The fold change was determined as $2^{-\Delta\Delta C_t}$, where Ct standard for the number of fractional cycle where the fluorescence of each sample passed the fixed threshold. All of the real-time PCR assays were performed with the Bio-Rad IQTM5 Multicolor Real-Time PCR Detection System (United States).

Statistical Analysis

All data was in the form of mean ± SEM or mean ± SD. All statistical analysis were performed using SPSS 19.0 software (IBM SPSS Inc., Chicago, IL, United States). Two-way repeated ANOVA was used to analyze the latency of MWM test. And two-way ANOVA and Bonferroni's *post hoc* tests were utilized to analyze the rest data. $p < 0.05$ was considered as statistically significant.

RESULTS

Spatial Learning and Memory Test

The general health conditions of the 3×Tg-AD mice during the fluoxetine treatment were carefully monitored during the trial period, and no significant changes were found in the body weight of the mice before and after the trial.

Spatial learning was evaluated by the length of the time to find the hidden platform (i.e., escape latency). The results of all mice during the water maze acquisition training could be found in **Figure 1A** ($p < 0.05$). From the perspective of daily escape latency, the spatial learning ability of the mice was effectively improved in both groups after the 5-day consecutive training period. Compared with the 3×Tg-AD mice group, a significantly shorter escape latency was observed for the fluoxetine-treated 3×Tg-AD mice ($p < 0.05$). However, in *post hoc* multiple comparisons, there was no significant differences across all groups regarding swimming speed (**Figure 1B**, $p > 0.05$). The data suggests that fluoxetine could have a significant influence in attenuating spatial learning deficits in 8-month-old 3×Tg-AD mice.

Following the 5-day training, probe trials were conducted to evaluate short-term (24 h later) and long-term (72 h later) memory on the 6th and 8th day, respectively (**Figures 1C,D**). Compared with the WT mice group, 3×Tg-AD mice group exhibited a longer path distance ($p < 0.01$) across all trial sessions (**Figures 1C,D**). Between the fluoxetine -treated group and the 3×Tg-AD mice group, a statistically significant difference was observed in both short-term and long-term memory test in terms of the length of time searching for target quadrant, and searching for non-target quadrants (**Figure 1C**, $p < 0.05$). When the 3×Tg-AD mice group was compared with WT group, the former spent significantly longer time than the latter group. Based on the assessment of the length of time searching for the pre-placed platform in both short-term and long-term memory test, a statistically significant improvement was observed in the fluoxetine treated group, compared with the 3×Tg-AD mice group (**Figure 1D**, $p < 0.05$). Mice in the treated groups were gender-matched, and no significant gender-specific differences in the results were observed. Compared three groups follow tracks, the fluoxetine treated 3×Tg-AD mice group and WT group were more similar (**Figure 1E**).

Fluoxetine Reduced the Production of Aβ in the Brains of 3×Tg-AD Mice

The effect of fluoxetine on Aβ burden in the brain was also investigated in the 3×Tg-AD mice. **Figures 2A,B** indicated the results of immunofluorescent staining and immunohistochemical staining for β-amyloid in the hippocampus of mice from all three groups. While little aggregation of β-amyloid was found in the WT mice, in the other

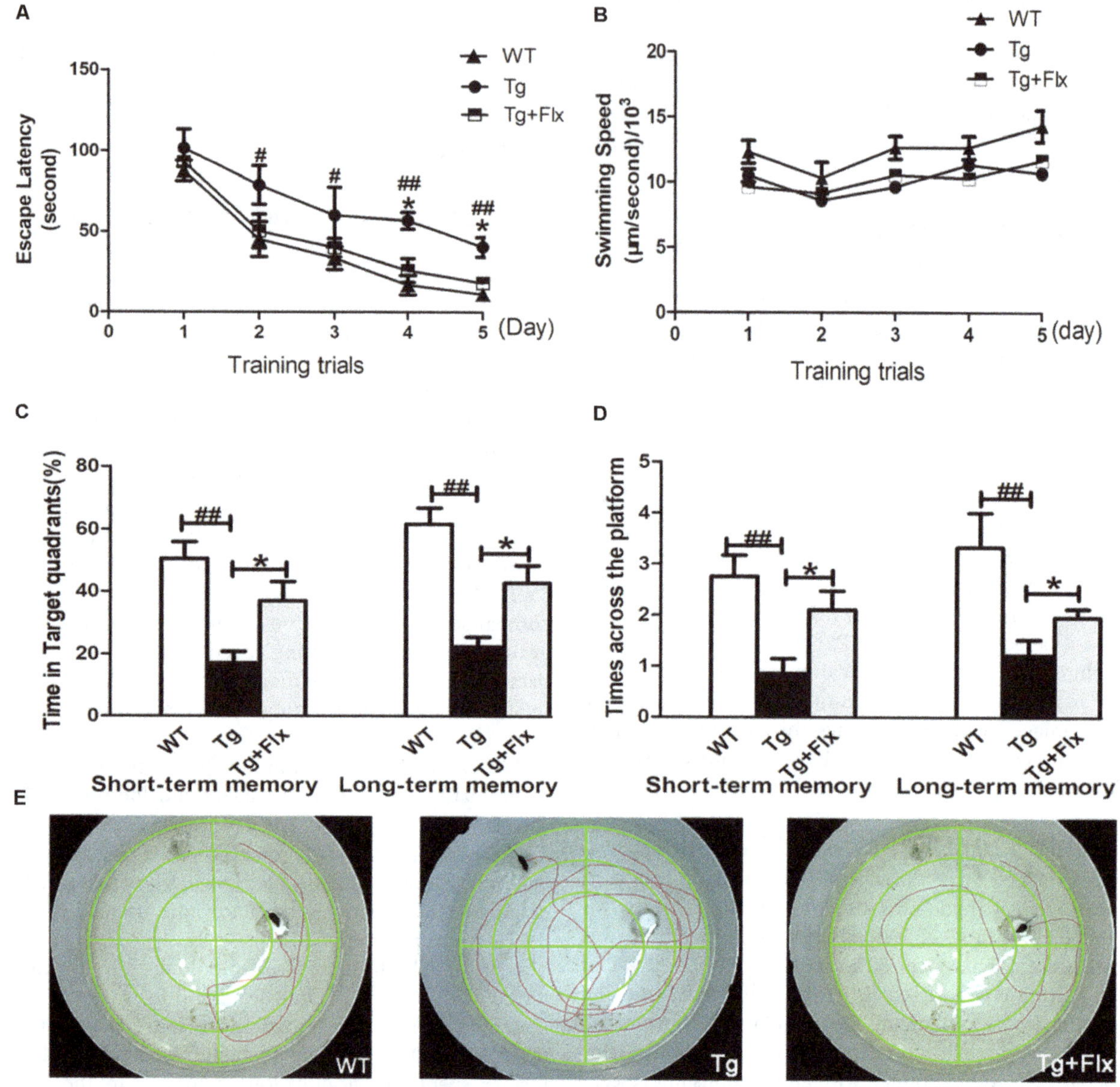

FIGURE 1 | Effects of fluoxetine on spatial learning and memory of 3×Tg-AD mice detected by the Morris water maze task. **(A)** In 5-day training trials, the escaping latencies of mice were measured to evaluate the three groups mouse memory ability. Based on the results, compared with vehicle control 3×Tg-AD mice. **(B)** Regarding the swimming speed, no significant differences were observed in all groups. **(C)** In the probe trail, the frequency that mice crossed the area where the submerged platform was placed in training trials was recorded. **(D)** In terms of the time spent searching for the pre-placed platform in the target quadrant, in both the short-term and long-term memory tests. **(E)** The swimming tracks the mice in the three groups made in the water tank on the last day of the test. WT, wild-type mice; Tg, 3×Tg-AD mice; Tg + FLX, fluoxetine treated 3×Tg-AD mice. Data were shown as mean ± SD, $n = 12$ animals/group. $^{\#}p < 0.05$, 3×Tg-AD group vs. WT group, $^{\#\#}p < 0.01$, 3×Tg-AD group vs. WT group. $^{*}p < 0.05$, fluoxetine treated 3×Tg-AD vs. 3×Tg-AD group.

two groups there could observe β-amyloid aggregation in the hippocampus (**Figures 2A,B**). Moreover, between the 3×Tg AD group and the 3×Tg AD + Flx group, the density of β-amyloid aggregating in the hippocampus was higher in the 3×Tg AD group, and the labeling for β-amyloid was also more intense (**Figure 2B**, $p < 0.05$). These findings were validated by ELISA test. The levels of Aβ42 and Aβ40 increased significantly in the hippocampus of 3×Tg AD mice, when compared with the WT mice. Treatment with fluoxetine could inhibit the level of Aβ42 and Aβ40 in the 3×Tg AD mice (**Figures 2C,D**, $p < 0.01$).

Fluoxetine Enhances Non-amyloidogenic Processing of APP in 3×Tg-AD Mice Brain

To explore the impacts of fluoxetine on APP processing, the study also measured the levels of APP protein in 3×Tg-AD mouse brain with a 4-month fluoxetine treatment. As shown in **Figure 3A**, there was a significant increase in the levels of APP protein in the hippocampus of 3×Tg AD mice, compared with that of the WT mice ($p < 0.01$). Treatment with fluoxetine could

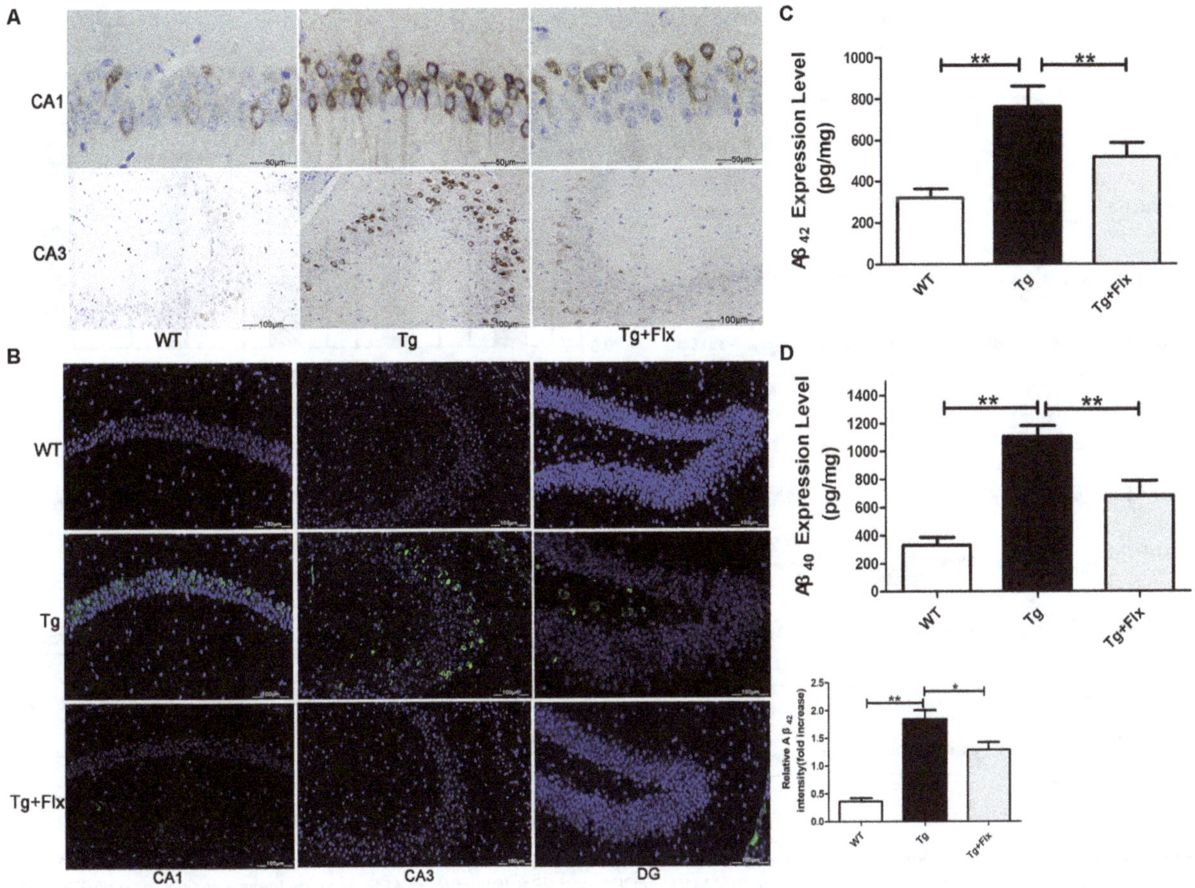

FIGURE 2 | Fluoxetine reduced the production of Aβ in the brains of 3×Tg-AD mice. Four-month old 3×Tg-AD mouse were treated with vehicle or fluoxetine (10 mg/kg/day) every day for 4 months and sacrificed for analysis. **(A)** Immunohistochemical staining for β-amyloid in the hippocampus of mice from the three groups. Scale bars: 100 μm. **(B)** Immunofluorescence of Aβ42 (green) in the hippocampi of mice from the three groups. Scale bars: 100 μm. **(C,D)** The levels Aβ42 and Aβ40 in the brains of three groups were detected by ELISA. WT, wild-type mice; Tg: 3×Tg-AD mice; Tg + FLX: fluoxetine treated 3×Tg-AD mice. Data were shown as mean ± SD, n = 12 animals/group.*$p < 0.05$, **$p < 0.01$.

reduce the level of APP protein in the 3×Tg AD mice (**Figure 3A**, $p < 0.05$). Then, it was investigated if fluoxetine was involved in APP cleavage. Western blot analysis was utilized to detect the APP cleavage enzymes and cleavage fragments in fluoxetine-treated 3×Tg-AD mouse brain (**Figure 3A**). Compared with that of WT mice, the protein levels of CTFs, BACE1, PS1, sAPPβ, and C99 in the hippocampus of 3×Tg AD mice were significantly higher. However, fluoxetine treatment could reduce the levels of protein-CTFs, BACE1, PS1, sAPPβ, and C99 in the hippocampus (**Figures 3A,B**) of the 3×Tg AD mice. We found that, compared with WT mice, 3×Tg AD mice had lower levels of ADAM10, sAPPα, and C83 in the hippocampus of, while fluoxetine treatment markedly enhanced the expression of ADAM10, sAPPα, and C83 in the hippocampus of 3×Tg AD mice.

The Promoting Effect of Fluoxetine on BDNF in the Brain of 3×Tg-AD Mice

The levels of BDNF in brain of three groups mice were measured. As indicated in **Figure 4A**, 3×Tg AD mice had remarkably lower levels of BDNF protein in the hippocampus than that of the WT mice ($p < 0.01$). Treatment with fluoxetine could have a positive impact on increasing the levels of BDNF protein in the 3×Tg AD mice ($p < 0.01$). **Figure 4B** indicated the results of immunofluorescent staining for NeuN in the hippocampus of mice from three groups, there was a decrease the number of cells stained with NeuN antibody in the 3×Tg AD mice compare with WT mice (**Figure 4B**, $p < 0.05$). Treatment with fluoxetine could increase the number of cells stained with NeuN antibody in the 3×Tg AD mice (**Figure 4B**, $p < 0.05$).

Fluoxetine Treatment Inhibited Apoptosis in Hippocampal Primary Neurons

As shown in **Figure 5A**, the 3×Tg AD primary neurons had a larger number of TUNEL-positive cells than the WT primary neurons ($p < 0.01$). Treatment of fluoxetine at 1 μM significantly reduced the number of TUNEL-positive cells ($p < 0.05$) in the 3×Tg AD primary neurons. As proved in previous research, the ratio between Bcl-2/Bcl-xl and Bax is correlated with

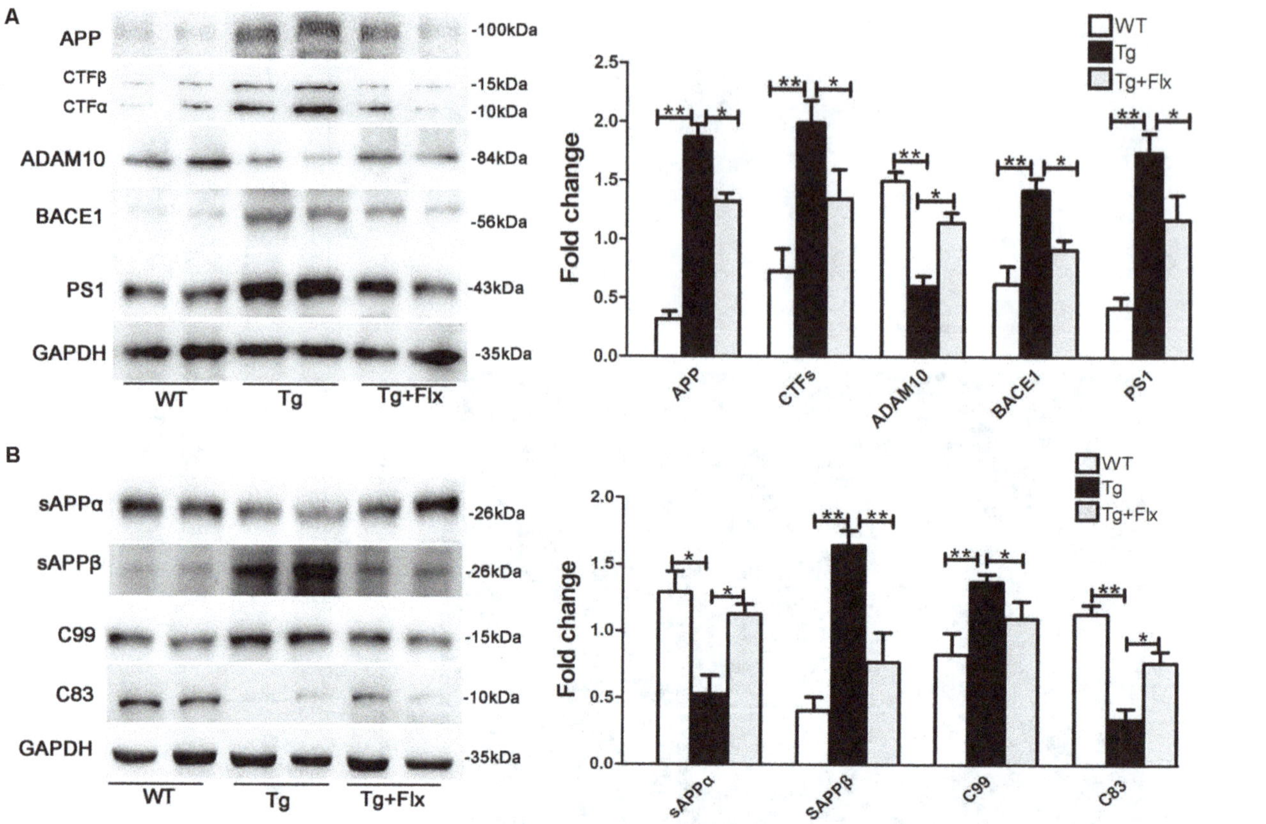

FIGURE 3 | Fluoxetine enhances the non-amyloidogenic pathway in 3×Tg-AD mice brain. **(A)** The western blot analysis was used to examine the expression levels of APP and APP cleavage enzymes, including APP, CTFβ, CTFα, ADAM10, BACE1, and PS1. **(B)** Levels of APP cleavage fragments, including sAPPα, sAPPβ, C83, and C99 generation, in the brain of three groups were assessed and quantified by immunoblotting. WT, wild-type mice; Tg: 3×Tg-AD mice; Tg + FLX: fluoxetine treated 3×Tg-AD mice. All data were shown as mean ± SD, n = 12 animals/group. $^{*}p < 0.05$, $^{**}p < 0.01$.

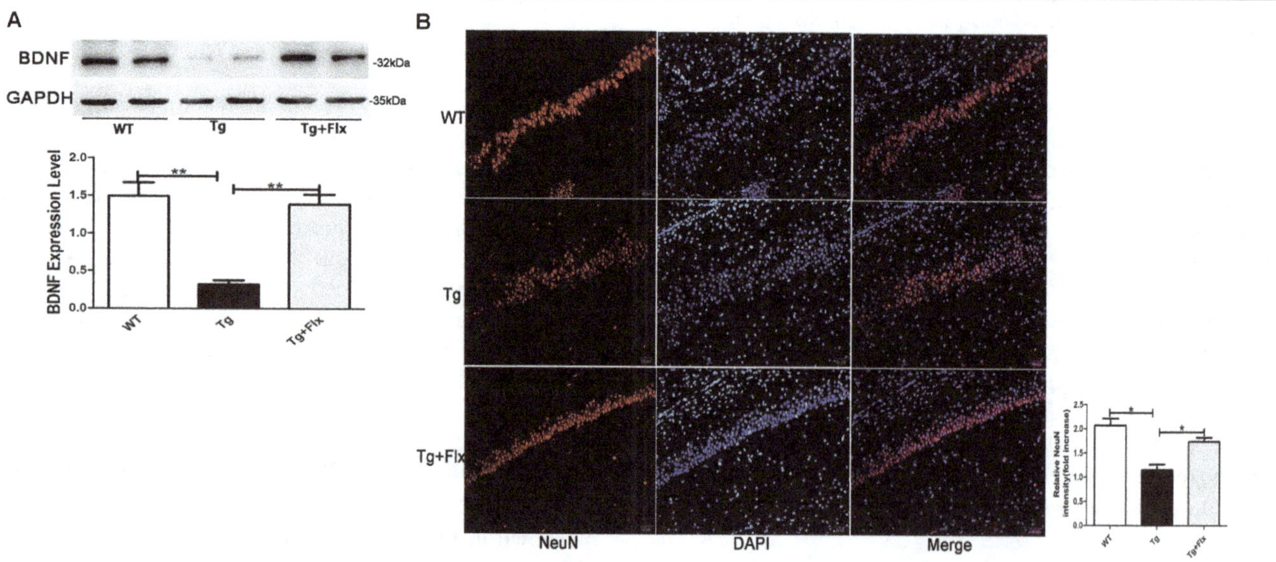

FIGURE 4 | Fluoxetine promotes BDNF in the brain of 3×Tg-AD mice. **(A)** The expression levels of BDNF were examined by western blot analysis. **(B)** Immunofluorescence of NeuN (red) in the hippocampi of mice from the three groups. Scale bars: 100 μm. WT, wild-type mice; Tg, 3×Tg-AD mice; Tg + FLX, fluoxetine treated 3×Tg-AD mice. Data were shown as mean ± SD, n = 12 animals/group. $^{*}p < 0.05$, $^{**}p < 0.01$.

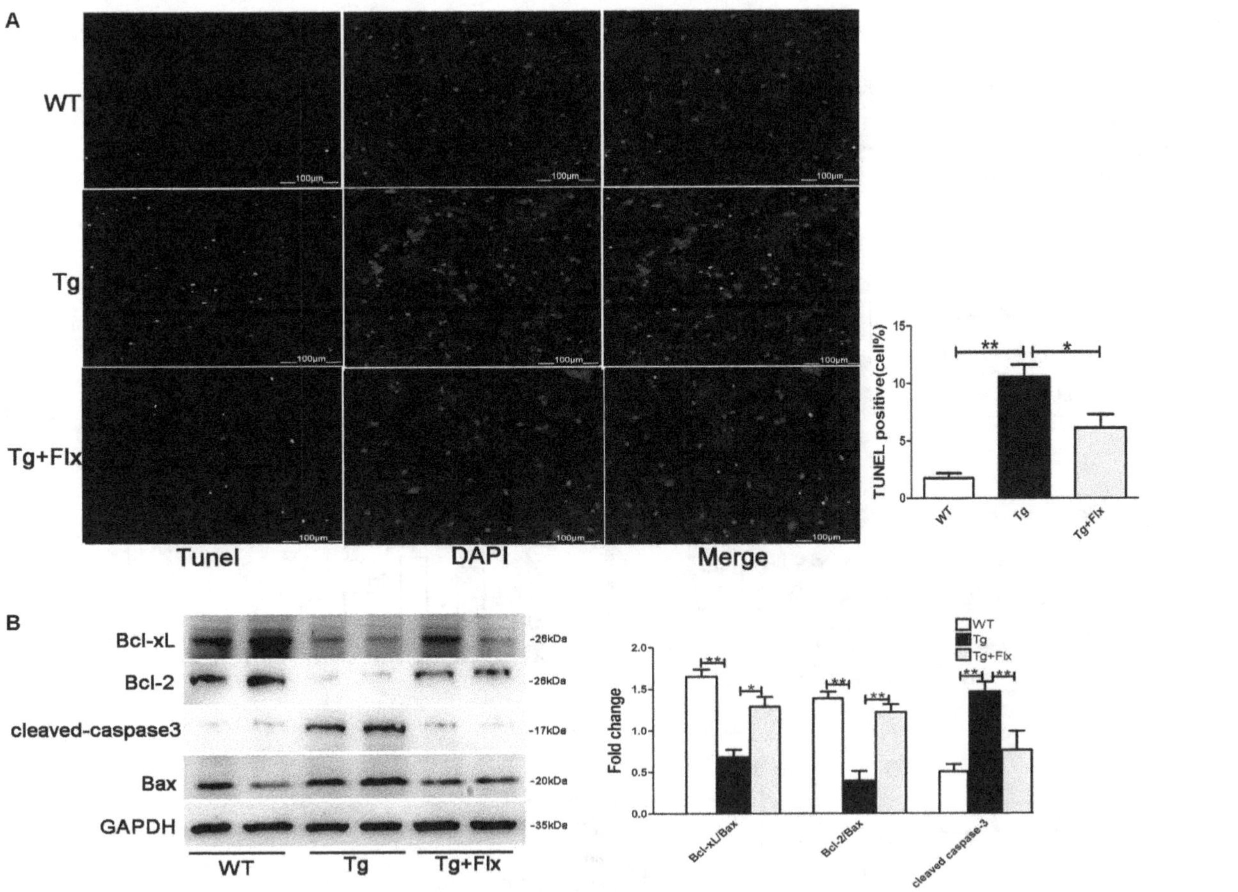

FIGURE 5 | Fluoxetine treatment inhibited apoptosis in hippocampal primary neurons. **(A)** The number of TUNEL-positive neurons (green). The number of TUNEL-positive neurons per 200× field in each group ($n = 6$) was averaged. $^{**}p < 0.001$ vs. control; Scale bar = 100 μm. **(B)** The western blot analysis was adopted to determine the Bcl-2, Bcl-xl cleaved-caspase 3, and Bax protein levels. WT, primarily cultured neurons of wild-type mice; Tg, primarily cultured neurons of 3×Tg-AD mice; Tg + FLX, primarily neurons of 3×Tg-AD mice treated with fluoxetine. Data were expressed as fold of control. $^{*}p < 0.05$ compared with control. $^{**}p < 0.01$ compared with control.

apoptosis (Liu et al., 2005). Thus, to investigate the molecular mechanism of the protective effect of fluoxetine in 3×Tg-AD primary neurons apoptosis, the expression of Bcl-2, Bcl-xl, and Bax was examined. Compared with the WT primary neurons, there could observe significant reduction in both Bcl-xl/Bax and Bcl-2/Bax expression ratio in the 3×Tg AD primary neurons. Treatment with fluoxetine significantly improved the Bcl-xl/Bax and Bcl-2/Bax expression ratio in the 3×Tg AD primary neurons. The levels of cleaved-caspase 3 were up-regulated in the 3×Tg AD primary neurons compared with the WT primary neurons (**Figure 5B**, $p < 0.01$). The results from the 3×Tg AD primary neurons demonstrated that treatment fluoxetine could significantly reverse this change (**Figure 5B**, $p < 0.01$).

Fluoxetine Targeted PP2A to Activate the Wnt/β-Catenin Signaling

The activity of PP2A would be inhibited by its phosphorylation at Tyr307 (Y307) residue of PP2A catalytic subunit (PP2Ac). Inversely, the ratio of PP2A-pY307/PP2Ac could reflect the activity of PP2A *in vivo*. It was observed that this ratio was significantly higher in 3×Tg AD mice than that in the WT mice (**Figure 6A**, $p < 0.05$). This implied that treatment with fluoxetine could reduce the ratio of PP2A pY307/PP2Ac in the 3×Tg AD mice (**Figure 6A**, $p < 0.05$). As the activity of GSK3β would require Y216 phosphorylation, the ratio of GSK3β pY216/GSK3β could then imply the activity of GSK3β *in vivo*. The research provided evidence that fluoxetine could significantly decrease the ratio of GSK3β pY216/GSK3β in the 3×Tg AD mice. A significant reduction in active β-catenin was observed in the hippocampus of 3×Tg AD mice when compared with the WT mice (**Figure 6B**, $p < 0.01$). Treatment with fluoxetine could increase the active β-catenin. The hippocampus of 3×Tg AD mice also demonstrated a significant higher level of active β-catenin, compared with that of WT mice (**Figure 6B**, $p < 0.01$). Thus, treatment with fluoxetine could decrease the inactive β-catenin. It implied that fluoxetine might be sufficient to enhance active β-catenin stabilization. To further confirm the protein expression of active β-catenin in the 3×Tg-AD mice brain,

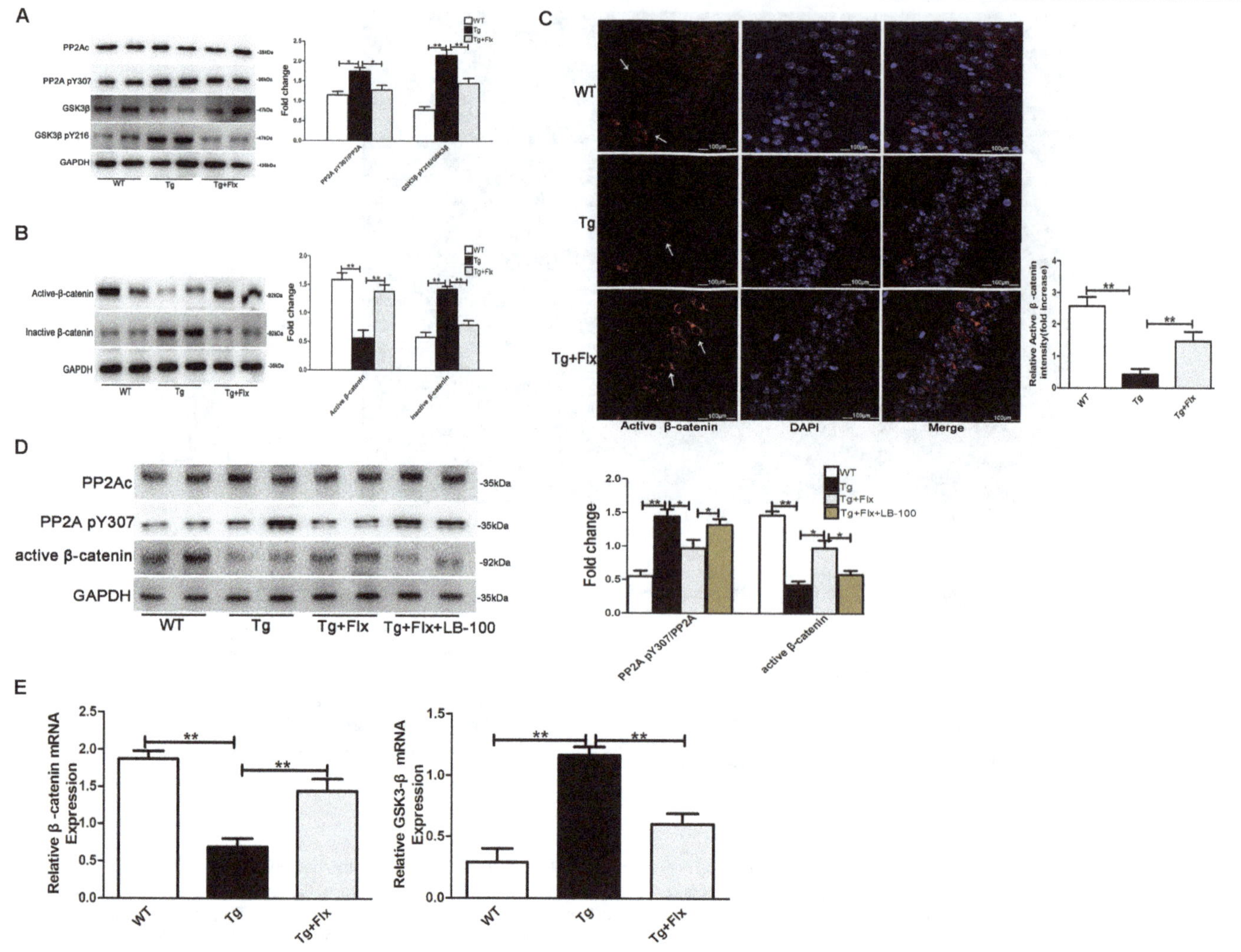

FIGURE 6 | (A) Western blots results that showed the expression levels of GSK3β and PP2A in the brains of mice. **(B)** Active β-catenin, and inactive β-catenin were studied through Western blot. **(C)** Immunofluorescence of β-catenin (red) and DAPI (blue) in the hippocampi of mice. WT, wild-type mice; Tg, 3×Tg-AD mice; Tg + FLX, fluoxetine treated 3×Tg-AD mice. **(D)** Analysis of primarily cultured neurons from mouse hippocampus. WT, primarily cultured neurons of wild-type mice; Tg, primarily cultured neurons of 3×Tg-AD mice; Tg + FLX, primarily neurons of 3×Tg-AD mice treated with fluoxetine. Tg + FLX+LB_100, primarily neurons of 3×Tg-AD mice treated with fluoxetine and LB_100 (an inhibitor of PP2A activity). **(E)** RT-PCR showed active β-catenin and GSK3β expression in the hippocampi of mice. Data are shown as mean ± SD, $n = 12$ animals/group. $^*p < 0.05$, $^{**}p < 0.01$.

an immunofluorescence analysis was performed (**Figure 6C**). Based on the immunofluorescence analysis, the level of active β-catenin in 3×Tg-AD mice was markedly increased in the treatment group ($p < 0.01$), compared with the 3×Tg-AD mice group (**Figure 6C**). Quantitative real-time (RT)-PCR analysis also confirmed that β-catenin mRNA expression was increased after fluoxetine treatment (**Figure 6D**, $p < 0.01$), while the mRNA levels of GSK3β were reduced (**Figure 6D**, $p < 0.01$) after fluoxetine treatment. The results suggested that fluoxetine treatment could efficiently activate Wnt/β-catenin signaling through inhibition of GSK3β in the 3×Tg-AD mice brain.

To further investigate if fluoxetine affected the Wnt/β-catenin signaling through PP2A activation, we isolated primarily cultured neurons, respectively, from the hippocampi of WT mouse and 3×Tg AD mouse. The cultured neurons from 3×Tg AD mouse were divided into three groups, which are 3×Tg AD, fluoxetine-treated 3×Tg AD, and fluoxetine-treated 3×Tg AD supplemented with LB-100(Tg+Flx+LB-100). LB-100, a specific inhibitor of PP2A, was used to suppress the activity of PP2A. As shown in **Figure 6E**, the 3×Tg AD primary neurons showed a significantly larger ratio of PP2A pY307/PP2Ac than the WT primary neurons. Treatment fluoxetine significantly decreased the ratio of PP2A pY307/PP2Ac in 3×Tg AD primary neurons, while adding LB-100 extensively eliminated the effect of fluoxetine. The remarkable reduction in active β-catenin between the 3×Tg AD and the WT primary neurons indicated that fluoxetine could raise the active β-catenin. Moreover, the data also demonstrated that adding LB-100 could extensively eliminate this impact from fluoxetine.

Fluoxetine Protection of Synapses

To determine the impact of fluoxetine treatment on synaptic functional protein expression, immunostaining analysis was performed in primary neurons, using synaptic marker PSD95 and MAP2, as shown in **Figure 7A**. A significant reduction in PSD95 was observed in the 3×Tg-AD primary neurons when compared with the WT primary neurons (**Figure 7A**). After fluoxetine treatment, PSD95 expression was partially recovered in the neuritis of 3×Tg-AD primary neurons. In addition, western blot was used to assay the level of synaptophysin and PSD95. Compared with the culture medium 3×Tg-AD primary neurons, the treatment with fluoxetine could increase the level of both synaptophysin (**Figure 7B**, $p < 0.05$) and PSD95 (**Figure 7B**, $p < 0.01$).

DISCUSSION

Although fluoxetine is a well-known neuroprotective agent (Qiao et al., 2016), there exists little information about how fluoxetine influences the Wnt/β-catenin signaling in the hippocampus of AD. Moreover, it remains unconfirmed if the activation of the Wnt/β-catenin signaling pathway has any anti-AD effect.

Utilizing 3×Tg-AD mice with an early-onset AD-like pathology, the study proved that regular administration of fluoxetine could stem the age-related cognitive impairments, as well as Aβ accumulation (Oddo et al., 2003b). Our research provides supports from multiple aspects that fluoxetine could have beneficial impacts on AD. First, utilizing the

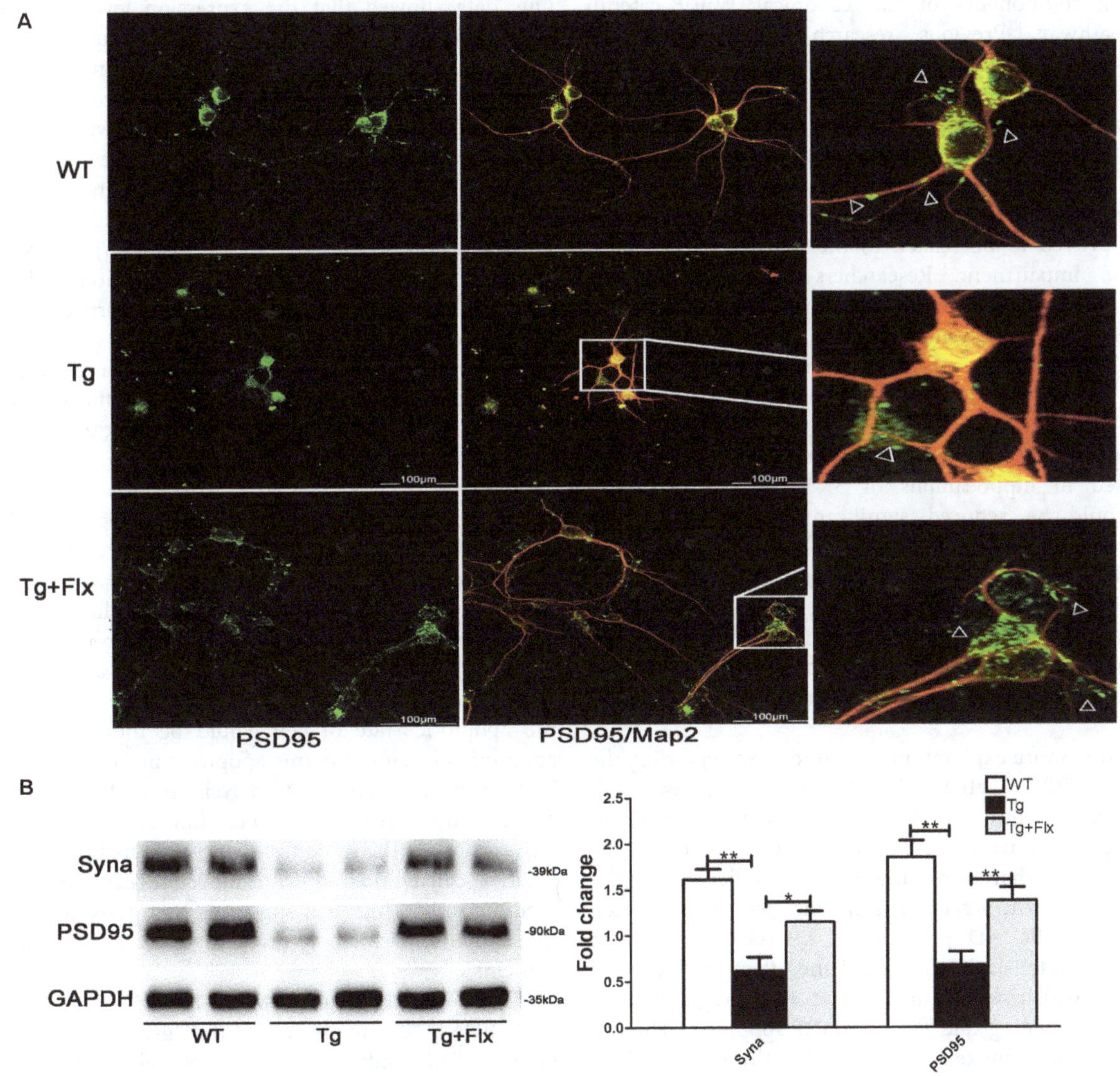

FIGURE 7 | Fluoxetine protection of synapses in 3×Tg-AD neurons. **(A)** Double-labeling analysis results for neurons from WT mice, 3×Tg-AD, and fluoxetine-treated 3×Tg-AD mice. Neuronal marker MAP2 (red) with post synaptic density protein 95 (PSD95) (green). Scale bar = 100 μm. **(B)** The levels of Syna and PSD95 expression were analyzed via Western blot assay. WT, primarily cultured neurons of wild-type mice; Tg, primarily cultured neurons of 3×Tg-AD mice; Tg + FLX, primarily neurons of 3×Tg-AD mice treated with fluoxetine. Data were shown as mean ± SD, $n = 12$ animals/group. $^{*}p < 0.05$, $^{**}p < 0.01$.

3×Tg-AD mouse model of AD, the study showed that fluoxetine could impact on brain Aβ levels, cognitive deficits, and amyloid neuropathology. Second, fluoxetine could prevent apoptosis in 3×Tg-AD primary neuronal cell. Third, fluoxetine could increase the expression of BDNF. Fourth, the study also demonstrates that fluoxetine could be able to protect neuron synapses. Moreover, our study proves evidence that fluoxetine would upregulates β-catenin expression and inhibits GSK3β expression *in vivo*. It suggests that there might be a correlation between neuroprotective effect of fluoxetine and the regulation of the Wnt signaling pathway in the AD brain.

It is widely accepted that Wnt/β-catenin signaling dysfunction plays a critical role in neurodegeneration process in the AD brain (Inestrosa and Toledo, 2008). GSK3β and β-catenin are two key components of the canonical Wnt/β-catenin signaling pathway. Previous research has demonstrated they could be considerably altered in the AD model mice brains (Zhang et al., 1998; Pei et al., 1999). Also, another study shows that activation of Wnt signaling can play a preventive impact on the neurodegeneration induced by Aβ fibrils (De Ferrari et al., 2003). The dysfunction of Wnt/β-catenin signaling induced by Aβ has been detected in AD and proved to be related to the neuron degeneration and synapse impairment. Researchers have detected the dysfunction of Wnt/β-catenin signaling induced by Aβ among AD. And this dysfunction has been proved to be associated with both neuron degeneration and synapse impairment (Thies and Bleiler, 2011; Inestrosa et al., 2012).

In this study, we showed that, when inactive β-catenin was increased in hippocampus of 3×Tg AD mice, active β-catenin could be reduced significantly. And the 3×Tg AD mouse demonstrated a remarkable reverse of these changes after treatment with fluoxetine. Meanwhile, the treatment of fluoxetine inhibited the cell apoptosis in the hippocampus of 3×Tg ADA primary neurons. These findings suggest that fluoxetine could be capable to activate the Wnt/β-catenin signaling to suppress the pathological hallmarks of AD.

Furthermore, more exploration was conducted regarding the relation across PP2A activity, Wnt/β-catenin signaling, and AD pathology, via utilizing the primarily cultured neurons from the hippocampus of 3×Tg AD mouse. Based on the results, we found that fluoxetine could significantly repair the function of Wnt/β-catenin signaling which had been impaired during the AD progression. LB-100, an inhibitor of PP2A, could extensively eliminated the effect of fluoxetine on β-catenin, which will result in the down-regulation of Wnt/β-catenin signaling and the neuronal apoptosis, Thus, it could be implied that fluoxetine could specifically activate PP2A to dephosphorylate β-catenin on S33/S37/T41 and GSK3β on Y216 for upregulation of Wnt/β-catenin signaling in 3×Tg AD mice.

Deposition of extracellular amyloid plagues in AD would also be subjected to PP2A regulation. PP2A could be capable of regulating the Aβ level through APP phosphorylation and BACE1 activity. Evidence from various aspects shows that APP could be cleaved within the sequence of the Aβ peptide and generate the sAPPα fragment through the α-secretase pathway (Esch et al., 1990). It would be beneficial for neuronal survival (Mattson et al., 1997; Wallace et al., 1997). However, through the β-secretase pathway, APP would be cleaved form neurotoxic Aβ and play a role in the pathogenesis of AD (Haass et al., 1992). This study focused on examining the role of fluoxetine in the APP process, based on the 3×Tg-AD mouse model of AD. The research found that expression level of APP proteins would be dramatically reduced in the fluoxetine-treated 3×Tg-AD mouse brain.

In this study, we examined the effects of fluoxetine on APP processing in the 3×Tg-AD mouse model of AD. Our data showed that the expression level of APP proteins would be dramatically reduced in the fluoxetine-treated 3×Tg-AD mouse brain. In this study, fluoxetine treatment could significantly enhance the expression level of ADAM10, a candidate of α-secretase. This was followed by an increase in the levels of both α-secretase-generated sAPPα and C83 fragments. Activation of the Wnt/β-catenin signaling reduced the transcription of BACE1. In our study, treatment with fluoxetine was shown to activate the Wnt/β-catenin signaling, which in term down regulated the expression of BACE1 in the hippocampus of 3×Tg AD mouse. These processes contributed to the decreased generation of Aβ. The results suggest that the Wnt/β-catenin signaling would play a significant part in regulating BACE1 expression, which then make Wnt/β-catenin signaling a core player in the formation of extracellular amyloid plagues.

Previous study has revealed that mitochondria could play a key role in regulating cell death, especially cell apoptosis (Yu et al., 2015). The dysfunction of mitochondria might become a hallmark of neuronal toxicity in AD (Xi et al., 2012; Zhang et al., 2012, 2016). Several researches also report that Bcl-2 family protein could play a certain role in regulating neuronal apoptotic cell death (Basu et al., 2006; Mancuso et al., 2008; Cartier et al., 2012). One of the key factors for the apoptotic state of cell would be the ratio between pro-apoptotic proteins and anti-apoptotic proteins (Yu et al., 2015). The result of western blot analysis shows that fluoxetine could significantly increase both expression ratios (Bcl-2/Bax and Bcl-xl/Bax) and, at the same time, decrease the number of TUNEL-positive cell compared with the culture treated with culture medium only. Thus, it is suggested that fluoxetine could inhibit the apoptosis, which involves the regulation of Bcl-2 family proteins.

BDNF is a neurotrophic factor, it is well known that BDNF is involved in the growth of neurites and synaptic plasticity (Sandhya et al., 2013). Fluoxetine might preserve synaptic protein expression, thus improve learning and memory abilities. After fluoxetine treatment, PSD95 and synaptic expression were partially recovered in the 3×Tg-AD neurons. The data above and the *in vivo* results together strongly implies that fluoxetine could be capable to abolish Aβ generation and preserve synaptic functional proteins.

CONCLUSION

Treatment with fluoxetine would significantly enhance the activity of PP2A and repress the pathology of AD significantly. After activated by fluoxetine, the PP2A could increase active β-catenin level and inhibit GSK3β activity in the hippocampus of 3×Tg AD mouse, which then could lead to signal the Wnt/β-catenin signaling. The treatment could relieve the APP cleavage and Aβ generation. Taking all these results into consideration, it could be concluded that fluoxetine could activate Wnt/β-catenin signaling via PP2A to repress the cross-talk among Aβ generation and neuronal apoptosis. These results suggest that fluoxetine could have a potential for the therapy of Alzheimer's disease through the activation of Wnt/β-catenin signaling.

AUTHOR CONTRIBUTIONS

MH, YL, and HC: conceived, designed, and performed the experiments. MH, YL, BX, CC, and PX: analyzed the data. MH: wrote the paper.

FUNDING

This work was supported by the National Natural Science Foundation of China (Grant No. 81503616) and the Project of Administration of Traditional Chinese Medicine of Guangdong Province of China (No.20181064).

REFERENCES

Basu, A., DuBois, G., and Haldar, S. (2006). Posttranslational modifications of Bcl2 family members–a potential therapeutic target for human malignancy. *Front. Biosci.* 11, 1508–1521. doi: 10.2741/1900

Billings, L. M., Oddo, S., Green, K. N., McGaugh, J. L., and LaFerla, F. M. (2005). Intraneuronal Aβ causes the onset of early Alzheimer's disease-related cognitive deficits in transgenic mice. *Neuron* 45, 675–688. doi: 10.1016/j.neuron.2005.01.040

Cartier, J., Marivin, A., Berthelet, J., and Dubrez, L. (2012). IAPs: a central element in the NF-κB activating signaling pathway. *Med. Sci.* 28, 69–75. doi: 10.1051/medsci/2012281019

Davidson, G., Wu, W., Shen, J. L., Bilic, J., Fenger, U., Stannek, P., et al. (2005). Casein kinase 1 gamma couples Wnt receptor activation to cytoplasmic signal transduction. *Nature* 438, 867–872. doi: 10.1038/nature04170

De Ferrari, G. V., Chacon, M. A., Barria, M. I., Garrido, J. L., Godoy, J. A., Olivares, G., et al. (2003). Activation of Wnt signaling rescues neurodegeneration and behavioral impairments induced by beta-amyloid fibrils. *Mol. Psychiatry* 8, 195–208. doi: 10.1038/sj.mp.4001208

Esch, F. S., Keim, P. S., Beattie, E. C., Blacher, R. W., Culwell, A. R., Oltersdorf, T., et al. (1990). Cleavage of amyloid beta peptide during constitutive processing of its precursor. *Science* 248, 1122–1124. doi: 10.1126/science.2111583

Haass, C., Schlossmacher, M. G., Hung, A. Y., Vigo-Pelfrey, C., Mellon, A., Ostaszewski, B. L., et al. (1992). Amyloid beta-peptide is produced by cultured cells during normal metabolism. *Nature* 359, 322–325. doi: 10.1038/359322a0

Inestrosa, N. C., Montecinos-Oliva, C., and Fuenzalida, M. (2012). Wnt signaling: role in Alzheimer disease and schizophrenia. *J. Neuroimmune Pharmacol.* 7, 788–807. doi: 10.1007/s11481-012-9417-5

Inestrosa, N. C., and Toledo, E. M. (2008). The role of *Wnt* signaling in neuronal dysfunction in Alzheimer's disease. *Mol. Neurodegener.* 3:9. doi: 10.1186/1750-1326-3-9

Inestrosa, N. C., and Varela-Nallar, L. (2014). Wnt signaling in the nervous system and in Alzheimer's disease. *J. Mol. Cell Biol.* 6, 64–74. doi: 10.1093/jmcb/mjt051

Li, W. L., Cai, H. H., Wang, B., Chen, L., Zhou, Q. G., Luo, C. X., et al. (2009). Chronic fluoxetine treatment improves ischemia-induced spatial cognitive deficits through increasing hippocampal neurogenesis after stroke. *J. Neurosci. Res.* 87, 112–122. doi: 10.1002/jnr.21829

Li, X., Zhu, W., Roh, M. S., Friedman, A. B., Rosborough, K., and Jope, R. S. (2004). *In vivo* regulation of glycogen synthase kinase-3beta (GSK3beta) by serotonergic activity in mouse brain. *Neuropsychopharmacology* 29, 1426–1431. doi: 10.1038/sj.npp.1300439

Liu, C. C., Tsai, C. W., Deak, F., Rogers, J., Penuliar, M., Sung, Y. M., et al. (2014). Deficiency in LRP6-mediated Wnt signaling contributes to synaptic abnormalities and amyloid pathology in Alzheimer's disease. *Neuron* 84, 63–77. doi: 10.1016/j.neuron.2014.08.048

Liu, R., and Wang, J. Z. (2009). Protein phosphatase 2A in Alzheimer's disease. *Pathophysiology* 16, 273–277. doi: 10.1016/j.pathophys.2009.02.008

Liu, Z., Lu, H., Jiang, Z., Pastuszyn, A., and Hu, C. A. (2005). Apolipoprotein l6, a novel proapoptotic Bcl-2 homology 3-only protein, induces mitochondria-mediated apoptosis in cancer cells. *Mol. Cancer Res.* 3, 21–31.

Ma, J., Gao, Y., Jiang, L., Chao, F. L., Huang, W., and Zhou, C. N. (2017). Fluoxetine attenuates the impairment of spatial learning ability and prevents neuron loss in middle-aged APPswe/PSEN1dE9 double transgenic Alzheimer's disease mice. *Oncotarget* 8, 27676–27692. doi: 10.18632/oncotarget.15398

Mancuso, M., Orsucci, D., Siciliano, G., and Murri, L. (2008). Mitochondria, mitochondrial DNA and Alzheimer's disease. What comes first? *Curr. Alzheimer Res.* 5, 457–468. doi: 10.2174/156720508785908946

Mattson, M. P., Barger, S. W., Furukawa, K., Bruce, A. J., Wyss-Coray, T., Mark, R. J., et al. (1997). Cellular signaling roles of TGF beta, TNF alpha and beta APP in brain injury responses and Alzheimer's disease. *Brain Res. Brain Res. Rev.* 23, 47–61. doi: 10.1016/S0165-0173(96)00014-8

Miller-Thomas, M. M., Sipe, A. L., Benzinger, T. L., McConathy, J., Connolly, S., and Schwetye, K. E. (2016). Multimodality review of amyloid-related diseases of the central nervous system. *Radiographics* 36, 1147–1163. doi: 10.1148/rg.2016150172

Modrego, P. J. (2010). Depression in Alzheimer's disease. Pathophysiology, diagnosis, and treatment. *J. Alzheimers Dis.* 21, 1077–1087. doi: 10.3233/JAD-2010-100153

Mowla, A., Mosavinasab, M., Haghshenas, H., and Borhani Haghighi, A. (2007). Does serotonin augmentation have any effect on cognition and activities of daily living in Alzheimer's dementia? A double-blind, placebo-controlled clinical trial. *J. Clin. Psychopharmacol.* 27, 484–487. doi: 10.1097/jcp.0b013e31814b98c1

Mueller, S. C., Temple, V., Oh, E., VanRyzin, C., Williams, A., Cornwell, B., et al. (2008). Early androgen exposure modulates spatial cognition in congenital adrenal hyperplasia (CAH). *Psychoneuroendocrinology* 33, 973–980. doi: 10.1016/j.psyneuen.2008.04.005

Oddo, S., Caccamo, A., Kitazawa, M., Tseng, B. P., and LaFerla, F. M. (2003a). Amyloid deposition precedes tangle formation in a triple transgenic model of Alzheimer's disease. *Neurobiol. Aging* 24, 1063–1070.

Oddo, S., Caccamo, A., Shepherd, J. D., Murphy, M. P., Golde, T. E., Kayed, R., et al. (2003b). Triple-transgenic model of Alzheimer's disease with plaques and tangles: intracellular Abeta and synaptic dysfunction. *Neuron* 39, 409–421. doi: 10.1016/S0896-6273(03)00434-3

Oulès, B., Del Prete, D., Greco, B., Zhang, X., Lauritzen, I., Sevalle, J., et al. (2012). Ryanodine receptors blockade reduces Amyloid-beta load and memory impairments in Tg2576 mouse model of Alzheimer disease. *J. Neurosci.* 32, 11820–11834. doi: 10.1523/JNEUROSCI.0875-12.2012

Patapoutian, A., and Reichardt, L. F. (2000). Roles of Wnt proteins in neural development and maintenance. *Curr. Opin. Neurobiol* 10, 392–399. doi: 10.1016/S0959-4388(00)00100-8

Pei, J. J., Braak, E., Braak, H., Grundke-Iqbal, I., Iqbal, K., Winblad, B., et al. (1999). Distribution of active glycogen synthase kinase 3beta (GSK-3beta) in brains staged for Alzheimer disease neurofibrillary changes. *J. Neuropathol. Exp. Neurol.* 58, 1010–1019. doi: 10.1097/00005072-199909000-00011

Pilar-Cuellar, F., Vidal, R., and Pazos, A. (2012). Subchronic treatment with fluoxetine and ketanserin increases hippocampal brain-derived neurotrophic factor, beta-catenin and antidepressant-like effects. *Br. J. Pharmacol.* 165, 1046–1057. doi: 10.1111/j.1476-5381.2011.01516.x

Qiao, J., Wang, J., Wang, H., Zhang, Y., Zhu, S., Adilijiang, A., et al. (2016). Regulation of astrocyte pathology by fluoxetine prevents the deterioration of Alzheimer phenotypes in an APP/PS1 mouse model. *GLIA* 64, 240–254. doi: 10.1002/glia.22926

Rosso, S. B., and Inestrosa, N. C. (2013). WNT signaling in neuronal maturation and synaptogenesis. *Front Cell Neurosci.* 7:103. doi: 10.3389/fncel.2013.00103

Sandhya, V. K., Raju, R., Verma, R., Advani, J., Sharma, R., Radhakrishnan, A., et al. (2013). A network map of BDNF/TRKB and BDNF/p75NTR signaling system. *J. Cell Commun. Signal.* 7, 301–307. doi: 10.1007/s12079-013-0200-z

Scharre, D. W., and Chang, S. I. (2002). Cognitive and behavioral effects of quetiapine in Alzheimer disease patients. *Alzheimer Dis. Assoc. Disord.* 16, 128–130. doi: 10.1097/00002093-200204000-00011

Seeling, J. M., Miller, J. R., Gil, R., Moon, R. T., White, R., and Virshup, D. M. (1999). Regulation of beta-catenin signaling by the B56 subunit of protein phosphatase 2A. *Science* 283, 2089–2091. doi: 10.1126/science.283.5410.2089

Selkoe, D. J. (2004). Cell biology of protein misfolding: the examples of Alzheimer's and Parkinson's diseases. *Nat. Cell Biol.* 6, 1054–1061. doi: 10.1038/ncb1104-1054

Sontag, E., Nunbhakdi-Craig, V., Sontag, J. M., Diaz-Arrastia, R., Ogris, E., Dayal, S., et al. (2007). Protein phosphatase 2A methyltransferase links homocysteine metabolism with tau and amyloid precursor protein regulation. *J. Neurosci.* 27, 2751–2759. doi: 10.1523/JNEUROSCI.3316-06.2007

Suh, Y. H., and Checler, F. (2002). Amyloid precursor protein, presenilins, and alphasynuclein: Molecular pathogenesis and pharmacological applications in Alzheimer's disease. *Pharmacol. Rev.* 54, 469–525. doi: 10.1124/pr.54.3.469

Sun, D. S., Gao, L. F., Jin, L., Wu, H., Wang, Q., Zhou, Y., et al. (2017). Fluoxetine administration during adolescence attenuates cognitive and synaptic deficits in adult 3 × TgAD mice. *Neuropharmacology* 126, 200–212. doi: 10.1016/j.neuropharm.2017.08.037

Thies, W., and Bleiler, L. (2011). Alzheimer's association report 2011 Alzheimer's disease facts and figures. *Alzheimers Dement.* 7, 208–244. doi: 10.1016/j.jalz.2011.02.004

Triaca, V., Sposato, V., Bolasco, G., Ciotti, M. T., Pelicci, P., Bruni, A. C., et al. (2016). NGF controls APP cleavage by downregulating APP phosphorylation at Thr668: relevance for Alzheimer's disease. *Aging Cell* 15, 661–672. doi: 10.1111/acel.12473

Vorhees, C. V., and Williams, M. T. (2006). Morris water maze: procedures for assessing spatial and related forms of learning and memory. *Nat. Protoc.* 1, 848–858. doi: 10.1038/nprot.2006.116

Voronkov, M., Braithwaite, S. P., and Stock, J. B. (2011). Phosphoprotein phosphatase 2A: a novel druggable target for Alzheimer's disease. *Future Med. Chem.* 3, 821–833. doi: 10.4155/fmc.11.47

Wallace, W. C., Akar, C. A., and Lyons, W. E. (1997). Amyloid precursor protein potentiates the neurotrophic activity of NGF. *Brain Res. Mol. Brain Res.* 52, 201–212. doi: 10.1016/S0169-328X(97)00258-1

Wang, J., Zhang, Y., Xu, H., Zhu, S., Wang, H., He, J., et al. (2014). Fluoxetine improves behavioral performance by suppressing the production of soluble β-amyloid in APP/PS1 mice. *Curr. Alzheimer Res.* 11, 672–680. doi: 10.2174/1567205011666140812114715

Xi, Y. D., Yu, H. L., Ding, J., Ma, W. W., Yuan, L. H., Feng, J. F., et al. (2012). Flavonoids protect cerebrovascular endothelial cells through Nrf2 and PI3Kfrom â-amyloid peptide-induced oxidative damage. *Curr. Neurovasc. Res.* 9, 32–41. doi: 10.2174/156720212799297092

Yu, T. X., Zhang, P., Guan, Y., Wang, M., and Zhen, M. Q. (2015). Protective effects of luteolin against cognitive impairment induced by infusion of Aβ peptide in rats. *Int. J.Clin. Exp. Pathol.* 8, 6740–6747.

Zeng, X., Huang, H., Tamai, K., Zhang, X. J., Harada, Y., Yokota, C., et al. (2008). Initiation of Wnt signaling: control of Wnt coreceptor Lrp6 phosphorylation/activation via frizzled, dishevelled and axin functions. *Development* 135, 367–375. doi: 10.1242/dev.013540

Zhang, Q., Huang, W. D., Lv, X. Y., and Yang, Y. M. (2012). Puerarin protects differentiated PC12 cells from H2O2-induced apoptosis through the PI3K/Akt signalling pathway. *Cell Biol. Int.* 36, 419–426. doi: 10.1042/CBI20100900

Zhang, X., Liang, D., Lian, X., Jiang, Y., He, H., Liang, W., et al. (2016). Berberine activates Nrf2 nuclear translocation and inhibits apoptosis induced by high glucose in renal tubular epithelial cells through a phosphatidylinositol 3-kinase/Akt-dependent mechanism. *Apoptosis* 21, 721–736. doi: 10.1007/s10495-016-1234-5

Zhang, Z., Hartmann, H., Do, V. M., Abramowski, D., Sturchler-Pierrat, C., Staufenbiel, M., et al. (1998). Destabilization of beta-catenin by mutations in presenilin-1 potentiates neuronal apoptosis. *Nature* 395, 698–702. doi: 10.1038/27208

Zuroff, L., Daley, D., Black, K. L., and Koronyo-Hamaoui, M. (2017). Clearance of cerebral Aβ in Alzheimer's disease: reassessing the role of microglia and monocytes. *Cell Mol. Life. Sci.* 74, 2167–2201. doi: 10.1007/s00018-017-2463-7

9

A Novel Early Diagnosis System for Mild Cognitive Impairment Based on Local Region Analysis

Fatma E. A. El-Gamal[1,2], *Mohammed M. Elmogy*[1,2], *Mohammed Ghazal*[2,3], *Ahmed Atwan*[1], *Manuel F. Casanova*[4], *Gregory N. Barnes*[5], *Robert Keynton*[6], *Ayman S. El-Baz*[2*†] *and Ashraf Khalil*[7†] *for the Alzheimer's Disease Neuroimaging Initiative* [‡]

[1] Faculty of Computers and Information, Information Technology Department, Mansoura University, Mansoura, Egypt, [2] BioImaging Laboratory, Department of Bioengineering, University of Louisville, Louisville, KY, United States, [3] Department of Electrical and Computer Engineering, College of Engineering, Abu Dhabi University, Abu Dhabi, United Arab Emirates, [4] School of Medicine, University of South Carolina, Greenville, SC, United States, [5] University of Louisville Autism Center, Department of Neurology, University of Louisville, Louisville, KY, United States, [6] Department of Bioengineering, University of Louisville, Louisville, KY, United States, [7] Department of Computer Science and Information Technology, College of Engineering, Abu Dhabi University, Abu Dhabi, United Arab Emirates

***Correspondence:**
Ayman S. El-Baz
aselba01@louisville.edu

[†] These authors have contributed equally to this work as senior authors.

[‡] Data used in preparation of this article were obtained from the Alzheimer's Disease Neuroimaging Initiative (ADNI) database (adni.loni.usc.edu). As such, the investigators within the ADNI contributed to the design and implementation of ADNI and/or provided data but did not participate in analysis or writing of this report. A complete listing of ADNI investigators can be found at: http://adni.loni.usc.edu/wp-content/uploads/how_to_apply/ADNI_Acknowledgement_List.pdf

Alzheimer's disease (AD) is an irreversible neurodegenerative disorder that accounts for 60–70% of cases of dementia in the elderly. An early diagnosis of AD is usually hampered for many reasons including the variable clinical and pathological features exhibited among affected individuals. This paper presents a computer-aided diagnosis (CAD) system with the primary goal of improving the accuracy, specificity, and sensitivity of diagnosis. In this system, PiB-PET scans, which were obtained from the ADNI database, underwent five essential stages. First, the scans were standardized and de-noised. Second, an Automated Anatomical Labeling (AAL) atlas was utilized to partition the brain into 116 regions or labels that served for local (region-based) diagnosis. Third, scale-invariant Laplacian of Gaussian (LoG) was used, per brain label, to detect the discriminant features. Fourth, the regions' features were analyzed using a general linear model in the form of a two-sample *t*-test. Fifth, the support vector machines (SVM) and their probabilistic variant (pSVM) were constructed to provide local, followed by global diagnosis. The system was evaluated on scans of normal control (NC) vs. mild cognitive impairment (MCI) (19 NC and 65 MCI scans). The proposed system showed superior accuracy, specificity, and sensitivity as compared to other related work.

Keywords: AD, CAD, PiB-PET, statistical analysis, personalized diagnosis

1. INTRODUCTION

Alzheimer's disease (AD) is a chronic neurodegenerative disorder marked by cognitive and behavioral impairments (Hodler et al., 2012; WHO, 2017). Statistically, 42% of AD sufferers are people over 85 years of age with the percentage decreasing to only 6% for people of 70–74 years old. Although the probability is small, younger individuals may also be affected (Brown, 2013).

AD is characterized by clinical symptoms and pathological features, both of which vary among patients (Lu and Bludau, 2011). In the clinical presentation, the patient faces progressive deficits in cognition as well as disturbances in thought, perception, and behavior. Neuropathological abnormalities include the formation of neurofibrillary tangles and neuritic plaques as well as neuronal loss and granulovacuolar degeneration. Indeed, the quantity and location of neurofibrillary tangles and neuritic plaques represent neurodegenerative features that distinguish AD from other types of dementia. Efforts to establish an early diagnosis of AD have been thwarted by the fact that pathological features of the disease occur 10–15 years before the emergence of clinical symptoms.

Mild cognitive impairment (MCI) can lead to AD. MCI can be defined as an impairment of cognition that is more severe than expected from normal aging and a persons education with objective evidence of impairment in one or more cognitive domains including memory, executive function, attention, language, or visuospatial skills. MCI does not interfere with his/her independence and daily activities including social or occupational functioning (Yaffe, 2013). In this regard, MCI represents an intermediate stage between the cognitive decline observed with normal aging and the severe impairment observed in dementia (Anderson et al., 2012; Yaffe, 2013). It is important to note that not all MCI cases proceed to AD, although studies have found that it increases the risk of later developing AD (Anderson et al., 2012; NIH, 2017). MCI due to AD is a progressive decline in cognition over months to years. MCI due to AD has a lack of significant vascular factors, vascular imaging findings, parkinsonism, visual hallucinations, prominent behavioral, or language disorders (Langa and Levine, 2014).

There are a number of tests that have to be considered when trying to establish a diagnosis of AD. These tests include: neuropsychological screening (to measure related cognitive impairments), patients medical history, and mental/physical examination. In addition, blood tests as well as brain imaging are usually evaluated to rule out other neurological or physiological disorders (Turkington and Harris, 2001; Wegrzyn and Rudolph, 2012). In general, these tests help to classify the subjects along the disease cascade into MCI, when the appearance of some cognitive decline does not fulfill dementia criteria, and other stages of AD (Wegrzyn and Rudolph, 2012). A recent meta-analysis of neuropsychological measures suggested that verbal memory measures and other language tests yield high predictive accuracy for those MCI subjects who will progress to AD. Other domains including executive function and visual memory showed better specificity than sensitivity (Belleville et al., 2017). These data show that there is a clinical need to identify biomarkers of neural circuits involved in MCI, which ultimately lead to the development of AD.

Brain biomarkers have been postulated to help in the diagnosis of AD throughout the diseases natural history. For example, Jack et al. (2010) presented a study in which positron emission tomography (PET) amyloid imaging and cerebrospinal fluid (CSF) amyloid beta 42 (Aβ42) revealed Aβ abnormalities in the brain. These abnormalities are the earliest pathological features observed in the AD-related disease cascade. Additionally, the study reported that both the increase in CSF tau and cerebral atrophy serve as biomarkers of neuronal injury and neurodegeneration. Finally, the decrease in 2-[^{18}F]fluoro-2-deoxy-D-glucose PET (FDG-PET), as demonstrated by the study, helps in revealing the synaptic dysfunction that accompanies the neurodegeneration. Therefore, according to this study, sMRI measures abnormalities of the brain's structure, and FDG-PET/CSF-tau identifies tau-mediated neuronal injury and dysfunction. The authors concluded that PET amyloid imaging could be considered an early identifier of AD-related abnormalities.

PET is a main scanning application of the emission computed tomography (ECT) methodology. Despite the role of the PET amyloid imaging in the early diagnosis of AD, arguments for and against the implementation of this scan modality in clinics should be carefully considered. False positive diagnoses of AD may occur since normal elderly subjects can have elevated Aβ levels. Fortunately, the introduction of carbon-11 labeled Pittsburgh compound B (^{11}C PiB), a neutral analog of the thioflavin T, caused a noteworthy conversion in studies related to AD (Johnson et al., 2013). The compound assists in visualizing the pathological hallmarks related to AD and consequently helps in quantitating the neuropathological burden during subsequent AD stages (Varghese et al., 2013).

Numerous research efforts have been proposed to help in the differentiation between normal control (NC), MCI, and AD utilizing PET scans. These efforts include studies focused on testing computer-aided diagnosis (CAD) systems, such as the automatic classification system proposed by Illán et al. (2010). For this purpose, principal component analysis (PCA) and support vector machines (SVM) were utilized. To evaluate the system, the PiB and FDG related scans were used to compare their results regarding early diagnosis. Although PiB and FDG showed similar accuracies, the PiB had a higher power of discrimination in the very early cases. Again, Illán et al. (2011) utilized PET scans to construct a CAD system that relied on eigenimage framework and composed of feature extraction, dimensionality reduction, and classification stages. In this system, PCA and independent component analysis (ICA) were utilized for image projection (feature reduction), eigenimage based decomposition for feature reduction, and SVM for classification. Through these stages, the system achieved an accuracy of 88.24%. Another study by Jiang et al. (2015) demonstrated a CAD system that improved the classification accuracy of AD using the PCA, ICA, and SVM. The PCA was used for dimension reduction, ICA for feature extraction, and SVM using linear and radial basis function (RBF) kernels for classification. The results of their study showed either better or equivalent performance as compared to the competitive CAD methods with higher accuracy than the traditional visual assessment methods.

In the same context, López et al. (2011) proposed a CAD system aimed at improving the accuracy of three-way classification between NC, MCI, and AD. The study used PCA and linear discriminant analysis/Fisher discriminant ratio for the feature selection process followed by artificial neural network/SVM for the classification purpose. Testing this methodology with FDG PET scans led to a classification accuracy of 89.52%. Martínez-Murcia et al. (2012) presented a CAD system composed of three stages: Mann-Whitney-Wilcoxon U-Test for voxel selection in order to exclude outliers, factor analysis for feature extraction, and linear SVM for classification. Testing this system on PET scans achieved an accuracy of 92.9%. Also,

Chaves et al. (2012) exploited association rule mining in a CAD system used in the early diagnosis of AD. Testing the system using two datasets, including PET scans, showed better results as compared to other related work. Padilla et al. (2012) introduced a CAD system to serve the early diagnosis of AD by combining nonnegative matrix factorization (NMF) for feature selection and reduction, and SVM with confidence bounds for classification. Application of the system led to an accuracy of 86%.

In addition to the aforementioned studies, various researchers have used voxel analysis for the early diagnosis of AD. For example, Morbelli et al. (2012) performed voxel-wise interregional correlations through statistical parametric mapping to extract relevant information. The study's results illustrated the association between the pathophysiological process of AD and alterations of the functional brain networks. According to the study, the default mode network (DMN) and memory function-related networks are the main causes of such alterations. Kemppainen et al. (2006) compared AD vs. NC subjects to find the brain regions that showed significant increases in the uptake of ^{11}C PiB by applying voxel-based analysis. A Statistical Parametric Mapping (SPM) analysis was performed using automated region of interest (ROI). The study found that the voxel-based analysis showed widespread distribution regarding the increased ^{11}C PiB uptake. Ziolko et al. (2006) statistically evaluated the amyloid imaging agents' (i.e., PiB) retention differences throughout the brain. In addition, they compared the PiB results with the FDG-based scans of glucose metabolism. The results revealed that the statistical significance of the PiB analysis was both greater than others and had a larger spatial extent. The results also showed that the PiB significance was retained after corrections of family-wise error and false discovery rate.

Forsberg et al. (2008) studied the amyloid deposition in patients with MCI. They used ^{11}C PiB and FDG based PET scans with AD, which were compared with NC scans. The analysis showed an intermediate retention of the mean cortical PiB in the MCI as compared to NC and AD. Also, the study found significantly higher PiB retention in the MCI conversion to AD group, comparable to that of AD patients ($p > 0.01$) and much less in MCI subjects who did not convert to AD. Shin et al. (2010) presented a voxel-based analysis relying on the FDG, PiB along with another tracer known as 2-(1-6-[(2-(^{18}F)fluoroethyl) (methyl) amino]-2-naphthylethylidene) malononitrile (FDDNP). These tracers were utilized to address the pathological hallmarks of AD, beta amyloid plaques, potential neurofibrillary tangles, and glucose metabolism related impairments. The experimental results demonstrated the available capacity to develop and test disease-modifying drugs targeting both tau and amyloid pathology, and/or energy metabolism when using the same subject based PET imaging with these three tracers.

Despite the achievements of the aforementioned investigations, the studies only supported a global diagnosis that indicate whether or not the subject belongs to a certain studied group. The main objectives of this paper are summarized in the following points. First, it provides a personalized diagnosis to help individualize diagnostic options as well as monitoring the disease progression. Second, it improves the final global diagnosis results as compared with previously published studies. To achieve these goals, our system utilized PiB PET scans due to the superior role of this brain imaging modality, as compared to other scanning modalities, when applied to the early diagnosis of the disease. Therefore, the paper is organized as follows. Section 2 (vide infra) starts by describing the materials used for the preparation of the paper and defines the methods used in the proposed CAD system. In section 3, different experimental results are presented to evaluate the performance as well as the efficiency of our system. Finally, the discussion of the applied tests and the future work are highlighted in section 4.

2. MATERIALS AND METHODS

2.1. Materials

A set of ^{11}C PiB-PET scans were used to validate the proposed framework. These scans were collected from the Alzheimer's Disease Neuroimaging Initiative (ADNI) database (adni.loni.usc.edu). The database of ADNI was initially launched in 2003 as a public-private partnership, led by principal investigator Michael Weiner, MD. The goal of demonstrating ADNI was to test whether serial MRI, PET, or other markers, in addition to clinical and neuropsychological assessment, can measure the progression of MCI and AD by combining them. For further advance information, please see www.adni-info.org. The used dataset was obtained from ADNI 1 where it contains a total number of 84 scans obtained from 19 NC and 65 MCI subjects. NC comprises those subjects who do not show any signs of depression, cognitive impairment, or dementia. The MCI group, in general, comprises those subjects with subjective memory concerns, whether self-reported or through an informant or a clinician. Those subjects display neither significant impairment levels in other cognitive domains nor signs of dementia. The Logical Memory II subtest of the Wechsler Memory Scale (WMS) was performed on the participants to document the normality/abnormality of their memory function with respect to their level of education. The demography of the used dataset is presented in **Table 1**.

2.2. Methods

The main aim of this article is to present local (i.e., region) based diagnosis of the MCI regarding AD, to assist clinicians in the personalized treatment of the disease. To achieve this goal, five main steps were performed, as illustrated in **Figure 1**. First, the scans were preprocessed through data standardization and de-noising. Data standardization aimed to prepare the scans for the labeling step, while the de-noising process aimed to improve the scan's quality and consequently the systems accuracy. Second, the atlas of Automated Anatomical Labeling (AAL) was used for brain parcellation to serve the local diagnosis goal. After labeling the brain, we used a Laplacian of Gaussian (LoG) with the automatic scale to extract the discriminant features from the scans. Then, a statistical analysis was performed to determine the significant brain regions to analyze rather than using all the labeled regions in the decision-making process. Finally, these regions were used to construct two decision-making levels using a probabilistic version of SVM (pSVM) and standard SVM to

TABLE 1 | The demographic data of the NC and MCI groups of the ^{11}C PiB-PET scans.

($N = 84$)	Average Age ± SD	Gender N (%)		WMS logical memory II results (based on years of education)		
		Male	Female	≥16 years	8–15 years	0–7 years
NC (19)	78.3 ± 5.01	11 (57.89)	8 (42.1)	≥ 9	≥ 5	≥ 3
MCI (65)	75.78 ± 7.67	44 (67.69)	21 (32.30)	≥ 8	≥ 4	≥ 2

provide local followed by global diagnosis. The details of the proposed system are presented in the following subsections.

2.2.1. Preprocessing

Scans underwent some preprocessing to orient the data and reduce noise. For orienting the data in a standard coordinate system, the SPM MATLAB toolbox (NeuroImaging, 2017) was used to perform re-orientation, co-registration, spatial normalization, and re-slicing. Noise reduction was accomplished through wavelet shrinkage. Details are as follows: PET scans' associated sMRI data were re-oriented so that the anterior-posterior axis coincides with the AC-PC line. This differs from the ADNI pipeline, which only ensures the axis is parallel to the AC-PC line. The associated PiB-PET scan was re-oriented to the resulting sMRI scan to produce a re-orientation matrix that was then used to re-orient the remaining PiB-PET scans. Precise co-registration between the PET scans and the previously used sMRI scan was performed using rigid body transformations (translations and rotations) to maximize the mutual information. Then, the spatial normalization and re-slicing were applied to the sMRI and PET scans to align the scans to the MNI-152 standard space. In this step, general affine transformation (translations, rotations, non-uniform scaling, and shears) was used, followed by nonlinear deformations. After data standardization, wavelet based de-noising was applied using the symlet8 mother wavelet with Steins unbiased risk estimate as a threshold selection rule and soft thresholding (Bagci and Mollura, 2013). The aim was to retain image detail while removing artifacts of image acquisition and/or transmission (Agrawal and Bahendwar, 2011). At this point, the scans were ready for voxel-wise comparison and labeling steps.

2.2.2. Brain Labeling

Due to the local diagnosis based goal of the proposed system, the brain labeling/partitioning needs to be performed. Through this aim, a detailed diagnosis of the subjects could be achieved. For this purpose, any of the detailed based brain atlases can be used, such as AAL, Talairach Daemon, and Brodmann areas atlases (Su et al., 2014; Zhang et al., 2015; Salas-Gonzalez et al., 2016). In this paper, the AAL atlas was used to label each of the preprocessed scans voxel's positions to the matched anatomical regions. The AAL atlas provides a total of 116 brain regions: 45 per cerebral hemisphere, 9 per cerebellar hemisphere, and 8 in the vermis of the cerebellum. AAL provides a detailed parcellation of the brain and is recommended for use with PET scans. To accomplish the labeling procedure, the xjView MATLAB toolbox (Alivelearn.net, 2017) was utilized.

2.2.3. Blob Detection Based Feature Extraction

Each of the labeled regions is individually fed to the scale-invariant blob detector, which employs LoG with automatic scale selection, for the purpose of feature extraction. Blob detection aims to separate structures (i.e., blobs) from the image background. Each blob is itself a radially symmetric distribution of image intensity about a local minimum or maximum (Toennies, 2012). Blobs corresponding to local maxima could reveal the targeted abnormalities, given that significantly greater retention of PiB in a brain region is linked with greater incidence of $A\beta$ plaques within that region (Shin et al., 2010). **Figure 2** shows a sample of the extracted features with a 3 Dimensional (3D) smoothed histogram showing the local maxima locations that are targeted through the detector.

2.2.4. Statistical Analysis

AAL regions where mean PiB uptake differs significantly in MCI with respect to NC was determined using two-sample t-tests. Each atlas region was tested independently. The Bonferroni method was applied to identify a region as "significant" when the p-value was less than 0.00043 (i.e., 0.05/116). Significant regions were subsequently used in building a classifier.

2.2.5. Diagnosis

A two-level diagnosis was performed to make local (region-specific abnormalities) and global (level of cognitive impairment) diagnoses. For this purpose, SVM and one of its variant (pSVM) were utilized. Standard SVM is an abstract machine learning technique where the training data are used for the learning followed by a generalization attempt for correct prediction on other novel data (Campbell and Ying, 2011). In SVM, a hyperplane (known as maximal margin hyperplane) is used for the binary separation of the labeled training data. The goal is to build a decision function $f: R^S \rightarrow \pm 1$, according to S-dimensional training patterns p_i and t_i, capable to perform classification for new example (p, t): $(p_1, t_1), (p_2, t_2), ..., (p_s, t_s) \in R^S \pm 1$. The decision hyperplanes in multidimensional feature space can be defined through either using a linear separation of the training data, using linear discriminant functions, or combining SVM with kernel techniques that produce a non-linear decision boundary (hyperplane) in the input space (Illán et al., 2011). Beside its classification power, a variation of SVM, which produces a posterior probability output of the classifier (pSVM), is useful to allow further post processes.

In the proposed system, a separate pSVM model was constructed, in the first diagnosis level, for each significant region. Each pSVM produces a probabilistic result for the

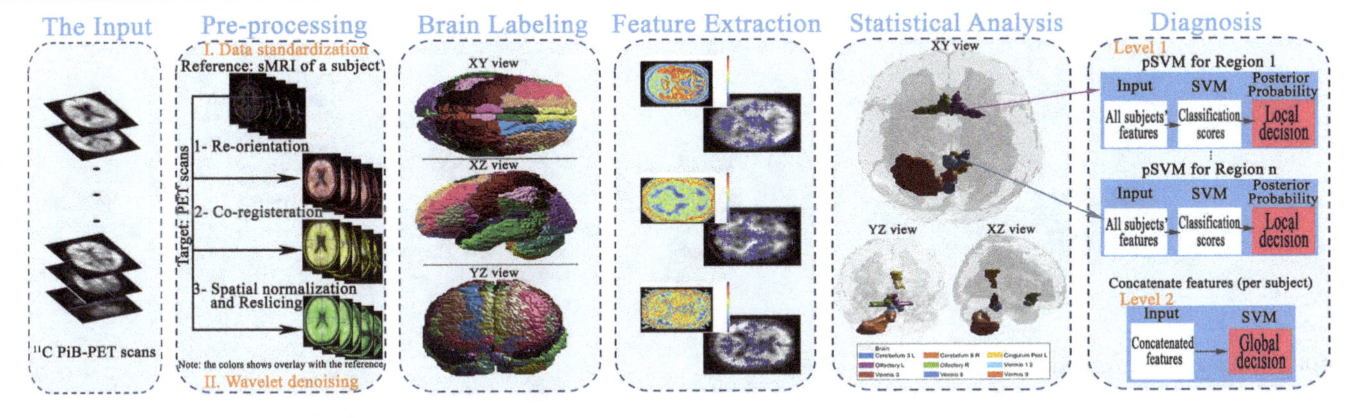

FIGURE 1 | The framework of the proposed early diagnosis system for AD based on local and global region analysis using ^{11}C PiB PET scans.

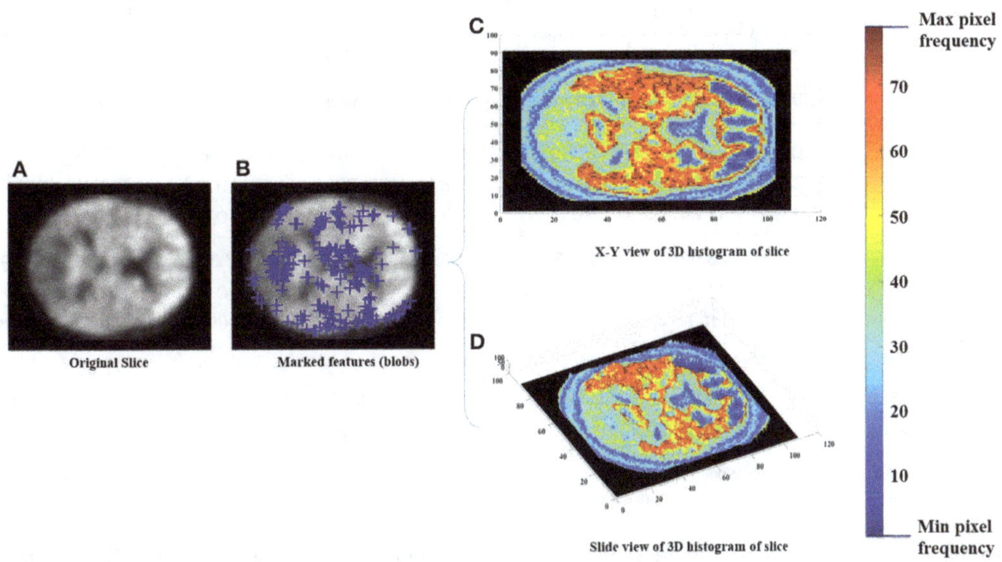

FIGURE 2 | An example of the feature extraction step, **(A)** the original slice, **(B)** the obtained features (blue pluses), **(C,D)** a 3D histogram representation of the slice to indicate the targeted local maxima/minima locations.

incidence of MCI given the features from its brain region independently of all others. In the second level, the scores obtained from the first level were fused with respect to each subject and used to train and test a single SVM model to produce the global diagnosis. Classifier performance, i.e., accuracy, sensitivity, and specificity, were estimated using both leave-one-subject-out (LOSO) and K-fold cross-validation, with two- and four-fold.

3. RESULTS

According to the Bonferroni corrected two-sample *t*-tests, the AAL brain regions of significance, nine regions, were Cerebelum_3_L (left alar central lobule), Cerebelum_8_R (right biventer lobule), Cingulum_Post_L (left posterior cingulate gyrus), Olfactory_L and Olfactory_R (bilateral olfactory cortex), plus Vermis_1_2, Vermis_3, Vermis_8, and Vermis_9 (lobules I, II, III, VIII, and IX of the vermis) as visualized in **Figure 3**. The performance of the resulting classifier was evaluated under a number of different kernels selected for the SVM, with best results being obtained when the linear kernel was used at both level 1 and level 2 (**Table 2**). This classifier was used to compare three cases, using data from all brain regions, using all regions except the significant ones, and using pre-selected, specific regions. The third case found to outperform the other two cases (**Table 3**).

The efficiency of the proposed system was compared to two other published methods (Chaves et al., 2012; Jiang et al., 2015). Our methodology was found to distinguish MCI from NC as well or better than either previous techniques (**Table 4**). Note that performance of the compared classifiers is taken directly from the respective publications since each of them used the same database (i.e., ^{11}PiB PET scans from ADNI), and LOSO cross-validation. Finally, **Figures 4**, **5** provide examples of the

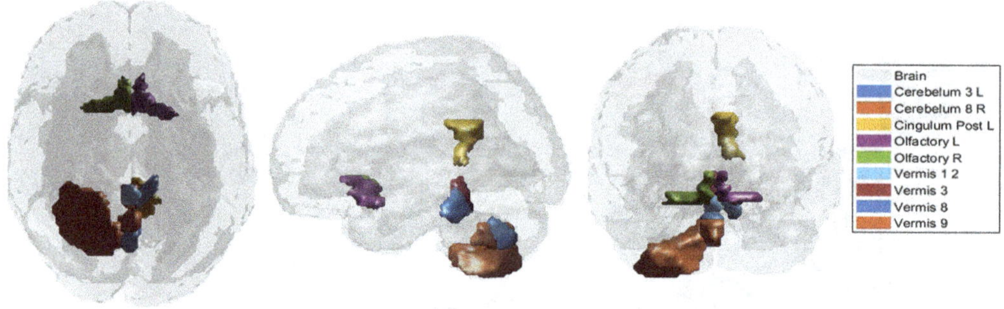

FIGURE 3 | The significant regions as obtained through the two sample *t*-test.

TABLE 2 | Evaluation of SVM classifier performance when different kernels are used.

			Level 2								
			LOSO			K-fold					
						$K = 2$			$K = 4$		
			RBF	Linear	Polynomial	RBF	Linear	Polynomial	RBF	Linear	Polynomial
Level 1	RBF	ACC	72.61	50	22.61	59.52	22.61	77.38	77.38	22.61	77.38
		Spec.	26.31	57.89	100	57.89	100	0	0	100	0
		Sens.	86.15	47.69	0	60	0	100	100	0	100
	Linear	ACC	77.38	**88.09**	95.23	77.38	**79.76**	77.38	77.38	**89.28**	77.38
		Spec.	0	**47.36**	78.94	0	**10.52**	0	0	**52.63**	0
		Sens.	100	**100**	100	100	**100**	100	100	**100**	100
	Polynomial	ACC	77.38	88.09	77.38	77.38	80.95	76.19	77.38	88.09	77.38
		Spec.	0	47.36	0	0	26.31	0	0	47.36	0
		Sens.	100	100	100	100	96.92	98.46	100	100	100

Classifier accuracy (ACC), sensitivity (Sens.) and specificity (Spec.), respectively in %, were estimated over all the labeled regions using LOSO and K-fold cross-validation. The bolded results (linear-pSVM linear-SVM) indicates the best combination of kernels used in the two levels.

local diagnostic results (i.e., the results of the first diagnosis level). **Figure 4** illustrates the local diagnosis of two NC and two MCI cases. While **Figure 5** shows examples of five different MCI subjects. The color bar in both figures represent the degree of abnormality starting from 0 (unaffected) to 1 (indicative of MCI). These examples indicate the varying abnormality effects in each significant region for each case independently. The implementation of the proposed CAD system can be found in the Supplementary Material.

4. DISCUSSION

This paper discusses a personalized MCI diagnosis system while improving the diagnostic performance as compared to other available methods. The personalized diagnosis is achieved through regional/local measurements, using the AAL atlas, which reflects how the disease affects different brain regions. To enhance this procedure, a statistical analysis was initially performed to determine the salient brain regions and consequently analyze the influence of the disease on them through the first diagnosis level, as shown in **Figures 4**, **5**. Apart from being the first stage of the MCI diagnosis procedure, the reported local diagnoses are helpful assistance in the personalized management of the disease. This has been represented through the color bar that shows the degree of abnormality from 0 (unaffected) to 1 (indicative of MCI) in each one of the nine significant regions separately. Finally, the system fuses the regional based probabilistic results obtained from the first diagnosis level to produce the final global diagnosis of each subject.

Regarding the cerebellar regions identified as significant, there have been several studies that focused on cerebellar abnormalities in dementia. Some of these studies were neuropathological-based studies that found that the neuronal shrinkage and loss represent well-known changes that accompany AD (Baldaçara et al., 2011). Morphological studies have targeted the prominent neuropathological AD-related hallmarks, like amyloid plaques (Cole et al., 1993; Wang et al., 2002). According to Wang et al. (2002), most AD-based pathological features that are found in the cerebellum include diffuse Aβ deposits. Considering the later finding and since the regions with increased Aβ plaques are represented as the high retention in the PiB, we could justify this finding in the early stage of AD. In addition to these findings

TABLE 3 | Using LOSO and K-fold cross-validation methods to evaluate the classification results, in %, (using linear-pSVM linear-SVMs) using the features of different cases of input regions: all the labeled regions, all the regions except the significant ones, and the significant regions only.

		LOSO	**K-fold**	
			$K = 2$	$K = 4$
All labeled regions	ACC	88.09	79.76	89.28
	Spec.	47.36	10.52	52.63
	Sens.	100	100	100
The resulting significant regions	ACC	100	97.61	98.80
	Spec.	100	94.73	94.73
	Sens.	100	98.46	100
Excluding the significant regions	ACC	82.14	77.38	83.33
	Spec.	21.05	0	26.31
	Sens.	100	100	100

and according to Sjöbeck and Englund (2001), structural based changes, mainly involved in the vermis, were judged to represent the progression of the disease.

Dysfunction in the olfactory cortex was found, through some studies, to probably be one of the earliest symptoms that are clinically obtained regarding AD (Serby et al., 1991; Devanand et al., 2000). According to Velayudhan (2015), the combination of the olfactory function tests along with the conventional diagnostic methods provides the ability to improve the sensitivity as well as the specificity of diagnosing AD. This consequently facilitates both the early recognition and diagnosis of AD. More details about the research progress and the future directions of the olfactory dysfunction in AD could be found in Zou et al. (2016).

Finally, as regards the posterior cingulate gyrus, some neuroimaging studies, which targeted several cortical regions, have identified that the posterior cingulate regions of the medial parietal cortex are among the earliest regions affected in AD (Scheff et al., 2015). These studies include one that supports the involvement of the posterior cingulate in the very early progression of AD (Rami et al., 2012).

In general, as shown in **Table 2**, the linear kernel shows best results either using it on both levels of the classifier or along with the polynomial kernel, while the RBF kernel performed poorly even when used conjointly with another kernel. The ability of the extracted features to differentiate the two groups (NC and MCI) and consequently make them linearly separate could justify the highest results of the linear kernel. For the polynomial as well as the RBF kernels, nonlinear kernels, the obtained separable features in addition to the small size of the dataset caused the outperformance of the polynomial kernel as compared to the RBF kernel that can show better results with large size of the dataset. According to these results and since linear-linear SVM-based classifiers show in general the best results, they were used to build the CAD system.

As expected, the significant region-based diagnostic performance outperforms that of the other two trial classifiers

TABLE 4 | The comparison of the proposed system's performance results, in %, against other related studies using LOSO cross-validation method.

	ACC	**Spec.**	**Sens.**
Chaves et al., 2012	90.48	100	87.69
Jiang et al., 2015	89.17	–	–
The proposed system	100	100	100

(**Table 3**) with a maximum performance of 100% of accuracy, specificity, and sensitivity. This finding could be due to the discrimination power of the features extractor in addition to the demonstration of alpha that helped in obtaining these salient regions. Regarding the two other tests, using all the labels shows better results than excluding the significant regions but worse than using the significant regions. This finding could be due to the presence of the labeled regions that are not significant enough to differentiate between the groups and consequently led to misclassification results that could finally affect the overall performance of the system. In addition, this is the same case when excluding the significant regions, but in addition to the presence of these not well significant regions, the significant regions are excluded causing this drop of performance results as compared with the other two tested cases.

The fact that our system improved performance with respect to other techniques while using the same dataset is of crucial consideration. The superior results of the proposed system over prior work (**Table 4**) could be justified through the capabilities of the combined components of the system that could extract the most discriminant features, identify the significant brains regions and then perform the classification using the SVM along with the linear kernel.

Since the primary goal of the paper was to provide local diagnosis, **Figures 4, 5** illustrated various examples that demonstrate the variability of the abnormality in each of the salient regions among the subjects. **Figure 4** showed sample cases of NC and MCI groups proving this point where the color bar indicates the degree of the diseases effect starting with the dark blue, no effect, to the dark red, total effect. **Figure 5** shows additional illustration source of the local diagnosis. The figure includes five different MCI subjects where the abnormalities' degree differ from one subject to another. Both figures demonstrate the power of the proposed system to reveal the local diagnosis of the disease on the significant brain regions. The analysis results that could be derived from the figures show the ability of the proposed analysis to reflect the current degree of the dysfunctionality that each region achieved through the disease. This visualization consequently can be considered an effective assistant for the individualized/personalized diagnosis process.

According to the above results, the proposed system may be of assistance in the diagnosis of MCI. In other words, the system offers a personalized diagnosis of the subjects in a short computation time using a subset of the brain's regions rather than using all regions. Additionally, the system provides high global diagnosis results compared to other related studies. Due

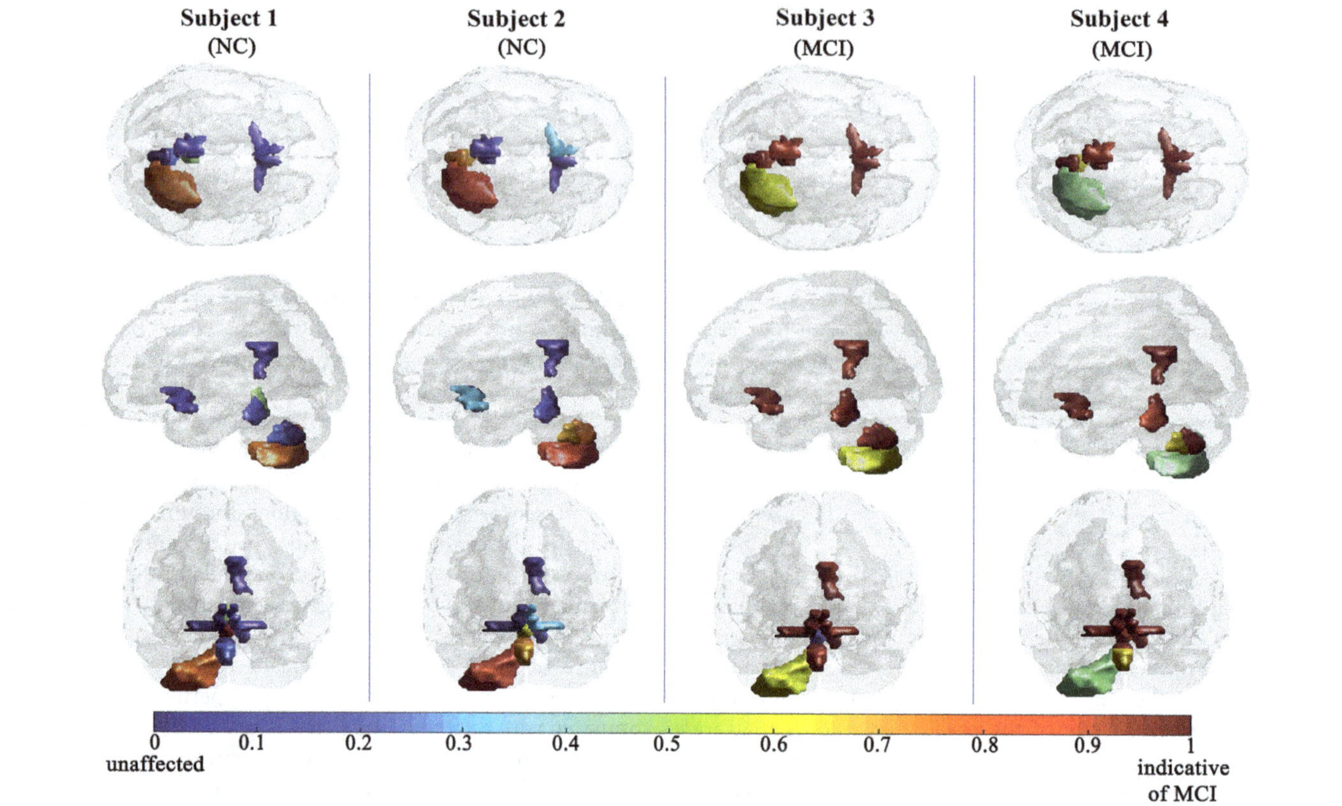

FIGURE 4 | Examples of local diagnosis results for NC vs. MCI classification problem.

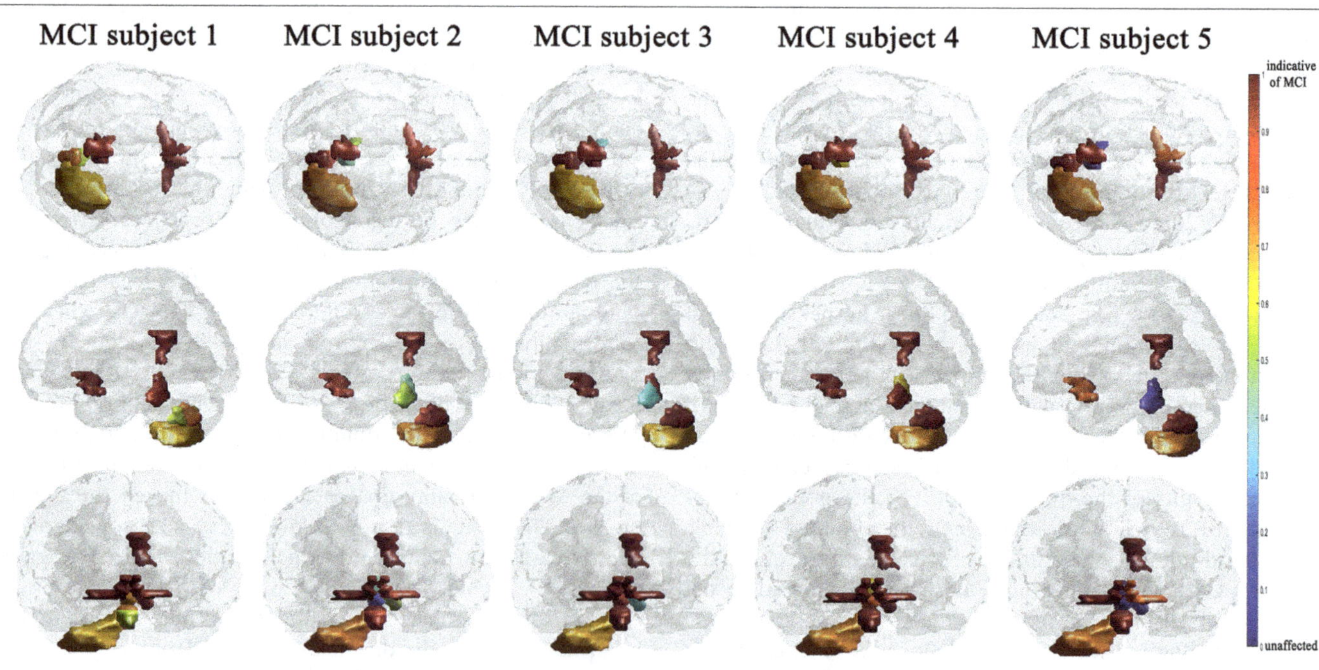

FIGURE 5 | Examples of local diagnosis results of different MCI subjects.

to the promising results of the proposed system and pilot nature of our data, we plan to examine two goals in the future work. First, the system's performance will be evaluated on larger PET scan datasets. Second, the results will be incorporated with other AD-related scanning modalities, to provide more analysis based assistance for the early diagnosis of AD.

AUTHOR CONTRIBUTIONS

FE-G: writing the manuscript and conducting the experiments. ME: advising, designing the experiments, developing the algorithm, and reviewing the entire paper. MG, RK, and AK: advising and financial support. AA: advising and reviewing the entire paper. MC: emphasizing the clinical aspect of the paper and reviewing the entire paper. GB: advising, reviewing the clinical aspect of the paper, reshaping the paper, and extensively editing it. AE-B: advising, designed the experiments, developing the algorithm, and reviewing the entire paper.

ACKNOWLEDGMENTS

The fund of the collected and shared data of this article was done by Alzheimer's Disease Neuroimaging Initiative (ADNI) (National Institutes of Health Grant U01 AG024904) and DOD ADNI (Department of Defense award number W81XWH-12-2-0012). ADNI is funded by the National Institute on Aging, the National Institute of Biomedical Imaging and Bioengineering, and through generous contributions from the following: AbbVie, Alzheimer's Association; Alzheimer's Drug Discovery Foundation; Araclon Biotech; BioClinica, Inc.; Biogen; Bristol-Myers Squibb Company; CereSpir, Inc.; Cogstate; Eisai Inc.; Elan Pharmaceuticals, Inc.; Eli Lilly and Company; EuroImmun; F. Hoffmann-La Roche Ltd and its affiliated company Genentech, Inc.; Fujirebio; GE Healthcare; IXICO Ltd.; Janssen Alzheimer Immunotherapy Research & Development, LLC.; Johnson & Johnson Pharmaceutical Research & Development LLC.; Lumosity; Lundbeck; Merck & Co., Inc.; Meso Scale Diagnostics, LLC.; NeuroRx Research; Neurotrack Technologies; Novartis Pharmaceuticals Corporation; Pfizer Inc.; Piramal Imaging; Servier; Takeda Pharmaceutical Company; and Transition Therapeutics. The Canadian Institutes of Health Research is providing funds to support ADNI clinical sites in Canada. Private sector contributions are facilitated by the Foundation for the National Institutes of Health (www.fnih.org). The grantee organization is the Northern California Institute for Research and Education, and the study is coordinated by the Alzheimer's Therapeutic Research Institute at the University of Southern California. ADNI data are disseminated by the Laboratory for Neuro Imaging at the University of Southern California.

The first author FE-G appreciates the financial support from the Cultural Affairs & Mission Sector, Ministry of Higher Education (MOHE), Egypt.

REFERENCES

Agrawal, S., and Bahendwar, Y. (2011). Denoising of MRI images using thresholding techniques through wavelet transform. *Int. J. Comput. Appl. Eng. Sci.* 1, 361–364.

Alivelearn.net (2017). *xjview | A Viewing Program for SPM.* Available online at: http://www.alivelearn.net/xjview/

Anderson, N., Murphy, K., and Troyer, A. (2012). *Living with Mild Cognitive Impairment: A Guide to Maximizing Brain Health and Reducing Risk of Dementia.* New York, NY: Oxford University Press.

Bagci, U., and Mollura, D. J. (2013). Denoising PET images using singular value thresholding and stein's unbiased risk estimate. *Int. Conf. Med. Image Comput. Comput. Assist. Interv.* 6(Pt 3), 115–122. doi: 10.1007/978-3-642-40760-4_15

Baldaçara, L., Borgio, J. G., Moraes, W. A., Lacerda, A. L., Montano, M. B., Tufik, S., et al. (2011). Cerebellar volume in patients with dementia. *Rev. Bras. Psiquiatr.* 33, 122–129. doi: 10.1590/S1516-44462011000200006

Belleville, S., Fouquet, C., Hudon, C., Zomahoun, H. T. V., Croteau, J., and Consortium for the Early Identification of Alzheimer's disease-Quebec. (2017). Neuropsychological measures that predict progression from mild cognitive impairment to Alzheimer's type dementia in older adults: a systematic review and meta-analysis. *Neuropsychol. Rev.* 27, 328–353. doi: 10.1007/s11065-017-9361-5

Brown, D. (2013). *Brain Diseases and Metalloproteins.* Singapore: Pan Stanford.

Campbell, C., and Ying, Y. (2011). *Learning with Support Vector Machines. Synthesis Lectures on Artificial Intelligence and Machine Learning.* Corvallis, OR: Morgan & Claypool.

Chaves, R., Ramirez, J., Górriz, J., Illán, I., and Salas-Gonzalez, D. (2012). "FDG and PIB biomarker PET analysis for the Alzheimer's disease detection using association rules," in *Nuclear Science Symposium and Medical Imaging Conference (NSS/MIC), 2012 IEEE* (Anaheim, CA), 2576–2579.

Cole, G., Neal, J. W., Singhrao, S. K., Jasani, B., and Newman, G. R. (1993). The distribution of amyloid plaques in the cerebellum and brain stem in down's syndrome and Alzheimer's disease: a light microscopical analysis. *Acta Neuropathol.* 85, 542–552.

Devanand, D., Michaels-Marston, K. S., Liu, X., Pelton, G. H., Padilla, M., Marder, K., et al. (2000). Olfactory deficits in patients with mild cognitive impairment predict Alzheimer's disease at follow-up. *Am. J. Psychiatry* 157, 1399–1405. doi: 10.1176/appi.ajp.157.9.1399

Forsberg, A., Engler, H., Almkvist, O., Blomquist, G., Hagman, G., Wall, A., et al. (2008). PET imaging of amyloid deposition in patients with mild cognitive impairment. *Neurobiol. Aging* 29, 1456–1465. doi: 10.1016/j.neurobiolaging.2007.03.029

Hodler, J., Schulthess, G., and Zollikofer, C. (2012). *Diseases of the Brain, Head & Neck, Spine 2012-2015: Diagnostic Imaging and Interventional Techniques.* Milan: Springer Science & Business Media.

Illán, I. A., Górriz, J. M., López, M. M., Ramírez, J., Salas-Gonzalez, D., Segovia, F., et al. (2011). Computer aided diagnosis of Alzheimer's disease using component based SVM. *Appl. Soft Comput.* 11, 2376–2382. doi: 10.1016/j.asoc.2010.08.019

Illán, I., Gorriz, J., Ramirez, J., Chaves, R., Segovia, F., López, M., et al. (2010). "Machine learning for very early Alzheimer's disease diagnosis; a 18 F-FDG and pib PET comparison," in *Nuclear Science Symposium Conference Record (NSS/MIC), 2010 IEEE* (Knoxville, TN), 2334–2337.

Illán, I., Górriz, J., Ramírez, J., Salas-Gonzalez, D., López, M., Segovia, F., et al. (2011). 18F-FDG PET imaging analysis for computer aided Alzheimer's diagnosis⋆. *Inform. Sci.* 181, 903–916.

Jack, C., Knopman, D., Jagust, W., Shaw, L., Aisen, P., Weiner, M., et al. (2010). Hypothetical model of dynamic biomarkers of the Alzheimer's pathological cascade. *Lancet Neurol.* 9, 119–128. doi: 10.1016/S1474-4422(09)70299-6

Jiang, J., Shu, X., Liu, X., and Huang, Z. (2015). "A computed aided diagnosis tool for Alzheimer's disease based on 11C-PIB PET imaging technique," in *IEEE International Conference on Information and Automation.*

Johnson, K., Minoshima, S., Bohnen, N., Donohoe, K., Foster, N., Herscovitch, P., et al. (2013). Appropriate use criteria for amyloid PET: a report of the amyloid imaging task force, the society of nuclear medicine and molecular imaging, and the alzheimer's association. *Alzheimer's Dement.* 9, E1–E16. doi: 10.1016/j.jalz.2013.01.002

Kemppainen, N., Aalto, S., Wilson, I., Någren, K., Helin, S., Brück, A., et al. (2006). Voxel-based analysis of PET amyloid ligand [11c] PIB uptake in Alzheimer disease. *Neurology* 67, 1575–1580. doi: 10.1212/01.wnl.0000240117.55680.0a

Langa, K. M., and Levine, D. A. (2014). The diagnosis and management of mild cognitive impairment: a clinical review. *JAMA* 312, 2551–2561. doi: 10.1001/jama.2014.13806

López, M., Ramírez, J., Górriz, J. M., Álvarez, I., Salas-Gonzalez, D., Segovia, F., et al. (2011). Principal component analysis-based techniques and supervised classification schemes for the early detection of Alzheimer's disease. *Neurocomputing* 74, 1260–1271. doi: 10.1016/j.neucom.2010.06.025

Lu, L., and Bludau, J. (2011). *Alzheimer's Disease, 1st Edn.* Westport, CT: ABC-CLIO.

Martínez-Murcia, F., Górriz, J., Ramírez, J., Puntonet, C., and Salas-González, D. (2012). Computer aided diagnosis tool for Alzheimer's disease based on Mann-Whitney-Wilcoxon U-test. *Expert Syst. Appl.* 39, 9676–9685. doi: 10.1016/j.eswa.2012.02.153

Morbelli, S., Drzezga, A., Perneczky, R., Frisoni, G. B., Caroli, A., van Berckel, B. N., et al. (2012). Resting metabolic connectivity in prodromal Alzheimer's disease. a european Alzheimer disease consortium (EADC) project. *Neurobiol. Aging* 33, 2533–2550. doi: 10.1016/j.neurobiolaging.2012.01.005

NeuroImaging, W. (2017). *Spm12 - Statistical Parametric Mapping. fil.ion.ucl.ac.uk.* Available online at: http://www.fil.ion.ucl.ac.uk/spm/software/spm12//

NIH (2017). *National Institute on Aging.* Available online at: http://www.nia.nih.gov/

Padilla, P., Lopez, M., Gorriz, J., Ramirez, J., Salas-Gonzalez, D., and Alvarez, I. (2012). NMF-SVM based CAD tool applied to functional brain images for the diagnosis of Alzheimer's disease. *IEEE Trans. Med. Imaging* 31, 207–216. doi: 10.1109/TMI.2011.2167628

Rami, L., Sala-Llonch, R., Solé-Padullés, C., Fortea, J., Olives, J., Lladó, A., et al. (2012). Distinct functional activity of the precuneus and posterior cingulate cortex during encoding in the preclinical stage of Alzheimer's disease. *J. Alzheimer's Dis.* 31, 517–526. doi: 10.3233/JAD-2012-120223

Salas-Gonzalez, D., Segovia, F., Martínez-Murcia, F. J., Lang, E. W., Gorriz, J. M., and Ramırez, J. (2016). An optimal approach for selecting discriminant regions for the diagnosis of Alzheimer's disease. *Curr. Alzheimer Res.* 13, 838–844. doi: 10.2174/1567205013666160415154852

Scheff, S. W., Price, D. A., Ansari, M. A., Roberts, K. N., Schmitt, F. A., Ikonomovic, M. D., et al. (2015). Synaptic change in the posterior cingulate gyrus in the progression of Alzheimer's disease. *J. Alzheimer's Dis.* 43, 1073–1090. doi: 10.3233/JAD-141518

Serby, M., Larson, P., and Kalkstein, D. (1991). The nature and course of olfactory deficits in Alzheimer's disease. *Am. J. Psychiatry* 148:357.

Shin, J., Lee, S.-Y., Kim, S. J., Kim, S.-H., Cho, S.-J., and Kim, Y.-B. (2010). Voxel-based analysis of Alzheimer's disease PET imaging using a triplet of radiotracers: PIB, FDDNP, and FDG. *Neuroimage* 52, 488–496. doi: 10.1016/j.neuroimage.2010.04.013

Sjöbeck, M., and Englund, E. (2001). Alzheimer's disease and the cerebellum: a morphologic study on neuronal and glial changes. *Dement. Geriatr. Cogn. Disord.* 12, 211–218. doi: 10.1159/000051260

Su, S.-S., Chen, K.-W., and Huang, Q. (2014). Discriminant analysis in the study of Alzheimer's disease using feature extractions and support vector machines in positron emission tomography with 18F-FDG. *J. Shanghai Jiaotong Univ.* 19, 555–560. doi: 10.1007/s12204-014-1540-4

Toennies, K. D. (2012). *Guide to Medical Image Analysis: Methods and Algorithms.* London: Springer Science & Business Media.

Turkington, C., and Harris, J. (2001). *The Encyclopedia of the Brain and Brain Disorders.* New York, NY: Infobase Pub.

Varghese, T., Sheelakumari, R., James, S. J., and Mathuranath, P. (2013). A review of neuroimaging biomarkers of Alzheimer's disease. *Neurol. Asia* 18, 239–248.

Velayudhan, L. (2015). Smell identification function and Alzheimer's disease: a selective review. *Curr. Opin. Psychiatry* 28, 173–179. doi: 10.1097/YCO.0000000000000146

Wang, H.-Y., D'Andrea, M. R., and Nagele, R. G. (2002). Cerebellar diffuse amyloid plaques are derived from dendritic aβ42 accumulations in purkinje cells. *Neurobiol. Aging* 23, 213–223. doi: 10.1016/s0197-4580(01)00279-2

Wegrzyn, R., and Rudolph, A. (2012). *Alzheimer's Disease: Targets for New Clinical Diagnostic and Therapeutic Strategies.* Boca Raton, FL: CRC Press.

WHO (2017). *World Health Organization.* Available online at: http://www.who.int/

Yaffe, K. (2013). *Chronic Medical Disease and Cognitive Aging: Toward a Healthy Body and Brain.* New York, NY: Oxford University Press.

Zhang, Y., Dong, Z., Phillips, P., Wang, S., Ji, G., Yang, J., et al. (2015). Detection of subjects and brain regions related to Alzheimer's disease using 3D MRI scans based on eigenbrain and machine learning. *Front. Comput. Neurosci.* 9:66. doi: 10.3389/fncom.2015.00066

Ziolko, S. K., Weissfeld, L. A., Klunk, W. E., Mathis, C. A., Hoge, J. A., Lopresti, B. J., et al. (2006). Evaluation of voxel-based methods for the statistical analysis of PIB PET amyloid imaging studies in Alzheimer's disease. *Neuroimage* 33, 94–102. doi: 10.1016/j.neuroimage.2006.05.063

Zou, Y.-M., Lu, D., Liu, L.-P., Zhang, H.-H., and Zhou, Y.-Y. (2016). Olfactory dysfunction in Alzheimer's disease. *Neuropsychiatr. Dis. Treat.* 12, 869–875. doi: 10.2147/NDT.S104886

10

Decreased Bilateral FDG-PET Uptake and Inter-Hemispheric Connectivity in Multi-Domain Amnestic Mild Cognitive Impairment Patients

Xiao Luo[1†‡], Kaicheng Li[1†], Qingze Zeng[1], Peiyu Huang[1], Yeerfan Jiaerken[1], Tiantian Qiu[1], Xiaojun Xu[1], Jiong Zhou[2], Jingjing Xu[1] and Minming Zhang[1*] for the Alzheimer's Disease Neuroimaging Initiative (ADNI)[§]

[1] Department of Radiology, The Second Affiliated Hospital of Zhejiang University School of Medicine, Hangzhou, China,
[2] Department of Neurology, The Second Affiliated Hospital of Zhejiang University School of Medicine, Hangzhou, China

***Correspondence:**
Minming Zhang
zhangminming@zju.edu.cn

† These authors have contributed equally to this work.

‡ orcid.org/0000-0003-1743-7842

§ The data used in the preparation of this article were obtained from the Alzheimer's Disease Neuroimaging Initiative (ADNI) database (adni.loni.usc.edu). As such, the investigators within the ADNI contributed to the design and implementation of ADNI and provided data but did not participate in the analysis or writing of this report.

Background: Amnestic mild cognitive impairment (aMCI) is a heterogeneous condition. Based on clinical symptoms, aMCI could be categorized into single-domain aMCI (SD-aMCI, only memory deficit) and multi-domain aMCI (MD-aMCI, one or more cognitive domain deficit). As core intrinsic functional architecture, inter-hemispheric connectivity maintains many cognitive abilities. However, few studies investigated whether SD-aMCI and MD-aMCI have different inter-hemispheric connectivity pattern.

Methods: We evaluated inter-hemispheric connection pattern using fluorine-18 positron emission tomography – fluorodeoxyglucose (^{18}F PET-FDG), resting-state functional MRI and structural T1 in 49 controls, 32 SD-aMCI, and 32 MD-aMCI patients. Specifically, we analyzed the 18^{F} PET-FDG (intensity normalized by cerebellar vermis) in a voxel-wise manner. Then, we estimated inter-hemispheric functional and structural connectivity by calculating the voxel-mirrored homotopic connectivity (VMHC) and corpus callosum (CC) subregions volume. Further, we correlated inter-hemispheric indices with the behavioral score and pathological biomarkers.

Results: We found that MD-aMCI exhibited more several inter-hemispheric connectivity damages than SD-aMCI. Specifically, MD-aMCI displayed hypometabolism in the bilateral middle temporal gyrus (MTG), inferior parietal lobe, and left precuneus (PCu) ($p < 0.001$, corrected). Correspondingly, MD-aMCI showed decreased VMHC in MTG, PCu, calcarine gyrus, and postcentral gyrus, as well as smaller mid-posterior CC than the SD-aMCI and controls ($p < 0.05$, corrected). Contrary to MD-aMCI, there were no neuroimaging indices with significant differences between SD-aMCI and controls, except reduced hypometabolism in bilateral MTG. Within aMCI patients, hypometabolism and reduced inter-hemispheric connectivity correlated with worse executive ability. Moreover, hypometabolism indices correlated to increased amyloid deposition.

Conclusion: In conclusion, patients with MD-aMCI exhibited the more severe deficit in inter-hemispheric communication than SD-aMCI. This long-range connectivity deficit may contribute to cognitive profiles and potentially serve as a biomarker to estimate disease progression of aMCI patients.

Keywords: mild cognitive impairment, cerebral metabolism, corpus callosum, resting-state functional MRI, voxel-mirrored homotopic connectivity

INTRODUCTION

The amnestic mild cognitive impairment (aMCI) represents an intermediate stage between normal aging and Alzheimer's disease (AD) (Petersen et al., 2014). According to impaired cognitive domains number, aMCI patients could be further categorized into two subtypes: single-domain aMCI (SD-aMCI), characterized by relatively selective memory impairment and the multi-domain aMCI (MD-aMCI), indicating extensive deficits involving at least one other domain (Winblad et al., 2004; Busse et al., 2006). Previous epidemiology study shows that MD-aMCI has a higher risk of clinical progression than the SD-aMCI (Golob et al., 2007). Therefore, to investigate the mechanism underlying these aMCI subtypes may efficiently facilitate clinical early intervention and management. Recently, neuroimaging studies pointed out that the MD-aMCI displays more diffuse gray matter atrophy (Haller et al., 2010; Zhang et al., 2012) and lower brain activity than the SD-aMCI, mainly involving default mode network (DMN) and frontoparietal regions (Li et al., 2014). Despite these studies shedding light into the aMCI pathological mechanism to some extent, it remains unclear whether SD-aMCI and MD-aMCI have different inter-hemispheric connection pattern.

Compared to the other neuroimaging indices, insufficient attention paid to the direct inter-hemispheric connectivity of aMCI patients. Anatomically, the connectivity between hemispheres is a core mode of the brain intrinsic functional architecture. Moreover, this bi-hemispheric communication procedure substantially affects many cognitive domains, including executive and memory functions (Salvador et al., 2008; Stark et al., 2008; Saar-Ashkenazy et al., 2016). Until now, only two functional MRI studies directly explored the inter-hemispheric functional connectivity in aMCI patients. However, two studies drew the entirely different conclusion. Specifically, Wang et al. (2015) demonstrated that MCI patients exhibited an enhanced inter-hemispheric functional connectivity in the sensorimotor cortex to resist the cognitive decline; however, another work reported the negative result between aMCI and controls (Qiu et al., 2016). Given that aMCI is a heterogeneous condition, we thus hypothesized that this inconsistency might attribute to the different damage pattern of inter-hemispheric connectivity between SD-aMCI and MD-aMCI patients.

Notably, some previous findings focusing on corpus callosum (CC) supported this hypothesis. Anatomically, CC acts as the most robust commissural white matter bundle to maintain the functional connectivity between the hemispheres (Roland et al., 2017). Specifically, some studies demonstrated that the AD and MCI patients exhibit the CC shape change, atrophy, and impaired diffusivity indices impairment, especially in the posterior part (Janowsky et al., 1996; Di Paola et al., 2010; Ardekani et al., 2014; Rasero et al., 2017). Subsequently, some studies further demonstrated patients with MD-aMCI, but not SD-aMCI, have reduced mean diffusivity (MD) in the whole CC compared to controls; moreover, decrease of MD in the CC body is associated with decreased general cognition and executive ability (Li et al., 2013). On the other hand, as a valid diagnostic biomarker in dementia studies, fluorine-18 fluorodeoxyglucose (^{18}F FDG) positron emission tomography (PET) research also shows more diffuse hypometabolism in MD-aMCI than the SD-aMCI. Interestingly, these hypometabolism regions are mostly located in the bilateral homotopic precuneus (PCu) and the temporoparietal cortex (Caffarra et al., 2008; Cerami et al., 2015). Considering the evidence of CC degeneration and bilateral homotopic hypometabolism, we inferred that different inter-hemispheric connectivity damage pattern might exist between aMCI subgroups.

To test this hypothesis, we analyzed the structural T1 image, resting-state functional MRI (rsfMRI), ^{18}F PET-FDG, neuropsychological scales, and pathological biomarkers in a relatively large aMCI sample from ADNI database. Firstly, we analyzed inter-hemispheric homotopic functional connectivity by using a voxel-wise method, namely voxel-mirrored homotopic connectivity (VMHC) (Zuo et al., 2010; Luo et al., 2018b). The potential inter-hemispheric structural connectivity was evaluated by estimating CC volume. We divided CC into five part due to its different anatomical connection [i.e., genus connects the frontal areas, while body and splenium part connects the temporal and parietal areas (Fischl, 2012)]. Moreover, to test whether regions with inter-hemispheric disruption accompanied by metabolic abnormalities, we also analyzed ^{18}F FDG-PET data in a voxel-wise manner. Additionally, we also correlated neuroimaging indices with cognition and pathological biomarkers (reflecting by CSF and amyloid imaging). Our study aims to (i) compare the alteration of the inter-hemispheric connectivity and the metabolism between aMCI subtypes; (ii) explore the possible interactions between different neuroimaging modalities; and (iii) explore the relationships between neuroimaging indices and cognition.

MATERIALS AND METHODS

Alzheimer's Disease Neuroimaging Initiative

Data used in this study were obtained from the Alzheimer's disease Neuroimaging Initiative (ADNI) database[1]. The ADNI was launched in 2003 by the National Institute on Aging (NIA),

[1] adni.loni.usc.edu

the National Institute of Biomedical Imaging and Bioengineering (NIBIB), the Food and Drug Administration (FDA), private pharmaceutical companies, and non-profit organizations, as a $60 million, 5-year public–private partnership. The primary goal of ADNI has been to test whether serial magnetic resonance imaging (MRI), PET, other biological markers, and clinical and neuropsychological assessment can be combined to measure the progression of mild cognitive impairment (MCI) and early Alzheimer's disease (AD). Determination of sensitive and specific markers of very early AD progression is intended to aid researchers and clinicians in developing new treatments and monitor their effectiveness, as well as lessen the time and cost of clinical trials.

Subjects

All procedures performed in studies involving human participants were following the ethical standards of the institutional and national research committee and with the 1975 Helsinki Declaration and its later amendments or comparable ethical standards. The ADNI project was approved by the Institutional Review Boards of all participating institutions, and all participants at each site signed informed consent. Based on ADNI GO and ADNI 2 database, we identified 49 healthy right-handed subjects (normal controls, NC) and 64 aMCI patients, who had undergone structural scans, rsfMRI scans, FDG-PET scans, and neuropsychological evaluation. We downloaded the study data from the ADNI publicly available database before April 15, 2017. According to ADNI protocol, to be classified as healthy controls, the Mini-Mental State Examination (MMSE) for the subject should be between 24 and 30 (inclusive), and clinical dementia rating (CDR) score should be 0. Besides, the subject has no signs of depression (Geriatric Depression Scale, GDS <6) or possible dementia. To be defined as aMCI, the subject had an MMSE score between 24 and 30 (inclusive), memory complaint, objective abnormal memory evidence, and a CDR score of 0.5. Besides, aMCI patients' general cognition preserved well (cannot meet AD diagnostic criteria). Also, there were no signs of depression (GDS score <6) in aMCI patients.

Followed by exclusion standards: the subject who has a history of apparent head trauma, other neurological or major psychiatric disorder, and alcohol/drug abuse. Additionally, subjects were also excluded if they exhibited a significant vascular disease risk history, defined as Hachinski Ischemia Scale (HIS) scores higher than 4.

Neuropsychological Evaluation and MCI Subtypes Diagnosis

All subjects underwent comprehensive neuropsychological tests. Content includes general mental status (MMSE score, Alzheimer's Disease Assessment Scale, ADAS) and other cognitive domain, including memory function (Auditory Verbal Learning Test, AVLT; Wechsler Memory Scale-Logical Memory, WMS-LM, including immediate and delayed score), processing speed (Trail-Making Test, Part A, TMT-A), visuospatial function (Clock-Drawing Test, CDT), executive function (Trail-Making Test, Part B, TMT-B), and language ability (Boston Naming Test, BNT). According to the previous studies, we used the composite scores for executive functioning and memory (Crane et al., 2012; Gibbons et al., 2012).

The aMCI patients were divided into two subtypes by the performance in cognitive domains (Shu et al., 2012). Specifically, SD-aMCI refers to aMCI patients having an impairment in memory alone; MD-aMCI refers to aMCI patients having an impairment in memory and other cognitive domain (at least one). We defined impairment as the presence of a test scoring 1.5 standard deviations (SD) below the average score, from age- and education-matched healthy controls from ADNI. Specifically, the total number of healthy controls from ADNI is 198, mean age is 73.03 ± 6.20, and mean education attainment is 16.47 ± 2.45. No significant difference existed in terms of age and education level ($p > 0.05$) between ADNI controls and aMCI subjects (mean age: 73.33 ± 5.69; education level: 15.84 ± 2.45). Finally, we enrolled 49 out of 198 ADNI controls who undergone structural scans, rsfMRI scans, and neuropsychological evaluation for subsequent analyses. Meanwhile, 32 MD-aMCI and 32 SD-aMCI patients entered the subsequent analyses.

CSF Data

We downloaded the CSF dataset from the ADNI database. Based on CSF samples, $A\beta_{1-42}$, total tau (t-tau) and phosphorylated tau (p-tau_{181}) were measured (Bittner et al., 2016). These CSF biomarkers, including $A\beta_{1-42}$, t-tau, and p-tau_{181}, are also useful candidates as they are intimately related to amyloid plaques, neuronal death, and accumulation of tangles, respectively (Jovicich et al., 2016). Moreover, the ratio of p-tau/$A\beta_{1-42}$ was also calculated due to its association with cognition and disease progression (Landau et al., 2010). Notably, not all subjects in the present study had the CSF samples due to the invasive procedure of lumbar puncture. Thus, the final CSF sample for analyses included 26 out of the 49 NC, 30 out of the 32 SD-aMCI, and 28 out of the 32 MD-aMCI patients.

Amyloid PET Data

Given that amyloid PET shows more potent than CSF markers for MCI prognosis, we further downloaded the results of ^{18}F-florbetapir PET data from the ADNI database, namely UCBERKELEYAV45_11_14_17.csv (Bouallègue et al., 2017). The detailed processing procedure was described previously (Landau et al., 2013). In the following analysis, we used the results of composite SUVR value (intensity-normalized by a whole cerebellum region).

Image Acquisition

The 3.0-Tesla Philips MRI scanner was used to scan all participants. Based on MPRAGE T1-weighted sequence, structural images were acquired with the following parameters: repetition time (TR) = 2300 ms; echo time (TE) = 2.98 ms; inversion time (TI) = 900 ms; 170 sagittal slices; within plane FOV = 256×240 mm^2; voxel size = $1.1 \times 1.1 \times 1.2$ mm^3; flip angle = 9°; and bandwidth = 240 Hz/pix. Based on echo-planar imaging sequence, rsfMRI images were acquired with the following parameters: time points = 140; TR = 3000 ms; TE = 30 ms; flip angle = 80°; the number of slices = 48; slice thickness = 3.3 mm; spatial resolution = 3.31 × 3.31 × 3.31 mm^3; and matrix = 64 × 64. Meanwhile, PET images were obtained by either a 30-min six frame scan acquired 30–60-min post-injection or a static 30-min single-frame scan acquired 30–60-min post-injection.

Image Preprocessing

The image data were preprocessed by using the Data Processing Assistant for rsfMRI, DPASF[2], based on the Statistical Parametric Mapping (SPM 12)[3] and rsfMRI Data Analysis Toolkit, REST[4]. Briefly, we removed the first 10 image volumes of rsfMRI scans were for the signal equilibrium and the subjects' adaptation to the machine noise. The remaining 130 image volumes were corrected for both timing differences and head motion (24 Friston; Friston et al., 1996). We excluded the data with more than 2.0 mm maximum displacement in any directions (*X*-, *Y*-, and *Z*-axis) and 2.0 degrees of any angular motion. Subsequently, the T1-weighted images were co-registered to the mean rsfMRI image based on a thorough rigid-body transformation and normalized to the Montreal Neurological Institute (MNI) space, subsequent resliced into of 3 mm × 3 mm × 3 mm cubic voxels. Besides, we performed linear trends and temporal filter (0.01 Hz $< f <$ 0.08 Hz). To remove any motion residual effects and other non-neuronal factors, we corrected covariates (including six head motion parameters, WM signal, CSF) in the following functional connectivity analysis. After preprocessing, we obtained each subject's 4D residual functional volume in native functional space. These 4D data were registered to the MNI152 space with 2 mm resolution (affine transformation). Due to the dispute of removing the global signal, we omit to regress out the global signal. Given the effect of the micro-motion artifact, we evaluated the frame-wise displacement (FD) value for each subject. Subjects were screened and excluded if FD value >0.5 mm on more than 35 volumes.

Voxel-Mirrored Homotopic Connectivity Analysis

For VMHC computation, firstly, the mean T1 image was generated from the average of 113 spatially normalized T1 images. Then, we flipped the left hemisphere along the midline of the *x*-axis to obtain the symmetric brain template, further, to create the final template. Subsequently, the each subject's T1 image was co-registered nonlinearly to the customized symmetric template. The same deformation field subsequently applied to the rsfMRI. More details regarding VMHC data processing are available in the literature (Anderson et al., 2010; Zuo et al., 2010). Based on Pearson's correlation, the homotopic RSFC between any pair of symmetrical inter-hemispheric voxels was estimated, then transformed to Fisher's *Z* map. Finally, we defined these resultant values as the VMHC and used it in following analyses.

[2]http://www.rfmri.org/DPARSF

[3]http://www.fil.ion.ucl.ac.uk/spm/

[4]http://www.resting-fmri.sourceforge.net/

Corpus Callosum Volume

We evaluated the CC volume and its subregions based on FreeSurfer software package (Version 5.1[5]) as described previously (Fischl, 2012; Reuter et al., 2012). In detail, FreeSurfer automatically segmented CC into five sections, with each section representing a fifth of the total area. We defined five segments as anterior (CC-A), mid-anterior (CC-MA), central (CC-C), mid-posterior (CC-MP), and posterior CC part (CC-P).

FDG-PET Voxel-Wise Analysis

We downloaded the ^{18}F FDG-PET data from the ADNI database in their most processed formats (PET Pre-processing protocol[6]). Specifically, pre-processed scans were generated following co-registration dynamic (to the first acquired frame), averaging frames, spatial re-orientation (AC–PC line), intensity normalization (within subject-specific mask), and smoothing (uniform isotropic spatial resolution 8 mm full width at half maximum kernel). The subsequent processing procedures of FDG-PET were conducted by combining T1 MRI images, which were similar to VMHC processing mentioned above. Firstly, each FDG-PET scan was co-registered to the individual's corresponding T1 MRI image in native space. Then, these structural scans were segmented, and the resulting GM partitions were spatially normalized using the SPM 12. The spatial normalization parameters (deformation fields) that had been estimated from the gray matter segment normalization were subsequently applied to the co-registered FDG-PET images so that both the GM, VMHC, and the FDG-PET images were in MNI space. To remove inter-individual nuisance variability in tracer metabolism, we intensity-normalized FDG-PET image via dividing it by the average FDG-PET value of the reference region (cerebellar vermis, defined by the AAL regions within the MNI atlas, manually checked by experienced radiologists, MMZ). Finally, we created the standardized uptake value ratio (SUVR) images for the following analysis.

Statistics

All statistical analyses were performed using IBM SPSS statistical software. The TMT-A, TMT-B, and ADAS-cog were log-transformed because of a positively skewed distribution. We used ANOVA to detect group differences in terms of age, education level, cognitive ability, and AD-related pathological results. We used the *post hoc* pairwise *t*-tests if ANOVA was significant ($p < 0.05$, corrected by Bonferroni).

Regarding VMHC results, the ANCOVA was used to explore different brain regions among the three groups, with controlling for age, education level, and gender. For the objective to explore, the threshold set at height $p < 0.05$ and cluster level $p < 0.05$ (Gaussian random field, GRF corrected). We performed the *post hoc* pairwise *t*-tests within the brain regions identified by the ANCOVA ($p < 0.005$ Bonferroni corrected). Regarding the FDG-PET SUVR image, we performed ANCOVA to explore metabolic differences, with controlling for age, education level,

[5]http://surfer.nmr.mgh.harvard.edu/

[6]http://adni.loni.usc.edu/methods/pet-analysis/pre-processing/

and gender [$p < 0.001$ at height and $p < 0.05$ at the cluster level (GRF corrected)]. Similarly, we performed the *post hoc* pairwise *t*-tests if ANCOVA was significant ($p < 0.005$, Bonferroni corrected). Also, we calculated the between-group CC subregions volume difference by using ANCOVA corrected by age, education level, gender, and total intracranial volume (TIV). We performed *post hoc* pairwise *t*-test if ANOVA was significant ($p < 0.05$, corrected by the least significant difference, LSD).

Further, we correlated imaging measures to cognitive abilities and also explored the possible interactions between neuroimaging modalities. To achieve the best visual effect, we overlapped between-group difference results of VMHC and FDG-PET SUVR image by the same statistical standard (ANCOVA, corrected by age, education level, and gender, $p < 0.05$ at height, $p < 0.05$ at the cluster level, GRF corrected). Meanwhile, to explore the possible interaction between CC subregions and other modalities, we performed voxel-wise regression analysis ($p < 0.05$ at height, $p < 0.05$ at the cluster level, GRF corrected). Notably, we calculated correlations limited to those indices having significant between-group differences.

RESULTS

Patient Characteristics

We displayed quantitative variables as the mean and its SD, and the categorical variable as absolute and relative frequency. **Table 1** shows the demographic characteristics, cognitive abilities, and pathological biomarkers for each group. There were no significant differences in terms of age, education level, and gender composition among the three groups. Regarding the general cognitive ability, we found that three groups exhibited the significant differences in the score of MMSE and ADAS-cog, with MD-aMCI displaying the worst performance. Regarding other cognitive domains, group effects were significant, with the best performance in NC and also the worst performance in MD-aMCI patients.

Regarding AD-related pathological biomarkers, MD-aMCI patients exhibited a significantly higher composite PET PiB SUVR value than NC ($p < 0.01$). Meanwhile, although MD-aMCI group presented a trend of the increased level of t-tau and p-tau$_{181}$ as well as decreased Aβ_{1-42}, no significant differences existed among groups ($p > 0.05$). Also, we also failed to detect the difference in the p-tau$_{181}$/Aβ_{1-42} ratio among groups.

Glucose Metabolism Differences

Three groups demonstrated the significant metabolic differences in the following regions: namely bilateral middle temporal gyrus (MTG), bilateral inferior parietal lobe (IPL), and left PCu. Subsequent pairwise group comparisons carried out on these clusters revealed that both aMCI patients exhibited a lower metabolism in bilateral MTG. Also, the MD-aMCI demonstrated a reduced metabolism in left PCu and bilateral IPL compared to the SD-aMCI and NC (**Figure 1** and **Table 2**).

Inter-Hemispheric Connection Differences

Among the three groups, we established the significant VMHC difference in these regions: namely middle MTG, PCu, postcentral gyrus (PCG), and calcarine gyrus (CG). As expected, subsequent pair-wise group comparisons suggested that MD-aMCI exhibited a decreased VMHC in MTG, CG, PCu, and PCG relative to SD-aMCI and NC ($p < 0.005$, corrected by Bonferroni); however, there were no significant differences of VMHC between SD-aMCI and NC (**Figure 2** and **Table 3**).

We observed the between-group effect on CC-MP subregion (**Figure 1**). Then, the *post hoc* *t*-test revealed that MD-aMCI exhibited the smallest CC-MP volume among groups, and no significant volume difference existed between SD-aMCI and NC ($p < 0.05$, corrected by LSD).

Neuroimaging Indices Correlate Cognitive Abilities and Pathological Biomarkers

All the correlation analyses we performed were within aMCI patients (**Figure 3**). We observed that reduced left IPL metabolism ($r = 0.27$) was related to worse executive ability ($p < 0.05$). In addition, regarding functional connectivity, we identified that reduced inter-hemispheric connection in PCu ($r = 0.39$), PCG ($r = 0.40$), and CG ($r = 0.54$) were related to worse composite score of executive functioning ($p < 0.001$). Also, the CC-MP volume was related to the composite score of executive functioning ($r = 0.40, p < 0.001$).

Regarding AD-related pathological biomarkers, we analyzed the correlation only within the indices having the between-group difference. Our results revealed that hypometabolism of left PCu ($r = -0.25$, $p < 0.05$) and right IPL ($r = -0.25$, $p < 0.05$) was related to the increased amyloid accumulation reflecting composite ^{18}F-florbetapir PET value.

Interaction Between Modalities

As expected, we noted that VMHC and PET-FDG SUVR between-group difference results overlapped well. Specifically, these overlapping included bilateral the MTG, the PCu, the IPL, and the PCG (Supplementary Material 1). Within these overlapping regions, we further observed that VMHC value related to SUVR uptake value within aMCI patient groups ($r = 0.27, p < 0.05$).

Within the aMCI patients, the mid-posterior CC volume was related to the bilateral MTG, PCu, CG, and insula ($p < 0.05$ at height and $p < 0.05$ at the cluster level, GRF-corrected Supplementary Material 2). However, we found no significance between mid-posterior CC volume and FDG SUVR uptake value ($p > 0.05$).

DISCUSSION

This study provides evidence that the MD-aMCI displayed simultaneous decreased bilateral metabolism and reduced inter-hemispheric functional connectivity in MTG, PCu, and

TABLE 1 | Comparison of demographic information, behavioral data, and pathological biomarkers.

	NC	SD-aMCI	MD-aMCI	F (χ^2)	P-value
Number	49	32	32		
Age	73.33 ± 4.60	72.43 ± 4.25	74.91 ± 5.27	2.29	0.11
Female	31	15	15	3.00	0.22
Education	16.24 ± 2.60	16.47 ± 2.24	15.25 ± 2.65	2.20	0.12
General mental status					
MMSE	29.02 ± 1.20	28.34 ± 1.68	27.16 ± 1.71	15.03	<0.001[bc]
Log-transformed ADAS	0.91 ± 0.17	1.07 ± 0.19	1.21 ± 0.20	24.21	<0.001[abc]
Spatial processing					
CDT	4.76 ± 0.48	4.75 ± 0.44	3.78 ± 1.18	19.69	<0.001[bc]
Language					
BNT	28.57 ± 1.44	28.09 ± 2.07	27.09 ± 11.36	0.55	0.58
Memory					
WMS-LM immediate	14.73 ± 2.76	9.88 ± 3.17	7.88 ± 2.83	60.49	<0.001[abc]
WMS-LM delayed	13.96 ± 2.99	7.97 ± 2.78	5.75 ± 3.06	84.93	<0.001[abc]
AVLT-Total	43.22 ± 9.01	37.34 ± 9.63	31.25 ± 8.78	16.85	<0.001[abc]
Processing speed					
Log-transformed TMTA	1.51 ± 0.12	1.47 ± 0.08	1.66 ± 0.15	23.82	<0.001[bc]
Executive function					
Log-transformed TMTB	1.86 ± 0.16	1.86 ± 0.13	2.18 ± 0.16	51.75	<0.001[bc]
Composite memory	1.05 ± 0.51	0.44 ± 0.59	0.06 ± 0.61	31.99	<0.001[abc]
Composite executive	0.80 ± 0.65	0.87 ± 0.51	−0.35 ± 0.51	47.82	<0.001[bc]
Pathological results					
$A\beta_{1-42}$ (pg/ml)	1222.19 ± 552.35	1132.06 ± 616.57	963.00 ± 438.94	1.85	0.16
t-tau (pg/ml)	248.52 ± 84.62	275.76 ± 90.51	300.33 ± 134.34	2.18	0.12
P-tau_{181} (pg/ml)	23.43 ± 9.46	25.69 ± 9.30	29.34 ± 15.01	2.30	0.11
p-tau/$A\beta_{1-42}$	0.03 ± 0.02	0.03 ± 0.02	0.04 ± 0.02	2.83	0.06
Composite PET-PiB	1.14 ± 0.19	1.20 ± 0.20	1.29 ± 0.25	4.54	0.01[b]

*Data are presented as means ± SD. Notably, the mean levels of $A\beta_{1-42}$, t-tau, and p-tau_{181} in **Table 1** only represent the subjects who had CSF samples. [a]Post hoc paired comparisons showed significant group differences between NC and SD-aMCI, after Bonferroni correction ($p < 0.05$). [b]Post hoc paired comparisons showed significant group differences between NC and MD-aMCI, after Bonferroni correction ($p < 0.05$). [c]Post hoc paired comparisons showed significant group differences between SD-aMCI and MD-aMCI, after Bonferroni correction ($p < 0.05$). MMSE, Mini-Mental State Examination; ADAS, the Alzheimer's Disease Assessment Scale-Cognitive Subscale; WMS-LM, Wechsler Memory Scale-Logical Memory; TMT, Trail-Making Test; CSF, cerebrospinal fluid; CDT, Clock-Drawing Test; AVLT, Auditory Verbal Learning Test; BNT, Boston Naming Test.*

parietal regions, accompanying with mid-posterior CC atrophy. However, except hypometabolism in bilateral MTG, no other differences existed between SD-aMCI and NC. Subsequently, the correlation analyses showed that these neuroimaging indices related to executive function across aMCI patients. Moreover, hypometabolism indices related to increased amyloid deposition. In summary, compared to SD-aMCI, the MD-aMCI exhibited the more severe deficit in inter-hemispheric communication. This long-range connectivity deficit may further contribute to cognitive abilities deficits and potentially serve as a biomarker to monitor the disease progression in aMCI patients.

Firstly, our findings suggested that both aMCI patients displayed hypometabolism in bilateral MTG, which is a region involving memory-related network (Ward et al., 2014; Munoz-Lopez et al., 2015). These deficits thus may contribute to the memory deficit in these patients. However, only the MD-aMCI simultaneously displayed inter-hemispheric functional connectivity decrease in MTG, supporting the notion that the MD-aMCI is a more advanced disease form than the SD-aMCI. Notably, one study pointed out that SD-aMCI displayed decreased regional activity in right MTG relative to NC (Luo et al., 2018a). Accordingly, we speculated that the intact inter-hemispheric connectivity in SD-aMCI might compensate its unilateral MTL impairment to some extent. Our neuropsychological results could support this interpretation, showing that MD-aMCI exhibited worse memory performance than SD-aMCI. Besides, other support evidence comes result from ^{18}F-florbetapir PET indicating that only the MD-aMCI has increased amyloid deposition than NC. Meanwhile, our findings validated previous studies, which reported that only MD-aMCI patients have cortical thinning, gray matter atrophy, and white matter tract deficit in MTG regions (Seo et al., 2007; Whitwell et al., 2007).

Many evidence suggests that amyloid accumulation preferentially starts in PCu, especially in the left side (Janke et al., 2001; Braak et al., 2006; Palmqvist et al., 2017). As expected, our results showed the MD-aMCI, but not the SD-aMCI, exhibited hypometabolism (left side) and reduced inter-hemispheric functional connection in PCu regions simultaneously. Moreover, we found that the reduced PCu inter-hemispheric functional

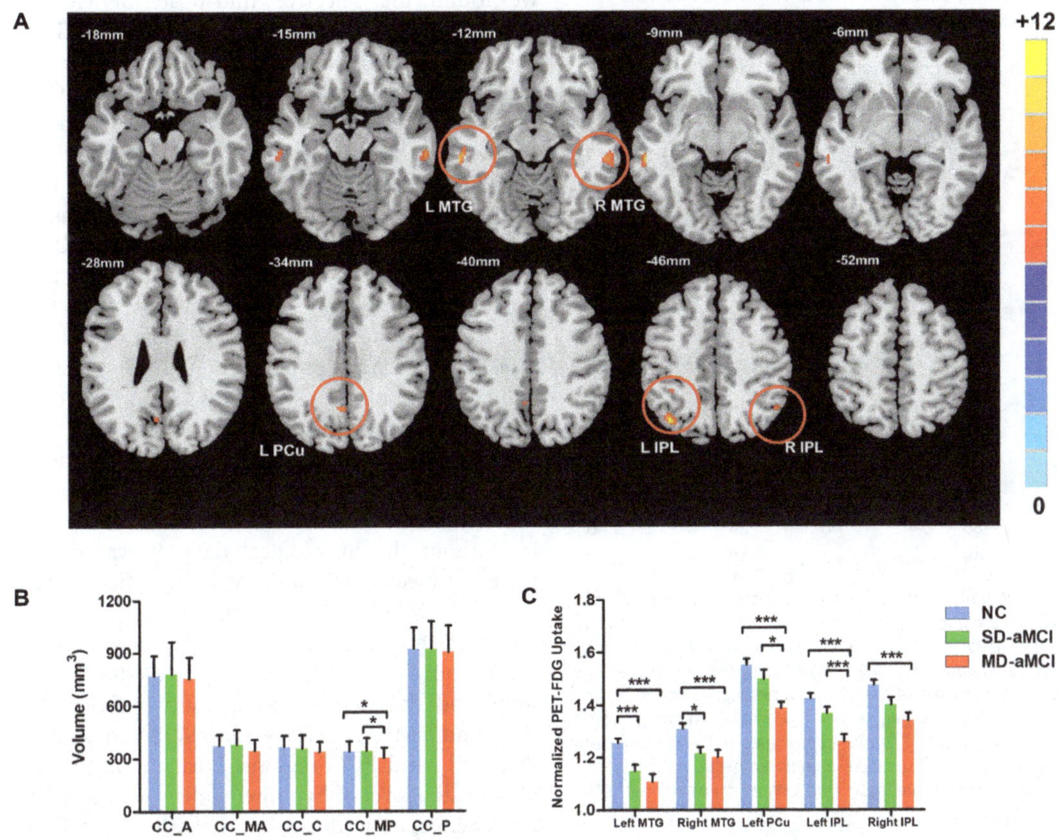

FIGURE 1 | Upper **(A)** shows the voxel-wise comparison result: brain areas with the significant difference of metabolism (normalized by cerebellum vermis) among NC, single-domain aMCI (SD-aMCI), and multi-domain aMCI (MD-aMCI), by controlling for age, education level, and gender. The threshold set $p < 0.001$ at height and $p < 0.05$ at the cluster level, GFR corrected. Lower figures show the histogram for MD-aMCI (red), SD-aMCI (green), and NCs (blue). Error bars represent SD. * represents $p < 0.05$ while *** represents $p < 0.001$, corrected for multiple comparisons. **(B)** The *post hoc* analyses were performed within the areas identified by the ANCOVA ($p < 0.05$). The MD-aMCI patients displayed the significantly decreased volume of the CC-MP compared to the other two groups. **(C)** We performed the *post hoc* analyses within the areas identified by the ANCOVA ($p < 0.005$). Among the three groups, the MD-aMCI patients exhibited the lowest metabolism in bilateral MTG, bilateral inferior parietal lobe (IPL), and left precuneus (L-PCu). Other abbreviation: A, anterior; MA, mid-anterior; C, central; MP, mid-posterior; and P, posterior.

connection associated with the worse executive function across aMCI patients. This relationship agrees with clinical manifestation in MD-aMCI patients, manifested by more than one cognitive domain impairment. Meanwhile, previous work also documented that MD-aMCI displayed impaired microstructure in PCu (Li et al., 2013). Specifically, by utilizing rsfMRI, one study demonstrated that the MD-aMCI exhibited lower regional activity in PCu than the SD-aMCI and NC. Coincidentally, their work also found that reduced PCu activity was related to worse executive ability (Li et al., 2014). As a central role in the primary executive networks, studies of the AD and MCI frequently reported that regional PCu deficit associated with the decreased executive ability (Sridharan et al., 2008; Chen et al., 2013; Luo et al., 2017a,b). Furthermore, we found that left PCu hypometabolism was related to amyloid deposition. Consequently, we speculated that amyloid-related neurotoxicity in unilateral PCu region might lead to the inter-hemispheric connectivity damage in corresponding areas.

Regarding the parietal cortex, the MD-aMCI exhibited hypometabolism in bilateral IPL and reduced inter-hemispheric PCG functional connectivity; additionally, we found that IPL hypometabolism was related to increased amyloid deposition. Therefore, we again interpreted that the hypometabolism in bilateral IPL may attribute to synaptic dysfunction caused by amyloid (Palop and Mucke, 2010; Tönnies and Trushina, 2017). Moreover, we observed that parietal cortex hypometabolism and inter-hemispheric dysfunction associated with worse executive ability. This relationship could attribute to the reason that both the IPL and PCG have extensive connections with the frontal region (i.e., frontoparietal circuit). Functionally, this circuit could send rich sensory information for processing speed and affect executive ability (Sullivan et al., 2001; Buckner et al., 2008; Luo et al., 2017b). Furthermore, some structural MRI studies support our results. One VBM study pointed out that patients with MD-aMCI exhibited GM reduction and increased mean diffusion in PCG (Li et al., 2013). Meanwhile, using diffusion spectrum

TABLE 2 | Brain areas with the significant difference of VMHC and PET-FDG among NCs, SD-aMCI, and MD-aMCI patients.

Regions	MNI coordinates			Cluster voxels	Peak intensity
	X	*Y*	*Z*		
VMHC					
Middle temporal gyrus	±51	−54	−3	128	8.30
Precuneus	±3	−57	60	133	7.60
Postcentral gyrus	±60	−21	24	317	8.86
Calcarine gyrus	±3	−75	9	195	9.60
PET-FDG					
L middle temporal gyrus	−60	−32	−10	59	11.08
	−44	−50	12	14	8.48
R middle temporal gyrus	62	−28	−14	52	9.37
L precuneus	−6	−54	38	38	8.86
L inferior parietal lobe	−38	−68	48	60	11.61
	−38	−42	48	24	9.46
R inferior parietal lobe	48	−58	44	13	8.60

Regarding VMHC results, the ANCOVA was used to explore differential brain regions among groups [controlling for age, education level, and gender, $p < 0.05$ at height and $p < 0.05$ at the cluster level, Gaussian random field (GRF) corrected]. Regarding the FDG-PET standardized uptake value ratio (SUVR) image, the ANCOVA was used to explore differential brain regions among the three groups (controlling for age, education level, and gender, $p < 0.001$ at height and $p < 0.05$ at cluster level, GRF corrected). The X, Y, and Z coordinates of the primary peak locations in the MNI space. MD-aMCI, multiple-domain amnestic mild cognitive impairment; SD-aMCI, single-domain amnestic mild cognitive impairment; MNI, Montreal Neurological Institute.

imaging (DSI), Chang et al. (2015) highlighted that the MD-aMCI groups have more impairment in the inferior cingulum bundle than the SD-aMCI groups, which anatomically connected with the parietal cortex.

Interestingly, MD-aMCI patients displayed reduced inter-hemispheric RSFC in CG, which is part of the extra-striate visual network and involved with the perception created by visual stimuli. Similarly, one rsfMRI study also illustrated that the MD-aMCI displayed decreased brain activity here (Li et al., 2014). On the other hand, most previous aMCI studies (without dividing into SD-aMCI and MD-aMCI) concluded that aMCI patients displayed increased intrinsic activity in CG (Han et al., 2011; Liu et al., 2012; Lou et al., 2016). This inconsistency may attribute to the aMCI heterogeneity. Besides, we found that decreased inter-hemispheric functional connectivity between bilateral CG was related to worse executive ability. Conceptually, the reaction time includes not only visual processing but also the time required for response execution (Thorpe et al., 1996). Moreover, optical encoding impairment could contribute to the reduction of processing speed (Brébion et al., 2015). Consequently, we interpreted this correlation as that the MD-aMCI patients were difficult to receive the information flows from visual sensors, further, exerting a negative influence on executive ability.

As the dominant white matter pathways, the CC links cortical hubs of the left and right hemispheres together. Here, we observed that MD-aMCI exhibited a smaller mid-posterior CC volume than the SD-aMCI and NC. Moreover, we found the selective mid-posterior CC degeneration in MD-aMCI corresponded well with the fMRI results discussed above. Specifically, regression analysis results showed that mid-posterior CC was significantly related to VMHC results, involving the bilateral MTG, PCu, CG, and PCG. In accord with our results, anatomical evidence showed that the bilateral MTG and PCu are strongly connected through the posterior CC (Cavanna and Trimble, 2006; van der Knaap and van der Ham, 2011; Wang et al., 2014). Additionally, we noted that smaller mid-posterior CC volume was related to worse executive function. This relationship suggests that CC degeneration might contribute to or even accelerate cognitive deficit (Agosta et al., 2015; Farrar et al., 2017; Luo et al., 2017b). Combined with the results of bilateral hypometabolism and inter-hemispheric disconnection, we hypothesized that mid-posterior CC atrophy may reflect the Wallerian degeneration secondary to neuronal loss caused by amyloid deposition (Bozzali et al., 2002).

Without the histological data, it was difficult to describe the exact mechanism underlying inter-hemispheric connectivity deficits in MD-aMCI patients. There are two reasons that may interpret the possible mechanism. Firstly, these deficits may result from the amyloid-related pathological process. Specifically, we found that the between-group difference results of PET-FDG and VMHC overlapped well, including the bilateral MTG, PCu, IPL, and PCG regions. Further, within these overlapping regions, the level of hypometabolism was significantly related to inter-hemispheric decrease. Nevertheless, only the metabolism indices were related to amyloid deposition. We, therefore, speculated that accumulated amyloid plaques in MD-aMCI patients might lead to synapse loss and hypometabolism, further, result in functional connectivity disruption with its contralateral regions (Tönnies and Trushina, 2017). Second, decreased inter-hemispheric functional connectivity may also result from the widespread white matter integrity disruption (White et al., 2009; Luo et al., 2016). Conclusively, these interpretations should be taken with caution due to the lack of animal study and diffusion tensor imaging (DTI) method, respectively.

Some limitations existed in our study. First, this cross-sectional study was failed to assess the long-term effects of hypometabolism and inter-hemispheric disconnection in the subsequent disease progression. Therefore, longitudinal studies are needed to explore the inter-hemispheric connection pattern following AD continuum, from healthy aging to clinical stages. Second, in accord with the inter-hemispheric functional connectivity results, correspondingly, MD-aMCI patients demonstrated selective mid-posterior CC degeneration. However, CC volume only identified the main inter-hemispheric connective tracts, rather than illustrating the precise definition of "inter-hemispheric structural connection." Therefore, future DTI studies by using tractography or network analysis are needed to provide more detailed information about inter-hemispheric white matter pathways in aMCI patients (Cavanna and Trimble, 2006; Rasero et al., 2017; Tucholka et al., 2018). In the current study, based on the ADNI 2 database, we noticed that subjects do not have both the DTI and the rsfMRI

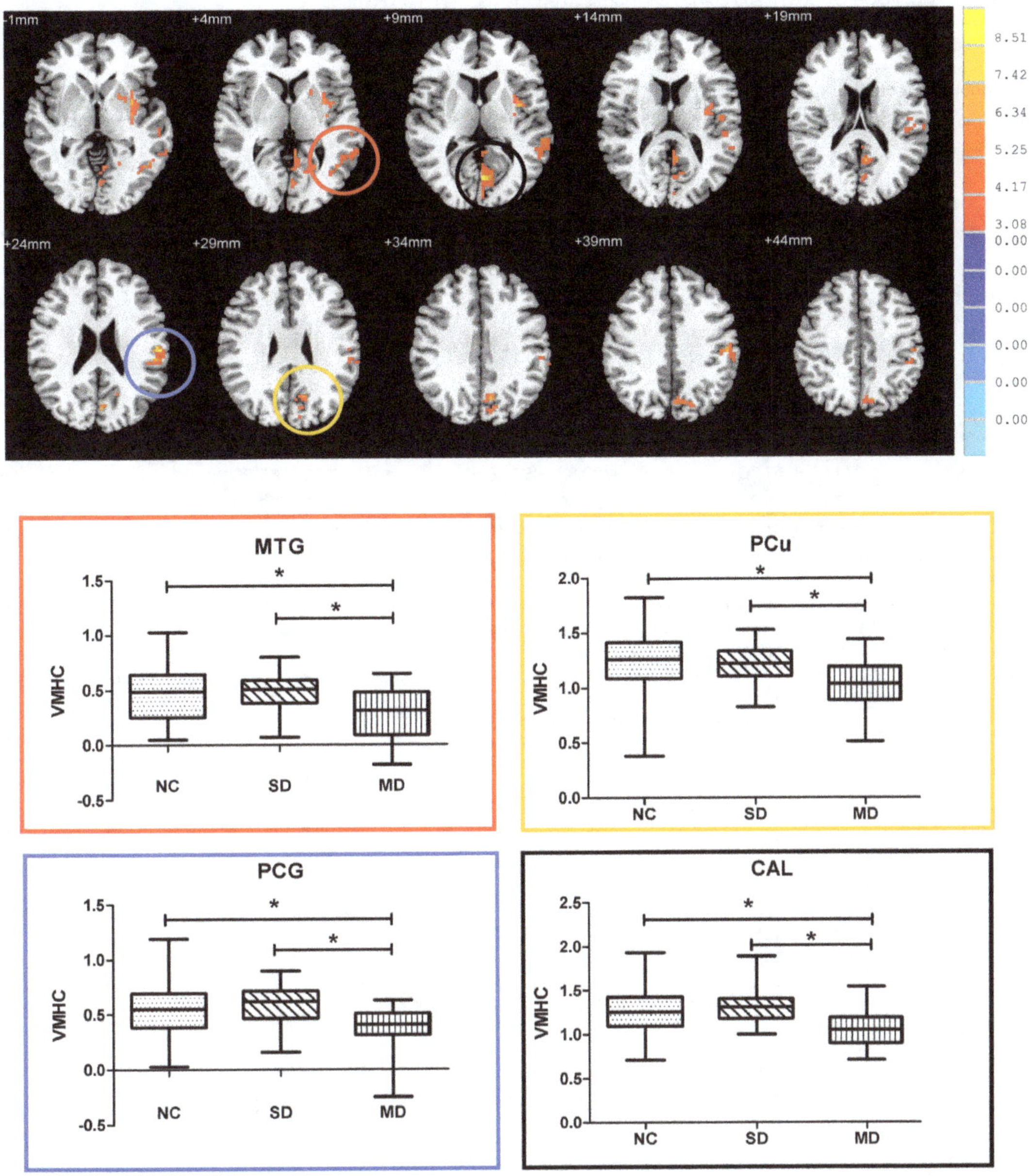

FIGURE 2 | Upper: brain areas with the significant difference of voxel-mirrored homotopic connectivity (VMHC) among normal control (NC), single-domain aMCI (SD-aMCI), and multi-domain aMCI (MD-aMCI), by controlling for age, education level, and gender. The threshold set $p < 0.05$ at height and cluster $p < 0.05$ at the cluster level, GFR corrected. Lower: we performed the *post hoc* analyses within the areas identified by the ANCOVA (corrected by Bonferroni). MD-aMCI patients displayed significantly decreased inter-hemispheric functional connectivity in bilateral middle temporal gyrus, precuneus (PCu), postcentral gyrus (PCG), and CG compared to NC and SD-aMCI patients ($p < 0.005$). But no significant difference existed between SD-aMCI patients and NC. Box graph displays mean VMHC value for middle temporal gyrus (MTG) (red), PCu (yellow), PCG (blue), and CG (black). *$p < 0.005$, Bonferroni corrected.

data. Finally, future studies with larger sample sizes are urgently required.

CONCLUSION

By using multi-modal neuroimaging methods, this study initially explored the mechanism underlying inter-hemispheric connection pattern in SD-aMCI and MD-aMCI patients. Firstly, our results support the notion that aMCI is heterogeneous. Specifically, MD-aMCI displayed more severe inter-hemispheric communication impairment while the SD-aMCI relatively preserved it. Moreover, our results demonstrate that different inter-hemispheric connectivity damage pattern contributes to distinct clinical symptoms in these two aMCI subtypes. Finally, our study shows that inter-hemispheric connectivity may serve as a potential biomarker to monitor disease progression in aMCI patients.

TABLE 3 | Comparisons of VMHC, FDG-PET SUVR, and corpus callosum subregions volume among groups.

	NC	SD-aMCI	MD-aMCI	*F*-value	*P*-value
Bi-hemispheric functional connectivity					
Middle temporal gyrus	0.48 ± 0.26	0.48 ± 0.17	0.28 ± 0.23	8.93	<0.001[bc]
Precuneus	1.23 ± 0.26	1.21 ± 0.17	1.02 ± 0.24	10.92	<0.001[bc]
Postcentral gyrus	0.54 ± 0.22	0.60 ± 0.18	0.37 ± 0.20	12.86	<0.001[bc]
Calcarine gyrus	1.25 ± 0.24	1.33 ± 0.20	1.06 ± 0.20	8.71	<0.001[bc]
Cerebral metabolism					
L Middle temporal gyrus	1.26 ± 0.12	1.14 ± 0.14	1.11 ± 0.16	11.72	<0.001[ab]
R Middle temporal gyrus	1.31 ± 0.14	1.22 ± 0.14	1.20 ± 0.15	6.94	<0.001[ab]
L Precuneus	1.55 ± 0.15	1.50 ± 0.20	1.39 ± 0.13	9.50	<0.001[bc]
L Inferior parietal lobe	1.42 ± 0.13	1.37 ± 0.13	1.26 ± 0.16	13.32	<0.001[bc]
R Inferior parietal lobe	1.48 ± 0.12	1.40 ± 0.16	1.34 ± 0.17	8.05	<0.001[b]
CC subregions volume					
CC-A	771.08 ± 113.95	781.06 ± 183.62	756.16 ± 120.71	0.26	0.77
CC-AP	374.65 ± 62.76	380.88 ± 87.48	343.75 ± 65.36	2.59	0.08
CC-C	367.82 ± 63.85	356.59 ± 77.61	337.59 ± 59.22	1.98	0.14
CC-MP	338.27 ± 61.17	342.06 ± 75.19	303.84 ± 56.78	3.61	0.03*
CC-P	921.65 ± 121.69	921.34 ± 157.03	904.50 ± 149.93	0.17	0.85

*[a]Post hoc paired comparisons showed significant group differences between NC and SD-aMCI, after Bonferroni correction ($p < 0.05$). [b]Post hoc paired comparisons showed significant group differences between NC and MD-aMCI, after Bonferroni correction ($p < 0.05$). [c]Post hoc paired comparisons showed significant group differences between SD-aMCI and MD-aMCI, after Bonferroni correction ($p < 0.05$). *Post hoc paired comparisons showed significant group differences between NC and MD-aMCI as well as SD-aMCI and MD-aMCI, corrected by the LSD ($p < 0.05$). Data are presented as means ± SD. CC, corpus callosum; A, anterior; MA, mid-anterior; C, central; MP, mid-posterior; P, posterior.*

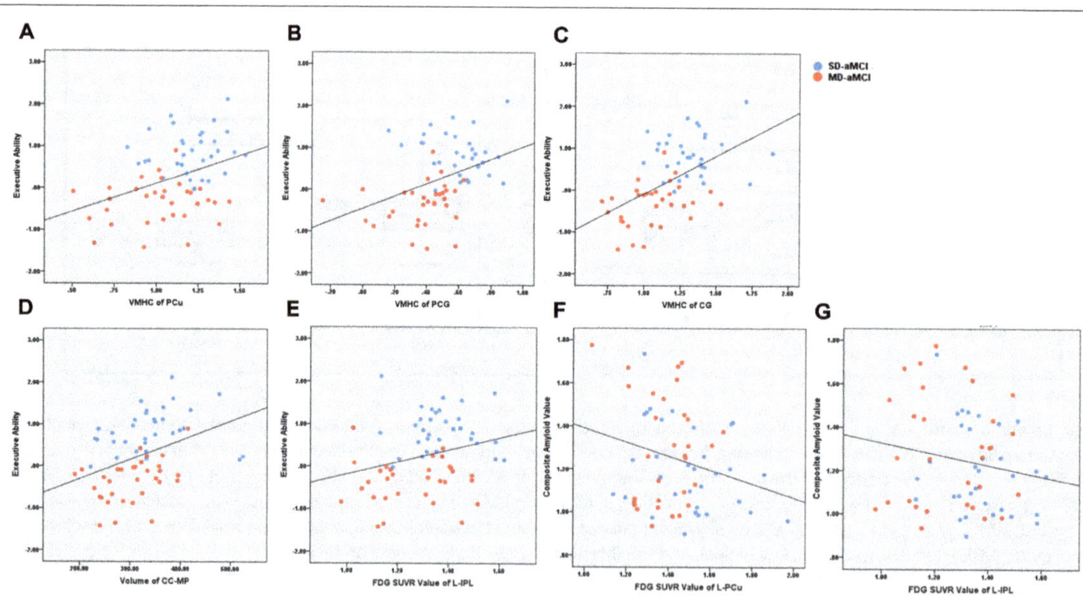

FIGURE 3 | It shows the scatter plot association between neuroimaging indices and behavioral/pathological data across aMCI patients. The blue and red dot represents the SD-aMCI and MD-aMCI patients, respectively. **(A–C)** Regarding functional connectivity, reduced inter-hemispheric functional connectivity in PCu ($r = 0.39$, $p < 0.001$), PCG ($r = 0.40$, $p < 0.001$), and CG ($r = 0.54$, $p < 0.001$) were related to the executive composite score. **(D)** The CC-MP volume was related to the executive composite score ($r = 0.40$, $p < 0.001$). **(E)** The PET-FDG SUVR uptake value in the left IPL ($r = 0.27$, $p < 0.05$) was related to executive function. **(F, G)** The PET-FDG SUVR uptake value in left PCu ($r = -0.25$, $p < 0.05$) and left IPL ($r = -0.25$, $p < 0.05$) were related to composite amyloid value reflecting by ^{18}F-florbetapir PET. Abbreviation: aMCI, amnestic mild cognitive impairment; PCu, precuneus; ITG, inferior temporal gyrus; AG, angular gyrus; CG, calcarine gyrus; PCG, postcentral gyrus; IPL, inferior parietal lobe; CC-MP, mid-posterior corpus callosum.

AUTHOR CONTRIBUTIONS

XL study design, analysis, interpretation, and writing. KL, QZ, and TQ analysis and interpretation of data, study concept, and design. PH, XX, MZ, YJ, JX, and JZ manuscript revision and statistical analysis.

FUNDING

This study was funded by National Key Research and Development Program of China (Grant No. 2016YFC1306600), Zhejiang Provincial Natural Science Foundation of China (Grant Nos. LZ14H180001 and Y16H090026), Young Research Talents Fund, Chinese Medicine Science, and Technology Project of Zhejiang Province (Grant No. 2018ZQ035). The data collection and sharing for this project were funded by the ADNI (National Institutes of Health Grant U01 AG024904) and DOD ADNI (Department of Defense Award No. W81XWH-12-2-0012). ADNI was funded by the NIA, the NIBIB, and through generous contributions from the following: AbbVie, Alzheimer's Association; Alzheimer's Drug Discovery Foundation; Araclon Biotech; Bio Clinica, Inc.; Biogen; Bristol-Myers Squibb Company; Cere Spir, Inc.; Eisai Inc.; Elan Pharmaceuticals, Inc.; Eli Lilly and Company; Euro Immun; F. Hoffmann-La Roche Ltd. and its affiliated company Genentech, Inc.; Fujirebio; GE Healthcare; IXICO Ltd.; Janssen Alzheimer Immunotherapy Research & Development, LLC.; Johnson & Johnson Pharmaceutical Research & Development LLC.; Lumosity; Lundbeck; Merck & Co., Inc.; MesoScale Diagnostics, LLC.; NeuroRx Research; Neurotrack Technologies; Novartis Pharmaceuticals Corporation; Pfizer Inc.; Piramal Imaging; Servier; Takeda Pharmaceutical Company; and Transition Therapeutics. The Canadian Institutes of Health Research is providing funds to support ADNI clinical sites in Canada. Private sector contributions are facilitated by the Foundation for the National Institutes of Health (www.fnih.org). The grantee organization is the Northern California Institute for Research and Education, and the study is coordinated by the AD Cooperative Study at the University of California, San Diego. ADNI data are disseminated by the Laboratory for Neuroimaging at the University of Southern California.

REFERENCES

Agosta, F., Caso, F., Mattavelli, D., Copetti, M., Magnani, G., Canu, E., et al. (2015). Grey matter and white matter MRI markers of cognitive progression in early and late onset variants of Alzheimer's disease (P4.090). *Przegląd Lekarski* 34, 28–66.

Anderson, J. S., Druzgal, T. J., Froehlich, A., DuBray, M. B., Lange, N., Alexander, A. L., et al. (2010). Decreased interhemispheric functional connectivity in autism. *Cereb. Cortex* 21, 1134–1146. doi: 10.1093/cercor/bhq190

Ardekani, B. A., Bachman, A. H., Figarsky, K., and Sidtis, J. J. (2014). Corpus callosum shape changes in early Alzheimer's disease: an MRI study using the OASIS brain database. *Brain Struct. Funct.* 219, 343–352. doi: 10.1007/s00429-013-0503-0

Bittner, T., Zetterberg, H., Teunissen, C. E., Ostlund, R. E., Militello, M., Andreasson, U., et al. (2016). Technical performance of a novel, fully automated electrochemiluminescence immunoassay for the quantitation of β-amyloid (1–42) in human cerebrospinal fluid. *Alzheimer's Dement.* 12, 517–526. doi: 10.1016/j.jalz.2015.09.009

Bouallègue, F. B., Mariano-Goulart, D., and Payoux, P. (2017). Comparison of CSF markers and semi-quantitative amyloid PET in Alzheimer's disease diagnosis and in cognitive impairment prognosis using the ADNI-2 database. *Alzheimer's Res. Ther.* 9:32. doi: 10.1186/s13195-017-0260-z

Bozzali, M., Falini, A., Franceschi, M., Cercignani, M., Zuffi, M., Scotti, G., et al. (2002). White matter damage in Alzheimer's disease assessed in vivo using diffusion tensor magnetic resonance imaging. *J. Neurol. Neurosurg. Psychiatry* 72, 742–746. doi: 10.1136/jnnp.72.6.742

Braak, H., Alafuzoff, I., Arzberger, T., Kretzschmar, H., and Del Tredici, K. (2006). Staging of Alzheimer disease-associated neurofibrillary pathology using paraffin sections and immunocytochemistry. *Acta Neuropathol.* 112, 389–404. doi: 10.1007/s00401-006-0127-z

Brébion, G., Stephan-Otto, C., Huerta-Ramos, E., Ochoa, S., Usall, J., Abellán-Vega, H., et al. (2015). Visual encoding impairment in patients with schizophrenia: contribution of reduced working memory span, decreased processing speed, and affective symptoms. *Neuropsychology* 29, 17–24. doi: 10.1037/neu0000104

Buckner, R. L., Andrewshanna, J. R., and Schacter, D. L. (2008). The brain's default network: anatomy, function, and relevance to disease. *Ann. N. Y. Acad. Sci.* 1124, 1–38. doi: 10.1196/annals.1440.011

Busse, A., Hensel, A., Gühne, U., Angermeyer, M. C., and Riedelheller, S. G. (2006). Mild cognitive impairment: long-term course of four clinical subtypes. *Neurology* 67, 2176–2185. doi: 10.1212/01.wnl.0000249117.23318.e1

Caffarra, P., Ghetti, C., Concari, L., and Venneri, A. (2008). Differential patterns of hypoperfusion in subtypes of mild cognitive impairment. *Open Neuroimage J.* 2, 20–28. doi: 10.2174/1874440000802010020

Cavanna, A. E., and Trimble, M. R. (2006). The precuneus: a review of its functional anatomy and behavioural correlates. *Brain* 129, 564–583. doi: 10.1093/brain/awl004

Cerami, C., Della Rosa, P. A., Magnani, G., Santangelo, R., Marcone, A., Cappa, S. F., et al. (2015). Brain metabolic maps in Mild Cognitive Impairment predict heterogeneity of progression to dementia. *Neuroimage* 7, 187–194. doi: 10.1016/j.nicl.2014.12.004

Chang, Y. L., Chen, T. F., Shih, Y. C., Chiu, M. J., Yan, S. H., and Tseng, W. Y. (2015). Regional cingulum disruption, not gray matter atrophy, detects cognitive changes in amnestic mild cognitive impairment subtypes. *J. Alzheimers Dis.* 44, 125–138.

Chen, A. C., Oathes, D. J., Chang, C., Bradley, T., Zhou, Z.-W., Williams, L. M., et al. (2013). Causal interactions between fronto-parietal central executive and default-mode networks in humans. *Proc. Natl. Acad. Sci. U.S.A.* 110, 19944–19949. doi: 10.1073/pnas.1311772110

Crane, P. K., Carle, A., Gibbons, L. E., Insel, P., Mackin, R. S., Gross, A., et al. (2012). Development and assessment of a composite score for memory in the Alzheimer's Disease Neuroimaging Initiative (ADNI). *Brain Imaging Behav.* 6, 502–516. doi: 10.1007/s11682-012-9186-z

Di Paola, M., Di Iulio, F., Cherubini, A., Blundo, C., Casini, A., Sancesario, G., et al. (2010). When, where, and how the corpus callosum changes in MCI and AD A multimodal MRI study. *Neurology* 74, 1136–1142. doi: 10.1212/WNL.0b013e3181d7d8cb

Farrar, D. C., Mian, A. Z., Budson, A. E., Moss, M. B., Koo, B. B., and Killiany, R. J. (2017). Retained executive abilities in mild cognitive impairment are associated with increased white matter network connectivity. *Eur. Radiol.* 28, 340–347. doi: 10.1007/s00330-017-4951-4

Fischl, B. (2012). FreeSurfer. *Neuroimage* 62, 774–781. doi: 10.1016/j.neuroimage.2012.01.021

Friston, K. J., Williams, S., Howard, R., Frackowiak, R. S., and Turner, R. (1996). Movement-related effects in fMRI time-series. *Magn. Reson. Med.* 35, 346–355. doi: 10.1002/mrm.1910350312

Gibbons, L. E., Carle, A. C., Mackin, R. S., Harvey, D., Mukherjee, S., Insel, P., et al. (2012). A composite score for executive functioning, validated in Alzheimer's Disease Neuroimaging Initiative (ADNI) participants with baseline mild cognitive impairment. *Brain Imaging Behav.* 6, 517–527. doi: 10.1007/s11682-012-9176-1

Golob, E. J., Irimajiri, R., and Starr, A. (2007). Auditory cortical activity in amnestic mild cognitive impairment: relationship to subtype and conversion to dementia. *Brain* 130(Pt 3), 740–752. doi: 10.1093/brain/awl375

Haller, S., Nguyen, D., Rodriguez, C., Emch, J., Gold, G., Bartsch, A., et al. (2010). Individual prediction of cognitive decline in mild cognitive impairment using support vector machine-based analysis of diffusion tensor imaging data. *J. Alzheimers Dis.* 22, 315–327. doi: 10.3233/JAD-2010-100840

Han, Y., Wang, J., Zhao, Z., Min, B., Lu, J., Li, K., et al. (2011). Frequency-dependent changes in the amplitude of low-frequency fluctuations in amnestic mild cognitive impairment: a resting-state fMRI study. *Neuroimage* 55, 287–295. doi: 10.1016/j.neuroimage.2010.11.059

Janke, A. L., Zubicaray, G. D., Rose, S. E., Griffin, M., Chalk, J. B., and Galloway, G. J. (2001). 4D deformation modeling of cortical disease progression in Alzheimer's dementia. *Magn. Reson. Med.* 46, 661–666. doi: 10.1002/mrm.1243

Janowsky, J. S., Kaye, J. A., and Carper, R. A. (1996). Atrophy of the corpus callosum in Alzheimer's disease versus healthy aging. *J. Am. Geriatr. Soc.* 44, 798–803. doi: 10.1111/j.1532-5415.1996.tb03736.x

Jovicich, J., Minati, L., Marizzoni, M., Bartresfaz, D., Nobili, F., Blin, O., et al. (2016). Impairment of resting-state functional connectivity in the default-mode network closely tracks CSF biomarkers in MCI. *Alzheimers Dement.* 12:34. doi: 10.1016/j.jalz.2016.06.049

Landau, S., Harvey, D., Madison, C., Reiman, E., Foster, N., Aisen, P., et al. (2010). Comparing predictors of conversion and decline in mild cognitive impairment. *Neurology* 75, 230–238. doi: 10.1212/WNL.0b013e3181e8e8b8

Landau, S. M., Lu, M., Joshi, A. D., Pontecorvo, M., Mintun, M. A., Trojanowski, J. Q., et al. (2013). Comparing positron emission tomography imaging and cerebrospinal fluid measurements of β-amyloid. *Ann. Neurol.* 74, 826–836. doi: 10.1002/ana.23908

Li, H., Liang, Y., Chen, K., Li, X., Shu, N., Zhang, Z., et al. (2013). Different patterns of white matter disruption among amnestic mild cognitive impairment subtypes: relationship with neuropsychological performance. *J. Alzheimers Dis.* 36, 365–376. doi: 10.3233/JAD-122023

Li, X., Cao, M., Zhang, J., Chen, K., Chen, Y., Ma, C., et al. (2014). Structural and functional brain changes in the default mode network in subtypes of amnestic mild cognitive impairment. *J. Geriatr. Psychiatry Neurol.* 27, 188–198. doi: 10.1177/0891988714524629

Liu, Z., Zhang, Y., Yan, H., Bai, L., Dai, R., Wei, W., et al. (2012). Altered topological patterns of brain networks in mild cognitive impairment and Alzheimer's disease: a resting-state fMRI study. *Psychiatry Res. Neuroimage* 202, 118–125. doi: 10.1016/j.pscychresns.2012.03.002

Lou, W., Shi, L., Wong, A., Chu, W. C. W., Mok, V., and Wang, D. (2016). Changes of cerebral perfusion and functional brain network organization in patients with mild cognitive impairment. *J. Alzheimer's Dis.* 54, 397–409. doi: 10.3233/JAD-160201

Luo, X., Jiaerken, Y., Huang, P., Xu, X. J., Qiu, T., Jia, Y., et al. (2018a). Alteration of regional homogeneity and white matter hyperintensities in amnestic mild cognitive impairment subtypes are related to cognition and CSF biomarkers. *Brain Imaging Behav.* 12, 188–200. doi: 10.1007/s11682-017-9680-4

Luo, X., Jiaerken, Y., Yu, X., Huang, P., Qiu, T., Jia, Y., et al. (2017a). Affect of APOE on information processing speed in non-demented elderly population: a preliminary structural MRI study. *Brain Imaging Behav.* 11, 977–985. doi: 10.1007/s11682-016-9571-0

Luo, X., Jiaerken, Y., Yu, X., Huang, P., Qiu, T., Jia, Y., et al. (2017b). Associations between APOE genotype and cerebral small-vessel disease: a longitudinal study. *Oncotarget* 8, 44477–44489. doi: 10.18632/oncotarget.17724

Luo, X., Li, K., Jia, Y., Zeng, Q., Jiaerken, Y., Qiu, T., et al. (2018b). Abnormal of inter-hemispheric functional connectivity in elderly subjects with overweight/obesity. *Obes. Res. Clin. Pract.* doi: 10.1016/j.orcp.2018.01.003 [Epub ahead of print].

Luo, X., Qiu, T., Xu, X., Huang, P., Gu, Q., Shen, Z., et al. (2016). Decreased inter-hemispheric functional connectivity in cognitively intact elderly APOE ?4 carriers: a preliminary study. *J. Alzheime's Dis.* 50, 1137–1148. doi: 10.3233/JAD-150989

Munoz-Lopez, M., Insausti, R., Mohedano-Moriano, A., Mishkin, M., and Saunders, R. (2015). Anatomical pathways for auditory memory II: information from rostral superior temporal gyrus to dorsolateral temporal pole and medial temporal cortex. *Front. Neurosci.* 9:158. doi: 10.3389/fnins.2015.00158

Palmqvist, S., Schöll, M., Strandberg, O., Mattsson, N., Stomrud, E., Zetterberg, H., et al. (2017). Earliest accumulation of β-amyloid occurs within the default-mode network and concurrently affects brain connectivity. *Nat. Commun.* 8:1214. doi: 10.1038/s41467-017-01150-x

Palop, J. J., and Mucke, L. (2010). Amyloid-β–induced neuronal dysfunction in Alzheimer's disease: from synapses toward neural networks. *Nat. Neurosci.* 13, 812–818. doi: 10.1038/nn.2583

Petersen, R. C., Caracciolo, B., Brayne, C., Gauthier, S., Jelic, V., and Fratiglioni, L. (2014). Mild cognitive impairment: a concept in evolution. *J. Intern. Med.* 275, 214–228. doi: 10.1111/joim.12190

Qiu, Y., Liu, S., Hilal, S., Loke, Y. M., Ikram, M. K., Xu, X., et al. (2016). Inter-hemispheric functional dysconnectivity mediates the association of corpus callosum degeneration with memory impairment in AD and amnestic MCI. *Sci. Rep.* 6:32573. doi: 10.1038/srep32573

Rasero, J., Amoroso, N., La Rocca, M., Tangaro, S., Bellotti, R., Stramaglia, S., et al. (2017). Multivariate regression analysis of structural MRI connectivity matrices in Alzheimer's disease. *PLoS One* 12:e0187281. doi: 10.1371/journal.pone.0187281

Reuter, M., Schmansky, N. J., Rosas, H. D., and Fischl, B. (2012). Within-subject template estimation for unbiased longitudinal image analysis. *Neuroimage* 61, 1402–1418. doi: 10.1016/j.neuroimage.2012.02.084

Roland, J. L., Snyder, A. Z., Hacker, C. D., Mitra, A., Shimony, J. S., Limbrick, D. D., et al. (2017). On the role of the corpus callosum in interhemispheric functional connectivity in humans. *Proc. Natl. Acad. Sci. U.S.A.* 114, 13278–13283. doi: 10.1073/pnas.1707050114

Saar-Ashkenazy, R., Veksler, R., Guez, J., Jacob, Y., Shelef, I., Shalev, H., et al. (2016). Breakdown of inter-hemispheric connectivity is associated with posttraumatic symptomatology and memory impairment. *PLoS One* 11:e0144766. doi: 10.1371/journal.pone.0144766

Salvador, R., Martínez, A., Pomarol-Clotet, E., Gomar, J., Vila, F., Sarró, S., et al. (2008). A simple view of the brain through a frequency-specific functional connectivity measure. *Neuroimage* 39, 279–289. doi: 10.1016/j.neuroimage.2007.08.018

Seo, S. W., Im, K., Lee, J. M., Kim, Y. H., Kim, S. T., Kim, S. Y., et al. (2007). Cortical thickness in single- versus multiple-domain amnestic mild cognitive impairment. *Neuroimage* 36, 289–297. doi: 10.1016/j.neuroimage.2007.02.042

Shu, N., Liang, Y., Li, H., Zhang, J., Li, X., Wang, L., et al. (2012). Disrupted topological organization in white matter structural networks in amnestic mild cognitive impairment: relationship to subtype. *Radiology* 265, 518–527. doi: 10.1148/radiol.12112361

Sridharan, D., Levitin, D. J., and Menon, V. (2008). A critical role for the right fronto-insular cortex in switching between central-executive and default-mode networks. *Proc. Natl. Acad. Sci. U.S.A.* 105, 12569–12574. doi: 10.1073/pnas.0800005105

Stark, D. E., Margulies, D. S., Shehzad, Z. E., Reiss, P., Kelly, A. M., Uddin, L. Q., et al. (2008). Regional variation in interhemispheric coordination of intrinsic hemodynamic fluctuations. *J. Neurosci.* 28, 13754–13764. doi: 10.1523/JNEUROSCI.4544-08.2008

Sullivan, M. O., Jones, D. K., Summers, P. E., Morris, R. G., Williams, S. C. R., and Markus, H. S. (2001). Evidence for cortical "disconnection" as a mechanism of age-related cognitive decline. *Neurology* 57, 632–638. doi: 10.1212/WNL.57.4.632

Thorpe, S., Fize, D., and Marlot, C. (1996). Speed of processing in the human visual system. *Nature* 381, 520–522. doi: 10.1038/381520a0

Tönnies, E., and Trushina, E. (2017). Oxidative stress, synaptic dysfunction, and Alzheimer's disease. *J. Alzheimer's Dis.* 57, 1105–1121. doi: 10.3233/JAD-161088

Tucholka, A., Grau-Rivera, O., Falcon, C., Rami, L., Sánchez-Valle, R., Lladó, A., et al. (2018). Structural connectivity alterations along the Alzheimer's Disease continuum: reproducibility across two independent samples and correlation with cerebrospinal fluid Amyloid-β and Tau. *J. Alzheimer's Dis.* 61, 1575–1587. doi: 10.3233/JAD-170553

van der Knaap, L. J., and van der Ham, I. J. (2011). How does the corpus callosum mediate interhemispheric transfer? A review. *Behav. Brain Res.* 223, 211–221. doi: 10.1016/j.bbr.2011.04.018

Wang, P. N., Chou, K. H., Chang, N. J., Lin, K. N., Chen, W. T., Lan, G. Y., et al. (2014). Callosal degeneration topographically correlated with cognitive function in amnestic mild cognitive impairment and Alzheimer's disease dementia. *Hum. Brain Mapp.* 35, 1529–1543. doi: 10.1002/hbm.22271

Wang, Z., Wang, J., Zhang, H., Mchugh, R., Sun, X., Li, K., et al. (2015). Interhemispheric functional and structural disconnection in Alzheimer's disease: a combined resting-state fMRI and DTI study. *PLoS One* 10:e0126310. doi: 10.1371/journal.pone.0126310

Ward, A. M., Schultz, A. P., Huijbers, W., Dijk, K. R., Hedden, T., and Sperling, R. A. (2014). The parahippocampal gyrus links the default-mode cortical network with the medial temporal lobe memory system. *Hum. Brain Mapp.* 35, 1061–1073. doi: 10.1002/hbm.22234

White, T., Magnotta, V. A., Bockholt, H. J., Williams, S., Wallace, S., Ehrlich, S., et al. (2009). Global white matter abnormalities in schizophrenia: a multisite diffusion tensor imaging study. *Schizophr. Bull.* 37, 222–232. doi: 10.1093/schbul/sbp088

Whitwell, J. L., Petersen, R. C., Negash, S., Weigand, S. D., Kantarci, K., Ivnik, R. J., et al. (2007). Patterns of atrophy differ among specific subtypes of mild cognitive impairment. *Arch. Neurol.* 64, 1130–1138. doi: 10.1001/archneur.64.8.1130

Winblad, B., Palmer, K., Kivipelto, M., Jelic, V., Fratiglioni, L., Wahlund, L. O., et al. (2004). Mild cognitive impairment beyond controversies, towards a consensus: report of the international working group on mild cognitive impairment. *J. Intern. Med.* 256, 240–246. doi: 10.1111/j.1365-2796.2004.01380.x

Zhang, H., Sachdev, P. S., Wen, W., Kochan, N. A., Crawford, J. D., Brodaty, H., et al. (2012). Gray matter atrophy patterns of mild cognitive impairment subtypes. *J. Neurol. Sci.* 315, 26–32. doi: 10.1016/j.jns.2011.12.011

Zuo, X.-N., Kelly, C., Di Martino, A., Mennes, M., Margulies, D. S., Bangaru, S., et al. (2010). Growing together and growing apart: regional and sex differences in the lifespan developmental trajectories of functional homotopy. *J. Neurosci.* 30, 15034–15043. doi: 10.1523/JNEUROSCI.2612-10.2010

11

Investigation of Gal-3 Expression Pattern in Serum and Cerebrospinal Fluid of Patients Suffering from Neurodegenerative Disorders

Ghulam M. Ashraf[1] and Saleh S. Baeesa[2]*

[1] King Fahd Medical Research Center, King Abdulaziz University, Jeddah, Saudi Arabia, [2] Division of Neurosurgery, College of Medicine, King Abdulaziz University, Jeddah, Saudi Arabia

***Correspondence:**
Ghulam M. Ashraf
ashraf.gm@gmail.com;
gashraf@kau.edu.sa

We performed this study to investigate the possibility of a definitive pattern of Galectin-3 (Gal-3) expression in the cerebrospinal fluid (CSF) and serum of Alzheimer's disease (AD) and Amyotrophic Lateral Sclerosis (ALS) patients. In our study, we collected the CSF and serum samples of 31 AD patients, 19 ALS patients and 50 normal healthy subjects (controls). Quantitative ELISA measured Gal-3 concentrations in CSF and serum samples. A comparative analysis was performed to analyze and understand the Gal-3 expression pattern. A number of neuropsychological assessments and statistical analyses were carried out to validate our findings. Recent researches have established the role of galectins in various neurodegenerative disorders (NDDs), but a definitive pattern of galectin expression is still elusive. A significant difference was observed in serum and CSF Gal-3 concentrations between AD patients and healthy controls. The difference in serum and CSF Gal-3 concentrations between ALS patients vs. controls was lesser as compared to AD patients vs. controls. The difference in serum and CSF Gal-3 concentrations of AD vs. ALS patients was not significant. The MMSE score and serum and CSF Gal-3 concentrations in AD and ALS patients, and controls exhibited a significant positive correlation. The findings of the present study are expected to provide an insight into the definitive pattern of Gal-3 expression in AD and ALS patients, and might thus establish Gal-3 as a strong biomarker. This in turn will open up new and promising research avenues targeting the expression of galectins to modulate the progression of NDDs, and pave the way for novel therapeutic options.

Keywords: Galectin-3, serum, cerebrospinal fluid, Alzheimer's disease, amyotrophic lateral sclerosis

INTRODUCTION

Galectins are mammalian class of an otherwise large family, lectin, and characterized as glycoproteins, which have been reported to be expressed in almost all vital organs and involved in almost all significant biological functions (Hasan et al., 2007; Viguier et al., 2014). Gal-3 has been reported to exhibit an altered pattern of expression in patients suffering from NDDs like AD, ALS,

---

Abbreviations: AD, Alzheimer's disease; AGEs, advanced glycation end products; ALS, amyotrophic lateral sclerosis; ANOVA, analysis of variance; CNS, central nervous system; CSF, cerebrospinal fluid; FOME, Fuld object memory evaluation; LSD, least square difference; MMSE, Mini Mental Status Examination; NDDs, neurodegenerative disorders; PD, Parkinson's disease; ROC, receiver operating characteristic; SE, sensitivity; SKT, short cognitive test; TBI, traumatic brain injury; TMT, trail making test; VaD, vascular dementia.

PD, and VaD. While the exact molecular mechanisms behind the pathogenesis of various NDDs remain elusive, the experimental findings from the samples obtained from the patients continue to generate remarkable inputs related to possible pathogenetic channels of these disorders. Gal-3 is present in intracellular (cytosol and nucleus) as well as extracellular spaces, and has been reported to be expressed by almost all cell types (Hasan et al., 2007; Fortuna-Costa et al., 2014). Gal-3 being a multifunctional protein has been reported to be involved in plethora of physiological functions like immune activation, apoptosis, angiogenesis and fibrosis, which in turn have been intricately associated with the development and progression of various NDDs (Ashraf et al., 2010b, 2011; Radosavljevic et al., 2012; Tam and Pasternak, 2012). Gal-3 has also been reported to inhibit the peripheral nerve generation post axotomy (Narciso et al., 2009; DeFrancesco-Lisowitz et al., 2015), act as cell surface receptor for AGEs (Yamamoto and Yamamoto, 2012; Chen H. et al., 2017), and exacerbate the CNS damage in experimental autoimmune encephalomyelitis (EAE) (Jiang et al., 2009; de Oliveira et al., 2015). Microglial Gal-3 has significant role in neuroinflammation process in chronic ALS and TBI (Lerman et al., 2012; Boza-Serrano et al., 2014; Yip et al., 2017). A detrimental role of Gal-3 has been established in inflammation associated with CNS related prion infections (Mok et al., 2007). Gal-3 elevation induced by microglia during the progression of Lewy body dementia and ALS can act as effective indicator of neurodegenerative immune response (Zhou et al., 2010; Surendranathan et al., 2015; Garden and Campbell, 2016). Moreover, onset of remyelination has been favored by microglial Gal-3, either by directly effecting the differentiation of oligodendrocytes or through M2 cell polarization (Cherry et al., 2014; Franco et al., 2015; Rinaldi et al., 2016). Elevated levels of Gal-3 have been observed in the CSF of patients with TBI, ALS and newborn infants after birth asphyxia (Wuolikainen et al., 2011; Sävman et al., 2013; Yip et al., 2017). Gal-3 deregulates hippocampus-dependent memory formation via intracellular as well as extracellular mechanisms (Chen Y.C. et al., 2017). Proteomics approaches has established Gal-3 as a candidate biomarker for ALS (Zhou et al., 2010). Gal-3 has also been reported to be involved in AD neuropathogenesis, and could be a potential biomarker for AD (Wang et al., 2015). Moreover, Gal-3 has been identified in central as well as peripheral nervous system in Schwann cells, endothelial cells, microglia/macrophages, and astrocytes; and the activation of endothelial cells and microglia has been intricately associated with AD pathogenesis (Zlokovic, 2008; Ottum et al., 2015). These studies proclaim elevated Gal-3 expression pattern in AD and ALS patients.

The idea of the proposed research study cropped from the above-mentioned reports suggesting altered expression level of Gal-3 in various NDDs. The detrimental role of Gal-3 in diseases like ALS and AD suggest that lysosomal dysfunctions combined with reduced autophagy can further stimulate neurodegeneration. Elevated levels of Gal-3 in serum and CSF might induce enhanced inflammation, apoptosis and neurodegeneration. There are few individual studies on either serum or CSF, which suggest Gal-3 as possible biomarker of NDDs. The findings of the present study suggesting a definitive Gal-3 expression pattern in serum as well as CSF samples of AD and ALS patients will firmly affirm the role of Gal-3 as potential biomarker for these diseases.

MATERIALS AND METHODS

Ethics Statement

This study was carried out in accordance with the recommendations of National Institute of Neurological and Communicative Disorders and Stroke AD and Related Disorders Association and International Classification of Diseases, Tenth Revision, Diagnostic and Statistical Manual of Mental Disorders (Third Edition) (McKhann et al., 1984). The KAUH (King Abdulaziz University Hospital) ethical committee approved the protocol. All subjects gave written informed consent in accordance with the Declaration of Helsinki.

Patients and Neuropsychological Assessment

The AD (31) and ALS (19) patients as well as healthy individuals (50) serving as controls were recruited from Division of Neurosurgery, College of Medicine, King Abdulaziz University, Jeddah, Saudi Arabia under the careful supervision of Prof. Saleh Baeesa. Each participant was requested to provide written informed consent. The clinical severity of cognitive status was assessed by the standard MMSE (Mini Mental Status Examination) (Folstein et al., 1975). All the neuropsychological assessments were carried out by trained MD (Neurosurgery) students under the supervision of Prof. Saleh Baeesa, and included tests like SKT (Lehfeld and Erzigkeit, 1997; Flaks et al., 2006), TMT (Tombaugh, 2004), and FOME (Fuld, 1980). The cut off scores of all neuropsychological tests were adjusted for educational level and age. The participants were assessed with 21-item Hamilton depressive scale and euthymia was defined as a score of less than 8 (Hamilton, 1960). To exclude metabolic and vascular etiologies, magnetic resonance imaging (MRI) studies and blood tests (blood chemistry, blood lipid profile, complete blood count, folic acid, thyroid function, vitamin B12 dosage and syphilis test) were carried out. A consensus was developed before the clinical diagnoses by taking into account all the laboratory and clinical informations.

Sample Collection

CSF as well as serum samples were collected from 31 patients with AD and 19 patients with ALS. The collected samples were frozen at −80°C until assayed. Samples were also collected from 50 healthy elderly individuals, which served as controls. For CSF sampling, lumbar puncture (LB) using 20G spinal needle was performed using a 20 Gauge, 3.5 inch Quincke point spinal needle (Becton, Dickinson and Company) under local anesthesia in recumbent position at the L3/L4 spine interspace or below of each subject. Every CSF sample collected was approximately 5–8 ml in volume. The CSF samples were collected in Falcon polypropylene tubes (BD Biosciences, Franklin Lakes, NJ, United States). The serum as well as CSF samples were collected early in the morning between 8 and 9 am. The collected CSF samples were centrifuged at 2500 rpm for 5 min to exclude blood contaminants. The samples were then aliquoted in smaller concentrations of 250 μl per aliquot and frozen instantly at −80°C until used for further analyses. While performing the experiments, we freeze thawed only the required number of aliquots as per the requirements of sample concentration needed for the experiment. All the patients and control individuals were fasting since the evening before at the time of LP, and were requested to abstain from smoking. Most of the CSF and serum samples were analyzed within 8 weeks of their collection. This duration was mainly attributed to the fact that before opening an ELISA kit, we made sure that we have collected at least 20 cumulative samples of CSF and serum.

Inclusion/Exclusion Criteria

- All the AD and ALS patients included in this study were diagnosed with the disease since at least 2 years.
- Only those patients and controls were included who gave their consent for the study either by themselves or with the help of their close kin.
- All the subjects under the prescription of NSAIDs or any other drugs interfering with the neuroinflammatory system at the time of sample collection were excluded.
- All the subjects reported for chain smoking were excluded; the information was confirmed by accompanying kin.

Limitations

- An important limitation of our study is relatively small sample size as compared with those used by large-scale multicentric studies.
- We collected the serum and CSF samples in a span of 2 years from almost all the NDDs patients like AD, PD, ALS, MCI, VaD, and MS based on their consent.
- For this study, we only selected the two group of patients with maximum number of samples, and those turned out to be AD (31 patients) and ALS (19 patients). The PD (7 patients), MCI (9 patients), VaD (7 patients) and MS (4 patients) were much lesser in number, and we chose to not include them in this study and wait for more samples to design an effective analyses.

Measurement of Gal-3 Concentrations in Serum, CSF and Control Samples

The concentrations of Gal-3 in serum, CSF and control samples were measured by Abcam's Galectin-3 *in vitro* SimpleStep ELISA^{TM} kit (ab188394). Briefly, 50 μL of all samples was added to respective wells of polystyrene 96-well plates which were pre-coated with antibodies against Gal-3 (i.e., anti-Gal-3-antibodies), followed by the addition of 50 μL antibody cocktail to each and every well. The treated plate was then sealed followed by incubation at RT (room temperature) for 1 h, and finally shaked at 400 rpm on a plate shaker at RT for 2 h. The plate was then washed three times with 350 μL wash buffer, the plate was inverted and blotted against clean paper towels to remove excess liquid. This was followed by the addition of 100 μL TMB substrate to every well, and incubation at 400 rpm on a plate shaker for 10 min in dark. In the last step, each well was added with 100 μL stop solution, and the plate was shaken for 1 min to mix the solutions. The endpoint reading was recorded at 450 nm in ELISA reader (ELx50, Biotek).

Data Interpretation and Statistical Analysis

The differences in cognitive performance, sociodemographic characteristics, and Gal-3 concentrations were analyzed by ANOVA test, with LSD tests for pairwise *post hoc* test between groups. Chi square tests were used to analyze the differences in gender distribution. The differences in scores of baseline and follow up neuropsychological tests for AD and ALS groups were analyzed by LSD test. ROC curves were built to determine the sensitivity (SE), specificity (SP), and area under the curve of Gal-3 biomarker for the discrimination between AD and controls, and ALS and controls.

RESULTS AND DISCUSSION

In relation to the present study, Gal-3 has been reported to be involved in the physiology of almost all types of immune cells (Rabinovich et al., 2012; Chung et al., 2013; Asayama et al., 2017). The information on the Gal-3 expression regulation, however, is quite limited and needs further elucidation. In the present study, we investigated the expression pattern of Gal-3 levels in serum and CSF of AD and ALS patients, and tried to explore the potential associations with the clinical symptoms of these disorders.

The AD patients were on average older than ALS patients were, and thus scored lower on MMSE test. No significant difference was found in years of education and gender distribution between AD, ALS and controls groups. The baseline characteristics and demographic parameters have been summarized in **Table 1**. The results of two consecutive neuropsychological evaluations performed at an interval of at least 1 year have been summarized in **Table 2**. In the ALS group, the scores in all neuropsychological tests remained stable over time, whereas in the AD group, there was a decline in TMT-A, FOME, and SKT scores in the same period.

Based on SE and SP values, ROC curves were drawn to determine the cutoff scores for serum as well as CSF Gal-3 concentrations (**Table 3**). Serum Gal-3 concentrations >8.32 ng/mL (SE = 87% and SP = 74%) and CSF Gal-3 concentrations >7.64 (SE = 83% and SP = 69%) best differentiated the AD, ALS and control groups. We also investigated whether the Gal-3 concentrations might alter the diagnostic accuracy. **Figure 1** represents the distribution of subjects according to the serum and

TABLE 1 | Demographic parameters and baseline characteristics.

Characteristics	AD	ALS	Control	P		
	(*n* = 31)	(*n* = 19)	(*n* = 50)	(AD vs. controls)	(ALS vs. controls)	(AD vs. ALS)
Age (years)	66.8 ± 7.8	64.1 ± 6.9	74.9 ± 7.3	0.06	0.07	0.03
Years of education	9.16 ± 5.67	10.65 ± 5.14	13.34 ± 6.12	0.03	0.04	0.38
Males	18	11	29	0.03	0.04	0.04
Females	13	8	21			
MMSE score	20.7 ± 5.2	23.4 ± 6.2	29.7 ± 0.8	<0.001	<0.001	<0.001
Serum Gal-3 (ng/mL)	11.19 ± 3.67	10.45 ± 3.48	8.76 ± 3.03	0.02	0.02	0.07
CSF Gal-3 (ng/mL)	8.37 ± 2.79	5.19 ± 2.23	7.92 ± 2.56	0.02	0.02	0.07

AD, Alzheimer's disease; ALS, amyotrophic lateral sclerosis; MMSE, Mini-Mental State Examination.

TABLE 2 | Neuropsychological performances of AD and ALS patients.

Test	ALS			AD		
	Baseline	Follow-up	P	Baseline	Follow-up	P
FOME	24.21 ± 6.26	24.19 ± 6.81	0.54	26.45 ± 5.84	21.2 ± 5.94	0.01
MMSE	21.86 ± 4.23	22.02 ± 4.16	0.62	24.84 ± 3.27	23.1 ± 3.96	0.65
TMT-A	68.2 ± 28.34	67.95 ± 24.2	0.12	70.55 ± 38.48	93.21 ± 41.22	0.05
TMT-B	144.28 ± 50.25	146.9 ± 54.23	0.51	159.75 ± 55.34	215 ± 88.65	0.06
SKT	2.95 ± 3.28	3.24 ± 4.19	0.43	5.84 ± 4.55	8.76 ± 5.18	0.02

AD, Alzheimer's disease; ALS, amyotrophic lateral sclerosis; FOME, Fuld object memory evaluation; MMSE, mini-mental state examination; TMT-A, trail making test A; TMT-B, trail making test B; SKT, short cognitive test.

TABLE 3 | Cutoff scores, sensitivity and specificity values of serum and CSF Gal-3 concentrations differentiating the AD patients from controls, ALS patients from controls, and AD patients and ALS patients.

	Cutoff	AD (*n* = 31) vs. controls (*n* = 50)		ALS (*n* = 19) vs. controls (*n* = 50)		AD (*n* = 31) vs. ALS (*n* = 19)	
		Sensitivity (%)	Specificity (%)	Sensitivity (%)	Specificity (%)	Sensitivity (%)	Specificity (%)
Serum Gal-3 (ng/mL)	>8.32	87	74	82	71	88	76
CSF Gal-3 (ng/mL)	>7.64	83	69	78	65	85	73

CSF Gal-3 concentrations in AD, ALS and control groups. Our findings suggested that the AD patients had a distribution almost similar those of ALS patients.

In order to incorporate the difference in age as a factor between AD and ALS patients, and controls; age was used as ANOVA covariate. Visible differences were observed in serum Gal-3 concentrations between the three different groups (AD, ALS, and healthy controls) (P = 0.005). Remarkable difference in the serum Gal-3 concentrations was observed between AD and ALS patients during the LSD test. **Figure 2** depicts that the difference in the serum Gal-3 concentrations between AD patients and healthy controls was significant [AD vs. controls (mean ± SD) 11.19 ± 3.67 vs. 8.76 ± 3.03 ng/mL; P = 0.02]. Similarly, **Figure 3** depicts that the difference in serum Gal-3 concentrations between ALS patients and controls was significant [ALS vs. controls (mean ± SD) 10.45 ± 3.48 vs. 8.76 ± 3.03 ng/mL; P = 0.02], but the difference was lesser as compared to AD vs. controls. **Figure 4** depicts that the difference in serum Gal-3 concentrations of AD and ALS patients was not significant [AD vs. ALS (mean ± SD) 11.19 ± 3.67 vs. 10.45 ± 3.48 ng/mL; P = 0.07]. **Figure 5** depicts that the MMSE score and serum Gal-3 concentrations in AD and ALS patients, and controls exhibited a significant positive correlation (P = 0.306; $P < 0.001$).

In order to incorporate the difference in age as a factor between AD and ALS patients, and controls; age was again used as ANOVA covariate. Visible differences were observed in CSF Gal-3 concentrations between the three different groups (AD, ALS, and healthy controls) (P = 0.005). Remarkable difference in the CSF Gal-3 concentrations was observed between AD and ALS patients during the LSD test. **Figure 6** depicts that the difference in the CSF Gal-3 concentrations between AD patients and healthy controls was significant [AD vs. healthy controls (mean ± SD) 8.37 ± 2.79 vs. 5.19 ± 2.23 ng/mL; P = 0.02]. Similarly, **Figure 7** depicts that the difference in CSF Gal-3 concentrations between ALS patients and controls was significant [ALS vs. healthy controls (mean ± SD) 7.92 ± 2.56 vs. 5.19 ± 2.23 ng/mL; P = 0.02], but the difference was lesser as compared to AD vs. controls. **Figure 8** depicts that the difference in CSF Gal-3 concentrations of AD and ALS patients was not significant

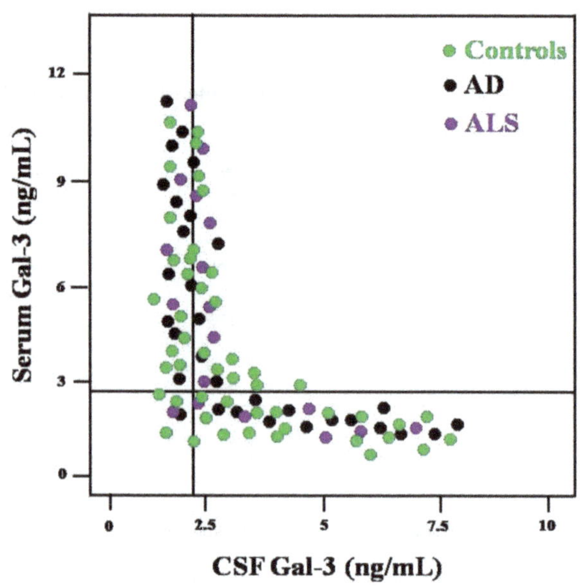

FIGURE 1 | Distribution of AD, ALS and control subjects according to the values of CSF Gal-3 (*x*-axis) and serum Gal-3 (*y*-axis).

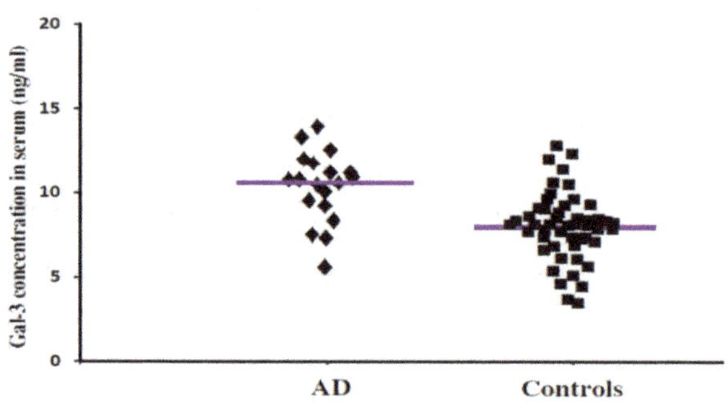

FIGURE 2 | The concentrations of Gal-3 in serum (ng/mL) of AD patients and healthy controls. AD patients showed enhanced Gal-3 concentrations in serum as compared to the healthy controls (AD vs. healthy controls [mean ± SD] 11.19 ± 3.67 vs. 8.76 ± 3.03 ng/mL; $P = 0.022$).

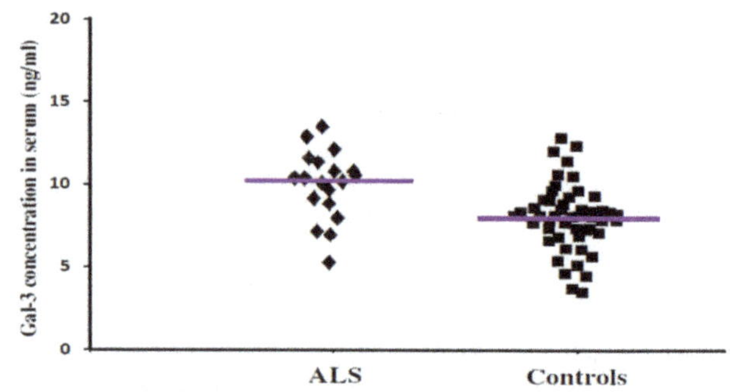

FIGURE 3 | The concentrations of Gal-3 in serum (ng/mL) of ALS patients and healthy controls. ALS patients showed enhanced Gal-3 concentrations in serum as compared to the healthy controls (ALS vs. healthy controls [mean ± SD] 10.45 ± 3.48 vs. 8.76 ± 3.03 ng/mL; $P = 0.019$).

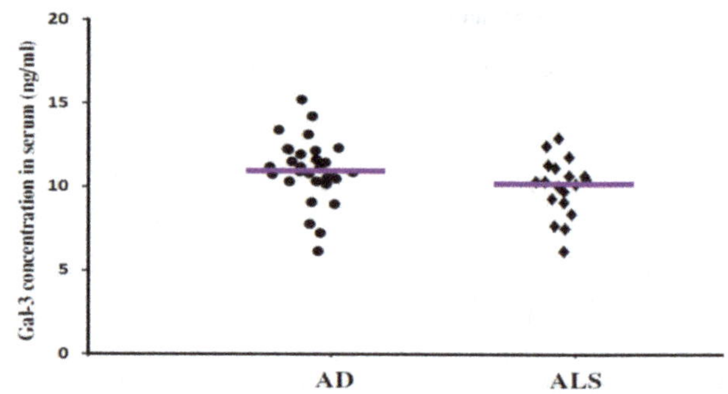

FIGURE 4 | The concentrations of Gal-3 in serum (ng/mL) of AD and ALS. There was no significant difference in the concentrations of Gal-3 in serum of AD and ALS patients (AD vs. ALS [mean ± SD] 11.19 ± 3.67 vs. 10.45 ± 3.48 ng/mL; $P = 0.719$).

[AD vs. ALS (mean ± SD) 8.37 ± 2.79 vs. 7.92 ± 2.56 ng/mL; $P = 0.07$]. **Figure 9** depicts that the MMSE score and CSF Gal-3 concentrations in AD and ALS patients, and controls exhibited a significant positive correlation ($P = 0.291$; $P < 0.001$).

The findings of our study demonstrated that the expression pattern of Gal-3 was significantly enhanced as compared to the controls in serum (**Figures 2, 3**) as well as CSF samples (**Figures 6, 7**) of AD and ALS patients. This enhanced expression of Gal-3 can be attributed to the activation and regulation of immune system in AD and ALS patients (Filer et al., 2009; Bauer et al., 2016; Yip et al., 2017). However, the difference in Gal-3 expression in serum (**Figure 4**) as well as CSF samples (**Figure 8**) between AD and ALS patients was not significant. This finding seems evident as the Gal-3 expression is altered to a considerable degree in AD as well as ALS patients, in reference to the control samples. This finding also suggests that Gal-3 is an aspecific marker that will discriminate every neurodegenerative/neuroinflammatory-related condition as opposed to a control population, and lacks specificity to discriminate between various dementias. A significant positive correlation between serum and CSF Gal-3 levels and MMSE score was observed (**Figures 5, 9** and **Table 1**). The scores of neuropsychological tests remained stable in ALS patients over time, whereas in the AD group, there was a decline in TMT-A, FOME, and SKT scores in the same period (**Table 2**). This finding is well received, as there is hardly any memory loss is ALS patients, whereas there is a rapid loss of memory and cognitive skills in AD patients.

To our knowledge, the findings that serum and CSF Gal-3 levels are elevated in AD as well as ALS patients are one of the first of its kind to be reported from Saudi Arabia. Gal-3 functional roles have been reported in CNS (Bresalier et al., 1997; Reichert and Rotshenker, 1999). Gal-3 inductions are evident in various pathological processes of brain diseases such as prion diseases, ALS, AD, ischemic brain lesions, and PD (Jin et al., 2007; Lerman et al., 2012; Ashraf et al., 2015). The possible physiological role of Gal-3 in AD and

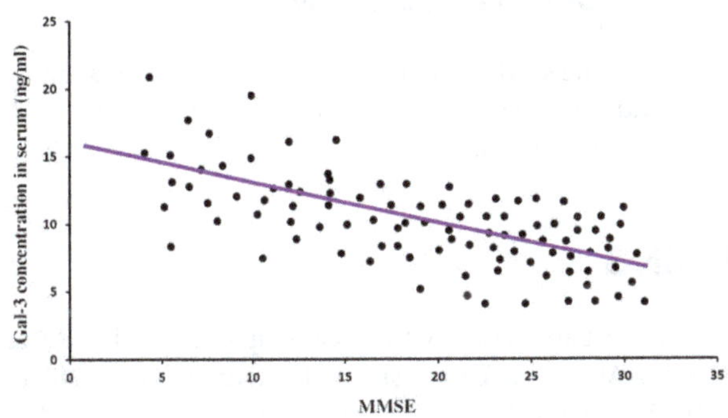

FIGURE 5 | Mini Mental Status Examination (MMSE) and serum Gal-3 concentrations. A significant correlation was observed between MMSE score as a measure of cognitive status and serum Gal-3 levels ($P = 0.306$; $P < 0.001$) in all the patients (AD = 31, ALS = 19, Controls = 50).

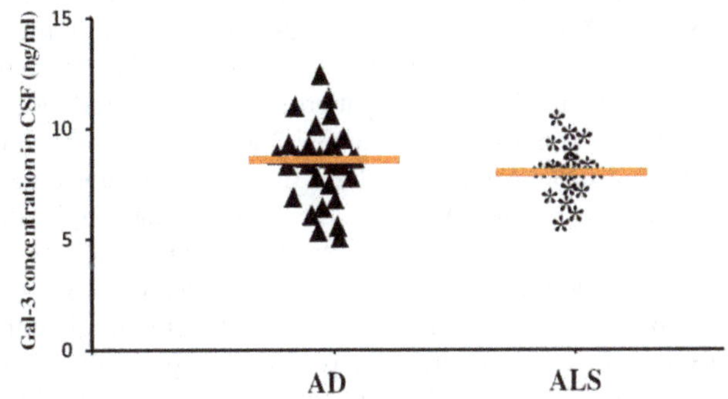

FIGURE 8 | The concentrations of Gal-3 in CSF (ng/mL) of AD and ALS. There was no significant difference in the concentrations of Gal-3 in CSF of AD and ALS patients (AD vs. ALS [mean ± SD] 8.37 ± 2.79 vs. 7.92 ± 2.56 ng/mL; $P = 0.734$).

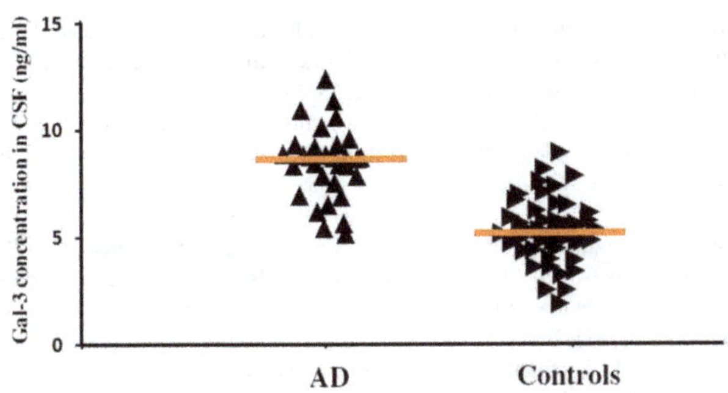

FIGURE 6 | The concentrations of Gal-3 in CSF (ng/mL) of AD patients and healthy controls. AD patients showed enhanced Gal-3 concentrations in CSF as compared to the healthy controls (AD vs. healthy controls [mean ± SD] 8.37 ± 2.79 vs. 5.19 ± 2.23 ng/mL; $P = 0.019$).

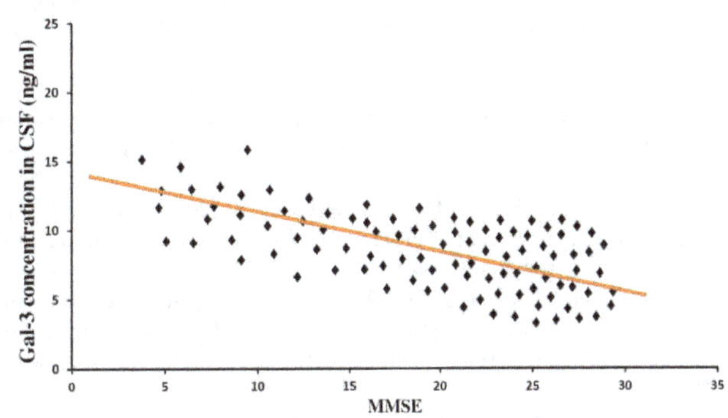

FIGURE 9 | Mini Mental Status Examination and CSF Gal-3 concentrations. A significant correlation was observed between MMSE score as a measure of cognitive status and CSF Gal-3 levels ($P = 0.306$; $P < 0.001$) in all the patients (AD = 31, ALS = 19, Controls = 50).

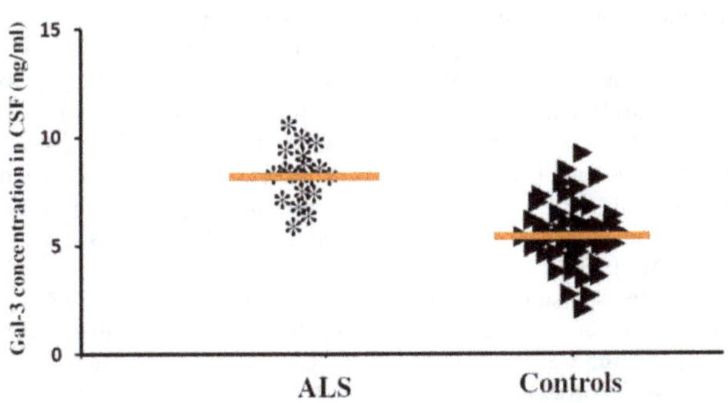

FIGURE 7 | The concentrations of Gal-3 in CSF (ng/mL) of ALS patients and healthy controls. ALS patients showed enhanced Gal-3 concentrations in CSF as compared to the healthy controls (ALS vs. healthy controls [mean ± SD] 7.92 ± 2.56 vs. 5.19 ± 2.23 ng/mL; $P = 0.017$).

ALS can be investigated by exploring its already established biological functions like their role in inflammation and apoptosis (extracellular Gal-3 being proapoptotic, and intracellular Gal-3 being anti-apoptotic) (Yu et al., 2002; Nangia-Makker et al., 2007; Henderson and Sethi, 2009; Ashraf et al., 2010a; Siwicki et al., 2016). The activation of Gal-3 dependent TLR4 induces a sustained microglia activation, which in turn prolongs the inflammatory response in the brain (Burguillos et al., 2015). Gal-3 generates an enhanced inflammatory response by suppressing the production of interleukin 10 (IL-10), which is anti-inflammatory neuroprotective cytokine released by microglia during the progression of AD (Zhou et al., 2010; Di Bona et al., 2012). In a recent study, Gal-3 levels in plasma were reported to be highly enhanced in ALS patients with limb onset of the disease (Yan et al., 2016). This effect was especially more pronounced in female ALS patients and was found to be positively correlated with disease duration. In another study, Gal-3 deletion exacerbated microglial activation and accelerated the disease progression and demise in SOD1(G93A) mouse model of ALS (Lerman et al., 2012). These findings suggest Gal-3 as a crucial factor associated with ALS.

Based on above discussions, the elevated levels of Gal-3 in serum and CSF samples of AD and ALS patients investigated in our study potentially suggests activation of inflammation and apoptosis, and impairment of neurodegenerative events in these patients. Our study successfully demonstrated a definitive association between the serum and CSF levels of Gal-3 and the cognitive status in AD and ALS patients and healthy individuals (controls). The secretory nature of Gal-3 and its detectable level in serum and CSF strongly proclaim this dynamic molecule as potential biomarker for AD and ALS in particular, and other NDDs in general. Our interesting findings suggest the need to explore and investigate the role of other galectins (Gal-1 to Gal-15) in various NDDs. These crucial findings strongly entail the need of future evaluation in prospective patient's cohort, which in turn can put galectins, especially Gal-3, in clinical trials.

AUTHOR CONTRIBUTIONS

GA conceived the study, performed all the experiments, analyzed the data, and compiled the whole manuscript. SB provided the CSF and serum samples.

FUNDING

This work was supported by the Deanship of Scientific Research (DSR), King Abdulaziz University, Jeddah, under Grant No. (141-764-D1435). The authors, therefore, gratefully acknowledge the DSR technical and financial support.

REFERENCES

Asayama, T., Tamura, H., Ishibashi, M., Kuribayashi-Hamada, Y., Onodera-Kondo, A., Okuyama, N., et al. (2017). Functional expression of Tim-3 on blasts and clinical impact of its ligand galectin-9 in myelodysplastic syndromes. *Oncotarget* 8, 88904–88917. doi: 10.18632/oncotarget.21492

Ashraf, G. M., Banu, N., Ahmad, A., Singh, L. P., and Kumar, R. (2011). Purification, characterization, sequencing and biological chemistry of galectin-1 purified from *Capra hircus* (goat) heart. *Protein J.* 30, 39–51. doi: 10.1007/s10930-010-9300-2

Ashraf, G. M., Bilal, N., Suhail, N., Hasan, S., and Banu, N. (2010a). Glycosylation of purified buffalo heart galectin-1 plays crucial role in maintaining its structural and functional integrity. *Biochemistry* 75, 1450–1457.

Ashraf, G. M., Rizvi, S., Naqvi, S., Suhail, N., Bilal, N., Hasan, S., et al. (2010b). Purification, characterization, structural analysis and protein chemistry of a buffalo heart galectin-1. *Amino Acids* 39, 1321–1332. doi: 10.1007/s00726-010-0574-7

Ashraf, G. M., Perveen, A., Tabrez, S., Jabir, N. R., Damanhouri, G. A., Zaidi, S. K., et al. (2015). Altered galectin glycosylation: potential factor for the diagnostics and therapeutics of various cardiovascular and neurological disorders. *Adv. Exp. Med. Biol.* 822, 67–84. doi: 10.1007/978-3-319-08927-0_10

Bauer, P. M., Zalis, M. C., Abdshill, H., Deierborg, T., Johansson, F., and Englund-Johansson, U. (2016). Inflamed in vitro retina: cytotoxic neuroinflammation and galectin-3 expression. *PLoS One* 11:e0161723. doi: 10.1371/journal.pone.0161723

Boza-Serrano, A., Reyes, J. F., Rey, N. L., Leffler, H., Bousset, L., Nilsson, U., et al. (2014). The role of Galectin-3 in α-synuclein-induced microglial activation. *Acta Neuropathol. Commun.* 2:156. doi: 10.1186/s40478-014-0156-0

Bresalier, R. S., Yan, P.-S., Byrd, J. C., Lotan, R., and Raz, A. (1997). Expression of the endogenous galactose-binding protein galectin-3 correlates with the malignant potential of tumors in the central nervous system. *Cancer* 80, 776–787. doi: 10.1002/(SICI)1097-0142(19970815)80:4<776::AID-CNCR17>3.0.CO;2-Q

Burguillos, M. A., Svensson, M., Schulte, T., Boza-Serrano, A., Garcia-Quintanilla, A., Kavanagh, E., et al. (2015). Microglia-secreted galectin-3 acts as a toll-like receptor 4 ligand and contributes to microglial activation. *Cell Rep.* 10, 1626–1638. doi: 10.1016/j.celrep.2015.02.012

Chen, H., Li, Y., Zhu, Y., Wu, L., Meng, J., Lin, N., et al. (2017). Advanced glycation end products promote ChREBP expression and cell proliferation in liver cancer cells by increasing reactive oxygen species. *Medicine* 96:e7456. doi: 10.1097/MD.0000000000007456

Chen, Y. C., Ma, Y. L., Lin, C. H., Cheng, S. J., Hsu, W. L., and Lee, E. H. (2017). Galectin-3 negatively regulates hippocampus-dependent memory formation through inhibition of integrin signaling and galectin-3 phosphorylation. *Front. Mol. Neurosci.* 10:217. doi: 10.3389/fnmol.2017.00217

Cherry, J. D., Olschowka, J. A., and O'Banion, M. K. (2014). Neuroinflammation and M2 microglia: the good, the bad, and the inflamed. *J. Neuroinflamm.* 11:98. doi: 10.1186/1742-2094-11-98

Chung, A. W., Sieling, P. A., Schenk, M., Teles, R. M., Krutzik, S. R., Hsu, D. K., et al. (2013). Galectin-3 regulates the innate immune response of human monocytes. *J. Infect. Dis.* 207, 947–956. doi: 10.1093/infdis/jis920

de Oliveira, F. L., Gatto, M., Bassi, N., Luisetto, R., Ghirardello, A., Punzi, L., et al. (2015). Galectin-3 in autoimmunity and autoimmune diseases. *Exp. Biol. Med.* 240, 1019–1028. doi: 10.1177/1535370215593826

DeFrancesco-Lisowitz, A., Lindborg, J. A., Niemi, J. P., and Zigmond, R. E. (2015). The neuroimmunology of degeneration and regeneration in the peripheral nervous system. *Neuroscience* 302, 174–203. doi: 10.1016/j.neuroscience.2014.09.027

Di Bona, D., Rizzo, C., Bonaventura, G., Candore, G., and Caruso, C. (2012). Association between interleukin-10 polymorphisms and Alzheimer's disease: a systematic review and meta-analysis. *J. Alzheimers Dis.* 29, 751–759. doi: 10.3233/JAD-2012-111838

Filer, A., Bik, M., Parsonage, G. N., Fitton, J., Trebilcock, E., Howlett, K., et al. (2009). Galectin 3 induces a distinctive pattern of cytokine and chemokine production in rheumatoid synovial fibroblasts via selective signaling pathways. *Arthritis Rheum.* 60, 1604–1614. doi: 10.1002/art.24574

Flaks, M. K., Yassuda, M. S., Regina, A. C., Cid, C. G., Camargo, C. H., Gattaz, W. F., et al. (2006). The short cognitive performance test (SKT): a preliminary study of its psychometric properties in Brazil. *Int. Psychogeriatr.* 18, 121–133. doi: 10.1017/S1041610205002577

Folstein, M. F., Folstein, S. E., and McHugh, P. R. (1975). Mini-mental state". A practical method for grading the cognitive state of patients for the clinician. *J. Psychiatr. Res.* 12, 189–198. doi: 10.1016/0022-3956(75)90026-6

Fortuna-Costa, A., Gomes, A. M., Kozlowski, E. O., Stelling, M. P., and Pavão, M. S. G. (2014). Extracellular galectin-3 in tumor progression and metastasis. *Front. Oncol.* 4:138. doi: 10.3389/fonc.2014.00138

Franco, P. G., Pasquini, L. A., Pérez, M. J., Rosato-Siri, M. V., Silvestroff, L., and Pasquini, J. M. (2015). Paving the way for adequate myelination: the contribution of galectin-3, transferrin and iron. *FEBS Lett.* 589, 3388–3395. doi: 10.1016/j.febslet.2015.08.001

Fuld, P. A. (1980). Guaranteed stimulus-processing in the evaluation of memory and learning. *Cortex* 16, 255–271. doi: 10.1016/S0010-9452(80)80061-X

Garden, G. A., and Campbell, B. M. (2016). Glial biomarkers in human central nervous system disease. *Glia* 64, 1755–1771. doi: 10.1002/glia.22998

Hamilton, M. (1960). A rating scale for depression. *J. Neurol. Neurosurg. Psychiatr.* 23, 56–62. doi: 10.1136/jnnp.23.1.56

Hasan, S. S., Ashraf, G. M., and Banu, N. (2007). Galectins – potential targets for cancer therapy. *Cancer Lett.* 253, 25–33. doi: 10.1016/j.canlet.2006.11.030

Henderson, N. C., and Sethi, T. (2009). The regulation of inflammation by galectin-3. *Immunol. Rev.* 230, 160–171. doi: 10.1111/j.1600-065X.2009.00794.x

Jiang, H.-R., Al Rasebi, Z., Mensah-Brown, E., Shahin, A., Xu, D., Goodyear, C. S., et al. (2009). Galectin-3 deficiency reduces the severity of experimental autoimmune encephalomyelitis. *J. Immunol.* 182, 1167–1173. doi: 10.4049/jimmunol.182.2.1167

Jin, J.-K., Na, Y.-J., Song, J.-H., Joo, H.-G., Kim, S., Kim, J.-I., et al. (2007). Galectin-3 expression is correlated with abnormal prion protein accumulation in murine scrapie. *Neurosci. Lett.* 420, 138–143. doi: 10.1016/j.neulet.2007.04.069

Lehfeld, H., and Erzigkeit, H. (1997). The SKT–a short cognitive performance test for assessing deficits of memory and attention. *Int. Psychogeriatr.* 9(Suppl. 1), 115–121. doi: 10.1017/S104161029700478X

Lerman, B. J., Hoffman, E. P., Sutherland, M. L., Bouri, K., Hsu, D. K., Liu, F.-T., et al. (2012). Deletion of galectin-3 exacerbates microglial activation and accelerates disease progression and demise in a SOD1 (G93A) mouse model of amyotrophic lateral sclerosis. *Brain Behav.* 2, 563–575. doi: 10.1002/brb3.75

McKhann, G., Drachman, D., Folstein, M., Katzman, R., Price, D., and Stadlan, E. M. (1984). Clinical diagnosis of Alzheimer's disease: report of the NINCDS-ADRDA Work Group under the auspices of department of health and human services task force on Alzheimer's Disease. *Neurology* 34, 939–944. doi: 10.1212/WNL.34.7.939

Mok, S. W., Riemer, C., Madela, K., Hsu, D. K., Liu, F.-T., Gültner, S., et al. (2007). Role of galectin-3 in prion infections of the CNS. *Biochem. Biophys. Res. Commun.* 359, 672–678. doi: 10.1016/j.bbrc.2007.05.163

Nangia-Makker, P., Nakahara, S., Hogan, V., and Raz, A. (2007). Galectin-3 in apoptosis, a novel therapeutic target. *J. Bioenerg. Biomembr.* 39, 79–84. doi: 10.1007/s10863-006-9063-9

Narciso, M. S., Mietto Bde, S., Marques, S. A., Soares, C. P., Mermelstein Cdos, D. S., El-Cheikh, M. C., et al. (2009). Sciatic nerve regeneration is accelerated in galectin-3 knockout mice. *Exp. Neurol.* 217, 7–15. doi: 10.1016/j.expneurol.2009.01.008

Ottum, P. A., Arellano, G., Reyes, L. I., Iruretagoyena, M., and Naves, R. (2015). Opposing roles of interferon-gamma on cells of the central nervous system in autoimmune neuroinflammation. *Front. Immunol.* 6:539. doi: 10.3389/fimmu.2015.00539

Peruzzotti-Jametti, L., Donegá, M., Giusto, E., Mallucci, G., Marchetti, B., and Pluchino, S. (2014). The role of the immune system in central nervous system plasticity after acute injury. *Neuroscience* 0, 210–221. doi: 10.1016/j.neuroscience.2014.04.036

Rabinovich, G. A., van Kooyk, Y., and Cobb, B. A. (2012). Glycobiology of immune responses. *Ann. N. Y. Acad. Sci.* 1253, 1–15. doi: 10.1111/j.1749-6632.2012.06492.x

Radosavljevic, G., Volarevic, V., Jovanovic, I., Milovanovic, M., Pejnovic, N., Arsenijevic, N., et al. (2012). The roles of Galectin-3 in autoimmunity and tumor progression. *Immunol. Res.* 52, 100–110. doi: 10.1007/s12026-012-8286-6

Reichert, F., and Rotshenker, S. (1999). Galectin-3/MAC-2 in experimental allergic encephalomyelitis. *Exp. Neurol.* 160, 508–514. doi: 10.1006/exnr.1999.7229

Rinaldi, M., Thomas, L., and Pasquini, L. A. (2016). Galectin-1 in myelin repair. *Oncotarget* 7, 81979–81980. doi: 10.18632/oncotarget.13455

Sävman, K., Heyes, M. P., Svedin, P., and Karlsson, A. (2013). Microglia/macrophage-derived inflammatory mediators galectin-3 and quinolinic acid are elevated in cerebrospinal fluid from newborn infants after birth asphyxia. *Transl. Stroke Res.* 4, 228–235. doi: 10.1007/s12975-012-0216-3

Siwicki, M., Engblom, C., and Pittet, M. J. (2016). Gal3 links inflammation and insulin resistance. *Cell Metab.* 24, 655–656. doi: 10.1016/j.cmet.2016.10.014

Surendranathan, A., Rowe, J. B., and O'Brien, J. T. (2015). Neuroinflammation in Lewy body dementia. *Parkinsonism Relat. Disord.* 21, 1398–1406. doi: 10.1016/j.parkreldis.2015.10.009

Tam, J. H., and Pasternak, S. H. (2012). Amyloid and Alzheimer's disease: inside and out. *Can. J. Neurol. Sci.* 39, 286–298. doi: 10.1017/S0317167100013408

Tombaugh, T. N. (2004). Trail making test A and B: normative data stratified by age and education. *Arch. Clin. Neuropsychol.* 19, 203–214. doi: 10.1016/S0887-6177(03)00039-8

Viguier, M., Advedissian, T., Delacour, D., Poirier, F., and Deshayes, F. (2014). Galectins in epithelial functions. *Tissue Barriers* 2:e29103. doi: 10.4161/tisb.29103

Wang, X., Zhang, S., Lin, F., Chu, W., and Yue, S. (2015). Elevated galectin-3 levels in the serum of patients with Alzheimer's Disease. *Am. J. Alzheimers Dis. Other Demen.* 30, 729–732. doi: 10.1177/1533317513495107

Wuolikainen, A., Moritz, T., Marklund, S. L., Antti, H., and Andersen, P. M. (2011). Disease-related changes in the cerebrospinal fluid metabolome in amyotrophic lateral sclerosis detected by GC/TOFMS. *PLoS One* 6:e17947. doi: 10.1371/journal.pone.0017947

Yamamoto, Y., and Yamamoto, H. (2012). Controlling the receptor for advanced glycation end-products to conquer diabetic vascular complications. *J. Diabetes Investig.* 3, 107–114. doi: 10.1111/j.2040-1124.2011.00191.x

Yan, J., Xu, Y., Zhang, L., Zhao, H., Jin, L., Liu, W.-G., et al. (2016). Increased expressions of plasma galectin-3 in patients with amyotrophic lateral sclerosis. *Chin. Med. J.* 129, 2797–2803. doi: 10.4103/0366-6999.194656

Yip, P. K., Carrillo-Jimenez, A., King, P., Vilalta, A., Nomura, K., Chau, C. C., et al. (2017). Galectin-3 released in response to traumatic brain injury acts as an alarmin orchestrating brain immune response and promoting neurodegeneration. *Sci. Rep.* 7:41689. doi: 10.1038/srep41689

Yu, F., Finley, R. L., Raz, A., and Kim, H. R. (2002). Galectin-3 translocates to the perinuclear membranes and inhibits cytochrome c release from the mitochondria. A role for synexin in galectin-3 translocation. *J. Biol. Chem.* 277, 15819–15827. doi: 10.1074/jbc.M200154200

Zhou, J.-Y., Afjehi-Sadat, L., Asress, S., Duong, D. M., Cudkowicz, M., Glass, J. D., et al. (2010). Galectin-3 is a candidate biomarker for ALS: discovery by a proteomics approach. *J. Proteome Res.* 9, 5133–5141. doi: 10.1021/pr100409r

Zlokovic, B. V. (2008). The blood-brain barrier in health and chronic neurodegenerative disorders. *Neuron* 57, 178–201. doi: 10.1016/j.neuron.2008.01.003

12

A Brainnetome Atlas Based Mild Cognitive Impairment Identification Using Hurst Exponent

Zhuqing Long [1†], Bin Jing [2†], Ru Guo [3†], Bo Li [4], Feiyi Cui [1], Tingting Wang [1] and Hongwen Chen [1]*

[1] Medical Apparatus and Equipment Deployment, Nanfang Hospital, Southern Medical University, Guangzhou, China, [2] School of Biomedical Engineering, Capital Medical University, Beijing, China, [3] Department of Tuberculosis, Beijing Chest Hospital Capital Medical University, Beijing, China, [4] Department of Traditional Chinese Medicine, Beijing Chest Hospital, Capital Medical University, Beijing Tuberculosis and Thoracic Tumor Research Institute, Beijing, China

***Correspondence:**
Hongwen Chen
chw47922@126.com

† These authors have contributed equally to this work.

Mild cognitive impairment (MCI), which generally represents the transition state between normal aging and the early changes related to Alzheimer's disease (AD), has drawn increasing attention from neuroscientists due that efficient AD treatments need early initiation ahead of irreversible brain tissue damage. Thus effective MCI identification methods are desperately needed, which may be of great importance for the clinical intervention of AD. In this article, the range scaled analysis, which could effectively detect the temporal complexity of a time series, was utilized to calculate the Hurst exponent (HE) of functional magnetic resonance imaging (fMRI) data at a voxel level from 64 MCI patients and 60 healthy controls (HCs). Then the average HE values of each region of interest (ROI) in brainnetome atlas were extracted and compared between MCI and HC. At last, the abnormal average HE values were adopted as the classification features for a proposed support vector machine (SVM) based identification algorithm, and the classification performance was estimated with leave-one-out cross-validation (LOOCV). Our results indicated 83.1% accuracy, 82.8% sensitivity and 83.3% specificity, and an area under curve of 0.88, suggesting that the HE index could serve as an effective feature for the MCI identification. Furthermore, the abnormal HE brain regions in MCI were predominately involved in left middle frontal gyrus, right hippocampus, bilateral parahippocampal gyrus, bilateral amygdala, left cingulate gyrus, left insular gyrus, left fusiform gyrus, left superior parietal gyrus, left orbital gyrus and left basal ganglia.

Keywords: mild cognitive impairment, range scaled analysis, Hurst exponent, brainnetome atlas, support vector machine

INTRODUCTION

Mild cognitive impairment (MCI), which is characterized by memory complaints, attention deficits and other reduced cognitive functions (Petersen, 2007; Han et al., 2011; Zhang et al., 2012), generally represents the transition state between normal aging and the early changes related to Alzheimer's disease (AD; Desikan et al., 2009; Wang et al., 2015).

Abbreviations: AD, Alzheimer's disease; BOLD, blood oxygen level dependent; fMRI, functional magnetic resonance imaging; HCs, healthy controls; HE, Hurst exponent; LOOCV, leave-one-out cross-validation; MCI, mild cognitive impairment; RBF, radial basis function; ROI, region of interest; rs-fMRI, resting-state functional magnetic resonance imaging; SVM, support vector machine.

Overall, MCI patients progress to AD at a rate of 10%–15% per year (Khazaee et al., 2016), and roughly half of them will evolve to AD within 3–5 years (Long et al., 2016). Recently, a great deal of attention from neuroscientists, neurologists and neuroradiologists has been paid to MCI due that efficient AD treatments need early initiation ahead of irreversible brain tissue damages (Davatzikos et al., 2008). Therefore, developing accurate and effective MCI identification methodologies that may be of great importance for clinical interventions of AD are desperately needed.

Functional magnetic resonance imaging (fMRI) has received increasing interests because it could provide a primary method of mechanism detection, diagnostic evaluation or therapeutic monitoring for MCI and AD (Fornito and Bullmore, 2010; Wang et al., 2015). Previous studies demonstrated that the aberrant and spontaneous neuronal activities in MCI or AD could be detected by resting-state fMRI (rs-fMRI; Zhang et al., 2012; Brier et al., 2014), and the abnormal brain regions mainly involved in hippocampus, parahippocampal gyrus, posterior cingulate gyrus and precuneus cortex, etc (Baron et al., 2001; He et al., 2007). In addition, many recent studies employed rs-fMRI data to identify MCI or AD from healthy controls (HCs) by extracting a single type of feature or multi-level characteristics (Chen et al., 2011; Dai et al., 2012; Zhang et al., 2012; Brier et al., 2014; Long et al., 2016), and the recognition accuracies were varied with a wide range, suggesting the MCI or AD discrimination needs to be continued. Generally, an effective rs-fMRI based MCI or AD discrimination method should: (I) exhibit an excellent discrimination accuracy between MCI or AD and HC; (II) specifically quantify fundamental characteristics of Alzheimer's pathology in individuals with MCI or AD.

Prior studies demonstrated that blood oxygen level dependent (BOLD) signals have been shown scale-free dynamics (Ciuciu et al., 2012; Wei et al., 2013), and the power spectrum of fMRI signals can be written as $S(f) \propto 1/|f|^{\beta}$ with $\beta < 1$ (where f represents frequency; Maxim et al., 2005; Gentili et al., 2015), suggesting that the fMRI signals have fractal or fractal-like properties. Hurst Exponent (HE), which has a direct linear relationship with the parameter $\beta = 2HE - 1$, could well display the fractal dynamics of fMRI signals via describing the self-similarity of a time series. In fact, the HE, an index ranging from 0 to 1, could divide the time series into three categories according to its values. A HE bigger than 0.5 indicates a persistent or positively correlated time series, meaning that the time series generally causes changes that fluctuate in the same direction along time. A HE equal to 0.5 stands for a random white noise. A HE smaller than 0.5 implies an anti-correlated or anti-persistent time series. In this case, the dynamics of a time series would keep a reversing pattern in time, and a decrease in the time series generally would be followed an increase and vice versa (Gentili et al., 2015). Recently, HE index has been utilized to measure the changes of BOLD signals related to major depressive disorder, normal and pathological aging, cholinergic modulation, AD, autism disorder and different personality traits (Maxim et al., 2005; Wink et al., 2006; Lai et al., 2010; Lei et al., 2013; Gentili et al., 2015; Jing et al., 2017). However, little information was known about the HE changes in MCI patients, and it still remains unknown whether the HE index could serve as an effective parameter for MCI classification.

In this article, the HE index of fMRI signals were first calculated using range scaled analysis at a voxel level. Then the average HE values of each region of interest (ROI) in brainnetome atlas, a newly structural and functional brain partition scheme, were extracted and compared between MCI and HC groups. At last, the abnormal HE values were adopted as the classification features for a proposed support vector machine (SVM)-based classification method to identify MCI patients from HC.

MATERIALS AND METHODS

Participants

Sixty-nine MCI patients and 63 HC subjects participated in the current study, and none of MCI patients had taken any medications that interfere with cognitive functions. All MCI patients were recruited from the memory outpatient clinic at Nanfang Hospital, and the clinical diagnosis of MCI was made by two experienced neurologists based on the following criteria: (1) memory complaints, confirmed by patient-self or their relatives; (2) normal or near normal performance on cognitive function; (3) normal or near normal activities of daily life; (4) Clinical Dementia Rate equals to 0.5; and (5) absence of dementia according to the DSM-IV (Diagnostic and Statistical Manual of Mental Disorders, 4th edition, revised). The HC participants matched well with MCI patients on gender, age and education level and were collected from local community by print advertisements, and the inclusions for all participants were: (1) no other nervous or psychiatric diseases that can intervene with cognitive functions, such as Parkinson's disease, depressive disorders and encephalitis, etc; (2) no history of stroke or dependence of alcohol; (3) no systemic diseases that cause cognitive impairments; and (4) no medication conditions that can influence cognitive performance. All subjects were undergone several clinical assessments including Clinical Dementia Rate, Mini-Mental State Examination (MMSE) and Auditory Verbal Learning Test (AVLT). This study was approved by the ethics committee of Nanfang Hospital affiliated to Southern Medical University, and the informed written consents from all subjects were obtained in accordance with the Declaration of Helsinki. Five MCI patients and three HC subjects were discarded due to excessive head motion during the scan, and the detailed clinical characteristics of the remaining participants were summarized in **Table 1**.

Data Acquisition

All images were collected on a 3 Tesla Siemens scanner with 8-channel radio frequency coil at Nanfang hospital. Headphones and a foam padding were utilized to reduce the scanner noise and limit the head motion during the scan, and all subjects were instructed to close their eyes, to keep mind relax, to not

TABLE 1 | Participants' demographic and clinical characteristics.

Characteristics	MCI	HC	*P* values
Gender (M/F)	64 (28/36)	60 (26/34)	0.96#
Age (years)	67.14 ± 7.33	65.27 ± 7.30	0.16*
Education (years)	9.73 ± 4.24	10.07 ± 4.27	0.66*
CDR	0.5	0	0*
MMSE	23.16 ± 2.77	27.40 ± 3.15	<0.001*
AVLT-immediate recall	7.99 ± 2.60	12.94 ± 2.94	<0.001*
AVLT-delay recall	3.64 ± 2.89	9.77 ± 2.79	<0.001*
AVLT-recognition	7.11 ± 3.55	11.58 ± 2.23	<0.001*

*Values are mean ± SD unless the SD was not calculated. M, male; F, female. CDR, Clinical Dementia Rating scale; MMSE, Mini-Mental State Examination; AVLT, Auditory Verbal Learning Test. #The P value was obtained by Chi-square test. *The P values were obtained by two-sample two-tailed-t-test.*

fall asleep and to not move their head. Resting-state fMRI were acquired using an echo-planar imaging sequence with the following parameters: repetition time = 2000 ms, echo time = 40 ms, flip angle = 90°, matrix size = 64 × 64, number of slices = 28, field of view = 240 × 240 mm^2, slice thickness = 4 mm, and voxel size = 3.75 × 3.75 × 4 mm^3. Two-hundred and thirty-nine volumes were collected for each subject within 478 s. T1-weighted structural images for all subjects were acquired by using magnetization-prepared rapid gradient echo sequence with the following parameters: repetition time = 1900 ms, echo time = 2.2 ms, inverse time = 900 ms, flip angle = 9°, matrix = 256 × 256, number of slices = 176, slice thickness = 1 mm, and voxel size = 1 × 1 × 1 mm^3.

Data Preprocessing

Data preprocessing for all images were carried out with Statistical Parametric Mapping (SPM8)[1]. The first 10 functional volumes were discarded due to signal equilibrium and participant's adaptation to the scanner environment, and the remaining 229 volumes were corrected for different acquisition time between slices. Then all volumes were realigned to the first volume by using a six-parameters rigid-body spatial transformation to compensate for head movement effects. Eight participants (five MCI patients and three HC subjects) were discarded because of excessive head motion (2 mm and 2°criteria). To improve the spatial normalization accuracy, the realigned images were normalized into the Montreal Neurological Institute space by using the parameters obtained from structural normalization, and all normalized functional images were re-sampled into a voxel size of 3 × 3 × 3 mm^3. Next, all the normalized images were detrended, and the spurious covariates including the six head motion parameters obtained from rigid-body transformation, signals of white matter and ventricular system were regressed. At last, a temporal band-pass filter (0.01–0.10 HZ) was carried out on the time series of each voxel to reduce the effects of low-frequency drifts and high-frequency cardiac and respiratory noise, and the filtered images were smoothed with a 4 mm full width at half maximum Gaussian kernel.

HE Calculation and Feature Selection

The range scaled analysis, which is an effective method to detect the temporal complexity of a time series, was utilized

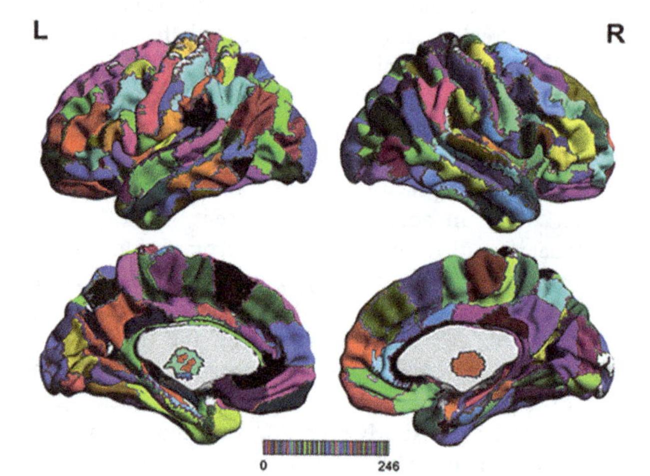

FIGURE 1 | The detailed brainnetome atlas which including 210 cortical sub-regions and 36 subcortical sub-regions.

to calculate the HE index of fMRI signals at a voxel level, and the detailed principle of HE calculation was reported in our previous study (Jing et al., 2017). In addition, the brainnetome atlas (**Figure 1**), which partitions the cerebral cortex into 246 ROIs including 210 cortical sub-regions and 36 subcortical sub-regions (Fan et al., 2016), was used to extract the HE index feature for the SVM-based classification algorithm. In this article, the average HE values of each ROI in brainnetome atlas were extracted as the candidate features. Considering that properly and correctly reducing the number of features could not only improve the classification performance but also speed up the computation (De Martino et al., 2008; Pereira et al., 2009). Thus a Fisher score method and two-sample two-tailed-*t*-test ($P < 0.05$, uncorrected) were utilized to select out the discriminative HE features between MCI patients and HC subjects. The detailed Fisher score criterion for each candidate feature is defined as:

$$FS = \frac{n_1(m_1 - m)^2 + n_2(m_2 - m)^2}{n_1\sigma_1^2 + n_2\sigma_2^2} \quad (1)$$

Here n_1 and n_2 are the number of the samples on each group, m_1 and m_2 are the respective mean value of the feature, m represents the mean value of the feature, σ_1^2 and σ_2^2 represent the

[1]http://www.fil.ion.ucl.ac.uk/spm

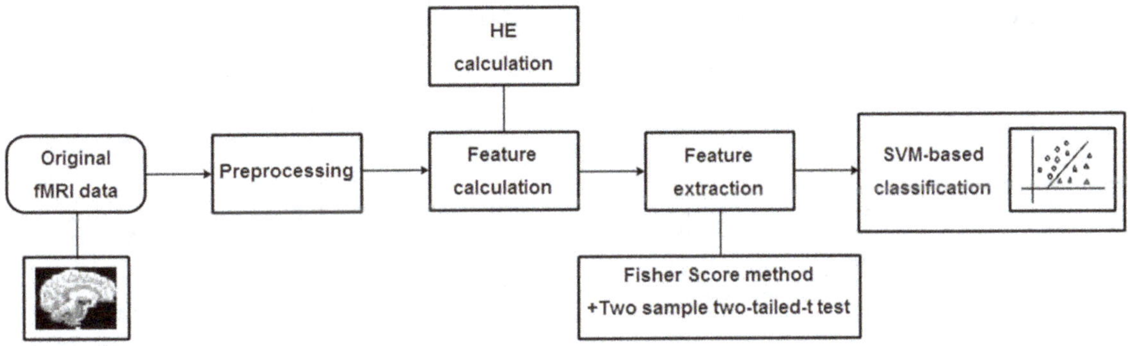

FIGURE 2 | A flowchart of the proposed support vector machine (SVM)-based classification method for mild cognitive impairment (MCI) identification.

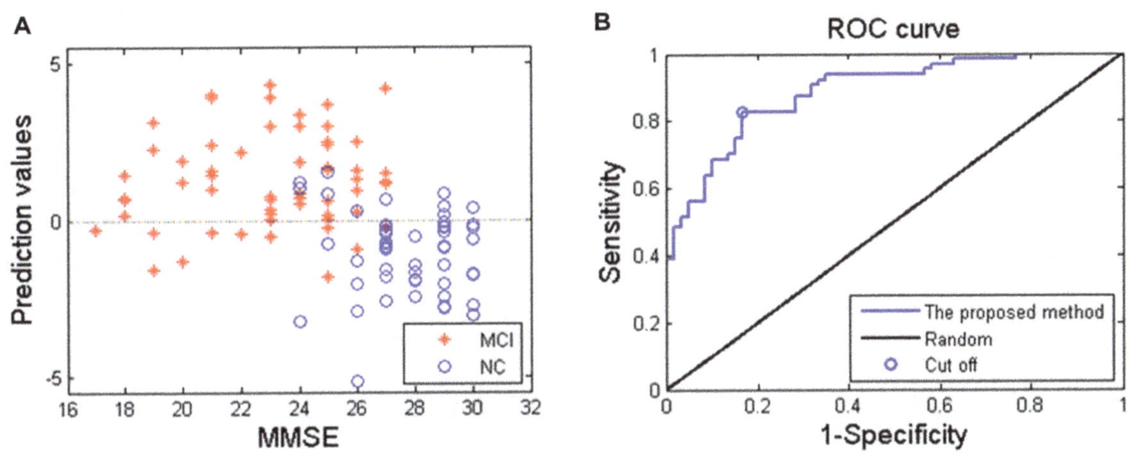

FIGURE 3 | (A) The relationship between the Mini-Mental State Examination (MMSE) score of MCI patients and prediction values; **(B)** receiver operating characteristics curve of the proposed classification method, and the area under curve is 0.88.

variance of the feature on each group. A high Fisher score value indicates a strong discriminative ability of the feature to some degree. At last, it's worth noting that the feature selection was only performed on the training set of per leave-one-out cross-validation (LOOCV) fold, which could reduce the overfitting of the classification algorithm.

SVM-Based Classification Method

The SVM algorithm, which has been widely utilized for its powerful recognition function as well as its simple theory and implementation, was originally proposed for binary classification problems based on statistical learning principles (Beheshti and Demirel, 2016). During the training process, the SVM algorithm seeks the optimal separation hyper-plane in the feature space where the input features were mapped into using a kernel function, and each divided subspace corresponds to one class of training set. In the same way, all the test samples could be labeled depending on which subspace they are mapped into after the training process (Magnin et al., 2009). In this article, the LibSVM toolbox[2] was utilized for SVM implementation.

The radial basis function (RBF) defined as $(X, X_i) \rightarrow K(X, X_i) = e^{\gamma|X-X_i|^2}$ was adopted as the kernel function for the SVM algorithm. To improve classification performance, a grid-search method was utilized to optimize two parameters: the parameter γ representing the width of RBF kernel and the punishment factor C adjusting the importance of error separation. In detail, at each pair of (γ, C), three steps including the above-mentioned feature selection, the training of the SVM-based algorithm and the prediction of the test samples were performed in succession, and the classification performance was estimated with LOOCV. It's worth noting that the feature selection was only carried out on the training set of each LOOCV fold. The whole classification process was repeatedly performed with (γ, C) varying along a grid with $\gamma = 2^{-8}$, $2^{-7.5}$,. . .,2^8 and $C = 2^{-8}$, $2^{-7.5}$,. . .,2^8, which is referred as the grid-search method. Considering that each pair of (γ, C)

[2]http://www.csie.ntu.edu.tw/~cjlin/libsvm

TABLE 2 | The number of features retained in per fold of leave-one-out cross-validation (LOOCV) with brainnetome atlas.

Fold	No. of features	Fold	No. of features	Fold	No. of features	Fold	No. of features
1	16	32	17	63	15	94	15
2	15	33	16	64	16	95	15
3	17	34	16	65	15	96	15
4	17	35	14	66	14	97	15
5	16	36	15	67	16	98	15
6	16	37	14	68	16	99	15
7	16	38	15	69	15	100	16
8	15	39	15	70	16	101	14
9	15	40	16	71	15	102	15
10	15	41	16	72	16	103	16
11	15	42	15	73	14	104	14
12	15	43	14	74	15	105	15
13	14	44	14	75	14	106	14
14	16	45	16	76	16	107	15
15	16	46	16	77	16	108	16
16	15	47	16	78	17	109	15
17	14	48	15	79	16	110	16
18	15	49	14	80	16	111	16
19	15	50	17	81	16	112	15
20	15	51	15	82	16	113	15
21	16	52	14	83	15	114	17
22	15	53	14	84	14	115	15
23	16	54	14	85	16	116	16
24	15	55	14	86	16	117	14
25	17	56	15	87	16	118	14
26	15	57	16	88	14	119	15
27	16	58	16	89	16	120	15
28	16	59	15	90	14	121	16
29	16	60	16	91	16	122	15
30	14	61	16	92	16	123	15
31	14	62	14	93	15	124	14

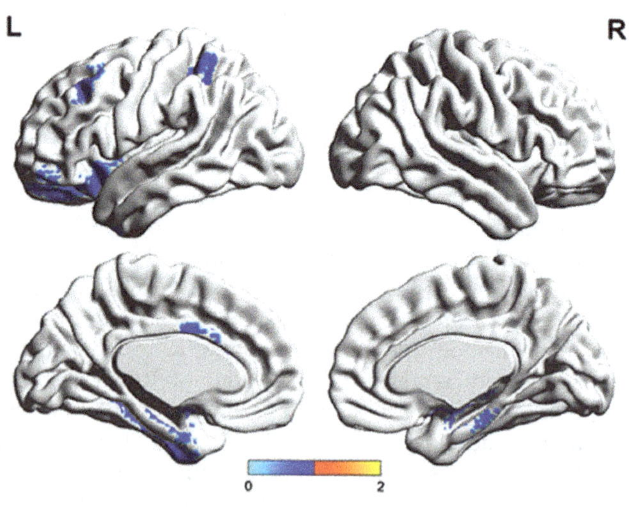

FIGURE 4 | The brain regions with abnormal hurst exponent (HE) values in MCI patients by using brainnetome atlas.

corresponds to an accuracy, the best accuracy rate on the grid of 33 × 33 was acquired as the classification accuracy of the classifier. A flowchart of the detailed classification process was shown in **Figure 2**.

RESULTS

Applying the proposed SVM-based classification method to identify MCI patients from HC subjects, our results indicated 83.1% accuracy, 82.8% sensitivity and 83.3% specificity. Besides, the receiver operating characteristics curve and the relationship between MMSE and prediction values were shown in **Figure 3**, and the area under curve of the classification algorithm is 0.88, indicating a powerful classification performance.

The number of features retained in per fold of LOOCV was shown in **Table 2**. In addition, the abnormal HE brain regions with the retained times of the HE features no less than 118 (124 × 0.95, 124 is the total number of the samples) in the whole LOOCV process were shown in **Figure 4**, and the Fisher score values of these abnormal HE features were displayed in **Figure 5**. Compared to HC subjects, these abnormal HE brain regions in MCI patients were predominately involved in left middle frontal gyrus, right hippocampus, bilateral parahippocampal gyrus, bilateral amygdala, left cingulate gyrus, left insular gyrus, left fusiform gyrus, left superior parietal gyrus, left orbital gyrus and left basal ganglia.

DISCUSSION

This study proposed an effective classification method to identify MCI patients from HC subjects using HE index of rs-fMRI.

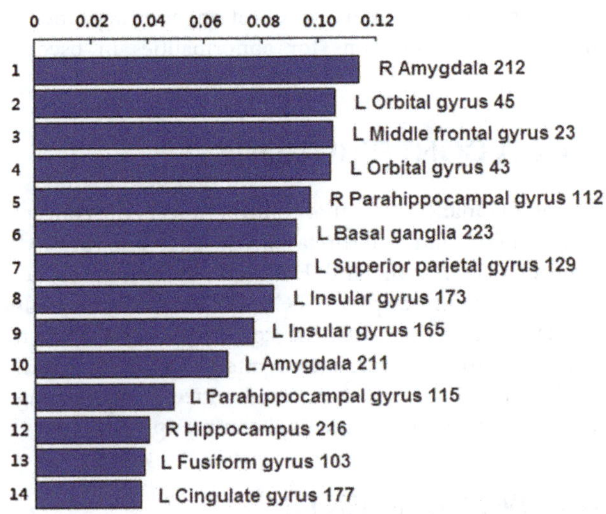

FIGURE 5 | The Fisher score values of these abnormal HE features which were retained no less than 118 times (124 × 0.95, 124 is the total number of the samples) in the whole leave-one-out cross-validation (LOOCV) process.

A promising classification performance was obtained with an accuracy of 83.1% and an area under curve value of 0.88, suggesting that the proposed SVM-based method was effective in identifying MCI from HC subjects, and the calculated HE index could serve as an effective feature for the SVM-based classification algorithm.

To obtain high discrimination accuracy for MCI classification, three steps were taken for the proposed classification method. First, previous studies demonstrated that properly reducing the number of features could not only improve the classification performance but also speed up the computation (Dosenbach et al., 2010; Dai et al., 2012). Thus two-sample two-tailed-*t*-test and Fisher score criteria were both utilized to select out the discriminative HE features in this article, and the classification performance was improved significantly compared to without feature selection. In fact, we firstly tried a total 246 HE features by using the proposed SVM-based algorithm, and the classification accuracy without feature selection was lower than 70%. It needs to note that the feature selection was only performed on the training set, which could reduce the overfitting of the classifier. Second, the RBF kernel function was adopted as the kernel function due that it could deal with the case when the relationship between labels and features is nonlinear (Hsu et al., 2003), which also has an important impact on classification performance. In this article, we also utilized the linear kernel function for MCI classification, and the discrimination rate was 78.2%, which was lower than that with RBF kernel. At last, the grid search method, which has a high learning accuracy and could be implemented with parallel processing (Long et al., 2016), was utilized to optimize the two parameters of SVM, which also improved the classification performance. In addition, to further validate the effectiveness of the proposed MCI classification method, the dataset was randomly split into two subsets including a training subset (42 MCI and 40 HC), a testing subset (22 MCI and 20 HC). The training subset was utilized to train the classification algorithm and optimize the two parameters through an internal cross-validation procedure which averagely divided the training set into two groups to train the algorithm with one group and then predict the other group mutually (Dyrba et al., 2015). Then the final performance of the classification algorithm was estimated with the testing subset. A promising accuracy of 85.71% was obtained, which also indicated that the proposed SVM-based method is effective in identifying MCI patients form HC subjects.

In this article, we found that the abnormal HE brain regions in MCI patients mainly involved in left middle frontal gyrus, right hippocampus, bilateral parahippocampal gyrus, bilateral amygdala, left cingulate gyrus, left insular gyrus, left fusiform gyrus, left superior parietal gyrus, left orbital gyrus and left basal ganglia. Almost all these brain regions were consistent with previous studies that analyzed the structural and functional data of MCI or AD patients with conventional statistical analysis (Hirata et al., 2005; Lerch et al., 2008; Xie et al., 2012). The middle frontal gyrus, hippocampus, parahippocampal gyrus, cingulate gyrus and orbital gyrus belong to the default mode network (Dai et al., 2012; De Vogelaere et al., 2012). Currently, the behavioral correlations of default mode network still remain uncharacterized although some investigators had proposed several potentially inclusive hypotheses that it mediates processes such as reviewing past knowledge and preparing for future actions (Greicius et al., 2004). The abnormal HE values in these brain regions supplementarily supported the abnormalities of default mode network in MCI patients. In addition, the amygdala and insular gyrus were labeled with significant atrophy in MCI patients in previous voxel-based morphometry studies (Hämäläinen et al., 2007), and the fusiform gyrus showed significantly aberrant amplitude of low-frequency fluctuations of BOLD signals in MCI (Wang et al., 2015). Furthermore, the basal ganglia was associated with cognitive functions such as mood swings or disorders (de Oliveira and de Oliveira, 2013). All the above-mentioned evidences suggested that these abnormal brain regions were related to the mechanisms underlying MCI patients.

The HE analysis has already been utilized to describe complex properties of biological signals including electroencephalogram and electrocardiogram (Costa and McCrae, 1992; Ignaccolo et al., 2010). By applying the HE analysis method to BOLD signals, some investigators found that the HE value of fMRI signals in gray matter was higher than in white gray (Maxim et al., 2005), and decreased with cholinergic transmission enhancement and augmented in hippocampus with aging (Wink et al., 2006). Nevertheless, these findings could not conclude that a higher HE value is associated with worse brain functioning. It seems to reflect some inherent patterns of spontaneous discharge and the HE could be modulated by different psychotic or psychological variables (Gentili et al., 2015). In this article, the HE analysis was applied in MCI patients, and some core brain regions were detected with HE abnormalities. It demonstrated that the persistent behavior of brain activities in these abnormal regions were changed, which may provide some information for the mechanisms underlying MCI patients. However, the physiological significance of HE index still remains unknown currently, and future studies should pay more attention to confirm it through the multi-modal imaging validation in animal models.

Several issues need to be addressed in this article. First, some other structural or functional brain partition atlases exist and these brain parcellation atlases could also be used for identifying different psychiatric disorders. Different parcellation schemes may lead to different classification results. Compared to the widely used automated anatomical labeling atlas, the brainnetome atlas that simultaneously combines information from structural and functional connections obtained better classification performance in differentiating major depressive disorder from HC in our previous study (Jing et al., 2017). Thus the brainnetome atlas was adopted to discriminate MCI from HC subjects in this work. Second, deep learning plays an increasing important role in identifying different psychiatric disorders as it could acquire powerful identification performance from high dimension feature data. Future studies could extract the HE features or other multi-level characteristics at a voxel level for deep learning algorithm to obtain better classification accuracy and more comprehensive explanations for abnormalities in psychiatric disorders.

AUTHOR CONTRIBUTIONS

ZL, BJ and RG made substantial contributions to the conception, design, analysis and interpretation of data and drafted the manuscript. ZL, BJ, BL and HC made contributions to the revision of the manuscript. ZL, FC and TW made contributions to the data acquisition. HC, the corresponding author, made contributions to conception and interpretation of data, and determined the final version to be submitted for publishing. All authors read and approved the final manuscript.

ACKNOWLEDGMENTS

There is no any competing interest among all authors, and thanks very much for all editors and reviewers of our manuscript. BJ was supported by the Beijing Natural Science Foundation (No.7174282).

REFERENCES

Baron, J. C., Chételat, G., Desgranges, B., Perchey, G., Landeau, B., Sayette, V., et al. (2001). *In vivo* mapping of gray matter loss with voxel-based morphometry in mild Alzheimer's disease. *Neuroimage* 14, 298–309. doi: 10.1006/nimg.2001.0848

Beheshti, I., and Demirel, H. (2016). Feature-ranking-based Alzheimer's disease classification from structural MRI. *Magn. Reson. Imaging* 34, 252–263. doi: 10.1016/j.mri.2015.11.009

Brier, M. R., Thomas, J. B., Fagan, A. M., Hassenstab, J., Holtzman, D. M., Benzinger, T. L., et al. (2014). Functional connectivity and graph theory in preclinical Alzheimer's disease. *Neurobiol. Aging* 35, 757–768. doi: 10.1016/j.neurobiolaging.2013.10.081

Chen, G., Ward, B. D., Xie, C., Li, W., Wu, Z., Jones, J. L., et al. (2011). Classification of Alzheimer disease, mild cognitive impairment, and normal cognitive status with large-scale network analysis based on resting-state functional MR imaging. *Radiology* 259, 213–221. doi: 10.1148/radiol.10100734

Ciuciu, P., Varoquaux, G., Abry, P., Sadaghiani, S., and Kleinschmidt, A. (2012). Scale-free and multifractal time dynamics of fMRI signals during rest and task. *Front. Physiol.* 3:186. doi: 10.3389/fphys.2012.00186

Costa, P. T., and McCrae, R. R. (1992). Normal personality assessment in clinical practice: the NEO personality inventory. *Psychol. Assess.* 4, 5–13. doi: 10.1037/1040-3590.4.1.5

Dai, Z., Yan, C., Wang, Z., Wang, J., Xia, M., Li, K., et al. (2012). Discriminative analysis of early Alzheimer's disease using multi-modal imaging and multi-level characterization with multi-classifier (M3). *Neuroimage* 59, 2187–2195. doi: 10.1016/j.neuroimage.2011.10.003

Davatzikos, C., Fan, Y., Wu, X., Shen, D., and Resnick, S. M. (2008). Detection of prodromal Alzheimer's disease via pattern classification of MRI. *Neurobiol. Aging* 29, 514–523. doi: 10.1016/j.neurobiolaging.2006.11.010

De Martino, F. D., Valente, G., Staeren, N., Ashburner, J., Goebel, R., and Formisano, E. (2008). Combining multivariate voxel selection and support vector machines for mapping and classification of fMRI spatial patterns. *Neuroimage* 43, 44–58. doi: 10.1016/j.neuroimage.2008.06.037

de Oliveira, J. R. M., and de Oliveira, M. F. (2013). Basal ganglia calcification as a putative cause for cognitive decline. *Dement. Neuropsychol.* 7, 151–154. doi: 10.1590/s1980-57642013dn70200003

Desikan, R. S., Cabral, H. J., Hess, C. P., Dillon, W. P., Glastonbury, C. M., Weiner, M. W., et al. (2009). Automated MRI measures identify individuals with mild cognitive impairment and Alzheimer's disease. *Brain* 132, 2048–2057. doi: 10.1093/brain/awp123

De Vogelaere, F., Santens, P., Achten, E., Boon, P., and Vingerhoets, G. (2012). Altered default-mode network activation in mild cognitive impairment compared with healthy aging. *Neuroradiology* 54, 1195–1206. doi: 10.1007/s00234-012-1036-6

Dosenbach, N. U., Nardos, B., Cohen, A. L., Fair, D. A., Power, J. D., Church, J. A., et al. (2010). Prediction of individual brain maturity using fMRI. *Science* 329, 1358–1361. doi: 10.1126/science.1194144

Dyrba, M., Grothe, M., Kirste, T., and Teipel, S. J. (2015). Multimodal analysis of functional and structural disconnection in Alzheimer's disease using multiple kernel SVM. *Hum. Brain Mapp.* 36, 2118–2131. doi: 10.1002/hbm.22759

Fan, L., Li, H., Zhuo, J., Zhang, Y., Wang, J., Chen, L., et al. (2016). The human brainnetome atlas: a new brain atlas based on connectional architecture. *Cereb. Cortex* 26, 3508–3526. doi: 10.1093/cercor/bhw157

Fornito, A., and Bullmore, E. T. (2010). What can spontaneous fluctuations of the blood oxygenation-level-dependent signal tell us about psychiatric disorders? *Curr. Opin. Psychiatry* 23, 239–249. doi: 10.1097/yco.0b013e328337d78d

Gentili, C., Vanello, N., Cristea, I., David, D., Ricciardi, E., and Pietrini, P. (2015). Proneness to social anxiety modulates neural complexity in the absence of exposure: a resting state fMRI study using hurst exponent. *Psychiatry Res.* 232, 135–144. doi: 10.1016/j.pscychresns.2015.03.005

Greicius, M. D., Srivastava, G., Reiss, A. L., and Menon, V. (2004). Default-mode network activity distinguishes Alzheimer's disease from healthy aging: evidence from functional MRI. *Proc. Natl. Acad. Sci. U S A* 101, 4637–4642. doi: 10.1073/pnas.0308627101

Hämäläinen, A., Tervo, S., Grau-Olivares, M., Niskanen, E., Pennanen, C., Huuskonen, J., et al. (2007). Voxel-based morphometry to detect brain atrophy in progressive mild cognitive impairment. *Neuroimage* 37, 1122–1131. doi: 10.1016/j.neuroimage.2007.06.016

Han, Y., Wang, J., Zhao, Z., Min, B., Lu, J., Li, K., et al. (2011). Frequency-dependent changes in the amplitude of low-frequency fluctuations in amnestic mild cognitive impairment: a resting-state fMRI study. *Neuroimage* 55, 287–295. doi: 10.1016/j.neuroimage.2010.11.059

He, Y., Wang, L., Zang, Y., Tian, L., Zhang, X., Li, K., et al. (2007). Regional coherence changes in the early stages of Alzheimer's disease: a combined structural and resting-state functional MRI study. *Neuroimage* 35, 488–500. doi: 10.1016/j.neuroimage.2006.11.042

Hirata, Y., Matsuda, H., Nemoto, K., Ohnishi, T., Hirao, K., Yamashita, F., et al. (2005). Voxel-based morphometry to discriminate early Alzheimer's disease from controls. *Neurosci. Lett.* 382, 269–274. doi: 10.1016/j.neulet.2005.03.038

Hsu, C. W., Chang, C. C., and Lin, C. J. (2003). A practical guide to support vector classification. Available online at: https://www.csie.ntu.edu.tw/~cjlin/papers/guide/guide.pdf

Ignaccolo, M., Latka, M., Jernajczyk, W., Grigolini, P., and West, B. J. (2010). The dynamics of EEG entropy. *J. Biol. Phys.* 36, 185–196. doi: 10.1007/s10867-009-9171-y

Jing, B., Long, Z., Liu, H., Yan, H., Dong, J., Mo, X., et al. (2017). Identifying current and remitted major depressive disorder with the hurst exponent: a comparative study on two automated anatomical labeling atlases. *Oncotarget* 8, 90452–90464. doi: 10.18632/oncotarget.19860

Khazaee, A., Ebrahimzadeh, A., and Babajani-Feremi, A. (2016). Application of advanced machine learning methods on resting-state fMRI network for identification of mild cognitive impairment and Alzheimer's disease. *Brain Imaging Behav.* 10, 799–817. doi: 10.1007/s11682-015-9448-7

Lai, M. C., Lombardo, M. V., Chakrabarti, B., Sadek, S. A., Pasco, G., Wheelwright, S. J., et al. (2010). A shift to randomness of brain oscillations in people with autism. *Biol. Psychiatry* 68, 1092–1099. doi: 10.1016/j.biopsych.2010.06.027

Lei, X., Zhao, Z., and Chen, H. (2013). Extraversion is encoded by scale-free dynamics of default mode network. *Neuroimage* 74, 52–57. doi: 10.1016/j.neuroimage.2013.02.020

Lerch, J. P., Pruessner, J., Zijdenbos, A. P., Collins, D. L., Teipel, S. J., Hampel, H., et al. (2008). Automated cortical thickness measurements from MRI can accurately separate Alzheimer's patients from normal elderly controls. *Neurobiol. Aging* 29, 23–30. doi: 10.1016/j.neurobiolaging.2006.09.013

Long, Z., Jing, B., Yan, H., Dong, J., Liu, H., Mo, X., et al. (2016). A support vector machine-based method to identify mild cognitive impairment with multi-level characteristics of magnetic resonance imaging. *Neuroscience* 331, 169–176. doi: 10.1016/j.neuroscience.2016.06.025

Magnin, B., Mesrob, L., Kinkingnéhun, S., Pélégrini-Issac, M., Colliot, O., Sarazin, M., et al. (2009). Support vector machine-based classification of Alzheimer's disease from whole-brain anatomical MRI. *Neuroradiology* 51, 73–83. doi: 10.1007/s00234-008-0463-x

Maxim, V., Sendur, L., Fadili, J., Suckling, J., Gould, R., Howard, R., et al. (2005). Fractional gaussian noise, functional MRI and Alzheimer's disease. *Neuroimage* 25, 141–158. doi: 10.1016/j.neuroimage.2004.10.044

Pereira, F., Mitchell, T., and Botvinick, M. (2009). Machine learning classifiers and fMRI: a tutorial overview. *Neuroimage* 45, S199–S209. doi: 10.1016/j.neuroimage.2008.11.007

Petersen, R. C. (2007). Mild cognitive impairment: current research and clinical implications. *Semin. Neurol.* 27, 022–031. doi: 10.1055/s-2006-956752

Wang, Y., Zhao, X., Xu, S., Yu, L., Wang, L., Song, M., et al. (2015). Using regional homogeneity to reveal altered spontaneous activity in patients with mild cognitive impairment. *Biomed Res. Int.* 2015:807093. doi: 10.1155/2015/807093

Wei, M., Qin, J., Yan, R., Li, H., Yao, Z., and Lu, Q. (2013). Identifying major depressive disorder using hurst exponent of resting-state brain networks. *Psychiatry Res.* 214, 306–312. doi: 10.1016/j.pscychresns.2013.09.008

Wink, A. M., Bernard, F., Salvador, R., Bullmore, E., and Suckling, J. (2006). Age and cholinergic effects on hemodynamics and functional coherence of human hippocampus. *Neurobiol. Aging* 27, 1395–1404. doi: 10.1016/j.neurobiolaging.2005.08.011

Xie, C., Bai, F., Yu, H., Shi, Y., Yuan, Y., Chen, G., et al. (2012). Abnormal insula functional network is associated with episodic memory decline in amnestic mild cognitive impairment. *Neuroimage* 63, 320–327. doi: 10.1016/j.neuroimage.2012.06.062

Zhang, Z., Liu, Y., Jiang, T., Zhou, B., An, N., Dai, H., et al. (2012). Altered spontaneous activity in Alzheimer's disease and mild cognitive impairment revealed by regional homogeneity. *Neuroimage* 59, 1429–1440. doi: 10.1016/j.neuroimage.2011.08.049

13

The Histamine H3 Receptor Antagonist DL77 Ameliorates MK801-Induced Memory Deficits in Rats

Nermin Eissa[1], *Nadia Khan*[1], *Shreesh K. Ojha*[1], *Dorota Łazewska*[2], *Katarzyna Kieć-Kononowicz*[2] *and Bassem Sadek*[1*]

[1] *Department of Pharmacology & Therapeutics, College of Medicine & Health Sciences, United Arab Emirates University, Al Ain, United Arab Emirates,* [2] *Department of Technology and Biotechnology of Drugs, Faculty of Pharmacy, Jagiellonian University-Medical College, Kraków, Poland*

***Correspondence:**
Bassem Sadek
bassem.sadek@uaeu.ac.ae

The role of Histamine H3 receptors (H3Rs) in memory, and the prospective of H3R antagonists in pharmacological control of neurodegenerative disorders, e.g., Alzheimer disease (AD) is well-accepted. For that reason, the procognitive effects of the H3R antagonist DL77 on cognitive impairments induced with MK801 were tested in an inhibitory passive avoidance paradigm (PAP) and novel object recognition (NOR) task in adult male rats, using donepezil (DOZ) as a standard drug. Acute systemic pretreatment with DL77 (2.5, 5, and 10 mg/kg, i.p.) significantly ameliorated memory deficits induced with MK801 in PAP (all $P < 0.05$, $n = 7$). The ameliorative effect of most promising dose of DL77 (5 mg/kg, i.p.) was reversed when rats were co-injected with the H3R agonist *R*-(α)-methylhistamine (RAMH, 10 mg/kg, i.p.) ($p = 0.701$ for MK801-amnesic group vs. MK801+DL77+RAMH group, $n = 6$). In the NOR paradigm, DL77 (5 mg/kg, i.p.) counteracted long-term memory (LTM) deficits induced with MK801 ($P < 0.05$, $n = 6$–8), and the DL77-provided effect was similar to that of DOZ ($p = 0.788$, $n = 6$–8), and was reversed when rats were co-injected with RAMH (10 mg/kg, i.p.) ($p = 0.877$, $n = 6$, as compared to the (MK801)-amnesic group). However, DL77 (5 mg/kg, i.p.) did not alter short-term memory (STM) impairment in NOR test ($p = 0.772$, $n = 6$–8, as compared to (MK801)-amnesic group). Moreover, DL77 (5 mg/kg) failed to modify anxiety and locomotor behaviors of animals innate to elevated-plus maze (EPM) ($p = 0.67$ for percentage of time spent exploring the open arms, $p = 0.52$ for number of entries into the open arms, $p = 0.76$ for percentage of entries into the open arms, and $p = 0.73$ number of closed arm entries as compared to saline-treated groups, all $n = 6$), demonstrating that the procognitive effects observed in PAP or NOR tests were unconnected to alterations in emotions or in natural locomotion of tested animals. These results signify the potential involvement of H3Rs in modulating neurotransmitters related to neurodegenerative disorders, e.g., AD.

Keywords: histamine H3 receptor, antagonist, learning and memory, Alzheimer's disease, neurodegeneration, passive avoidance paradigm, novel object recognition, behavioral research

INTRODUCTION

Alzheimer's disease (AD) is a life long-lasting brain disorder that is considered by its cognitive deficits, memory impairment, and dementia (Khunnawutmanotham et al., 2016; Shaik et al., 2016). Following a recent report, around 36 million people worldwide were diagnosed with dementia in recent years, and the number is estimated to significantly increase by the double every two decades, ultimately leading to more than 100 million people with AD after four decades (Khunnawutmanotham et al., 2016). The pathogenesis of AD is still complex, though several theories have been established. The multifaceted pathophysiological alterations include deficient cholinergic neurotransmission, malfunctioning metabolic status of β-amyloid protein, irregularities of numerous central neurotransmitters including glutamate, norepinephrine, serotonin and dopamine, and the contribution of neuroinflammation and high oxidative stress to the progression of AD (Doraiswamy, 2002; Khan et al., 2015; Sadek et al., 2016a). Brain histamine is an established neurotransmitter in the central nervous system (CNS) (Arrang et al., 1983, 1985, 1987a,b, 1988, 2007; Schwartz et al., 1986), exerting its biological activities through interaction with four histamine receptor (HR) subtypes (H1-H4R) that belong to the family of G-protein coupled receptors (Schneider and Seifert, 2009; Panula et al., 2015). H1R and H2R are present in the brain and periphery, whereas H4Rs are predominately expressed in mast cells and leukocytes (Schneider and Seifert, 2009; Panula et al., 2015). Contrary, H3Rs are abundant in the CNS (Arrang et al., 1983, 1985, 1987a,b, 1988, 2007; Panula et al., 2015). Moreover, H3Rs acting as auto-receptors in the CNS are coupled to $G\alpha_{i/o}$-proteins and are capable of controlling the synthesis and release of histamine (Arrang et al., 1983, 1985, 1987a,b, 1988, 2007). Furthermore, H3Rs operating as hetero-receptors located on non-histaminergic neurons in different brain regions can also moderate the release of other neurotransmitters including acetylcholine, glutamate, GABA, norepinephrine, serotonin, dopamine (Brown et al., 2001, 2013). Previous preclinical experiments have proposed H3R antagonists to be of characteristic feature by their possible memory-enhancing effects (Panula et al., 1998, 2015; Panula and Nuutinen, 2011; Sadek and Stark, 2015; Sadek et al., 2016b). Accordingly, several H3R antagonists improved cognitive deficits induced with ketamine and MK801 in numerous animal models (Browman et al., 2004), suggesting that these H3R antagonists may also be effective in neurodegenerative disorders, e.g., AD (Witkin and Nelson, 2004; Bardgett et al., 2010; Charlier et al., 2013; Sadek and Stark, 2015; Sadek et al., 2016b). Among a wide range of H3R antagonists investigated so far, H3R antagonists ABT-239 and A-431404 were found to ameliorate cognitive deficits induced by ketamine and MK-801 in rodents, demonstrating enhanced procognitive effects of these compounds compared to standard drugs, e.g., DOZ (Brown et al., 2013). Therefore, the central H3Rs embodies an attractive target for the development of novel H3R antagonists with the prospective therapeutic future in neurodegenerative disorders (Yokoyama et al., 1993; Yokoyama, 2001; Harada et al., 2004; Witkin and Nelson, 2004; Uma Devi et al., 2010; Bhowmik et al., 2012, 2014; Sadek and Stark, 2015; Sadek et al., 2016b). Regardless of the abovementioned experimental observations for the role for H3Rs in the modulation of memory deficits and related behaviors, targeting H3Rs in the CNS is not commonly proposed as a future strategy to treat AD.

In the current study and as a continuation of our research efforts, the procognitive effects of the non-imidazole H3R antagonist, namely DL77 [1-(3-(4-*tert*-pentylphenoxy)propyl)piperidine dihydrogenoxalate], with high *in vitro* selectivity to human H3R, high antagonist affinity in the subnanomolar concentration range and a pK_i-value of 8.03, and high H3R antagonist *in vivo* potency with an ED_{50} value of 2.1 ± 0.2 mg/kg, per oral (p.o.) (Łazewska et al., 2006) has been explored on its procognitive effects on memory deficits induced with MK801 in PAP and NOR paradigms in adult male rats applying DOZ as a reference drug. Moreover, the effects of DL77 on anxiety and locomotor behaviors in EPM was assessed, since anxiety and locomotion could influence the performance of rats in PAP or NOR. Furthermore, the abrogative effects of the histamine H3R agonist RAMH on the memory-enhancing effects provided with DL77 in PAP and NOR paradigms were examined. The non-imidazole H3R antagonist DL77 was selected for testing in the current studies as it in an earlier study proved to exhibit (5–15 mg/kg, i.p.) anticonvulsant properties and procognitive effects on acquisition, consolidation and retrieval in the same animal species (Sadek et al., 2016c). Also, a previous study showed a promising effects of DL77 (3–30 mg/kg, i.p.) on alcohol intake and preference in adult C57BL/6 mice (Bahi et al., 2015).

EXPERIMENTAL PROCEDURES

Animals

Male Wistar rats (inbred of Central Animal Facility of the UAE University, aged 6–8 weeks) of body weight 180–220 g were used for the study. The animals were retained in an air-conditioned animal facility room with controlled temperature (24 ± 2°C) and humidity (55 ± 15%) under a 12 h light/dark cycle, and were provided free access to food and water. Experiments were carried out between 9:00 and 13:00 h, and all procedures were approved by the Institutional Animal Ethics Committee of College of Medicine and Health Sciences/United Arab Emirates University (A30-13). All efforts were made to minimize animal suffering, to reduce the number of animals used. Also, all behavioral studies were conducted in a blinded fashion and by the same experimenter.

Drugs

R-(α)-methylhistamine dihydrochloride (RAMH), donepezil hydrochloride (DOZ), and MK801 hydrogen maleate were purchased from Sigma-Aldrich (St Louis, Missouri, USA). The H3R antagonist 1-(3-(4-*tert*-pentylphenoxy)propyl)piperidine dihydrogenoxalate (DL77, 2.5, 5, 10, mg/kg) was synthesized by

Abbreviations: AD, Alzheimer disease; H3Rs, histamine H3 receptors; RAMH, *R*-(α)-methyl-histamine; DOZ, donepezil; MK801, dizocilpine; PAP, passive avoidance paradigm; STL, step-through latency; NOR, novel object recognition; STM, short-term memory; LTM, long-term memory; EPM, elevated plus maze; p.o., per oral; i.p., intraperitoneal.

us in the Department of Technology and Biotechnology of Drugs (Kraków, Poland) as described previously (Meier et al., 2001; Łazewska et al., 2006). All drugs were dissolved in isotonic saline and injected intraperitoneal (i.p.) at a volume of 1 ml/kg, and all doses were expressed in terms of the free base.

Behavioral Tests

Inhibitory PAP Test

Male adult Wistar rats were tested in a two compartment step-through passive avoidance apparatus (Step-through Cage, 7550, Ugo Basile, Comerio, Italy) as described previously (Izquierdo et al., 1999; Bernaerts et al., 2004; da Silva et al., 2009; Goshadrou et al., 2013; Khan et al., 2015; Sadek et al., 2016a,c; Alachkar et al., 2017; Sultan et al., 2017), with minor modifications. The test was conducted in an automatically operated commercial passive avoidance apparatus as previously described (Khan et al., 2015; Sadek et al., 2016a,c; Alachkar et al., 2017). The experiment consisted of two trials (training and testing) separated by a 24 h interval. Each rat in the first trial was placed in the white compartment (facing the auto guillotine door) and after a 30-s habituation period the door was raised automatically. The rat was given a 60 s cut-off time to step-through to the dark compartment. Rats that failed to move within this time period were excluded from the test session on the following day. Once the rat moved into the dark compartment, the sliding door was lowered and a scrambled foot shock (0.4 mA, 20 Hz, 8.3 ms) was delivered to the grid floor for a duration of 3 s. The power of the delivered foots-hock was designated following confirming the sensitivity threshold that yields the minimal vocalization and jumping responses in tested rats. The rat was removed from the dark chamber directly after receiving the foot-shock, returned to its home cage, and both compartments were cleaned. The animals were trained for 3 consecutive days; in which they were injected with saline i.p. 30–45 min before each training session, with the only modification that the cut-off latency was put at 300 s to move to the dark compartment without delivery of scrambled foot-shock (Khan et al., 2015; Sadek et al., 2016a,c). Rats that did not move into the dark compartment during the training, despite the practices carried out during training sessions, were excluded from the current test. For each separate experiment, 9–11 animals of the same age and weight average were trained on the step-through latency (STL) paradigm. Approximately 2–4 rats failed to demonstrate enhanced performance in a cut-off time of 60 s. In the current series of behavioral experiments, a group of 7 animals was used for each STL task conducted for the PAP. In the test session, animals were turned amnesic with acute systemic injection of MK801 (0.1 mg/kg, i.p.) 30–45 min prior to test session, and the animals were allowed to move to the dark compartment for a maximum period of 300 s. In this test session, the STL time for each rat to enter the dark compartment in 300 s was measured.

Dose regimen

Six groups of seven rats each were used, and were pretreated with Saline+Saline, MK801+Saline, MK801+DL77 (2.5, 5, and 10 mg/kg, i.p.), or MK801+DOZ (1 mg/kg, i.p.) 30–45 min before the test session, and the procognitive effects DL77 (2.5, 5, and 10 mg/kg, i.p.) on amnesia induced with acute systemic injection of MK801 (0.1 mg/kg, i.p.) was investigated by determining the STLs to move into the dark compartment. In an additional experiment, a single group of seven rats received two injections; the first injection contained the most effective dose of DL77 and was administered 30–45 min before the PAP test, and the second injection contained RAMH (10 mg/kg, i.p.) which was administered 15–20 min prior PAP test. The CNS penetrant H3R agonist RAMH was injected 15–20 min before the start of test conduction to ensure its presence in the CNS, as RAMH shows fast metabolism (Krause et al., 2001). Doses of DL77, DOZ, and RAMH were chosen according to previously published results in the same species of rodents (Orsetti et al., 2001, 2002; Khan et al., 2015; Sadek et al., 2016a,c) (**Figures 1, 2**).

NOR Test

Recognition memory was assessed in a novel object recognition (NOR) test as previously described (Ennaceur and Delacour, 1988; Izquierdo et al., 1999; de Lima et al., 2005; Karasawa et al., 2008; Alachkar et al., 2017). The experiments were conducted in a black open field box (50 × 35 ×50 cm), and the experimental procedure included two sessions of habituation of 1 h interval, whereby the animals were provided 3 min time to explore the apparatus. On the test day and after a 3 min exploration of the apparatus, two novel objects were introduced in two corners (∼30 cm apart from each other). The objects (9 × 5 × 9 cm) used in this study were wood blocks and existed in different shape and color, but were of the same size. They appeared devoid of natural

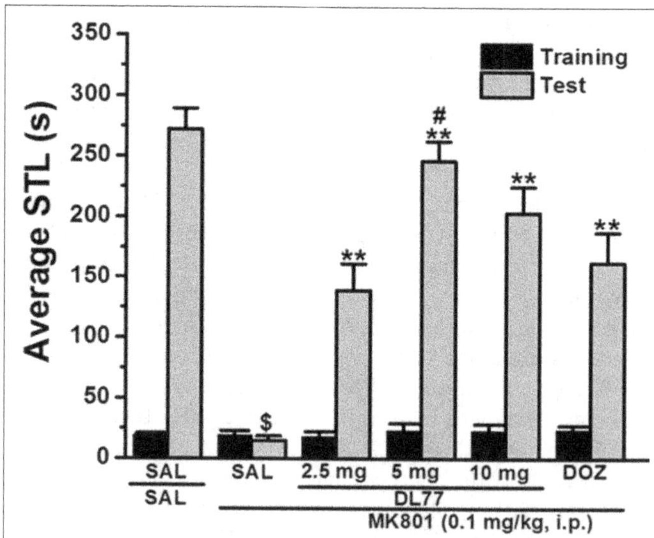

FIGURE 1 | Effects of DL77 on MK801-induced memory deficits in an inhibitory PAP in rats. Gray columns represent the mean STLs measured during the training trial before the delivery of the foot-shock (pre-shock latencies) and black columns the mean STLs measured during the retention test (test latencies). Rats were injected with DL77 (2.5, 5, or 10 mg/kg, i.p.) or donepezil (DOZ, 1 mg/kg, i.p.) 30 min before the test session. $^{\$}P < 0.001$ for mean STLs vs the value of the (saline)-treated group. $^{**}P < 0.001$ for mean STLs vs. the value of the (MK801)-treated group. $^{\#}P < 0.05$ for mean STLs vs. the value of MK801+DOZ-treated group. Data are expressed as mean ± SEM ($n = 7$).

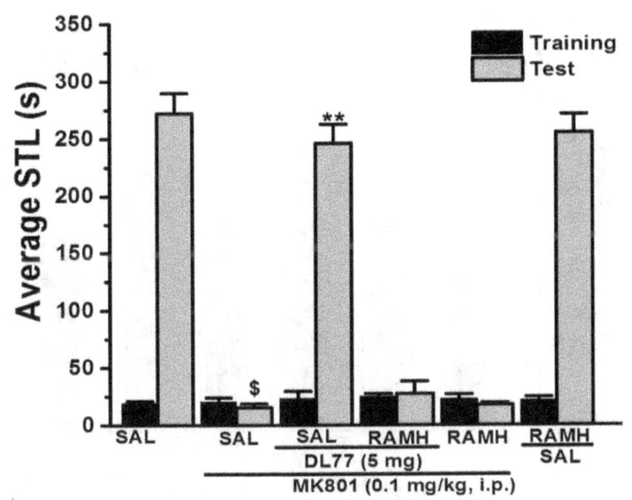

FIGURE 2 | Effect of vehicle, DL77, and RAMH on MK801-induced deficit in an inhibitory PAP in rats. Gray columns represent the mean STLs measured during the training trial before the delivery of the foot-shock (pre-shock latencies) and black columns the mean STLs measured during the retention test (test latencies). Rats were injected with DL77 (5 mg/kg, i.p.), RAMH, or a combination of RAMH (10 mg/kg)+DL77 (5 mg/kg) 15 min (RAMH) or 30 min (DL77) before the test session. $^{\$}P < 0.001$ for mean STLs vs. the value of the (Saline)-treated group. $^{**}P < 0.001$ for mean STLs vs. the value of the (MK801)-treated group. Data are expressed as mean ± SEM ($n = 7$).

significance for the animals and had never been linked with reinforcement. They were adequately heavy to be not displaced by the tested rats. The experimental session consisted of two trials T1 and T2, each lasting for 3 min. In T1, rats were exposed to two identical objects, and those exploring the objects for less than 10 s during T1 were excluded from the tests. In T2, performed 120 min (for STM) or 24 h (for LTM) later, rats were exposed to two objects, one of which was a duplicate of familiar object in order to exclude olfactory traits, and another novel object. The role (familiar or novel object) as well as the relative position of the two objects were counterbalanced and arbitrarily permuted during T2. The principle measure was the time spent by the rat for exploring objects during both trials, namely T1 and T2. The test box as well as all used objects were thoroughly cleaned with 70% (volume/volume; v/v) alcoholic solution. All sessions of NOR test were executed during the light phase (8:00–12:00 a.m.). In order to detect procognitive effects of test compound, MK801 and test compound were dissolved in isotonic saline and injected i.p. at a volume of 1 ml/kg 30–45 min. following T1. The control groups received an equivalent volume of saline injection. The choice of doses and pretreatment times for each compound was decided according to the results of most promising dose in PAP and was derived from previously reported procognitive studies (Bernaerts et al., 2004; da Silva et al., 2009; Goshadrou et al., 2013; Khan et al., 2015; Sadek et al., 2016c; Alachkar et al., 2017; Sultan et al., 2017).

Dose regimen

Six groups of six to eight rats each were used for the detection of a procognitive effect in STM. The groups were injected with Saline, MK801, MK801+DL77 (5 mg/kg, i.p.), MK801+DL77(5 mg/kg)+RAMH (10 mg/kg, i.p.), MK801+DOZ (1 mg/kg, i.p.), or MK801+RAMH (10 mg/kg, i.p.) 30–45 min before T2, respectively, and the counteracting effects of DL77 on cognitive deficits induced with MK801 were assessed by measuring the time spent by the rat in exploring objects in both trials T1 and T2 for STM (**Figure 3**). In an additional experiment, the procognitive effect of DL77 on MK801-induced memory impairments was confirmed by abrogative study in which the respective promising dose (5 mg/kg, i.p.) of DL77 and RAMH (10 mg/kg, i.p.) were co-administered to a separate group of six rats 30–45 min prior to T2 and 24 h after T1. The latter experiment was carried out to confirm the procognitive effect for LTM, whereas control groups received comparable saline injections (**Figure 4**). Doses of MK801, RAMH, and DOZ were chosen according to previous experimental protocols of NOR (Bernaerts et al., 2004; de Lima et al., 2005; da Silva et al., 2009; Goshadrou et al., 2013; Khan et al., 2015; Sadek et al., 2016c; Alachkar et al., 2017; Sultan et al., 2017).

EPM Test

Anxiety-like behaviors were evaluated in an EPM as previously described (Jiang et al., 2016; Alachkar et al., 2017). The EPM apparatus consisted of several parts including one central part (8 × 8 cm), two opposing open and closed arms (30 × 8 cm), and nontransparent walls (30 cm in height). Between every session, both the plat form and the wall were thoroughly cleaned using 10% alcoholic spray. Animals were placed individually in the center arena of the maze (50 cm above the floor) facing an open arm, and test sessions took place in the light phase (9:00–12:00 a.m.). The amount of time spent with head and forepaws on the open arms and closed arms of the maze as well as the number of entries into each arm was manually scored for a session of 5 min. The maze was thoroughly cleaned between sessions using a tissue dampened with 70% (volume/volume; v/v) alcohol to remove the odor after each rat was tested. The total number of entries into the closed arms is usually used as an index of locomotor activity in the test.

Dose regimen

Rats were divided into two groups of six rats each. One group received saline injection i.p. 30–45 min before the test and test group received the H3R antagonist DL77 (5 mg/kg, i.p.) for testing its modulating effects on anxiety and locomotion (**Figure 5**).

Statistical Analysis

IBM® SPSS Statistics® version 24 software (IBM Middle East, Dubai, United Arab Emirates) was used for all statistical comparisons. The results of NOR were expressed as the means and standard errors (SEM) of the exploratory time spent by the rat exploring both objects in T1 and T2. The results of the EPM test were expressed as the means and SEM of the percentage time spent on open arms, number of entries into the open arms, the percentage of entries into the open arms, and number of entries into closed arms. Results of NOR and EPM were analyzed by using a two-way analysis of variance

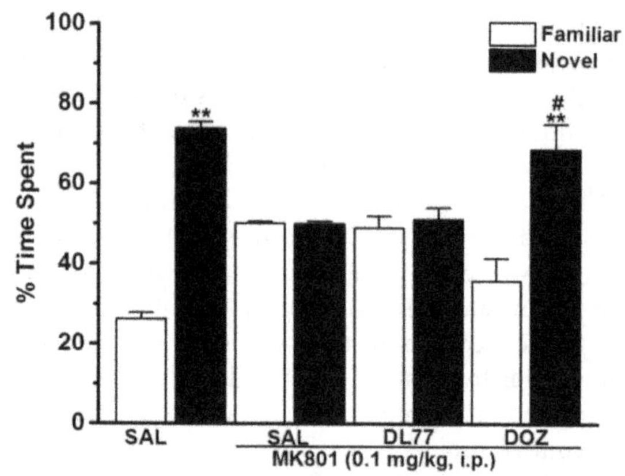

FIGURE 3 | Effects of DL77 on MK801-induced STM cognitive deficits in NOR paradigm in rats. Following training session T1, DL77 (5 mg/kg) or DOZ (1 mg/kg) was administrated i.p., followed 30 min later by i.p. administration of MK801 at a dose of 0.1 mg/kg. The test session T2 was performed 120 min (STM) after the training session T1. Results are calculated as individual percentage of time spent exploring familiar (white columns) and novel (black columns) objects. Data represent mean ± SEM ($n = 6$). **$P < 0.001$ vs. respective familiar object. #$P < 0.05$ vs. MK801-treated group.

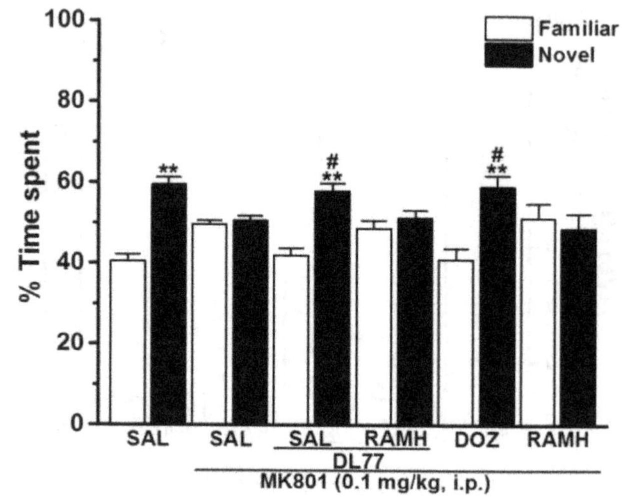

FIGURE 4 | Effects of DL77 on MK801-induced LTM cognitive deficits in NOR paradigm in rats. Following training session T1, DL77 (5 mg/kg) or DOZ (1 mg/kg) was administrated i.p., followed 30 min later by i.p. injection of MK801 at a dose of 0.1 mg/kg. The test session T2 was performed 24 h (LTM) after the training session T1. Results are calculated as individual percentage of time spent exploring familiar (white columns) and novel (black columns) objects. Data represent mean ±SEM ($n = 6$). **$P < 0.001$ vs. respective familiar object. #$P < 0.05$ vs. MK801-treated group.

(ANOVA). When relevant *post-hoc* comparisons were performed with *Bonferroni's* test in case of a significant main effect. STLs observed in PAP test were expressed as means and SEM. Because of the arbitrary cutoff latency used, the results were evaluated by using nonparametric Kruskal–Wallis ANOVA, and the differences between groups were estimated by individual Mann–Whitney *U*-tests. The criterion for statistical significance was set at *P*-value of <0.05.

RESULTS

Memory-Enhancing Effects of H3R Antagonist DL77 and Standard Drug DOZ on Memory Deficits Induced with MK801 in PAP Task

The effect of acute systemic injection of DL77 at three different doses, namely 2.5, 5, and 10 mg/kg, and DOZ (1 mg/kg) on memory deficits induced with MK801 in an inhibitory PAP test in rats are shown in **Figure 1**. Statistical analysis of observed results indicated that acute systemic pretreatment with the three doses of DL77, and DOZ (1 mg/kg) prior to retention test exhibited a significant memory-enhancing effect on STLs [$H_{(5)} = 28.29$; $P < 0.001$; **Figure 1**]. As shown following pairwise comparisons, MK801 (0.1 mg/kg) decreased STL time when compared to the (saline)-treated control group with ($U = 28.00$, $P < 0.05$). Moreover, DL77 tested in three different doses (2.5, 5, and 10 mg/kg) showed significant improving effect on STLs time when compared to (MK801)-treated group with (all $P < 0.05$). However, pretreatment with DL77 (5 mg/kg, i.p.) was found to be not significantly different from (Saline)-treated control rats ($U = 38.50$, $p = 0.073$) (**Figure 1**). Furthermore, DL77 (5 mg/kg) showed signicantly higher improving effects on STL when compared with the DOZ(1 mg)-provided memory-enhancing efects with ($U = 5.00$, $P < 0.05$) (**Figure 1**).

Abrogative Effects of RAMH on the Memory Improvement Provided with DL77 in MK801-Induced Deficits in PAP Task

For this experiment, a group of seven animals was injected with the most promising dose of DL77 (5 mg/kg, i.p.) 30–45 min prior to test, and also adminstered with the H3R agonist RAMH (10 mg/kg, i.p.) 15 min before the test session (**Figure 2**). As shown in **Figure 2**, statistical analysis revealed that this factor had a significant effect on the STL time [$H_{(5)} = 31.32$; $P < 0.001$]. Moreover, pairwise comparisons indicated that acute systemic pretreatment with DL77 (5 mg/kg, i.p.) enhanced STL time when compared to the (MK801)-amnesic group with ($U = 49.00$; $P < 0.05$). Interestingly, the improvmemnt of observed STL time provided with DL77 was abrogated following acute co-injection of RAMH ($U = 49.00$; $p = 0.701$: MK801-amnesic group vs. MK801+DL77+RAMH group, **Figure 2**). Noteably, acute systemic administration of RAMH (10 mg/kg, i.p.) alone failed to affect the observed STL time in MK801-amnesic group as well as in Saline group with no significant differences ($U = 30.50$; $p = 0.442$) and ($U = 20.50$; $p = 0.620$), respectively (**Figure 2**).

Modulating Effects of H3R Antagonist DL77 and DOZ on the STM Deficits Induced with MK801 in NOR Task

The results observed for the total time exploring both objects during T1 and T2 were not significantly different when comparing groups pretreated with saline and those injected with MK801 (**Table 1**). The latter experimental observation is substantial to exclude any confounding factors, e.g., that the post-training treatment with the amnesic compound MK801 in the first experiment did not modify sensorimotor considerations such as locomotor activity and motivations of tested animals. Furthermore, statistical results revealed that no significant differences were present in exploratory times between the two identical objects during T1 for each respective experimental group of animals (**Table 1**). The observed results, also, showed that acute systemic pretreatment with DL77 (5 mg/kg, i.p.) and standard drug DOZ (1 mg/kg, i.p.) significantly counteracted time spent exploring objects in T2 with [$F_{(3, 20)} = 13.76$; $P < 0.001$] when injected 30–45 min after T1 (**Figure 3**). As revealed by conducted post hoc analyses, MK801 (0.1 mg/kg, i.p.) decreased memory toward the novel object in T2 when compared to the (saline)-treated group with [$F_{(1, 10)} = 140.96$; $P < 0.001$], and DOZ (1 mg/kg, i.p.) significantly counteracted this memory deficit in STM in T2 when compared to (MK801)-amnesic group [$F_{(1, 10)} = 7.02$; $P < 0.05$)]. Contrary, acute systemic administration of DL77 (5 mg/kg, i.p.) did not counteract the decreased STM when compared to (MK801)-amnesic group with [$F_{(1, 10)} = 0.08$; $p = 0.772$].

Modulating Effects of H3R Antagonist DL77 and DOZ on the LTM Deficits Induced with MK801 in NOR Task

The results showed that H3R antagonist DL77 (5 mg/kg, i.p.) and standard drug DOZ (1 mg/kg, i.p.) when injected 30–45 min before T2 exhibited a significant counteracting effect on time spent exploring objects in T2 with [$F_{(5, 30)} = 2.67$; $P < 0.05$] (**Figure 4**). Moreover, subsequent *post-hoc* analyses revealed that MK801 (0.1 mg/kg, i.p.) decreased memory for the novel object in T2 when compared to the (MK801)-amnesic

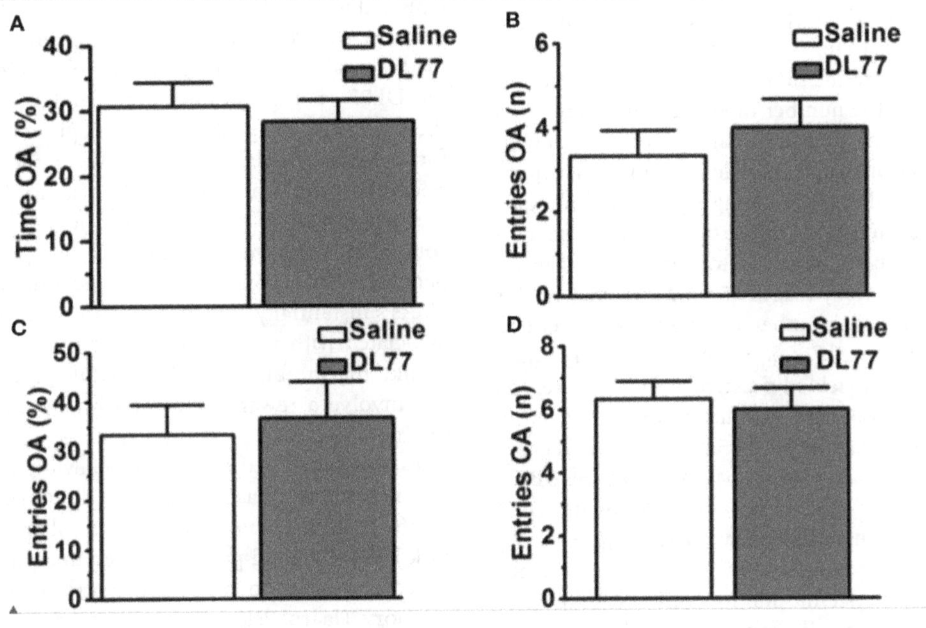

FIGURE 5 | Effects of acute systemic administration of DL77 on exploratory behavior in EPM. DL77 (5 mg/kg) did not alter the percentage of time spent on the open arms of the EPM **(A)**, increase the number of entries into the open arms **(B)** and the percentage of entries into the open arms **(C)**. Acute systemic pretreatment with the H3R antagonist/inverse agonist DL77 (5 mg/kg, i.p.) did not affect the number of closed arm entries **(D)**. Data are expressed as mean ± SEM (*n* = 6).

TABLE 1 | Effects of DL77 on MK801-induced total exploratory time spent with both objects during training and test session in NOR in rats.

Group		Time exploring objects (s)			
	n	Training session STM	Test session STM	Training session LTM	Test session LTM
Saline	6	37.50 ± 3.2	41.83 ± 2.67	36.67 ± 2.93	38.17 ± 3.86
MK801	8	36.00 ± 2.73	42.25 ± 1.57	23.63 ± 2.73	28.88 ± 2.32
MK801 + DL77(5 mg/kg)	8	24.88 ± 2.73	28.17 ± 3.57	23.50 ± 1.71	23.63 ± 2.73
MK801+DL77(5 mg/kg)+RAMH(10 mg/kg)	6	ND	ND	23.63 ± 2.73	23.33 ± 4.87
MK801+DOZ(1 mg/kg)	6	24.83 ± 1.72	25.33 ± 1.88	23.00 ± 3.34	25.33 ± 1.68
MK801+RAMH(10 mg/kg)	6	ND	ND	21.67 ± 1.74	22.67 ± 2.35

Data are expressed as mean ±SEM of 6 or 8 animals per experimental group. There were no significant differences in total exploratory times among treated groups.

group with [$F_{(1, 10)} = 13.92$; $P < 0.05$]. However, acute systemic administration with the H3R antagonist DL77 (5 mg/kg, i.p.) significantly counteracted the induced memory deficits in LTM when compared to (MK801)-amnesic group with [$F_{(1, 10)} = 9.05$; $P < 0.05$] (**Figure 4**). Moreover, the LTM-enhancing procognitive effect provided by DL77 (5 mg/kg, i.p.) was reversed when rats were co-administered with RAMH (10 mg/kg, i.p., i.p.) as compared to the (MK801)-amnesic group with [$F_{(1, 10)} = 0.03$; $p = 0.877$]. Notably, the significant LTM enhancing effect provided with DL77 (5 mg/kg, i.p.) was comparable to the effects observed by the standard drug DOZ (1 mg/kg, i.p.) in T2 with [$F_{(1, 10)} = 0.08$; $p = 0.788$]. Also and similar to the results observed in STM, statistical analyses revealed that RAMH (10 mg/kg, i.p.) alone did not alter LTM in T2 when compared to the MK801-amnesic group with [$F_{(1, 10)} = 0.20$; $p = 0.67$] (**Figure 4**).

Effect of DL77 on Rat Anxiety and Locomotor Activity in EPM Test

Figure 5 shows the observed effects of acute systemic injection of Saline or H3R antagonist DL77 (5 mg/kg, i.p.) on the anxiety parameters of rats exposed to the EPM, namely the percentage of time spent in open arms, the number of entries into open arms, the percentage entries into open arms, and locomotor activity expressed as the number of entries into closed arms. Subsequent *post-hoc* analyses showed that DL77 (5 mg/kg, i.p.) did not alter the percentage of time spent exploring the open arms of the maze during a 5 min session when compared to saline-treated group with [$F_{(1, 10)} = 0.19$, $p = 0.67$] (**Figure 5A**). Moreover, further analyses of data describing the number and percentage of entries into the open arms of the maze [$F_{(1, 10)} = 0.45$, $p = 0.52$; $F_{(1, 10)} = 0.10$, $p = 0.76$, respectively] yielded practically the same results. As depicted in **Figures 5B,C**, no significant differences were obtained between the results in the DL77(5 mg/kg)-treated group and those observed in the saline-treated group (**Figures 5B,C**). Interestingly, the number of closed arm entries following DL77 injection was not significantly changed with [$F_{(1, 10)} = 0.12$, $p = 0.73$], demonstrating that locomotor activity as such was not modulated following acute systemic administration with the H3R antagonist DL77 (5 mg/kg, i.p.) (**Figure 5D**).

DISCUSSION

In the current series of experiments, acute systemic injection of 2.5, 5, and 10 mg/kg of DL77 ameliorated the memory deficits induced by MK801 in an inhibitory PAP in rats. The observed results revealed that DL77 significantly reversed the memory deficits induced by MK801 (**Figure 1**). Since MK801 is a very well-known NMDA receptor antagonist and NMDA receptors were confirmed with their important role in both consolidation and retrieval processes, it is likely that DL77 partially counteracted memory deficits induced with MK801 through direct interaction and activation of NMDA receptors by the increased release of central histamine as a consequence of antagonistic activity of DL77 at histamine H3-auto-receptors. These latter results are in agreement with earlier studies in which histamine enhanced NMDA receptor-mediated neurotransmission in cultured hippocampal cells, indicating that the interaction between histamine and NMDA receptors might facilitate the histamine's capability to counteract MK801-induced amnesic effect (Vorobjev et al., 1993; Xu et al., 2005; Brabant et al., 2013; Sadek et al., 2016a). Notably, the procognitive effect provided by DL77 was dose-dependent, as DL77 at a dose of 5 mg/kg provided significantly higher counteracting effect on decreased STL time when compared to the lower as well as higher dose (2.5 and 10 mg/kg), respectively, indicating that an optimum of DL77-provided memory-enhancing effect might have been reached with a dose of 5 mg/kg, and that off-targets effects could have been present following acute systemic administration of DL77 at a dose of 10 mg/kg (**Figure 1**). Interestingly, the latter observations for the dose dependency are, also, similar to those observed in previous preclinical experiments in rodents (Benetti and Izquierdo, 2013; Benetti et al., 2013; Sadek et al., 2016c). Moreover, the results observed in regard to dose dependency strongly support our previous results detected for the effects of H3R antagonist DL77 (2.5, 5, and 10 mg/kg, i.p.) on different memory stages, namely acquisition, consolidation, and retrieval (Sadek et al., 2016c). Notably, the observed procognitive effects for DL77 (5 mg/kg) were comparable to those obtained for the reference drug DOZ, a procognitive compound available for memory-enhancing effect, since there is up to date no reference drug which is targeting H3Rs (**Figure 1**). Moreover, the procognitive effects found for DL77 (5 mg/kg) were completely reversed when animals were pretreated with the CNS penetrant H3R agonist RAMH, indicating clearly that blockade of H3Rs substantially contributes in the central neurotransmissions associated with retrieval processes of tested animals (**Figure 2**). Unlike the inhibitory PAP, the NOR paradigm in rodents does not involve a reward or a punishment, and it takes advantage of their innate interest for exploring their environment, as it is established on the natural behavior of rodents. Therefore, the behavioral reaction of tested animals is not biased by reinforcement/response interactions of tested rats. Also, the NOR task is a behavioral paradigm used in animal models to evaluate aspects related to cognitive performance, e.g., recognition memory (Jaaro-Peled, 2009; Tseng et al., 2009; Brown et al., 2013; Callahan et al., 2017). Furthermore, previous preclinical studies revealed that NOR paradigm can be utilized in cognitive related experiments due to its sensitivity to both agents capable of impairing (Ennaceur and Delacour, 1988; Ennaceur and Meliani, 1992a,b) as well as enhancing cognition (Lebrun et al., 2000; Barak and Weiner, 2011) following acute systemic pre- and/or post-training administration of the individual agent (King et al., 2004; de Lima et al., 2005; Pichat et al., 2007). In the current study, acute systemic post-training injection of DL77 (5 mg/kg, the most promising dose in PAP test) significantly improved the exploratory time spent with the novel object compared with the familiar objects (**Figure 3**). These observations are in consensus with previous reports revealing that various H3R antagonists belonging to the imidazole-based class, e.g., thioperamide and clobenpropit (Giovannini et al., 1999), and to the non-imidazole-based class, e.g., pitolisant (Ligneau et al., 2007); GSK189254 (Giannoni et al., 2010); SAR110894 (Griebel et al., 2012), and

ABT-239 (Provensi et al., 2016) counteracted the memory-impairing effects of MK801 and scopolamine in NOR tests using different rodents. In our conducted experiments, DL77 potently counteracted the LTM-impairing effects induced with MK801, and these DL77-provided effects were entirely reversed when rats were co-injected with the H3R agonist RAMH (**Figure 3** and **Table 1**). The latter observations are in agreement with an earlier study in which RAMH abolished the memory-enhancing effects provided by H3R antagonist ciproxifan on LTM (Pascoli et al., 2009). Unlike the results observed for DL77 on LTM, acute systemic post-training administration of DL77 did not increase the exploratory time spent with the novel objects in STM when compared with the familiar objects (**Figure 4** and **Table 1**). The latter results are in discrepancy with earlier studies in which H3R antagonist ABT-239 enhanced STM in mice (Provensi et al., 2016). The discrepancy in the results observed in STM might be explained with the different species used or the differences in doses used or in the conduct of experiments. Accordingly, acute systemic post-training administration of MK801 was used in the current study to induce amnesia, whereas natural memory decline as well as presence or absence of histaminergic neurotransmission were examined in the study conducted by Provensi et al. (2016). Moreover, the current experimental findings in NOR obviously point toward profound contribution of histaminergic H3Rs in neuronal circuits associated with the DL77-provided procognitive effects in LTM (**Figure 4** and **Table 1**). The lack of memory-enhancing activity of DL77 in STM is in agreement with previous reports in which no differences were found in time spent exploring novel object in wild type (intact brain histamine) and histidine decarboxylase-knocked out mice (lack of brain histamine) when tested 2 h post-training (STM), but not when testing 24 h post-training (LTM), indicating that histaminergic neurotransmission is more involved the neural circuits which modulate the LTM (Acevedo et al., 2006, 2007; Provensi et al., 2016). Interestingly, several H3R antagonists have in earlier preclinical studies been designated as talented candidates for AD and were suggested to be of possible novel therapeutics due to their capability to interact with H3 auto- and hetero-receptors, modulating the synthesis and release of numerous brain neurotransmitters critical for cognition, including histamine, dopamine, and acetylcholine (Brioni et al., 2011; Sadek and Stark, 2015; Sadek et al., 2016b). The EPM test is considered to be one of the most used animal tests in neuroscience to assess emotionality-related behaviors, e.g., anxiety, based on the innate tendency of animals to avoid open spaces in favor of protected areas, while measuring percent and/or number of closed arms entries reportedly ensures that behavior observed in the maze did not simply reflect drug-induced alterations in locomotor activity (Fernandes and File, 1996; Hogg, 1996; Alachkar et al., 2017). Notably, DL77 at the dose (5 mg/kg) that exhibited the most encouraging procognitive effect in PAP and NOR paradigms did not affect anxiety levels of the adult male Wistar rats (**Figures 5A–D**). Also, DL77 administered at the same dose (5 mg/kg) did not affect the number of closed arm entries, indicating that DL77 failed to modify locomotion of tested rats, demonstrating that enhanced memory performance in PAP as well as NOR is not related to modified emotional responses or altered spontaneous locomotor activity considered as confounding factors when assessing memory-enhancing effects in PAP and NOR (**Figure 5D**) (McGaugh and Roozendaal, 2009; Charlier et al., 2013). The latter results are, also, in line with our earlier results in which acute systemic injection of DL77 (2.5, 5, and 10 mg/kg, i.p.) did not affect spontaneous locomotion of the same animal species when tested in the open field task (Sadek et al., 2016c). Therefore, it is unlikely that acute systemic injection of DL77 (5 mg/kg, i.p.) in the post-training sessions provided memory-enhancing effects in PAP and NOR paradigms due to a nonspecific effect rather than improved learning tasks conducted in the training sessions of both paradigms.

CONCLUSION

The results show that the non-imidazole H3R antagonist DL77 ameliorated cognitive deficits induced by the NMDA receptor antagonist MK801 in an inhibitory PAP and in NOR paradigms in rats (**Figure 6**). Moreover, the results observed in PAP as well as LTM of NOR indicated that DL77 ameliorated cognitive deficits through blockade of H3Rs, demonstrating the therapeutic prospective of H3R antagonists in the future treatment of neurodegenerative diseases, e.g., AD. However, additional preclinical experiments in other behavioral test

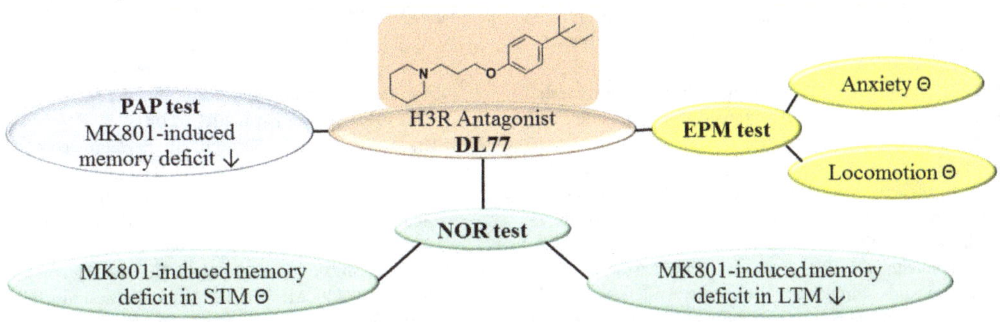

FIGURE 6 | Schematic representation of proposed ameliorative effects for H3R antagonist DL77 in MK801-induced memory deficit in PAP, NOR, and EPM. PAP, passive avoidance paradigm; NOR, novel object recognition; EPM, elevated plus maze; ⊖, no effect; ↓, ameliorates.

models and with several rodent species are still warranted to comprehend the translational validity of the prospective use of H3R antagonists in future therapy of neurodegenerative diseases.

AUTHOR CONTRIBUTIONS

BS was responsible for the study concept, design, acquisition, and analysis of animal data; NK provided technical support to the conducted behavioral experiments; NE and NK conducted behavioral experiments; KK-K and DŁ were responsible for the generation, synthesis, and pharmacological *in vitro* characterization the H3R antagonist DL77; BS and NE drafted the manuscript; KK-K, DŁ, and SO provided critical revision for the manuscript; All authors critically reviewed content and approved final version for publication.

ACKNOWLEDGMENTS

The Office of Graduate Studies and Research of UAE University as well as ADEK Award for Research Excellence (AARE) 2017 are highly thanked for the support provided to BS in form of intermural College of Medicine and Health Sciences as well as extramural funds from ADEK. The authors, also, acknowledge the partial support of National Science Center granted on the basis of decision numbers DEC-2011/02/A/NZ4/00031. Support was kindly provided by the EU COST Actions CA151315 (KK-K; DŁ).

REFERENCES

Acevedo, S. F., de Esch, I. J., and Raber, J. (2007). Sex- and histamine-dependent long-term cognitive effects of methamphetamine exposure. *Neuropsychopharmacology* 32, 665–672. doi: 10.1038/sj.npp.1301091

Acevedo, S. F., Pfankuch, T., Ohtsu, H., and Raber, J. (2006). Anxiety and cognition in female histidine decarboxylase knockout (Hdc(-/-)) mice. *Behav. Brain Res.* 168, 92–99. doi: 10.1016/j.bbr.2005.10.016

Alachkar, A., Łazewska, D., Kiec' -Kononowicz, K., and Sadek, B. (2017). The histamine H3 receptor antagonist E159 reverses memory deficits induced by dizocilpine in passive avoidance and novel object recognition paradigm in rats. *Front. Pharmacol.* 8:709. doi: 10.3389/fphar.2017.00709

Arrang, J. M., Devaux, B., Chodkiewicz, J. P., and Schwartz, J. C. (1988). H3-receptors control histamine release in human brain. *J. Neurochem.* 51, 105–108. doi: 10.1111/j.1471-4159.1988.tb04841.x

Arrang, J. M., Garbarg, M., Lancelot, J. C., Lecomte, J. M., Pollard, H., Robba, M., et al. (1987a). Highly potent and selective ligands for histamine H3-receptors. *Nature* 327, 117–123. doi: 10.1038/327117a0

Arrang, J. M., Garbarg, M., and Schwartz, J. C. (1983). Auto-inhibition of brain histamine release mediated by a novel class (H3) of histamine receptor. *Nature* 302, 832–837. doi: 10.1038/302832a0

Arrang, J. M., Garbarg, M., and Schwartz, J. C. (1985). Autoregulation of histamine release in brain by presynaptic H3-receptors. *Neuroscience* 15, 553–562. doi: 10.1016/0306-4522(85)90233-7

Arrang, J. M., Garbarg, M., and Schwartz, J. C. (1987b). Autoinhibition of histamine synthesis mediated by presynaptic H3-receptors. *Neuroscience* 23, 149–157. doi: 10.1016/0306-4522(87)90279-X

Arrang, J. M., Morisset, S., and Gbahou, F. (2007). Constitutive activity of the histamine H3 receptor. *Trends Pharmacol. Sci.* 28, 350–357. doi: 10.1016/j.tips.2007.05.002

Bahi, A., Sadek, B., Nurulain, S. M., Lazewska, D., and Kiec-Kononowicz, K. (2015). The novel non-imidazole histamine H receptor antagonist DL77 reduces voluntary alcohol intake and ethanol-induced conditioned place preference in mice. *Physiol. Behav.* 151, 189–197. doi: 10.1016/j.physbeh.2015.07.012

Barak, S., and Weiner, I. (2011). Putative cognitive enhancers in preclinical models related to schizophrenia: the search for an elusive target. *Pharmacol. Biochem. Behav.* 99, 164–189. doi: 10.1016/j.pbb.2011.03.011

Bardgett, M. E., Davis, N. N., Schultheis, P. J., and Griffith, M. S. (2010). Ciproxifan, an H3 receptor antagonist, alleviates hyperactivity and cognitive deficits in the APP Tg2576 mouse model of Alzheimer's disease. *Neurobiol. Learn. Mem.* 95, 64–72. doi: 10.1016/j.nlm.2010.10.008

Benetti, F., Baldi, E., Bucherelli, C., Blandina, P., and Passani, M. B. (2013). Histaminergic ligands injected into the nucleus basalis magnocellularis differentially affect fear conditioning consolidation. *Int. J. Neuropsychopharmacol.* 16, 575–582. doi: 10.1017/S1461145712000181

Benetti, F., and Izquierdo, I. (2013). Histamine infused into basolateral amygdala enhances memory consolidation of inhibitory avoidance. *Int. J. Neuropsychopharmacol.* 16, 1539–1545. doi: 10.1017/S1461145712001514

Bernaerts, P., Lamberty, Y., and Tirelli, E. (2004). Histamine H3 antagonist thioperamide dose-dependently enhances memory consolidation and reverses amnesia induced by dizocilpine or scopolamine in a one-trial inhibitory avoidance task in mice. *Behav. Brain Res.* 154, 211–219. doi: 10.1016/j.bbr.2004.02.017

Bhowmik, M., Khanam, R., and Vohora, D. (2012). Histamine H3 receptor antagonists in relation to epilepsy and neurodegeneration: a systemic consideration of recent progress and perspectives. *Br. J. Pharmacol.* 167, 1398–1414. doi: 10.1111/j.1476-5381.2012.02093.x

Bhowmik, M., Saini, N., and Vohora, D. (2014). Histamine H3 receptor antagonism by ABT-239 attenuates kainic acid induced excitotoxicity in mice. *Brain Res.* 1581, 129–140. doi: 10.1016/j.brainres.2014.06.012

Brabant, C., Charlier, Y., and Tirelli, E. (2013). The histamine H(3)-receptor inverse agonist pitolisant improves fear memory in mice. *Behav. Brain Res.* 243, 199–204. doi: 10.1016/j.bbr.2012.12.063

Brioni, J. D., Esbenshade, T. A., Garrison, T. R., Bitner, S. R., and Cowart, M. D. (2011). Discovery of histamine H3 antagonists for the treatment of cognitive disorders and Alzheimer's disease. *J. Pharmacol. Exp. Ther.* 336, 38–46. doi: 10.1124/jpet.110.166876

Browman, K. E., Komater, V. A., Curzon, P., Rueter, L. E., Hancock, A. A., Decker, M. W., et al. (2004). Enhancement of prepulse inhibition of startle in mice by the H3 receptor antagonists thioperamide and ciproxifan. *Behav. Brain Res.* 153, 69–76. doi: 10.1016/j.bbr.2003.11.001

Brown, J. W., Whitehead, C. A., Basso, A. M., Rueter, L. E., and Zhang, M. (2013). Preclinical evaluation of non-imidazole histamine H3 receptor antagonists in comparison to atypical antipsychotics for the treatment of cognitive deficits associated with schizophrenia. *Int. J. Neuropsychopharmacol.* 16, 889–904. doi: 10.1017/S1461145712000739

Brown, R. E., Stevens, D. R., and Haas, H. L. (2001). The physiology of brain histamine. *Prog. Neurobiol.* 63, 637–672. doi: 10.1016/S0301-0082(00)00039-3

Callahan, P. M., Bertrand, D., Bertrand, S., Plagenhoef, M. R., and Terry, A. V. Jr. (2017). Tropisetron sensitizes alpha7 containing nicotinic receptors to low levels of acetylcholine *in vitro* and improves memory-related task performance in young and aged animals. *Neuropharmacology* 117, 422–433. doi: 10.1016/j.neuropharm.2017.02.025

Charlier, Y., Brabant, C., Serrano, M. E., Lamberty, Y., and Tirelli, E. (2013). The prototypical histamine H3 receptor inverse agonist thioperamide improves multiple aspects of memory processing in an inhibitory avoidance task. *Behav. Brain Res.* 253, 121–127. doi: 10.1016/j.bbr.2013.07.016

da Silva, A. L., Silva Martins, B., Linck Vde, M., Herrmann, A. P., Mai, N., Nunes, D. S., et al. (2009). MK801- and scopolamine-induced amnesias are reversed by an Amazonian herbal locally used as a "brain tonic". *Psychopharmacology* 202, 165–172. doi: 10.1007/s00213-008-1272-y

de Lima, M. N., Laranja, D. C., Bromberg, E., Roesler, R., and Schroder, N. (2005). Pre- or post-training administration of the NMDA receptor blocker MK-801 impairs object recognition memory in rats. *Behav. Brain Res.* 156, 139–143. doi: 10.1016/j.bbr.2004.05.016

Doraiswamy, P. M. (2002). Non-cholinergic strategies for treating and preventing Alzheimer's disease. *CNS Drugs* 16, 811–824. doi: 10.2165/00023210-200216120-00003

Ennaceur, A., and Delacour, J. (1988). A new one-trial test for neurobiological studies of memory in rats. 1: behavioral data. *Behav. Brain Res.* 31, 47–59. doi: 10.1016/0166-4328(88)90157-X

Ennaceur, A., and Meliani, K. (1992a). Effects of physostigmine and scopolamine on rats' performances in object-recognition and radial-maze tests. *Psychopharmacology* 109, 321–330. doi: 10.1007/BF02245880

Ennaceur, A., and Meliani, K. (1992b). A new one-trial test for neurobiological studies of memory in rats. III. Spatial vs. non-spatial working memory. *Behav. Brain Res.* 51, 83–92. doi: 10.1016/S0166-4328(05)80315-8

Fernandes, C., and File, S. E. (1996). The influence of open arm ledges and maze experience in the elevated plus-maze. *Pharmacol. Biochem. Behav.* 54, 31–40. doi: 10.1016/0091-3057(95)02171-X

Giannoni, P., Medhurst, A. D., Passani, M. B., Giovannini, M. G., Ballini, C., Corte, L. D., et al. (2010). Regional differential effects of the novel histamine H3 receptor antagonist 6-[(3-cyclobutyl-2,3,4,5-tetrahydro-1H-3-benzazepin-7-yl)oxy]-N-methyl-3-pyridine carboxamide hydrochloride (GSK189254) on histamine release in the central nervous system of freely moving rats. *J. Pharmacol. Exp. Ther.* 332, 164–172. doi: 10.1124/jpet.109.158444

Giovannini, M. G., Bartolini, L., Bacciottini, L., Greco, L., and Blandina, P. (1999). Effects of histamine H3 receptor agonists and antagonists on cognitive performance and scopolamine-induced amnesia. *Behav. Brain Res.* 104, 147–155. doi: 10.1016/S0166-4328(99)00063-7

Goshadrou, F., Kermani, M., Ronaghi, A., and Sajjadi, S. (2013). The effect of ghrelin on MK-801 induced memory impairment in rats. *Peptides* 44, 60–65. doi: 10.1016/j.peptides.2013.03.022

Griebel, G., Pichat, P., Pruniaux, M. P., Beeske, S., Lopez-Grancha, M., Genet, E., et al. (2012). SAR110894, a potent histamine H(3)-receptor antagonist, displays procognitive effects in rodents. *Pharmacol. Biochem. Behav.* 102, 203–214. doi: 10.1016/j.pbb.2012.04.004

Harada, C., Hirai, T., Fujii, Y., Harusawa, S., Kurihara, T., and Kamei, C. (2004). Intracerebroventricular administration of histamine H3 receptor antagonists decreases seizures in rat models of epilepsia. *Methods Find. Exp. Clin. Pharmacol.* 26, 263–270.

Hogg, S. (1996). A review of the validity and variability of the elevated plus-maze as an animal model of anxiety. *Pharmacol. Biochem. Behav.* 54, 21–30. doi: 10.1016/0091-3057(95)02126-4

Izquierdo, I., Medina, J. H., Vianna, M. R., Izquierdo, L. A., and Barros, D. M. (1999). Separate mechanisms for short- and long-term memory. *Behav. Brain Res.* 103, 1–11. doi: 10.1016/S0166-4328(99)00036-4

Jaaro-Peled, H. (2009). Gene models of schizophrenia: DISC1 mouse models. *Prog. Brain Res.* 179, 75–86. doi: 10.1016/S0079-6123(09)17909-8

Jiang, Y. M., Li, X. J., Meng, Z. Z., Liu, Y. Y., Zhao, H. B., Li, N., et al. (2016). Effects of xiaoyaosan on stress-induced anxiety-like behavior in rats: involvement of CRF1 receptor. *Evid. Based Complement. Alternat. Med.* 2016:1238426. doi: 10.1155/2016/1238426

Karasawa, J., Hashimoto, K., and Chaki, S. (2008). D-Serine and a glycine transporter inhibitor improve MK-801-induced cognitive deficits in a novel object recognition test in rats. *Behav. Brain Res.* 186, 78–83. doi: 10.1016/j.bbr.2007.07.033

Khan, N., Saad, A., Nurulain, S. M., Darras, F. H., Decker, M., and Sadek, B. (2015). The dual-acting H3 receptor antagonist and AChE inhibitor UW-MD-71 dose-dependently enhances memory retrieval and reverses dizocilpine-induced memory impairment in rats. *Behav. Brain Res.* 297, 155–164. doi: 10.1016/j.bbr.2015.10.022

Khunnawutmanotham, N., Chimnoi, N., Saparpakorn, P., and Techasakul, S. (2016). Synthesis and anti-acetylcholinesterase activity of scopoletin derivatives. *Bioorg. Chem.* 65, 137–145. doi: 10.1016/j.bioorg.2015.12.002

King, M. V., Sleight, A. J., Woolley, M. L., Topham, I. A., Marsden, C. A., and Fone, K. C. (2004). 5-HT6 receptor antagonists reverse delay-dependent deficits in novel object discrimination by enhancing consolidation–an effect sensitive to NMDA receptor antagonism. *Neuropharmacology* 47, 195–204. doi: 10.1016/j.neuropharm.2004.03.012

Krause, M., Stark, H., and Schunack, W. (2001). Azomethine prodrugs of (R)-alpha-methylhistamine, a highly potent and selective histamine H3-receptor agonist. *Curr. Med. Chem.* 8, 1329–1340. doi: 10.2174/0929867013372274

Łazewska, D., Ligneau, X., Schwartz, J. C., Schunack, W., Stark, H., and Kiec-Kononowicz, K. (2006). Ether derivatives of 3-piperidinopropan-1-ol as non-imidazole histamine H3 receptor antagonists. *Bioorg. Med. Chem.* 14, 3522–3529. doi: 10.1016/j.bmc.2006.01.013

Lebrun, C., Pillière, E., and Lestage, P. (2000). Effects of S 18986-1, a novel cognitive enhancer, on memory performances in an object recognition task in rats. *Eur. J. Pharmacol.* 401, 205–212. doi: 10.1016/S0014-2999(00)00429-5

Ligneau, X., Perrin, D., Landais, L., Camelin, J. C., Calmels, T. P., Berrebi-Bertrand, I., et al. (2007). BF2.649 [1-{3-[3-(4-Chlorophenyl)propoxy]propyl}piperidine, hydrochloride], a nonimidazole inverse agonist/antagonist at the human histamine H3 receptor: preclinical pharmacology. *J. Pharmacol. Exp. Ther.* 320, 365–375. doi: 10.1124/jpet.106.111039

McGaugh, J. L., and Roozendaal, B. (2009). Drug enhancement of memory consolidation: historical perspective and neurobiological implications. *Psychopharmacology* 202, 3–14. doi: 10.1007/s00213-008-1285-6

Meier, G., Apelt, J., Reichert, U., Grassmann, S., Ligneau, X., Elz, S., et al. (2001). Influence of imidazole replacement in different structural classes of histamine H_3-receptor antagonists. *Eur. J. Pharm. Sci.* 13, 249–259. doi: 10.1016/S0928-0987(01)00106-3

Orsetti, M., Ferretti, C., Gamalero, R., and Ghi, P. (2002). Histamine H3-receptor blockade in the rat nucleus basalis magnocellularis improves place recognition memory. *Psychopharmacology* 159, 133–137. doi: 10.1007/s002130100892

Orsetti, M., Ghi, P., and Di Carlo, G. (2001). Histamine H(3)-receptor antagonism improves memory retention and reverses the cognitive deficit induced by scopolamine in a two-trial place recognition task. *Behav. Brain Res.* 124, 235–242. doi: 10.1016/S0166-4328(01)00216-9

Panula, P., Chazot, P. L., Cowart, M., Gutzmer, R., Leurs, R., Liu, W. L., et al. (2015). International union of basic and clinical pharmacology. XCVIII. Histamine Receptors. *Pharmacol. Rev.* 67, 601–655. doi: 10.1124/pr.114.010249

Panula, P., and Nuutinen, S. (2011). Histamine and H3 receptor in alcohol-related behaviors. *J. Pharmacol. Exp. Ther.* 336, 9–16. doi: 10.1124/jpet.110.170928

Panula, P., Rinne, J., Kuokkanen, K., Eriksson, K. S., Sallmen, T., Kalimo, H., et al. (1998). Neuronal histamine deficit in Alzheimer's disease. *Neuroscience* 82, 993–997. doi: 10.1016/S0306-4522(97)00353-9

Pascoli, V., Boer-Saccomani, C., and Hermant, J. F. (2009). H3 receptor antagonists reverse delay-dependent deficits in novel object discrimination by enhancing retrieval. *Psychopharmacology* 202, 141–152. doi: 10.1007/s00213-008-1171-2

Pichat, P., Bergis, O. E., Terranova, J. P., Urani, A., Duarte, C., Santucci, V., et al. (2007). SSR180711, a novel selective alpha7 nicotinic receptor partial agonist: (II) efficacy in experimental models predictive of activity against cognitive symptoms of schizophrenia. *Neuropsychopharmacology* 32, 17–34. doi: 10.1038/sj.npp.1301188

Provensi, G., Costa, A., Passani, M. B., and Blandina, P. (2016). Donepezil, an acetylcholine esterase inhibitor, and ABT-239, a histamine H3 receptor antagonist/inverse agonist, require the integrity of brain histamine system to exert biochemical and procognitive effects in the mouse. *Neuropharmacology* 109, 139–147. doi: 10.1016/j.neuropharm.2016.06.010

Sadek, B., Khan, N., Darras, F. H., Pockes, S., and Decker, M. (2016a). The dual-acting AChE inhibitor and H3 receptor antagonist UW-MD-72 reverses amnesia induced by scopolamine or dizocilpine in passive avoidance paradigm in rats. *Physiol. Behav.* 165, 383–391. doi: 10.1016/j.physbeh.2016.08.022

Sadek, B., Saad, A., Sadeq, A., Jalal, F., and Stark, H. (2016b). Histamine H3 receptor as a potential target for cognitive symptoms in neuropsychiatric diseases. *Behav. Brain Res.* 312, 415–430. doi: 10.1016/j.bbr.2016.06.051

Sadek, B., Saad, A., Subramanian, D., Shafiullah, M., Łazewska, D., and Kieć-Kononowiczc, K. (2016c). Anticonvulsant and procognitive properties of the non-imidazole histamine H3 receptor antagonist DL77 in male adult rats. *Neuropharmacology* 106, 46–55. doi: 10.1016/j.neuropharm.2015.10.023

Sadek, B., and Stark, H. (2015). Cherry-picked ligands at histamine receptor subtypes. *Neuropharmacology* 106, 56–73. doi: 10.1016/j.neuropharm.2015.11.005

Schneider, E. H., and Seifert, R. (2009). Histamine H(4) receptor-RGS fusion proteins expressed in Sf9 insect cells: a sensitive and reliable approach for the functional characterization of histamine H(4) receptor ligands. *Biochem. Pharmacol.* 78, 607–616. doi: 10.1016/j.bcp.2009.05.015

Schwartz, J. C., Arrang, J. M., Garbarg, M., and Korner, M. (1986). Properties and roles of the three subclasses of histamine receptors in brain. *J. Exp. Biol.* 124, 203–224.

Shaik, J. B., Palaka, B. K., Penumala, M., Kotapati, K. V., Devineni, S. R., Eadlapalli, S., et al. (2016). Synthesis, pharmacological assessment, molecular modeling and *in silico* studies of fused tricyclic coumarin derivatives as a new family of multifunctional anti-Alzheimer agents. *Eur. J. Med. Chem.* 107, 219–232. doi: 10.1016/j.ejmech.2015.10.046

Sultan, A., Yang, K. S., Isaev, D., Nebrisi, E. E., Syed, N., Khan, N., et al. (2017). Thujone inhibits the function of alpha7-nicotinic acetylcholine receptors and impairs nicotine-induced memory enhancement in one-trial passive avoidance paradigm. *Toxicology* 384, 23–32. doi: 10.1016/j.tox.2017.04.005

Tseng, K. Y., Chambers, R. A., and Lipska, B. K. (2009). The neonatal ventral hippocampal lesion as a heuristic neurodevelopmental model of schizophrenia. *Behav. Brain Res.* 204, 295–305. doi: 10.1016/j.bbr.2008.11.039

Uma Devi, P., Manocha, A., Khanam, R., and Vohora, D. (2010). Beneficial interaction between clobenpropit and pyridoxine in prevention of electroshock-induced seizures in mice: lack of histaminergic mechanisms. *Hum. Exp. Toxicol.* 30, 84–88. doi: 10.1177/0960327110372398

Vorobjev, V. S., Sharonova, I. N., Walsh, I. B., and Haas, H. L. (1993). Histamine potentiates N-methyl-D-aspartate responses in acutely isolated hippocampal neurons. *Neuron* 11, 837–844. doi: 10.1016/0896-6273(93)90113-6

Witkin, J. M., and Nelson, D. L. (2004). Selective histamine H3 receptor antagonists for treatment of cognitive deficiencies and other disorders of the central nervous system. *Pharmacol. Ther.* 103, 1–20. doi: 10.1016/j.pharmthera.2004.05.001

Xu, L. S., Yang, L. X., Hu, W. W., Yu, X., Ma, L., Liu, L. Y., et al. (2005). Histamine ameliorates spatial memory deficits induced by MK-801 infusion into ventral hippocampus as evaluated by radial maze task in rats. *Acta Pharmacol. Sin.* 26, 1448–1453. doi: 10.1111/j.1745-7254.2005.00229.x

Yokoyama, H. (2001). The role of central histaminergic neuron system as an anticonvulsive mechanism in developing brain. *Brain Dev.* 23, 542–547. doi: 10.1016/S0387-7604(01)00261-3

Yokoyama, H., Onodera, K., Iinuma, K., and Watanabe, T. (1993). Effect of thioperamide, a histamine H3 receptor antagonist, on electrically induced convulsions in mice. *Eur. J. Pharmacol.* 234, 129–133. doi: 10.1016/0014-2999(93)90717-V

14

An Algorithm for Preclinical Diagnosis of Alzheimer's Disease

*Tapan K. Khan**

Center for Neurodegenerative Diseases, Blanchette Rockefeller Neurosciences Institute, West Virginia University, Morgantown, WV, United States

***Correspondence:**
Tapan K. Khan
tkhan@hsc.wvu.edu

Almost all Alzheimer's disease (AD) therapeutic trials have failed in recent years. One of the main reasons for failure is due to designing the disease-modifying clinical trials at the advanced stage of the disease when irreversible brain damage has already occurred. Diagnosis of the preclinical stage of AD and therapeutic intervention at this phase, with a perfect target, are key points to slowing the progression of the disease. Various AD biomarkers hold enormous promise for identifying individuals with preclinical AD and predicting the development of AD dementia in the future, but no single AD biomarker has the capability to distinguish the AD preclinical stage. A combination of complimentary AD biomarkers in cerebrospinal fluid ($A\beta_{42}$, tau, and phosphor-tau), non-invasive neuroimaging, and genetic evidence of AD can detect preclinical AD in the *in-vivo* ante mortem brain. Neuroimaging studies have examined region-specific cerebral blood flow (CBF) and microstructural changes in the preclinical AD brain. Functional MRI (fMRI), diffusion tensor imaging (DTI) MRI, arterial spin labeling (ASL) MRI, and advanced PET have potential application in preclinical AD diagnosis. A well-validated simple framework for diagnosis of preclinical AD is urgently needed. This article proposes a comprehensive preclinical AD diagnostic algorithm based on neuroimaging, CSF biomarkers, and genetic markers.

Keywords: Alzheimer's disease, neuroimaging (anatomic and functional), CSF, diagnosis, differential, preclinical Alzheimer's disease

INTRODUCTION

Therapeutic interventions for Alzheimer's disease (AD) will have a better chance of success if initiated at the earliest stage (preclinical), before the synaptic loss and neuronal death occur. Therefore, an effective disease-modifying clinical trial should target the stage before the manifestation of clinical symptoms of memory loss and cognitive impairment. The term preclinical AD is initially described to classify cognitively normal individuals with evidence of amyloid plaques and hyperphosphorylated tau (p-tau) tangles (hallmarks of AD pathology) at time of brain autopsy (Hubbard et al., 1990). This definition of preclinical AD was built on the existing AD mechanistic hypothesis. Several longitudinal studies predicted the conversion of mild cognitive impairment (MCI) to AD when there is amyloid plaques and p-tau tangles in the brain (Petersen et al., 1999, 2001; Grand et al., 2011). In preclinical familial AD cases, Fox et al. (1999) were the first to use serial structural magnetic resonance imaging (MRI) to detect cerebral atrophy in a longitudinal study of asymptomatic individuals (no cognitive impairment) at high risk of the familial AD (autosomal dominant early-onset before 65 years of age). Since that study, several groups have examined the predictive capacity of various brain biomarkers, such as noninvasive neuroimaging modalities, and invasive cerebrospinal fluid (CSF) biomarkers ($A\beta_{42}$, tau, and p-tau). These studies concluded that patients who are positive for various AD biomarkers in the preclinical AD stage are at higher risk of progressing to AD dementia (Mintun et al., 2006; Villemagne et al., 2008; Johnson et al., 2012; Dubois et al., 2016). Non-invasive neuroimaging modalities, such as positron emission tomography (PET), functional MRI (fMRI), diffusion tensor imaging (DTI) MRI, and arterial spin labeling (ASL) MRI hold enormous promise for identifying preclinical AD (Mintun et al., 2006; Mosconi et al., 2006; Villemagne et al., 2008; Johnson et al., 2012; Ewers et al., 2013; Dubois et al., 2016) (**Table 2**). CSF biomarkers can predict decreasing cognitive ability in studies of conversion of MCI to AD (Frölich et al., 2017) and predicting memory deficit in longitudinal studies of normal individuals (Fagan et al., 2007; Gustafson et al., 2007; Stomrud et al., 2007; Jansen et al., 2015). AD is a multifactorial disease with several genetic biomarkers are found to be involved (http://www.alzgene.org) in the pathogenesis of AD. Those genes increase the predictability of conversion of preclinical AD to MCI and finally AD. In this perspective review, we describe the utility of combining neuroimaging, CSF, and genetic AD biomarker in the diagnosis of preclinical AD and propose a comprehensive preclinical AD diagnostic algorithm.

Preclinical Stage of Alzheimer's Disease

The National Institute on Aging and Alzheimer's Association (NIA-AA) (2011) introduced the concept of "preclinical AD" that arises before MCI and advanced stages of AD. The most recent definition of preclinical AD, proposed in a joint meeting of NIA-AA and the International Working Group (IWG) in 2015 (Dubois et al., 2016), is the simplest: preclinical AD starts the day that pathological AD lesions appear without any clinical symptoms. The NIA-AA guideline (2011) divides the progression of AD into distinct phases, taking into account both AD pathobiology and clinical symptoms: preclinical, asymptomatic pre-dementia; symptomatic pre-dementia (MCI); and dementia due to AD (McKhann et al., 2011; Sperling et al., 2011). Before that, preclinical stage AD biomarkers were categorized as Stage 1: amyloidosis by PET and CSF $A\beta_{42}$ analysis, and Stage 2: Neurodegeneration by PET and CSF tau (Jack et al., 2010). The preclinical phase can also be separated into "pre-symptomatic" and "asymptomatic at risk" suggested by IGW–2014 (Dubois et al., 2014). The pre-symptomatic preclinical AD refers to individuals with familial AD who will develop AD in the future. Individuals with pre-symptomatic preclinical AD show no clinical symptoms but have at least one mutation in the familial AD genes (APP, PSEN1, PSEN2). Asymptomatic at risk refers to preclinical AD in individuals without clinical symptoms, but positive for AD biomarkers (decreased level of $A\beta_{42}$, increased the level of tau p-tau in CSF) or positive in Aβ-PET (Dubois et al., 2014). According to the NIA-AA (2011) progressive preclinical AD pathological trajectory can be divided into three distinguishable stages: in the first stage, there is evidence of abnormality in Aβ, and individuals in this stage would be positive for Aβ, no dementia or neurodegeneration. The second stage consists of positive for Aβ, plus higher CSF tau (neurodegeneration). In the third stage, individuals begin exhibiting evidence of memory problems along with abnormalities in CSF biomarkers and neuroimaging, but all evidence of memory problems is less than MCI cases (Sperling et al., 2011).

CRITICAL EVALUATION OF IGW AND NIA-AA PRECLINICAL ALZHEIMER'S DISEASE CRITERIA

AD pathology is a continuum process spanning many years of underlying changes in brain morphology due to preclinical AD stage to a clinical AD phase. Hippocampus volume loss, temporoparietal hypometabolism, and neocortical Aβ deposition are the first to be affected in brain areas due to preclinical AD pathology. Metabolic brain networks of these areas are affected by age as well as by preclinical AD. White matter brain network is the primary area that is also affected in preclinical AD. On the cellular level, the synaptic and the axonal degenerations start to occur, but such degenerations would not affect the overall memory at the preclinical AD stage. The critical point is how and when the *in-vivo* AD-related pathology that determines preclinical AD can be measured by AD-biomarkers. The revised IWG definition of a preclinical AD: no clinical sign of AD but has at least one positive pathological AD biomarker (Dubois et al., 2016). In a critical viewpoint, it will be very difficult to distinguish preclinical AD by only one AD-biomarker. On the other hand, the NIA-AA definition of preclinical AD is more generalized (not specific): evidence of amyloidosis and neurodegeneration (Sperling et al., 2011). Here also we need the more specific definition of the role and applicability of AD *in-vivo* pathological biomarkers. The revised IWG definition of preclinical AD is too simplified to find the right condition to diagnose preclinical AD. Therefore, neither of them are perfect for determining *in-vivo* preclinical AD by AD pathological biomarkers. Both IGW and NIA-AA definition of preclinical AD considered amyloidosis ahead of tauopathy. There is evidence that neurodegeneration due to high tau or tauopathy started before amyloidosis (Jack and Holtzman, 2013; Jack et al., 2013). The phenomenon of mixed pathologies (AD with non-AD dementia) underlying the preclinical AD stage of neurodegeneration has been completely ignored by both (IGW and NIA-AA) the definitions of preclinical AD.

HYPOTHETICAL MODEL OF PRECLINICAL ALZHEIMER'S DISEASE AND PROGRESSION OF ALZHEIMER'S DISEASE

A hypothetical model of AD progression in relation to aging and disease severity is shown in **Figure 1**. The disease severity increases as age increases, because age is the most important risk factor for AD dementia. Two trajectories of AD progression are shown, one based on changes in brain morphology (red) and the other is the onset of clinical symptoms of neurodegeneration (blue). Neurodegeneration due to normal aging is shown as a

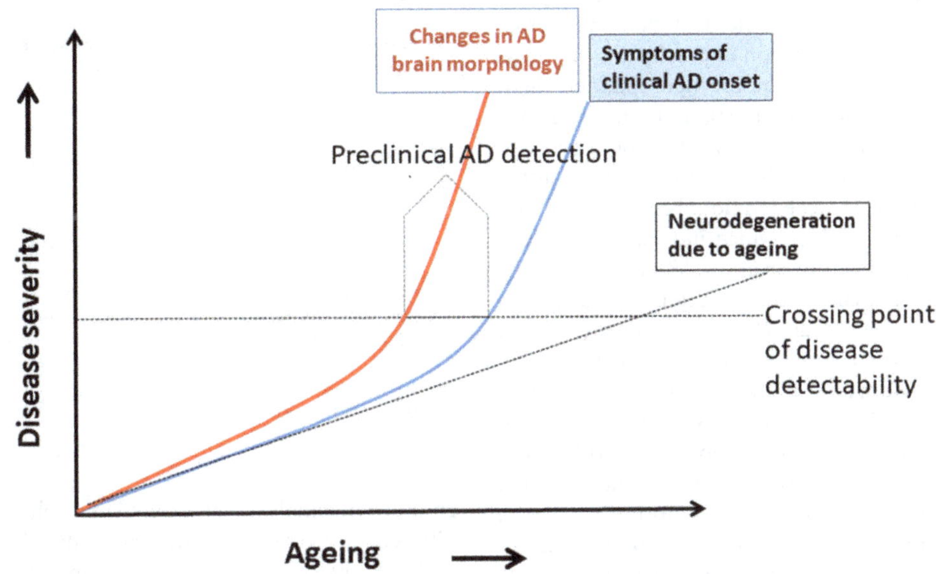

FIGURE 1 | A hypothetical model for detecting preclinical Alzheimer's disease (AD). Disease severity increases with aging, the major risk factor for an AD. Two disease trajectories represent brain morphology changes (red) and clinical AD symptoms (blue). Neurodegeneration due to aging shown by the broken black line. The model shows the hypothetical deviation of the changes in brain morphology trajectory and symptoms trajectory, and where they cross a horizontal line of disease detectability. The preclinical AD can be detected before the onset of AD symptoms (modified from Khan, 2016).

broken black line. The model shows deviations of the brain morphology trajectory and the clinical symptoms trajectory as they cross a hypothetical line of disease detectability. The trajectory of neurodegeneration due to normal aging crosses this line much later in life. Note that the changes in brain morphology increased much earlier than clinical symptoms; this indicates that the pathological changes and abnormalities in brain cell signaling (neuronal network function) occur earlier in disease progression than symptoms, such that CSF biomarkers, for example, would be detectable even in the absence of symptoms. Preclinical AD could thus be detected before the onset of AD symptoms (**Figure 1**). Preclinical diagnosis of AD is possible when brain morphology due to AD pathology started to change (box "Preclinical AD detection" in **Figure 1**), (subtle changes in brain white matters, minute changes in brain metabolites, and abnormalities in the neuronal network by functional MRI) and biomarkers of brain morphology changes can detect such signals. It is at this point in disease progression that advanced non-invasive neuroimaging of morphologic biomarkers with modalities, such as rs-fMRI, DTI MRI, ASL MRI, and PET, have enormous potential for diagnosis of preclinical AD.

The abnormalities in the brain due to the onset of AD pathology start 10–20 years before symptoms of cognitive deficiencies appear in genetically susceptible cases (Morris, 2005; Reiman et al., 2012). In one study, brain MRI was used to image brain atrophy in individuals classified as asymptomatic AD mutation carriers (presymptomatic preclinical). A recent study found that brain atrophy could be detected 1–8 years before the clinical symptoms of familial AD appeared (Kinnunen et al., 2017). A similar approach to detecting preclinical AD based on MRI-measured brain atrophy over time is not as simple for sporadic AD, however. More research is necessary to validate the preclinical AD category of "asymptomatic at risk." Brain amyloidosis (higher Aβ deposition) in a cognitively normal individual has a higher likelihood of progression from preclinical stages to symptomatic stages of AD.

APPLICABILITY OF CEREBROSPINAL FLUID (CSF) BIOMARKERS IN PRECLINICAL ALZHEIMER'S DISEASE DIAGNOSIS

Widely researched CSF AD biomarkers are low $A\beta_{42}$, high tau, and high p-tau (phosphorylated tau) levels compared to age-matched non-demented controls. Three CSF biomarkers represent three different aspects of AD brain pathology, respectively. Low levels of $A\beta_{42}$ reflects higher amyloid plaques (amylolysis), high levels of tau represents neurodegeneration, and high p-tau level correlates with high levels of neurofibrillary tangles (NFTs) in the AD brain. As a single test CSF biomarkers are not accurate to detect conversion of MCI to AD; however, negative CSF results in MCI cases can accurately predict conversion of non-Alzheimer's disease (Ritchie et al., 2017). Moreover, an evaluation of CSF biomarkers found them to have the ability to predict memory decline in individuals with aging (Fagan et al., 2007; Gustafson et al., 2007; Stomrud et al., 2007; Jansen et al., 2015). Therefore, CSF biomarkers can be used as part of a preclinical biomarker panel that can predict developing AD in the future.

CSF biomarker patterns of preclinical AD were found to be different in middle aged asymptomatic cases in a recent longitudinal study (Sutphen et al., 2015). Besides established AD CSF, ($A\beta_{42}$, tau, and p-tau) there are other CSF biomarkers that are more close to the neurodegeneration in preclinical AD stage. Such recently studied CSF biomarkers are neurofilament light chain, neurogranin, inflammatory markers, and tau fragments. Levels of CSF neurogranin are high in AD and progressive AD cases (Kester et al., 2015). Higher levels of neurogranin represent synaptic dysfunction and neurodegeneration. Neurogranin level was correlated with tau but not Aβ, which indicates it can be a measure of neurodegeneration, not levels of Aβ deposition. The levels of neurofilament light chain concentration were also high in AD progression (Zetterberg et al., 2016). Neurofilament light chain is a measure of axonal degeneration due to underlying preclinical AD. CSF inflammatory markers such as IL-15, MCP-1, VEGFR-1, sICAM1, sVCAM-1, and VEGF-D were found to correlate with the levels of tau and p-tau (Popp et al., 2017). More research and validation is needed for these newly incorporated CSF biomarkers before considering them definitive preclinical AD biomarkers. Longitudinal follow-up of CSF biomarkers in individuals in risk cohort will be more effective than cross-sectional cohort for determining preclinical AD progression.

ADVANCED MRI AND PET-BASED NEUROIMAGING FOR THE DIAGNOSIS OF PRECLINICAL ALZHEIMER'S DISEASE

Non-invasive imaging of the brain is a promising tool for the early detection of AD. The most widely researched neuroimaging biomarkers of AD are summarized in **Table 1**. Advanced neuroimaging techniques are most promising in detecting the disease at its earliest stage for initiating therapeutic intervention and finding individuals at risk of AD. In fact, hippocampus volume is one of the first brain areas affected due to preclinical AD pathology. Advanced MRI-based neuroimaging techniques and protocols have been introduced to detect more subtle changes in brain tissues at the microscopic level (**Table 2**). Tissues and cell damage that precede neurodegeneration include loss of synapses, loss of axonal integrity, demyelination, loss of microtubule assembly, and minute changes in levels of brain metabolites. Resting-state functional MRI (rs-fMRI), DTI, and ASL MRI have been developed to detect these preclinical AD biomarkers and are described here. Longitudinal follow-up of imaging biomarkers in individuals in an at risk cohort will be more effective than a cross-sectional cohort for determining preclinical AD progression.

Resting-State Functional MRI (rs-fMRI)

Resting-state functional MRI was first developed by Biswal et al. (1995) to detect low-frequency fluctuations in the resting brain. In principle, it measures changes in paramagnetic properties of oxyhemoglobin/deoxy-hemoglobin in blood flowing through different brain regions influenced by changes in neuronal network activity. In the resting brain, the neuronal network is linearly dependent on spontaneous low-frequency fluctuations of the blood oxygen-dependent (BOLD) signals detected by fMRI in different brain areas. In a task-free state, functional connectivity analysis can detect subtle changes in brain network differences between individuals with the early-stage disease and healthy controls. The neuronal network and synaptic activities are beginning to change in preclinical AD, before the symptomatic manifestation of AD. Thus, rs-fMRI enables functional connectivity analysis to detect subtle brain network abnormalities in the very beginning of AD pathology in the brain. Recently, lower functional connectivity measured by rs-fMRI has also been demonstrated to be an indicator of pre-MCI and pre-dementia due to AD in longitudinal studies of individuals with preclinical AD (Buckley et al., 2017) (**Table 2**).

TABLE 1 | Neuroimaging biomarkers in Alzheimer's disease.

Neuroimaging biomarker	Biomarker readout associated with AD
MRI*	Atrophy
fMRI	Disrupted neural network
^{11}C-PIB PET*	Increased amyloid plaque binding to PIB
^{18}F-Aβ-binding compound-PET**	Higher amount of amyloid in brain
^{18}FDG-PET*	Low brain metabolism measured by decreased glucose uptake

Aβ, amyloid beta; AD, Alzheimer's disease; FDG, fluoro-2-deoxy-D-glucose; fMRI, functional MRI; MRI, magnetic resonance imaging; PET, positron emission tomography; PIB, Pittsburgh compound B.

**Included in the NIA-2011 and IWG–2014 criteria to support diagnosis of AD for research purposes.*

*** Approved by FDA and EMA.*

Diffusion Tensor Imaging (DTI) With sMRI

DTI, sometimes called diffusion-weighted imaging (DWI), was developed in the last decade of the twentieth century (Moseley et al., 1990; Beaulieu and Allen, 1994; Pierpaoli and Basser, 1996; Pierpaoli et al., 1996). In principle, it measures the probability distribution of diffusion of water molecules in the brain in terms of the diffusion tensor. In the ideal case, if there are no hindrances, the probability distribution of diffusion of water molecules should be isotropic. A brain has nerve fibers and tightly associated axonal bundles; therefore, the distribution of water molecules should be highly anisotropic in non-demented normal brains. The phenomenon of white matter loss starts at the preclinical AD stage. This loss of white matter decreases the anisotropic nature of the diffusion of the water molecules. DTI calculates two measurable quantities from the anisotropic nature of diffusion of water molecules by sMRI in the region of interest in the brain. Those two quantities are fractional anisotropy (FA) and mean diffusion coefficient (MD). Increased MD and decreased FA values indicate loss of white matter in AD and MCI brains indicating that MD and FA may be potential neuroimaging biomarkers of early-stage AD. Several studies have shown that DTI has the ability to distinguish between AD, MCI, and age-matched control case (Chua et al., 2009; a meta-analysis of 41 DTI studies by Sexton et al., 2011) (**Table 2**).

Expanding on this work, DTI technology combined with novel mathematical tools has been used recently to identify preclinical AD cases. New evidence suggests that white matter alterations begin in preclinical AD and can be measured by

TABLE 2 | Preclinical Alzheimer's disease neuroimaging biomarkers.

Modality	Parameter	Values in preclinical AD	Notes	References
rs-fMRI	Paramagnetic property of oxy-hemoglobin/deoxy-hemoglobin in blood flow	Low-frequency spontaneous fluctuation of BOLD signal Reduced functional connectivity	rs-fMRI can detect abnormalities before brain volume loss No regulatory guidelines by FDA or EMA	Machulda et al., 2011; Sheline and Raichle, 2013; Buckley et al., 2017
DTI with sMRI	Diffusion of water molecules in brain	Higher overall mean diffusivity of water molecules Lower fractional anisotropy	Region specificity Detectable abnormality in WM networks in preclinical AD No regulatory guidelines by FDA or EMA	Sexton et al., 2011; Racine et al., 2014; Fischer et al., 2015; Nedelska et al., 2015
ASL/sMRI	CBF traced by magnetically labeled water molecules	Decreased blood flow in brain	Consistent with vascular hypothesis of AD Could be useful biomarker for tracking disease severity and progression No radiotracer or contrast reagents No regulatory guidelines by FDA or EMA	Alsop et al., 2010; Wang et al., 2013; Wierenga et al., 2014; Hays et al., 2016
Aβ-PET	Radiotracer binding to amyloid beta in specific brain regions	Presence of Aβ detected with ^{11}C-PIB or ^{18}F-labeled amyloid-binding agents	Amyloid accumulation occurs before brain atrophy and is hypothesized to be the first pathological event in AD It is not correlated with AD clinical severity and neurodegeneration Can be used for differential diagnosis per FDA or EMA	Jack et al., 2009; Jagust et al., 2009; Scheinin et al., 2009; Okamura et al., 2014
^{18}FDG-PET	Glucose uptake in different brain regions	Glucose uptake using ^{18}FDG	Useful for differential diagnosis of AD and FTD Brain region-specific differentiation capability Can be used for differential diagnosis per FDA or EMA	Mosconi et al., 2006; Ewers et al., 2013, 2014
Tau-^{18}F-T807-PET	Region specific distribution of tau deposition	^{18}F-T807	Progression of AD related to neurodegeneration due to tau deposition	Johnson et al., 2016

Aβ, amyloid beta; AD, Alzheimer's disease; ASL MRI, arterial spin-labeled magnetic resonance imaging; BOLD, blood oxygen level-dependent; CBF, cerebral blood flow; DTI, diffusion tensor imaging; EMA, European Medical Agency; FDA, Food and Drug Administration; FTD, frontotemporal dementia; FDG, fluoro-2-deoxy-D-glucose; fMRI, functional MRI; MRI, magnetic resonance imaging; ^{18}F-T807-PET, Fluorinated tau PET ligand; PET, positron emission tomography; PIB, Pittsburgh Compound B; rs-fMRI, resting state functional MRI; sMRI, structural MRI; WM, white matter.

DTI (Racine et al., 2014; Kantarci et al., 2017). White matter primarily consists of axon and myelin sheets that is altered by AD pathology. Axonal degeneration and deformation of myelin sheets are early events that occur before the wide-spread neuronal loss in the AD brain. Among the neuroimaging techniques, DTI is the best suited to assess degeneration of myelinated nerve fibers in the brain. By applying tractography and graph theory in DTI, a study reported alterations within the entire white matter network in preclinical AD, even before structural markers of significant neurodegeneration, such as atrophy by MRI and reduced cortical glucose utilization by ^{18}FDG-PET, were detected (Fischer et al., 2015). Moreover, the alteration of DTI parameters (FA and MD) were correlated with common risk factors of sporadic AD (Adluru et al., 2014).

Arterial Spin Labeling (ASL) MRI

ASL/MRI imaging of AD is consistent with the hypothesis of vascular abnormality of the AD. ASL was first developed in 1992 for imaging the rat brain using magnetically labeled blood water (arterial spin labeling) followed by MRI (Detre et al., 1992). The principle of ASL is based on imaging magnetically labeled blood water in brain tissues of a region of interest by applying a 180° radio-frequency pulse (Detre et al., 2009, 2012). In the next step, the local changes of magnetization in brain tissue by blood flow with magnetically labeled water are measured by scanning with normal MRI sequence scanning mode. It has the ability to identify vascular factors in neurodegenerative diseases such as AD and vascular dementias (Detre et al., 2012). Cerebral blood flow (CBF) is a possible biomarker of AD that can be measured by ASL MRI. Typical CBF images by ASL MRI measure reduced CBF in AD, and can even differentiate between MCI, and age-matched control groups (Wang et al., 2013). Reduced CBF values measured by ASL MRI were found to be region specific AD patients compared to age-matched control cases. Reduced CBF occurs in the lateral prefrontal cortex, posterior cingulate, precuneus, and inferior parietal areas of AD brains (Alsop et al., 2000, 2010; Johnson et al., 2005; Dai et al., 2009) (**Table 2**). CBF is easy to follow over time and imaging a biomarker can be useful to follow the disease's condition and prognosis. It has been hypothesized that abnormality in CBF occurs much earlier than cognitive deficits appear in AD, possibly earlier than wide-spread brain atrophy or plaque/tangle formation. Recent studies showed that ASL MRI can be extended to detect preclinical AD, at least for research purposes (Wierenga et al., 2014; Hays et al., 2016).

AD BRAIN IMAGING BY POSITRON EMISSION TOMOGRAPHY (PET)

Amyloid Imaging by PET as AD Biomarker

Aβ deposition can be found in the neocortical area of the brain, one of the first areas affected due to preclinical AD pathology. Imaging of amyloid as a biomarker of AD is based on the popular yet controversial "amyloid cascade hypothesis" of AD (Hardy and Allsop, 1991; Hardy and Higgins, 1992). According to this oversimplified hypothesis, toxic deposition of amyloid in the AD brain causes synaptic loss and neuronal apoptosis; thus, measuring Aβ aggregates in antemortem AD brain imaging by PET would give the right AD diagnosis (**Table 2**). This hypothesis also supports the idea that amyloid plaque deposition is the primary pathophysiologic change that occurs in preclinical AD. Since fibrillary tau deposition is common in another neurodegenerative disease (Tauopathy, Frontotemporal dementia, Corticobasal degeneration), amyloid imaging by tau would have higher specificity. Klunk et al. (2004) were first to develop ^{11}C-PIB (2-(4′-[11C] methylaminophenyl)-6-hydroxybenzothiazole or Pittsburgh compound B) as an Aβ PET imaging agents (Klunk et al., 2004). The ^{11}C-PIB-PET imaging biomarker has a limitation in terms of sensitivity specificity. A study found ^{11}C-PIB-PET positive in about 20–30% of cases of cognitively normal individuals (Pike et al., 2007). On the other hand, a report demonstrated that ~16% of patients with probable AD were PIB PET negative (Shimada et al., 2011). As Aβ plaque is not associated with dementia in AD, the earliest event in preclinical AD, synaptic loss, would not be expected to correlate with ^{11}C-PIB-PET alone. A longitudinal study of PIB-PET found no correlation of PIB uptake depending their dementia status in age-matched control, MCI, and AD individuals (Jack et al., 2009). Therefore, ^{11}C-PIB-PET may provide evidence of amyloid deposit in the brain but may not be useful for diagnosing preclinical AD alone. Another Aβ PET imaging compound, ^{18}F-florbetapir demonstrated greater specificity than CSF Aβ_{42} (Mattsson et al., 2014). The half-life of positron-emitting ^{11}C-PIB (20.33 min) is much lower than that of ^{18}F (109.77 min). While ^{18}F compounds provide a shorter window for conducting an imaging study, this also means that the ^{18}F radiotracer must be made in-house using a cyclotron, or within a range consistent with the 20-min half-life. Other well studied Aβ radiotracers are ^{11}C-BF227 and ^{18}F-NAV4694. A recent study found that Aβ-PET is suitable for defining preclinical AD along with CSF biomarkers (Dubois et al., 2016). Moreover ante mortem ^{11}C-PIB-PET scanning results were correlated with the Thal amyloid deposition stages (Murray et al., 2015). Amyloid plaque score in terms of Thal stage has been incorporated in NIA-AA (2011) AD neuropathological criteria (Hyman et al., 2012).

Biomarker of Glucose Metabolism in AD by PET

Dysfunctional brain glucose metabolism is another hypothesis of AD pathogenesis. Temporoparietal hypometabolism is one of the brain areas first affected due to preclinical AD pathology. [^{18}F]-fluoro-2-deoxy-D-glucose (^{18}FDG) has been extensively used as the PET agent for region-specific brain imaging. ^{18}FDG-PET imaging outcomes from AD patients were appropriately correlated with the mini-mental score examination (MMSE) (Jagust et al., 2009). In fact, among the PET imaging techniques, ^{18}FDG-PET is the most widely researched imaging biomarker for AD. ^{18}FDG-PET showed consistent low signal in the parietal-temporal area and posterior cingulate cortex. In severe AD, the frontal cortex showed lower signal; however, other brain areas unaffected by AD pathologies such as the cerebellum, striatum basal ganglia and the visual and sensory cortex remained unchanged. A differential low glucose metabolism detected at different brain region by ^{18}FDG-PET can be used for differential AD and non-AD dementia diagnosis (Silverman et al., 2001; Mosconi et al., 2008). ^{18}FDG-PET can be used for differential AD diagnosis vs. other non-AD dementia suggested by important regulatory authorities, such as FDA and EMA. In addition to that, International panels for AD diagnostic criteria have included ^{18}FDG-PET as one of the AD biomarkers (Sperling et al., 2011; Dubois et al., 2014). The Centers for Medicare and Medicaid Services (CMS) have allowed the use of ^{18}FDG-PET to establish the diagnosis of dementia due to AD and frontotemporal dementia (FTD). ^{18}FDG-PET also has potential to predict preclinical AD pathology (Ito et al., 2015).

Biomarkers of tau Imaging in AD by PET

The hyperphosphorylated paired helical filament (PHF) that forms NFTs quantified by Braak stages are better correlated with AD severity and neuronal atrophy than amyloid plaques (Bierer et al., 1995; Nelson et al., 2007). Both tau and phosphorylated tau (p-tau) are increased in AD pathology considered to be the measure of neuronal injury. Some studies even showed that neuronal injuries due to tau and p-tau are earlier than abnormalities in amyloidosis (Jack and Holtzman, 2013; Jack et al., 2013). CSF tau is not the same as deposition of NFTs in the AD brain. Moreover, the dynamic ranges of tau and p-tau in CSF AD biomarkers are lower than Aβ_{42}. Therefore, tau imaging by PET as AD preclinical should have a higher implication.

Tau-PET imaging for AD was initiated with^{18}FDDNP (a radiofluorinated derivative of the 2-(1-[6-(dimethylamino)-2-naphthyl]ethylidene) malononitrile) showing higher binding in AD and MCI cases (Small et al., 2006). The first human trial of tau radiotracer ^{18}F-T807 by Siemens Molecular Imaging Biomarker Research (Culver City, CA) found higher tau levels in brain areas rich in PHF and very low in white matter (Chien et al., 2013). There are several other new tau-PET tracers that have been developed based on quinolone derivatives (^{18}F-THK-523, ^{18}F-THK-5105, and ^{18}F-THK-5117) (Fodero-Tavoletti et al., 2011; Harada et al., 2013; Okamura et al., 2014). Longitudinal tau-PET cohorts in patients with high-risk preclinical AD provided special distribution of deposition of tau that can allow to staging *in-vivo* neurodegeneration according to tau levels in preclinical AD (Johnson et al., 2016). Special distribution of tau deposition by tau-PET would serve a very important role in determining preclinical AD cases. For example, tau-PET ligand uptake in the neocortex and increase amyloidosis with time in longitudinal studies can find underlining preclinical AD pathology. Tau-PET uptake in the medial temporal lobe can be due to non-AD pathology preclinical FTD (frontotemporal dementia), CBD (corticobasal degeneration), PSP (progressive supranuclear palsy), or age-related tauopathy (Crary et al., 2014). Tau-PET binding in medial temporal lobe is not useful for preclinical AD diagnosis since it cannot differentiate control from MCI cases. Moreover, Tau-PET binding occurs in media temporal lobe even in asymptomatic elderly cases up to Braak stage 2.

APPLICABILITY OF BRAIN NEUROIMAGING MODALITIES FOR DETECTION OF BIOMARKERS IN PRECLINICAL ALZHEIMER'S DISEASE

A comparison of the different neuroimaging modalities used to detect preclinical AD biomarkers is shown in **Table 3**. ^{18}FDG-PET imaging outcome determines region-specific subtle metabolic changes in the brain. According to metabolic dysfunction hypothesis AD, pathologic changes first occur in the metabolic pathway of a preclinical AD brain. While ^{18}FDG-PET correlates strongly with AD and AD progression, it has the potential to distinguish AD vs. other non-AD dementia, and it strongly correlates with MMSE. Therefore, ^{18}FDG-PET has the capability to distinguish preclinical AD. There will be some disadvantages using ^{18}FDG-PET for the diagnosis of preclinical AD. The ^{18}FDG-PET signal can be affected by inflammation, local ischemia, and the behavior state of the subject (Duara et al., 2010; Shipley et al., 2013). The diagnostic criteria for the preclinical AD by IWG-AA (2015) does not list either MRI or ^{18}FDG-PET as suitable modalities for defining preclinical AD (Dubois et al., 2016). However, IWG-AA recommends^{18}FDG-PET for tracking progress in clinical AD in individuals with asymptomatic preclinical AD (Dubois et al., 2016).

rs-fMRI can detect abnormalities before brain volume loss (atrophy as determined by sMRI). It can be used to detect reduced functional connectivity in the preclinical stage of AD. However, there are no regulatory guidelines by FDA or EMA. DTI/sMRI has the potential to detect abnormalities in white matter networks in preclinical AD. In addition, it has the capability to detect region specificity to detect a specific region affected by preclinical AD. ASL/MRI can detect the abnormality in CBF in the preclinical AD. While Aβ-PET imaging can only be a signature of an amount of Aβ levels in the preclinical AD brain, it may not be used to detect the level of neurodegeneration (**Table 3**).

RISK FACTORS IN PRECLINICAL ALZHEIMER'S DISEASE

Preclinical AD can be classified in terms of degree of the risk factor of developing preclinical AD (except age). Such risk factors are positive amyloidosis, positive neurodegeneration, abnormalities in synaptic function by fMRI, and positive genetic AD risk factors. Individuals with high-risk factors should be included in a longitudinal follow-up in a cohort to find the relationship between risk factor and development of preclinical AD. A longitudinal cohort study showed CSF AD biomarkers ($A\beta_{42}$ and tau) and Aβ-PET can distinguish preclinical AD as high risk and low-risk categories (Vos et al., 2013). In future patients in a high-risk AD category and preclinical categories can be advised to change their lifestyle and food habits to delay the disease. Longitudinal changes with different risk factor in preclinical AD follow-up until cognitively impaired will allow for estimating positive and negative predictive values of the use of AD biomarkers in an at-risk population.

NEED FOR DIAGNOSTIC GUIDELINES FOR PRECLINICAL AD

Ample evidence shows that AD has long prodromal stages (preclinical AD → MCI due to AD pathology → AD-dementia) before the real clinical manifestation of dementia. The earlier treatment of AD begins in the disease course, the more effective it is at slowing the progression of the disease. Therefore, the detection of preclinical AD in asymptomatic individuals has become a major AD research focus. A simple definition of preclinical AD by the International panel (IWG-2014): No clinical symptoms of AD but positive AD biomarker values (in CSF: decreased $A\beta_{42}$, increased tau and/or p-tau in CSF; or in brain imaging: increased fibrillary amyloid on PET; Dubois et al., 2014). This simplistic definition needs more extensive diagnostic guidelines for preclinical AD. Deposition of amyloid plaques in the brain begins decades before clinical manifestation of AD, and the NIA-AA (2011) defines preclinical AD on the basis of pathological changes in the brain that occur before a demonstration of cognitive deficits. Later, IWG and NIA-AA (2015) simplified the definition of preclinical AD as the period of time between the first evidence of neuropathological lesions in the brain to the date of first clinical symptoms of AD. Now the challenge is to find validated biomarkers capable of detecting the first evidence of neuropathological lesions in the brain. Extensive research of AD biomarkers over the last couple decades has shown that preclinical AD is more likely to be diagnosed using multi-modal criteria. There is a need for evidence-based guidance on how to combine validated tests and imaging modalities to diagnose AD before the widespread synaptic loss and irreversible neuronal damage occur.

A combination of early Aβ-PET, ^{18}FDG-PET, and DTI MRI and/or fMRI to detect neurodegeneration, supported by genetic tests of the mutated APP, PSEN1, PSEN2, and APOE4, may be appropriate for preclinical AD diagnosis. Positive Aβ-PET, low ^{18}FDG-PET, and the presence of subtle neurodegeneration on MRI has been detected in familial AD prior to clinical symptoms. In sporadic AD, it would be reasonable to categories individuals with APOE4, positive Aβ-PET, low ^{18}FDG-PET, and subtle neurodegeneration by MRI as having a preclinical AD. Diagnosis of preclinical AD in an individual without genetic markers but with positive Aβ-PET, low ^{18}FDG-PET, and subtle evidence of neurodegeneration on MRI would have to wait until subtle evidence of cognitive decline appears that is not yet equivalent to the level indicative of MCI.

TABLE 3 | Comparison of preclinical Alzheimer's disease neuroimaging modalities.

Neuroimaging modalities	Differences	References
Tau-^{18}F-T807-PET vs. ^{13}C-PIB-PET	Region specific distribution of tau deposition	Johnson et al., 2016
Tau-^{18}F-THK5317-PET vs. ^{18}FDG-PET	Progression of AD is better tracked by ^{18}FDG-PET	Chiotis et al., 2017
^{18}FDG-PET vs. DTI with sMRI	Whole-brain white matter network properties in preclinical AD can be detected by DTI with sMRI before structural markers of significant neurodegeneration such as atrophy (by MRI) or reduced cortical glucose utilization (by ^{18}FDG-PET)	Fischer et al., 2015
^{18}FDG-PET vs. ASL\MRI	ASL MRI is not invasive ^{18}FDG-PET is more expensive than ASL/MRI ASL/MRI operation is simple	Wolk and Detre, 2012

Aβ, amyloid beta; AD, Alzheimer's disease; ASL MRI, arterial spin-labeled magnetic resonance imaging; DTI, diffusion tensor imaging; FDG, fluoro-2-deoxy-D-glucose; fMRI, functional MRI; ^{18}F-T807-PET, Fluorinated tau PET ligand; Tau-^{18}F-THK5317, Fluorinated tau PET ligand; MRI, magnetic resonance imaging; PET, positron emission tomography; PIB, Pittsburgh compound B.

A POSSIBLE ALGORITHM FOR COMPREHENSIVE PRECLINICAL ALZHEIMER'S DISEASE DIAGNOSIS

How and at what point in the lifespan can we begin to detect clear-cut signs of the ongoing neurodegenerative process of AD pathology that is distinct from normal aging? A multidimensional "panel" of preclinical AD biomarkers presents the best chance for a diagnosis and prediction of progression to AD dementia. A combination of three sets of evidence is recommended: (1) neuroimaging to detect early evidence of neurodegeneration in brain areas susceptible to AD pathology; (2) the genetic risk markers that predict AD onset; and (3) evidence of abnormalities in AD biomarkers (e.g., CSF Aβ_{42}, tau, and p-tau) (**Figure 2**). Major exclusion criteria would not be useful for preclinical AD diagnosis. Only deposition of tau at the medial temporal lobe by tau-PET can be used as an exclusion of preclinical AD from other tau related preclinical non-AD dementia (preclinical FTD, CBD or age-related tauopathy). Preclinical AD diagnostic algorithm has been proposed based on this combinatorial approach of neuroimaging, genetic testing, and CSF biomarker tests (**Table 4**). Incorporation of biomarkers and genetic information into the preclinical AD diagnostic scheme may also permit prediction of the *in vivo* physiological changes occurring in the brain before a clinical AD diagnosis.

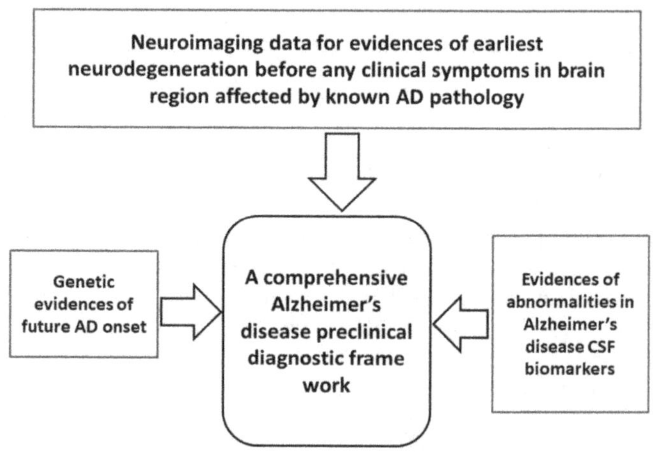

FIGURE 2 | A simple framework for comprehensive diagnosis preclinical Alzheimer's disease (AD). The framework includes three diagnostic modalities: neuroimaging to detect the earliest evidence of neurodegeneration in brain areas susceptible to AD pathology, genetic markers associated with an AD, and biomarker testing to detect abnormalities associated with an AD.

Validation of this framework will require accurate identification of an asymptomatic cohort at risk of AD. Longitudinal follow-up of different risk factors in preclinical AD will allow estimating accuracy, sensitivity, specificity, positive, and negative predictive values of the use of a particular AD biomarker at-risk population. The applicability of this diagnostic algorithm for screening of preclinical case needs extensive validation. Predicting positive and negative predictive values and false positives will depend on how preclinical AD cases will be selected. Standardization of operating procedure, thresholds, and cutoff values of CSF and neuroimaging biomarkers are needed to minimize between-lab and between-batch variability. Despite these challenges, the use of biomarkers holds great promise for the detection of the preclinical AD and the initiation of therapy at earlier stages to slow the progression of the disease. CSF sample collection is highly invasive and neuroimaging biomarkers are expensive; therefore, the ultimate goal for this research area is to find peripheral preclinical biomarkers for AD.

ISSUES CONCERNING PRECLINICAL AD BIOMARKERS

There are several necessary issues of preclinical AD biomarkers to be addressed before application. Most important issues are diagnostic accuracy, patient selection in clinical trial, universal standardization of diagnostic protocols, cost of diagnosis, the complexity of patient selection in clinical trials, and ethical challenges.

TABLE 4 | Algorithm for preclinical Alzheimer's disease diagnosis.

Approach	Preclinical AD biomarkers	Preclinical AD diagnosis
Pre-symptomatic genetic risk factors of familial AD	Familial AD genes: APP, PSEN1, PSEN2	Definite preclinical AD
Combination of sporadic AD risk factor genes (APOE4), CSF biomarkers, and neuroimaging biomarkers	APOE4, TOMM40: Yes CSF: low $A\beta_{42}$, high tau and p-tau Neuroimaging: high Aβ by PET, neurodegeneration by low ^{18}FDG-PET	Highly probable preclinical AD
Combination of sporadic AD risk factor genes (APOE4), CSF biomarkers, and neuroimaging biomarkers	APOE4: No CSF: low $A\beta_{42}$, high tau and p-tau Neuroimaging: high Aβ by PET, neurodegeneration by low ^{18}FDG-PET	Probable preclinical AD
Combination of sporadic AD risk factor genes from Alzgen data base, CSF biomarkers, and neuroimaging biomarkers	Susceptible gene: Alzgene database CSF: low $A\beta_{42}$, high tau and p-tau Neuroimaging: high Aβ by PET, neurodegeneration by low ^{18}FDG-PET, deposition of tau in cortical region by ^{18}F-T807-PET	Probable preclinical AD
Combination of sporadic AD risk factor genes (APOE4), CSF biomarkers, and neuroimaging biomarkers	APOE4: No CSF: low $A\beta_{42}$, high tau and p-tau Neuroimaging: high Aβ by PET, no neurodegeneration by ^{18}FDG-PET, deposition of tau in cortical region by 18F-T807-PET	Suspected preclinical AD
Combination of sporadic AD risk factor genes (APOE4), CSF biomarkers, and neuroimaging biomarkers	APOE4: No CSF: no $A\beta_{42}$, high tau and p-tau Neuroimaging: low or no Aβ by PET, neurodegeneration by low ^{18}FDG-PET	Suspected preclinical non-AD pathophysiology

Alzgene (http://www.alzgene.org/); Aβ, amyloid beta; APOE, apolipoprotein; CSF, cerebrospinal fluid; FDG, fluoro-2-deoxy-D-glucose; ^{18}F-T807-PET, Fluorinated tau PET ligand; PET, positron emission tomography; TOMM40, translocate of outer mitochondrial membrane 40.

Diagnostic Accuracy and Patient Selection

Improved diagnostic accuracy (sensitivity, specificity, positive predictive value, negative predictive value) and universally accepted unified standard operating procedures (SOP; for sample collection, cut-off values, analysis) are urgently required. The diagnostic sensitivity (SN), specificity (SP), positive likely-hood ratio (LR+), and negative likely-hood ratio (LR–) of all three core CSF biomarkers ($A\beta_{42}$: SN = 79%, SP = 63%, LR+ = 2, and LR– = 0.3; tau: SN = 76%, SP = 58%, LR+ = 2, and LR– = 0.4; p-tau: SN = 78%, SP = 56%, LR+ = 2, and LR– = 0.4; combination of three: $A\beta_{42}$: SN = 84%, SP = 63%, LR+ = 2, and LR– = 0.3) for MCI conversion to AD were found to be moderate by a systemic meta-analysis (Ferreira et al., 2014). The diagnostic sensitivity, specificity, positive likely-hood ratio, and negative likely-hood ratio of ^{18}F-labeled Aβ-PET imaging biomarkers (Florbetapir: SN = 89.6%, SP = 87.2%, LR+ = 7.9 and LR– = 0.108; Florbetaben: SN = 89.3%, SP = 87.6%, LR+ = 6.06 and LR– = 0.141) for distinguishing AD with non-demented control were found to be considerably higher by a systemic meta-analysis (Yeo et al., 2015). The progression of AD in non-demented elderly individuals was predicted with considerable accuracy (SN = 82% and SP = 93%) by studying brain metabolic states by FDG-PET (Ewers et al., 2014). ^{11}C-PIB-PET has higher SN (96%), low SP (58%), moderate LR+ (2.3), and LR– (0.07) for the conversion of MCI-AD (Zhang et al., 2014).

One of the main issues of concern of using this proposed algorithm is how to select potential patients to be screened. The selection of patients should be conducted as described in **Table 4**.

Universal Standardization Diagnostic Protocols

Standard methods of sample collection, reference standards, universal cut-off values for diagnostic tests, and standard operating procedures (SOP) are urgently needed for most advanced AD biomarkers (CSF core biomarkers, Aβ-PET, FDG-PET, and tau-PET). A significant amount of work has been done by an IWG for a universal standardization of AD diagnostic biomarkers (Mattsson and Zetterberg, 2012; Mattsson et al., 2012, 2013; https://aibl.csiro.au/wp-content/uploads/2014/01/sperling.pdf).

Estimated Costs of AD Diagnosis Tests

No doubt, there will be several thousand dollar cost for selecting each patient, and more cost would be during longitudinal follow up. An estimated cost of MRI ($1,694–$3,624) is higher than CSF biomarkers (http://www.comparemricost.com/. Study of 10 cities in the USA show that (Orlando, FL Dallas, TX—MRI Testing Facility A MRI and Dallas, TX—MRI Testing Facility B, San Diego, CA, Salt Lake City, UT, Detroit, MI, New York, NY—MRI Testing Facility A, New York, NY—MRI Testing Facility B, Raleigh, NC, Omaha, NE) fMRI costs are even higher than MRI. Specialized bio-informatics personals with expensive equipment are the main reason for the higher cost of modern neuroimaging AD biomarkers. Moderately invasive PET imaging costs $825–$6,800 (http://www.newchoicehealth.com/procedures/pet-scan-brain: National PET Scan Brain Procedure Pricing Summary). Highly invasive CSF biomarker tests are moderately expensive (~$450-$1,000 per test) (Fiandaca et al.,

2014; Valcárcel-Nazco et al., 2014), because highly skilled personals are required in specialized medical centers for CSF sample collection (lumbar puncture), three ELISA kits are necessary for (Aβ_{42}, tau, and p-tau), and the cost of CSF biomarker tests are much higher than blood-based diagnostic tests. Neuroimaging biomarkers are expensive because modality is a technical sophistication that needs technically trained expert teams of neuroscientists, radiologists, and bioinformatics specialists. A panel of a combination of CSF and neuroimaging biomarkers would increase the predicting power of preclinical AD diagnosis. However, the cost of diagnosis of such AD biomarkers will be much higher. Peripheral AD diagnosis in preclinical AD phase is the best way to decrease this enormous cost.

The Complexity of Patient Selection for Preclinical AD Clinical Trials

A homogeneous set of patients with preclinical AD certainly would not be available by its own characteristic feature of heterogeneity. Therefore, several subgroups of patients with preclinical AD can be separated according to their initial baseline preclinical AD biomarker values and follow longitudinally for a longer time (5–10 years). Such sub-groups are A. genetic sub-group: Asymptomatic high genetic risk with APOE4 and TOMM40 alleles, B. Neurodegeneration subgroup: Asymptomatic neurodegeneration by brain hypometabolism/tau deposition/atrophy, and C. Asymptomatic high-risk Aβ deposition by Aβ-PET and low CSF Aβ_{42} values. Because of longtime follow-up, preclinical AD longitudinal clinical trials should be expensive. Other drawbacks of such clinical trial are patient withdrawal, interference of comorbidity, and lifestyle changes of patients during the longitudinal long follow-up.

Ethical Challenges

Ethical issues to a conclusion and disclosure of a preclinical AD is very complex. The main ethical concerns for an individual are emotional, social, and economical. Emotional issues are feelings, fears, impact on personal motivation, and behavior to family members. A Metlife Foundation survey in 2011 found Americans middle aged and older ($\geq$55 years) are afraid of AD (31%), more than diabetes, heart disease, or stroke and less than cancer (41%) (Metlife Foundation, 2011). Preclinical AD disclosure may induce anxiety and depression. Social issues, such as the social stigma of future development of AD and withdrawal from social events, are an impact on friendship networks. The economic impact will be enormous to an individual with a preclinical AD diagnosis. Health insurance companies may increase the insurance premium. An individual working in higher cognitive performing jobs, such as pilot, clinical practitioners, and nurses need to be reported to a higher authority. Regulatory authorities should develop suitable guidelines for ethical issues for informing individuals about preclinical AD diagnosis.

Keeping all of these issues in mind, one can look at the positive aspect of the disclosure of preclinical AD. More than 90% responded in a survey that they wanted to adopt a healthier lifestyle if they knew they were at risk of AD (Caselli et al., 2014). Individuals who want to take a positive outlook of preclinical AD diagnosis should be influenced to increase social contact, healthy food, and mental exercises such as numerical problem solving, meditation, and yoga.

Feasibility and Utility of the Preclinical AD Diagnostic Algorithm

The main challenge remains how to choose individuals for preclinical AD diagnostic clinical trials. We proposed four different categories of probable preclinical AD cases and definitive preclinical AD category of pre-symptomatic genetic risk factors (**Table 4**) to be longitudinally tested in clinical trials by proposed preclinical AD biomarkers. In longitudinal follow-up trials will produce four different categories of biomarkers results (amyloid+ and neurodegenerative+, amyloid+ and neurodegenerative-, amyloid-and neurodegenerative+, amyloid-and neurodegenerative– (Pereira et al., 2017), and cognitive impairment due to AD. Those results will be complied in a comprehensive AD preclinical diagnostic framework presented in **Figure 2** to generate correlation of AD converters and AD non-converters with preclinical AD biomarkers.

Although challenges of cost, positive predictive values, and ethical issues are substantial this algorithm will provide a frame work of preclinical AD diagnosis, like lipid profiling for an individual in risk of heart disease. In the future individual with a risk of a preclinical AD from this framework should have suggestion from doctors to follow a healthy lifestyle.

AUTHOR CONTRIBUTIONS

The author confirms being the sole contributor of this work and approved it for publication.

ACKNOWLEDGMENTS

Financial assistance from the Intramural Research Program of the Blanchette Rockefeller Neurosciences Institute at West Virginia University, Morgantown, WV (TK), is gratefully acknowledged. The author is indebted to Ms. Cassandra George for assisting in the preparation of this manuscript. The author is grateful to the honorable editor and reviewers for their valuable comments for the improvement of this article.

REFERENCES

Adluru, N., Destiche, D. J., Lu, S. Y., Doran, S. T., Birdsill, A. C., Melah, K. E., et al. (2014). White matter microstructure in late middle-age: effects of apolipoprotein E4 and parental family history of Alzheimer's disease. *Neuroimage Clin.* 4, 730–742. doi: 10.1016/j.nicl.2014.04.008

Alsop, D. C., Dai, W., Grossman, M., and Detre, J. A. (2010). Arterial spin labeling blood flow MRI: its role in the early characterization of Alzheimer's disease. *J. Alzheimers Dis.* 20, 871–880. doi: 10.3233/JAD-2010-091699

Alsop, D. C., Detre, J. A., and Grossman, M. (2000). Assessment of cerebral blood flow in Alzheimer's disease by spin-labeled magnetic resonance imaging. *Ann. Neurol.* 47, 93–100. doi: 10.1002/1531-8249(200001)47:1<93::AID-ANA15>3.0.CO;2-8

Beaulieu, C., and Allen, P. S. (1994). Determinants of anisotropic water diffusion in nerves. *Magn. Reson. Med.* 31, 394–400. doi: 10.1002/mrm.1910310408

Bierer, L. M., Hof, P. R., Purohit, D. P., Carlin, L., Schmeidler, J., Davis, K. L., et al. (1995). Neocortical neurofibrillary tangles correlate with dementia severity in Alzheimer's disease. *Arch. Neurol.* 52, 81–88. doi: 10.1001/archneur.1995.00540250089017

Biswal, B., Yetkin, F. Z., Haughton, V. M., and Hyde, J. S. (1995). Functional connectivity in the motor cortex of resting human brain using echo-planar MRI. *Magn. Reson. Med.* 34, 537–541. doi: 10.1002/mrm.1910340409

Buckley, R. F., Schultz, A. P., Hedden, T., Papp, K. V., Hanseeuw, B. J., Marshall, G., et al. (2017). Functional network integrity presages cognitive decline in preclinical Alzheimer disease. *Neurology* 89, 29–37. doi: 10.1212/WNL.0000000000004059

Caselli, R. J., Langbaum, J., Marchant, G. E., Lindor, R. A., Hunt, K. S., Henslin, B. R., et al. (2014). Public perceptions of presymptomatic testing for Alzheimer disease. *Mayo Clin. Proc.* 89, 1389–1396. doi: 10.1016/j.mayocp.2014.05.016

Chien, D. T., Bahri, S., Szardenings, A. K., Walsh, J. C., Mu, F., Su, M. Y., et al. (2013). Early clinical PET imaging results with the novel PHF-tau radioligand [F-18]-T807. *J. Alzheimers Dis.* 34, 457–468. doi: 10.3233/JAD-122059

Chiotis, K., Saint-Aubert, L., Rodriguez-Vieitez, E., Leuzy, A., Almkvist, O., Savitcheva, I., et al. (2017). Longitudinal changes of tau PET imaging in relation to hypometabolism in prodromal and Alzheimer's disease dementia. *Mol. Psychiatry.* doi: 10.1038/mp.2017.108. [Epub ahead of print].

Chua, T. C., Wen, W., Chen, X., Kochan, N., Slavin, M. J., Trollor, J. N., et al. (2009). Diffusion tensor imaging of the posterior cingulate is a useful biomarker of mild cognitive impairment. *Am. J. Geriatr. Psychiatry* 17, 602–613. doi: 10.1097/JGP.0b013e3181a76e0b

Crary, J. F., Trojanowski, J. Q., Schneider, J. A., Abisambra, J. F., Abner, E. L., Alafuzoff, I., et al. (2014). Primary age-related tauopathy (PART): a common pathology associated with human aging. *Acta Neuropathol.* 128, 755–766. doi: 10.1007/s00401-014-1349-0

Dai, W., Lopez, O. L., Carmichael, O. T., Becker, J. T., Kuller, L. H., and Gach, H. M. (2009). Mild cognitive impairment and Alzheimer disease: patterns of altered cerebral blood flow at MR imaging. *Radiology* 250, 856–866. doi: 10.1148/radiol.2503080751

Detre, J. A., Leigh, J. S., Williams, D. S., and Koretsky, A. P. (1992). Perfusion imaging. *Magn. Reson. Med.* 23, 37–45. doi: 10.1002/mrm.1910230106

Detre, J. A., Rao, H., Wang, D. J., Chen, Y. F., and Wang, Z. (2012). Applications of arterial spin labeled MRI in the brain. *J. Magn. Reson. Imaging* 35, 1026–1037. doi: 10.1002/jmri.23581

Detre, J. A., Wang, J., Wang, Z., and Rao, H. (2009). Arterial spin-labeled perfusion MRI in basic and clinical neuroscience. *Curr. Opin. Neurol.* 22, 348–355. doi: 10.1097/WCO.0b013e32832d9505

Duara, R., Loewenstein, D. A., Greig-Custo, M. T., Raj, A., Barker, W., Potter, E., et al. (2010). Diagnosis and staging of mild cognitive impairment, using a modification of the clinical dementia rating scale: the mCDR. *Int. J. Geriatr. Psychiatry* 25, 282–289. doi: 10.1002/gps.2334

Dubois, B., Feldman, H. H., Jacova, C., Hampel, H., Molinuevo, J. L., Blennow, K., et al. (2014). Advancing research diagnostic criteria for Alzheimer's disease: the IWG-2 criteria. *Lancet Neurol.* 13, 614–629. doi: 10.1016/S1474-4422(14)70090-0

Dubois, B., Hampel, H., Feldman, H. H., Scheltens, P., Aisen, P., Andrieu, S., et al. (2016). Preclinical Alzheimer's disease: definition, natural history, and diagnostic criteria. *Alzheimers Dement.* 12, 292–323. doi: 10.1016/j.jalz.2016.02.002

Ewers, M., Brendel, M., Rizk-Jackson, A., Rominger, A., Bartenstein, P., Schuff, N., et al. (2014). Reduced FDG-PET brain metabolism and executive function predict clinical progression in elderly healthy subjects. *Neuroimage Clin.* 4, 45–52. doi: 10.1016/j.nicl.2013.10.018

Ewers, M., Insel, P. S., Stern, Y., and Weiner, M. W. (2013). Cognitive reserve associated with FDG-PET in preclinical Alzheimer disease. *Neurology* 80, 1194–1201. doi: 10.1212/WNL.0b013e31828970c2

Fagan, A. M., Roe, C. M., Xiong, C., Mintun, M. A., Morris, J. C., and Holtzman, D. M. (2007). Cerebrospinal fluid tau/beta-amyloid (42) ratio as a prediction of cognitive decline in nondemented older adults. *Arch. Neurol.* 64, 343–349. doi: 10.1001/archneur.64.3.noc60123

Ferreira, D., Perestelo-Pérez, L., Westman, E., Wahlund, L. O., Sarría, A., and Serrano-Aguilar, P. (2014). Meta-review of CSF core biomarkers in Alzheimer's disease: the state-of-the-art after the new revised diagnostic criteria. *Front. Aging Neurosci.* 6:47. doi: 10.3389/fnagi.2014.00047

Fiandaca, M. S., Mapstone, M. E., Cheema, A. K., and Federoff, H. J. (2014). The critical need for defining preclinical biomarkers in Alzheimer's disease. *Alzheimers Dement.* 10(Suppl. 3), S196–S212. doi: 10.1016/j.jalz.2014.04.015

Fischer, F. U., Wolf, D., Scheurich, A., and Fellgiebel, A. (2015). Altered whole-brain white matter networks in preclinical Alzheimer's disease. *Neuroimage Clin.* 8, 660–666. doi: 10.1016/j.nicl.2015.06.007

Fodero-Tavoletti, M. T., Okamura, N., Furumoto, S., Mulligan, R. S., Connor, A. R., McLean, C. A., et al. (2011). 18F-THK523: a novel *in vivo* tau imaging ligand for Alzheimer's disease. *Brain* 134, 1089–1100. doi: 10.1093/brain/awr038

Fox, N. C., Warrington, E. K., and Rossor, M. N. (1999). Serial magnetic resonance imaging of cerebral atrophy in preclinical Alzheimer's disease. *Lancet* 353, 2125–2125. doi: 10.1016/S0140-6736(99)00496-1

Frölich, L., Peters, O., Lewczuk, P., Gruber, O., Teipel, S. J., Gertz, H. J., et al. (2017). Incremental value of biomarker combinations to predict progression of mild cognitive impairment to Alzheimer's dementia. *Alzheimers Res. Ther.* 9:84. doi: 10.1186/s13195-017-0301-7

Grand, J. H., Caspar, S., and Macdonald, S. W. (2011). Clinical features and multidisciplinary approaches to dementia care. *J. Multidiscip. Healthc.* 4, 125–147. doi: 10.2147/JMDH.S17773

Gustafson, D. R., Skoog, I., Rosengren, L., Zetterberg, H., and Blennow, K. (2007). Cerebrospinal fluid beta-amyloid 1-42 concentration may predict cognitive decline in older women. *J. Neurol. Neurosurg. Psychiatr.* 78, 461–464. doi: 10.1136/jnnp.2006.100529

Harada, R., Okamura, N., Furumoto, S., Tago, T., Maruyama, M., Higuchi, M., et al. (2013). Comparison of the binding characteristics of [18F]THK-523 and other amyloid imaging tracers to Alzheimer's disease pathology. *Eur. J. Nucl. Med. Mol. Imaging* 40, 125–132. doi: 10.1007/s00259-012-2261-2

Hardy, J. A., and Higgins, G. A. (1992). Alzheimer's disease: the amyloid cascade hypothesis. *Science* 256, 184–185. doi: 10.1126/science.1566067

Hardy, J., and Allsop, D. (1991). Amyloid deposition as the central event in the aetiology of Alzheimer's disease. *Trends Pharmacol. Sci.* 12, 383–388. doi: 10.1016/0165-6147(91)90609-V

Hays, C. C., Zlatar, Z. Z., and Wierenga, C. E. (2016). The utility of cerebral blood flow as a biomarker of preclinical Alzheimer's disease. *Cell. Mol. Neurobiol.* 36, 167–179. doi: 10.1007/s10571-015-0261-z

Hubbard, B. M., Fenton, G. W., and Anderson, J. M. (1990). A quantitative histological study of early clinical and preclinical Alzheimer's disease. *Neuropathol. Appl. Neurobiol.* 16, 111–121.

Hyman, B. T., Phelps, C. H., Beach, T. G., Bigio, E. H., Cairns, N. J., Carrillo, M. C., et al. (2012). National Institute on Aging-Alzheimer's Association guidelines for the neuropathologic assessment of Alzheimer's disease. *Alzheimers Dement.* 8, 1–13. doi: 10.1016/j.jalz.2011.10.007

Ito, K., Fukuyama, H., Senda, M., Ishii, K., Maeda, K., Yamamoto, Y., et al. (2015). Prediction of outcomes in mild cognitive impairment by using 18F-FDG-PET: a multicenter study. *J. Alzheimers Dis.* 45, 543–552. doi: 10.3233/JAD-141338

Jack, C. R. Jr, and Holtzman, D. M. (2013). Biomarker modeling of Alzheimer's disease. *Neuron* 80, 1347–1358. doi: 10.1016/j.neuron.2013.12.003

Jack, C. R. Jr, Knopman, D. S., Jagust, W. J., Shaw, L. M., Aisen, P. S., Weiner, M. W., et al. (2010). Hypothetical model of dynamic biomarkers of the Alzheimer's pathological cascade. *Lancet Neurol.* 9, 119–128. doi: 10.1016/S1474-4422(09)70299-6

Jack, C. R. Jr, Lowe, V. J., Weigand, S. D., Wiste, H. J., Senjem, M. L., Knopman, D. S., et al. (2009). Serial PIB and MRI in normal, mild cognitive impairment and Alzheimer's disease: implications for sequence of pathological events in Alzheimer's disease. *Brain* 132, 1355–1365. doi: 10.1093/brain/awp062

Jack, C. R. Jr., Wiste, H. J., Weigand, S. D., Knopman, D. S., Lowe, V., Vemuri, P., et al. (2013). Amyloid-first and neurodegeneration-first profiles characterize incident amyloid PET positivity. *Neurology* 81, 1732–1740. doi: 10.1212/01.wnl.0000435556.21319.e4

Jagust, W. J., Landau, S. M., Shaw, L. M., Trojanowski, J. Q., Koeppe, R. A., Reiman, E. M., et al. (2009). Relationships between biomarkers in aging and dementia. *Neurology* 73, 1193–1199. doi: 10.1212/WNL.0b013e3181bc010c

Jansen, W. J., Ossenkoppele, R., Knol, D. L., Tijms, B. M., Scheltens, P., Verhey, F. R., et al. (2015). Prevalence of cerebral amyloid pathology in persons without dementia: a meta-analysis. *JAMA* 313, 1924–1938. doi: 10.1001/jama.2015.4668

Johnson, K. A., Fox, N. C., Sperling, R. A., and Klunk, W. E. (2012). Brain imaging in Alzheimer disease. *Cold Spring Harb. Perspect. Med.* 2:a006213. doi: 10.1101/cshperspect.a006213

Johnson, K. A., Schultz, A., Betensky, R. A., Becker, J. A., Sepulcre, J., Rentz, D., et al. (2016). Tau positron emission tomographic imaging in aging and early Alzheimer disease. *Ann. Neurol.* 79, 110–119. doi: 10.1002/ana.24546

Johnson, N. A., Jahng, G. H., Weiner, M. W., Miller, B. L., Chui, H. C., Jagust, W. J., et al. (2005). Pattern of cerebral hypoperfusion in Alzheimer disease and mild cognitive impairment measured with arterial spin-labeling MR imaging: initial experience. *Radiology* 234, 851–859. doi: 10.1148/radiol.2343040197

Kantarci, K., Murray, M. E., Schwarz, C. G., Reid, R. I., Przybelski, S. A., Lesnick, T., et al. (2017). White-matter integrity on DTI and the pathologic staging of Alzheimer's disease. *Neurobiol. Aging* 56, 172–179. doi: 10.1016/j.neurobiolaging.2017.04.024

Kester, M. I., Teunissen, C. E., Crimmins, D. L., Herries, E. M., Ladenson, J. H., Scheltens, P., et al. (2015). Neurogranin as a cerebrospinal fluid biomarker for synaptic loss in symptomatic Alzheimer disease. *JAMA Neurol.* 72, 1275–1280. doi: 10.1001/jamaneurol.2015.1867

Khan, T. K. (2016). *Biomarkers in Alzheimer's Disease*. London: Academic Press, 37.

Kinnunen, K. M., Cash, D. M., Poole, T., Frost, C., Benzinger, T. L. S., Ahsan, R. L., et al. (2017). Presymptomatic atrophy in autosomal dominant Alzheimer's disease: a serial MRI study. *Alzheimers Dement.* 14, 43–53. doi: 10.1016/j.jalz.2017.06.2268

Klunk, W. E., Engler, H., Nordberg, A., Wang, Y., Blomqvist, G., Holt, D. P., et al. (2004). Imaging brain amyloid in Alzheimer's disease with Pittsburgh Compound-B. *Ann. Neurol.* 55, 306–319. doi: 10.1002/ana.20009

Machulda, M. M., Jones, D. T., Vemuri, P., McDade, E., Avula, R., Przybelski, S., et al. (2011). Effect of APOE epsilon4 status on intrinsic network connectivity in cognitively normal elderly subjects. *Arch. Neurol.* 68, 1131–1136. doi: 10.1001/archneurol.2011.108

Mattsson, N., and Zetterberg, H. (2012). What is a certified reference material. *Biomark. Med.* 6, 369–370. doi: 10.2217/bmm.12.37

Mattsson, N., Andreasson, U., Persson, S., Carrillo, M. C., Collins, S., Chalbot, S., et al. (2013). CSF biomarker variability in the Alzheimer's Association quality control program. *Alzheimers Dement.* 9, 251–261. doi: 10.1016/j.jalz.2013.01.010

Mattsson, N., Insel, P. S., Landau, S., Jagust, W., Donohue, M., Shaw, L. M., et al. (2014). Diagnostic accuracy of CSF Aβ42 and florbetapir PET for Alzheimer's disease. *Ann. Clin. Transl. Neurol.* 1, 534–543. doi: 10.1002/acn3.81

Mattsson, N., Zegers, I., Andreasson, U., Bjerke, M., Blankenstein, M. A., Bowser, R., et al. (2012). Reference measurement procedures for Alzheimer's disease cerebrospinal fluid biomarkers: definitions and approaches with focus on amyloid β42. *Biomark. Med.* 6, 409–417. doi: 10.2217/bmm.12.39

McKhann, G. M., Knopman, D. S., Chertkow, H., Hyman, B. T., Jack, C. R. Jr, Kawas, C. H., et al. (2011). The diagnosis of dementia due to Alzheimer's disease: recommendations from the National Institute on Aging-Alzheimer's Association workgroups on diagnostic guidelines for Alzheimer's disease. *Alzheimers Dement.* 7, 263–269. doi: 10.1016/j.jalz.2011.03.005

Metlife Foundation (2011). *What America Thinks: MetLife Foundation Alzheimer's Survey*. New York, NY: Harris Interactive.

Mintun, M. A., Larossa, G. N., Sheline, Y. I., Dence, C. S., Lee, S. Y., Mach, R. H., et al. (2006). [11C]PIB in a nondemented population: potential antecedent marker of Alzheimer disease. *Neurology* 67, 446–452. doi: 10.1212/01.wnl.0000228230.26044.a4

Morris, J. C. (2005). Early-stage and preclinical Alzheimer's disease. *Alzheimer Dis. Assoc. Disord.* 19, 163–165. doi: 10.1097/01.wad.0000184005.22611.cc

Mosconi, L., Sorbi, S., de Leon, M. J., Li, Y., Nacmias, B., Myoung, P. S., et al. (2006). Hypometabolism exceeds atrophy in presymptomatic early-onset familial Alzheimer's disease. *J. Nucl. Med.* 47, 1778–1786.

Mosconi, L., Tsui, W. H., Herholz, K., Pupi, A., Drzezga, A., Lucignani, G., et al. (2008). Multicenter standardized 18F-FDG PET diagnosis of mild cognitive impairment, Alzheimer's disease, and other dementias. *J. Nucl. Med.* 49, 390–398. doi: 10.2967/jnumed.107.045385

Moseley, M. E., Cohen, Y., Kucharczyk, J., Mintorovitch, J., Asgari, H. S., Wendland, M. F., et al. (1990). Diffusion-weighted MR imaging of anisotropic water diffusion in cat central nervous system. *Radiology* 176, 439–445. doi: 10.1148/radiology.176.2.2367658

Murray, M. E., Lowe, V. J., Graff-Radford, N. R., Liesinger, A. M., Cannon, A., Przybelski, S. A., et al. (2015). Clinicopathologic and 11C-Pittsburgh compound B implications of Thal amyloid phase across the Alzheimer's disease spectrum. *Brain* 138, 1370–1381. doi: 10.1093/brain/awv050

Nedelska, Z., Schwarz, C. G., Boeve, B. F., Lowe, V. J., Reid, R. I., Przybelski, S. A., et al. (2015). White matter integrity in dementia with Lewy bodies: a voxel-based analysis of diffusion tensor imaging. *Neurobiol. Aging* 36, 2010–2017. doi: 10.1016/j.neurobiolaging.2015.03.007

Nelson, P. T., Jicha, G. A., Schmitt, F. A., Liu, H., Davis, D. G., Mendiondo, M. S., et al. (2007). Clinicopathologic correlations in a large Alzheimer disease center autopsy cohort: neuritic plaques and neurofibrillary tangles "do count" when staging disease severity. *J. Neuropathol. Exp. Neurol.* 66, 1136–1146. doi: 10.1097/nen.0b013e31815c5efb

Okamura, N., Furumoto, S., Fodero-Tavoletti, M. T., Mulligan, R. S., Harada, R., Yates, P., et al. (2014). Non-invasive assessment of Alzheimer's disease neurofibrillary pathology using 18F-THK5105 PET. *Brain* 137, 1762–1771. doi: 10.1093/brain/awu064

Pereira, J. B., van Westen, D., Stomrud, E., Strandberg, T. O., Volpe, G., Westman, E., et al. (2017). Abnormal structural brain connectome in individuals with preclinical Alzheimer's disease. *Cereb. Cortex*. doi: 10.1093/cercor/bhx236. [Epub ahead of print].

Petersen, R. C., Doody, R., Kurz, A., Mohs, R. C., Morris, J. C., Rabins, P. V., et al. (2001). Current concepts in mild cognitive impairment. *Arch. Neurol.* 58, 1985–1992. doi: 10.1001/archneur.58.12.1985

Petersen, R. C., Smith, G. E., Waring, S. C., Ivnik, R. J., Tangalos, E. G., and Kokmen, E. (1999). Mild cognitive impairment: clinical characterization and outcome. *Arch. Neurol.* 56, 303–308. doi: 10.1001/archneur.56.3.303

Pierpaoli, C., and Basser, P. J. (1996). Toward a quantitative assessment of diffusion anisotropy. *Magn. Reson. Med.* 36, 893–906. doi: 10.1002/mrm.1910360612

Pierpaoli, C., Jezzard, P., Basser, P. J., Barnett, A., and Di Chiro, G. (1996). Diffusion tensor MR imaging of human brain. *Radiology* 201, 637–648. doi: 10.1148/radiology.201.3.8939209

Pike, K. E., Savage, G., Villemagne, V. L., Ng, S., Moss, S. A., Maruff, P., et al. (2007). β-amyloid imaging and memory in non-demented individuals: evidence for preclinical Alzheimer's disease. *Brain* 130, 2837–2844. doi: 10.1093/brain/awm238

Popp, J., Oikonomidi, A., Tautvydaite, D., Dayon, L., Bacher, M., Migliavacca, E., et al. (2017). Markers of neuroinflammation associated with Alzheimer's disease pathology in older adults. *Brain Behav. Immun.* 62, 203–211. doi: 10.1016/j.bbi.2017.01.020

Racine, A. M., Adluru, N., Alexander, A. L., Christian, B. T., Okonkwo, O. C., Oh, J., et al. (2014). Associations between white matter microstructure and amyloid burden in preclinical Alzheimer's disease: a multimodal imaging investigation. *Neuroimage Clin.* 4, 604–614. doi: 10.1016/j.nicl.2014.02.001

Reiman, E. M., Quiroz, Y. T., Fleisher, A. S., Chen, K., Velez-Pardo, C., Jimenez-Del-Rio, M., et al. (2012). Brain imaging and fluid biomarker analysis in young adults at genetic risk for autosomal dominant Alzheimer's disease in the presenilin 1 E280A kindred: a case-control study. *Lancet Neurol.* 11, 1048–1056. doi: 10.1016/S1474-4422(12)70228-4

Ritchie, C., Smailagic, N., Noel-Storr, A. H., Ukoumunne, O., Ladds, E. C., and Martin, S. (2017). CSF tau and the CSF tau/ABeta ratio for the diagnosis of Alzheimer's disease dementia and other dementias in people with mild cognitive impairment (MCI). *Cochrane Database Syst. Rev.* 3:CD010803. doi: 10.1002/14651858.CD010803.pub2

Scheinin, N. M., Aalto, S., Koikkalainen, J., Lötjönen, J., Karrasch, M., Kemppainen, N., et al. (2009). Follow-up of [11C] PIB uptake and brain volume in patients with Alzheimer disease and controls. *Neurology* 73, 1186–1192. doi: 10.1212/WNL.0b013e3181bacf1b

Sexton, C. E., Kalu, U. G., Filippini, N., Mackay, C. E., and Ebmeier, K. P. (2011). A meta-analysis of diffusion tensor imaging in mild cognitive impairment and Alzheimer's disease. *Neurobiol Aging* 32, 2322.e5–2322.e18. doi: 10.1016/j.neurobiolaging.2010.05.019

Sheline, Y. I., and Raichle, M. E. (2013). Resting state functional connectivity in preclinical Alzheimer's disease. *Biol. Psychiatry* 74, 340–347. doi: 10.1016/j.biopsych.2012.11.028

Shimada, H., Ataka, S., Takeuchi, J., Mori, H., Wada, Y., Watanabe, Y., et al. (2011). Pittsburgh Compound B-negative dementia–a possibility of misdiagnosis of patients with non-Alzheimer disease-type dementia as having AD. *J. Geriatr. Psychiatry Neurol.* 24, 123–126. doi: 10.1177/0891988711409410

Shipley, S. M., Frederick, M. C., Filley, C. M., and Kluger, B. M. (2013). Potential for misdiagnosis in community-acquired PET scans for dementia. *Neurol. Clin. Pract.* 3, 305–312. doi: 10.1212/CPJ.0b013e318296f2df

Silverman, D. H., Small, G. W., Chang, C. Y., Lu, C. S., Kung De Aburto, M. A., Chen, W., et al. (2001). Positron emission tomography in evaluation of dementia: regional brain metabolism and long-term outcome. *JAMA* 286, 2120–2127. doi: 10.1001/jama.286.17.2120

Small, G. W., Kepe, V., Ercoli, L. M., Siddarth, P., Bookheimer, S. Y., Miller, K. J., et al. (2006). PET of brain amyloid and tau in mild cognitive impairment. *N. Engl. J. Med.* 355, 2652–2663. doi: 10.1056/NEJMoa054625

Sperling, R. A., Aisen, P. S., Beckett, L. A., Bennett, D. A., Craft, S., Fagan, A. M., et al. (2011). Toward defining the preclinical stages of Alzheimer's disease: recommendations from the National Institute on Aging-Alzheimer's Association workgroups on diagnostic guidelines for Alzheimer's disease. *Alzheimers Dement.* 7, 280–292. doi: 10.1016/j.jalz.2011.03.003

Stomrud, E., Hansson, O., Blennow, K., Minthon, L., and Londos, E. (2007). Cerebrospinal fluid biomarkers predict decline in subjective cognitive function over 3 years in healthy elderly. *Dement. Geriatr. Cogn. Disord.* 24, 118–124. doi: 10.1159/000105017

Sutphen, C. L., Jasielec, M. S., Shah, A. R., Macy, E. M., Xiong, C., Vlassenko, A. G., et al. (2015). Longitudinal cerebrospinal fluid biomarker changes in preclinical Alzheimer disease during middle age. *JAMA Neurol.* 72, 1029–1042. doi: 10.1001/jamaneurol.2015.1285

Valcárcel-Nazco, C., Perestelo-Pérez, L., Molinuevo, J. L., Mar, J., Castilla, I., and Serrano-Aguilar, P. (2014). Cost-effectiveness of the use of biomarkers in cerebrospinal fluid for Alzheimer's disease. *J. Alzheimers Dis.* 42, 777–788. doi: 10.3233/JAD-132216

Villemagne, V. L., Pike, K. E., Darby, D., Maruff, P., Savage, G., Ng, S., et al. (2008). Abeta deposits in older non-demented individuals with cognitive decline are indicative of preclinical Alzheimer's disease. *Neuropsychologia* 46, 1688–1697. doi: 10.1016/j.neuropsychologia.2008.02.008

Vos, S. J., Xiong, C., Visser, P. J., Jasielec, M. S., Hassenstab, J., Grant, E. A., et al. (2013). Preclinical Alzheimer's disease and its outcome: a longitudinal cohort study. *Lancet. Neurol.* 12, 957–965. doi: 10.1016/S1474-4422(13)70194-7

Wang, Z., Das, S. R., Xie, S. X., Arnold, S. E., Detre, J. A., and Wolk, D. A. (2013). Arterial spin labeled MRI in prodromal Alzheimer's disease: a multi-site study. *Neuroimage Clin.* 2, 630–636. doi: 10.1016/j.nicl.2013.04.014

Wierenga, C. E., Hays, C. C., and Zlatar, Z. Z. (2014). Cerebral blood flow measured by arterial spin labeling MRI as a preclinical marker of Alzheimer's disease. *J. Alzheimers Dis.* 42(Suppl. 4), S411–S419. doi: 10.3233/JAD-141467

Wolk, D. A., and Detre, J. A. (2012). Arterial spin labeling MRI: an emerging biomarker for Alzheimer's disease and other neurodegenerative conditions. *Curr. Opin. Neurol.* 25, 421–428. doi: 10.1097/WCO.0b013e328354ff0a

Yeo, J. M., Waddell, B., Khan, Z., and Pal, S. (2015). A systematic review and meta-analysis of ^{18}F-labeled amyloid imaging in Alzheimer's disease. *Alzheimers Dement.* 1, 5–13. doi: 10.1016/j.dadm.2014.11.004

Zetterberg, H., Skillbäck, T., Mattsson, N., Trojanowski, J. Q., Portelius, E., Shaw, L. M., et al. (2016). Association of cerebrospinal fluid neurofilament light concentration with Alzheimer disease progression. *JAMA Neurol.* 73, 60–67. doi: 10.1001/jamaneurol.2015.3037

Zhang, S., Smailagic, N., Hyde, C., Noel-Storr, A. H., Takwoingi, Y., McShane, R., et al. (2014). (11)C-PIB-PET for the early diagnosis of Alzheimer's disease dementia and other dementias in people with mild cognitive impairment (MCI). *Cochrane Database Syst. Rev.* 7:CD010386. doi: 10.1002/14651858.CD010386.pub2

15

Identification of a Novel Hemizygous SQSTM1 Nonsense Mutation in Atypical Behavioral Variant Frontotemporal Dementia

Lin Sun [1†], Zhouyi Rong [2†], Wei Li [1], Honghua Zheng [2,3], Shifu Xiao [1*] and Xia Li [1*]*

[1] Shanghai Mental Health Center, Alzheimer's Disease and Related Disorders Center, Shanghai Jiao Tong University School of Medicine, Shanghai, China, [2] Fujian Provincial Key Laboratory of Neurodegenerative Disease and Aging Research, Institute of Neuroscience, College of Medicine, Xiamen University, Xiamen, China, [3] Department of Neuroscience, Shenzhen Research Institute of Xiamen University, Shenzhen, China

***Correspondence:**
Honghua Zheng
honghua@xmu.edu.cn
Shifu Xiao
xiaoshifu@msn.com
Xia Li
ja_1023@hotmail.com

† These authors have contributed equally to this work.

Frontotemporal dementia includes a large spectrum of neurodegenerative disorders. *SQSTM1*, coding for p62 protein, plays a vital role in the pathogenesis of FTD. Here, we report a case of a female patient with *SQSTM1* mutation S224X, who was 59 years old when she initially exhibited memory decline, mild personality changes, and subtle atrophy of frontal/temporal lobes in magnetic resonance imaging (MRI). Genetic testing revealed a nonsense mutation of the *SQSTM1* gene (S224X), resulting in premature termination of protein synthesis and a predicted truncated protein 217 amino acids shorter than the normal protein. Moreover, neither intact nor truncated SQSTM1 proteins was detectable in *SQSTM1* S224X mutant overexpressing HEK-293T cells. We assayed for *SQSTM1* cDNA in samples from the patient's peripheral leucocytes, and did not detect its mutation. The test of quantitative PCR showed significant decreased level of *SQSTM1* mRNA from peripheral leucocytes of the patient compared to five dementia controls. Our results identify a novel pathogenic *SQSTM1* S224X mutation in an atypical FTD patient accompanied with loss of SQSTM1/p62 protein expression probably due to *SQSTM1* gene haploinsufficiency.

Keywords: Frontotemporal dementia, FTD, *SQSTM1*, p62, S224X, nonsense mutation

INTRODUCTION

Frontotemporal dementia is the second common form of neurodegenerative dementia in presenile population, characterized by atrophy of frontal and/or temporal lobes, and is frequently linked to genetic mutations (Miller et al., 2015; Luis et al., 2016). The three primary clinical FTD subtypes include behavioral variant FTD (bvFTD), nonfluent variant primary progressive aphasia (nfvPPA), and semantic variant primary progressive aphasia (svPPA) (Miller et al., 2015; O'Connor et al., 2016). As the most common presentation, bvFTD presents as a progressive change in personality with abnormalities in social-emotional behavior, and its diagnosis remains difficult, with patients being erroneously considered as having Alzheimer's disease or psychiatric disorders (Pottier et al., 2016; Tosun et al., 2016). The definite diagnosis is based on three major pathological subtypes characterized by the presence of 43 kDa TAR DNA-binding protein (TDP43), tau, or fused in sarcoma (FUS) positive neuronal inclusions (Boutoleau-Bretonniere et al., 2015). Approximately 30–50% of FTD patients have a positive family history, and 10% exhibit an autosomal dominant mode of inheritance. Mutations in the genes that encode microtubule associated protein tau (MAPT), progranulin and C9orf72 are the most common causes of FTD (Sun et al., 2017). Sequestosome 1 (SQSTM1), coding for p62 protein, is an adaptor protein that contains several protein-protein interaction motifs and serves as a signaling hub in a variety of key cellular processes including cell differentiation, transcriptional regulation, apoptosis, and oxidative stress response (Rea et al., 2014). SQSTM1, which has been identified in FTD in 2012 (Rubino et al., 2012), suggesting a role in the pathogenesis of neurodegenerative disease (Boutoleau-Bretonniere et al., 2015), is initially considered as a monogenic cause of Paget disease of bone (PDB) in 2002 (Laurin et al., 2002) and amyotrophic lateral sclerosis in 2011 (Fecto et al., 2011). Mutation in the *SQSTM1* gene is a rare cause of FTD and ALS (van der Zee et al., 2014). Rubino et al. only identified 3 missense mutations in the *SQSTM1* gene in 3 of 170 Italian patients with FTD, and 3 missense variants in 3 of 124 Italian patients with ALS (Rubino et al., 2012).

Here we report an atypical bvFTD patient with memory decline as an initial symptom and mild personality change emerging gradually, carried a novel pathogenic variant of the *SQSTM1* gene causing absent expression of SQSTM1/p62 protein.

MATERIALS AND METHODS

Genetic Procedures

Total genomic DNA was prepared and amplified from peripheral blood according to standard procedures. The quality of DNA was assessed by Qubit 3.0 (Thermo Fisher, USA) and agarose gel electrophoresis. Then the sequencing library was prepared according to the SureSelectXT Target Enrichment System Manual (Agilent, USA), and whole exome sequencing was performed by HiSeq X Ten (Illumina, USA). After this next-generation sequencing and bio-information analysis of the sequencing data, especially AD and FTD related genes including *APP, PSEN1, PSEN2, MAPT, GRN, CHMP2B, C9ORF72, VCP, FUS, SQSTM1, TREM2, TYROBP* etc., we found that there was a nonsense mutation in *SQSTM1* gene. The nonsense mutation of *SQSTM1* gene were analyzed by Sanger sequencing (forward primer: 5′-AGCGTCTGCCCAGACTACGA-3′ and reverse primer: 5′-CAGGCACTTAGGCACCTCAG-3′, the values of Tm were 63.4 and 61.0 respectively, and the length of amplified product is 547 bp). Moreover, we detected *APOE* genotyping at locus of rs429358 and rs7412. The software of Mutation Taster was applied to predict the pathogenicity of the detected mutations (http://www.mutationtaster.org/).

Analysis of SQSTM1 Mutant Protein Expression

Plasmid DNA for wild type *SQSTM1* was prepared by inserting coding sequence of the human *SQSTM1* gene (NM_003900) into the pcDNA3.1/Myc-His vector, and the *SQSTM1* S224X mutation was obtained by PCR-based site-directed mutagenesis with c.671C>A. All constructs were verified by sequencing (Minbo Biotech, Xiamen, China). Human embryonic kidney cells (HEK 293T) were grown to 80% confluence and transfected with vectors by Turbofect Transfection Reagent (Thermo Fisher, USA) according to the manufacturer's instructions. Media were then replaced with fresh DMEM containing 10% FBS. Cells were then collected 24 h later for western blotting. Equal amounts of total proteins (20 μg) were subjected to SDS-PAGE and transferred to PVDF membrane (Millipore, USA). Membranes were incubated with antibodies specific for SQSTM1 Gly162 (Cell Signaling Technology, 8025, USA), SQSTM1 Gly410 (Cell Signaling Technology, 5114, USA), Myc (Proteintech, 16282-1-AP, USA), or GAPDH (Abcam, ab181602, USA). Proteins were quantified using ImageJ Software.

Characterization of SQSTM1 Gene Expression

The mutation S224X (c.671 C>A) of *SQSTM1* cDNA amplicons were obtained from the patient's mRNA sample by RT-PCR reaction. The cycling parameters of RT-PCR were 3 min at 95°C, followed by 30 s at 94°C, followed by 35 cycles of 60°C for 30 s, 72°C for 30 s, and a final extension of 72°C for 5 min. The pair of PCR primer sequence included the forward primer 5′-CTGTCTGAGGGCTCTCGC-3′ and reverse primer 5′-TCAACTTAATGCCCAGAGG-3′. The pyrosequencing and Sanger sequencing were performed following the manufacturer's protocols (Sangon, China). The analysis was used through PyroMark Software 1.0.11 software environment (Sangon, China).

Total cellular RNA was extracted from cell culture using TRIzol (Invitrogen, USA) according to manufacturer's procedures. Real-time PCR analysis was performed using 7900HT PCR instrument (ABI, USA). PCR conditions were at 95°C for 1 min, followed by 40 cycles at 95°C for 15 s, and 60°C for 30 s. For each biological replicate, three technical replicates were performed. The pair of PCR primer sequence included the forward primer 5′-TGGCGGAGCAGATG AGGAAG-3′ and reverse primer 5′-GGACTGGAGTTCACCTGTAGACG-3′.

Statistical Analysis

All data are presented as mean ± standard error of mean. The data were analyzed by one-way analysis of variance (ANOVA). Results were considered to be statistically different when $p < 0.05$.

Ethics and Patient Consent

We received approval from the regional ethical standards committee on human experimentation for our experiments using human materials. We also received written informed consent for research from the participants and guardians.

RESULTS

Case Report

The patient underwent a clinical evaluation at our institution and was then enrolled in the Foundation of China Alzheimer's disease and related disorders study. Additional data from the proband and her relatives were collected and analyzed.

A 65-year-old, right-handed female with 15 years of school education was first seen in our geriatric psychiatry department in December 2016 for memory difficulties over 6 years combined with mild personality change over 1 year. She received surgical treatment for oophoroma in 2005 and drug treatment for hyperthyroidism in 2015, and gained full control of both diseases.

Her caregiver described the patient's forgetfulness at age 59, which had developed insidiously. She was referred to hospital because of memory decline and depression, and was prescribed antidepressant drugs. The patient refused to take the medications, and went on to care for her sick mother. At 5 years post-onset of symptoms, she began to lose her way and fall occasionally. In June 2015, she fell, resulting in cracking her head and bleeding. Her family brought her to hospital for testing. The brain computed tomography (CT) revealed cerebral atrophy, and electromyogram/ nerve conduction velocity (EMG/NCV) showed no positive finding. Subsequently, therapy with huperzine A was initiated. However, the patient took the medication irregularly, and her condition gradually aggravated. In May 2016, her family noticed her daytime somnolence, sluggishness, and reticence. Magnetic resonance imaging (MRI) showed mild atrophy of the cerebral cortex. Subsequently, combination therapy with Exelon and Escitalopram was started. In December 2016, the patient was brought to our department, and standard blood tests were normal. The neurological evaluation showed slow gait, normal muscular tension, brisk tendon reflexes, positive sign of bilateral palm-chin reflex, and negative Babinski sign. Her Mini Mental State Examination (MMSE) score was 20/30 and Montreal Cognitive Assessment (MoCA) score 15/30 (**Figures 1A,B**). Brain MRI in Dec 2016 revealed subtle atrophy in frontal and temporal lobes (**Figure 1C**). Although these findings did not lead to a definitive diagnosis, Memantine, Exelon, and Sertraline were administered as therapy. After 10 months, she was referred to our department again, and complained more serious memory decline. Her MMSE score was 12/30, and MoCA 10/30 (**Figures 1A,B**). However, brain MRI in Oct 2017 revealed no significant difference when compared with the last MRI (**Figure 1D**).

The family history is summarized in **Figure 2B**. There are no similar manifestations in the relatives of the patient.

Genetic Analysis

The mutation c.671 C>A, p. S224X of *SQSTM1* was detected by whole exome sequencing, and validated in gDNA by Sanger Sequencing (**Figure 2A**). This mutation has not been reported as pathogenic elsewhere, and is predicted to lead to premature termination of protein synthesis. The pathogenicity prediction of the nonsense mutation by Mutation Taster software was disease causing with a probability equal to 1. The Combined Annotation Dependent Depletion (CADD) predicted that Raw score was 6.91 and PHRED was 33. The mutation was not found in the dbSNP, 1000G, HGMD, or ExAC database. At the same time, we didn't detect the same mutation in 200 normal Chinese individuals. The mutation site of the *SQSTM1* gene was also assessed by evaluating the patient's unaffected younger sister, who did not carry the same mutation. Because the patient's father and mother were deceased, we could not determine whether the mutation was hereditary. The p.S224X heterozygous nonsense mutation is located at highly conserved position, as shown by a comparison of the corresponding sequences of 10 vertebrates (**Figure 2C**). The *APOE* genotype of the patient was *ε3/ε4*.

Analysis of SQSTM1 Mutant Protein Expression

HEK 293T cells were transfected with an empty-vector control or plasmids encoding either wild type or S224X mutant Myc-His tagged *SQSTM1* for 24 h. SQSTM1 was recognized in western blotting by different antibodies, which were SQSTM1 Gly162 and SQSTM1 Gly410 directed upstream and downstream, respectively, of the SQSTM1 mutation site (S224X). The SQSTM1

A

MMSE Category	2016.12 (6 year post onset)	2017.10 (6 year and 10 month post onset
orientation	7	4
attention and calculation	3	1
recall	3	3
language	5	3
execution	2	1
visual construction	0	0
total	20	12

B

MoCA Category	2016.12 (6 year post onset)	2017.10 (6 year and 10 month post onset)
visual-construction	1	1
alternate line	0	0
recall	0	0
attention and calculation	6	4
language	2	0
abstraction	1	1
orientation	5	4
Total	15	10

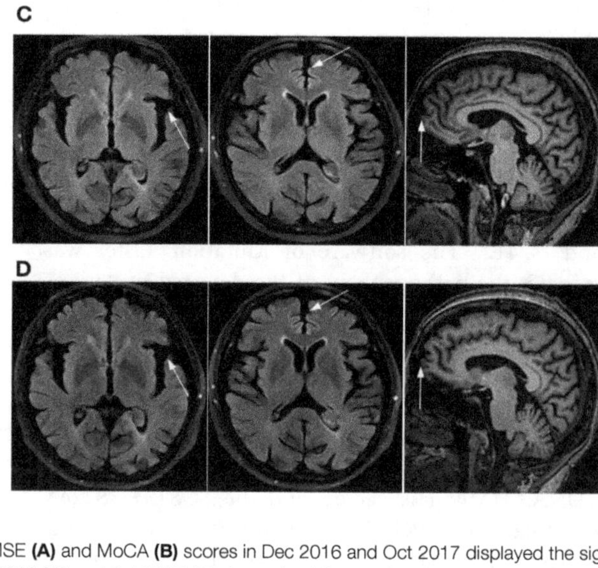

FIGURE 1 | Summary of MMSE and MoCA, and imaging data. Summary of MMSE **(A)** and MoCA **(B)** scores in Dec 2016 and Oct 2017 displayed the significant damage in cognitive function and decline trend with time. The brain MRI in Dec 2016 **(C)** and Oct 2017 **(D)** showed subtle atrophy of frontal and temporal lobes on transverse FLAIR weighted and sagittal T1 weighted sequences.

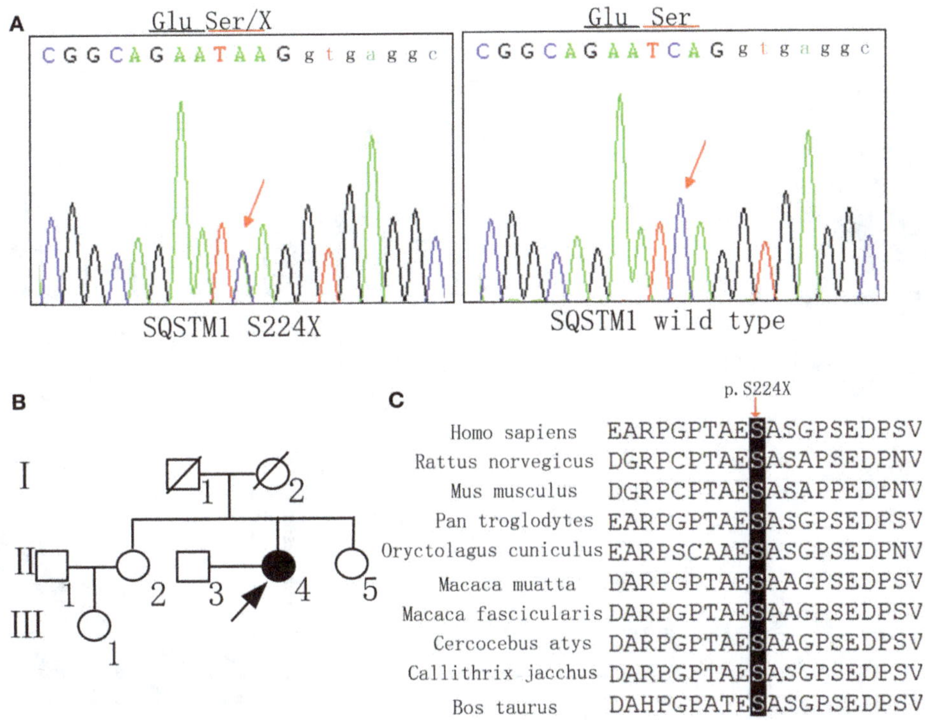

FIGURE 2 | DNA sequence, pedigree of the family, and gene conservation. **(A)** DNA sequence at codon 224 of *SQSTM1* gene from the patient and a control. The arrow indicates a mutated hemizygous site and a normal homozygous site, respectively. **(B)** The proband is indicated by an arrow (II-4). Her younger sister (II-5) also received the gene test and did not carry the same mutation. **(C)** The p.S224X heterozygous nonsense mutation occurs at highly conserved position, as shown by a comparison of the corresponding sequences of 10 vertebrates.

Gly162 antibody was used to detect truncated and intact SQSTM1 protein, and Gly410 to detect intact SQSTM1 protein (**Figure 3A**). Western blotting demonstrated that the levels of intact or truncated SQSTM1 protein in the S224X mutation group were all significantly reduced compared to wild type, similar to the vehicle ($p < 0.01$) (**Figure 3B**). Western blotting of Myc protein demonstrated no detectable Myc protein in the vehicle or S224X mutation group, only in the *SQSTM1* wild type group (**Figure 3A**).

Analysis of SQSTM1 Gene Expression

SQSTM1 cDNA was amplified by RT-PCR from mRNA extracted from peripheral blood leucocytes of the patient. We did not find the same mutation in *SQSTM1* cDNA (**Figures 3C,D**) through pyrosequencing or Sanger sequencing, which was inconsistent with DNA sequencing result. For analyzing the gene transcription differences between the *SQSTM1* S224X mutation and *SQSTM1* wild type, we included another five dementia controls (female: 3, male: 2, and age matched) without the *SQSTM1* mutation. The relative transcription of *SQSTM1* normalized to β-actin was analyzed using the concept of the threshold cycle (Ct) comparative method. Although the small sized of the samples adopted in the present study, it seemed that all dementia controls without *SQSTM*1 mutation presented an increased relative transcription level of *SQSTM1* mRNA (up to 3.06 ± 0.88-fold) with regards to the patient ($p < 0.05$) (**Figure 3E**).

DISCUSSION

The patient exhibited early-onset dementia combined with the initial symptom of memory decline, a gradual appearance of mild personality change, subtle atrophy of frontal/temporal lobes in MRI, negative appearance in EMG/NCV, and rapidly progressive course. The data of whole exome sequencing showed that AD related genes were all negative. These findings suggested an atypical bvFTD. The *SQSTM1* mutation (S224X) was found in the patient, which produced a stop codon and resulted in a predicted truncated protein 217 amino acids shorter than the normal SQSTM1 protein. *SQSTM1* has been reported to be associated with FTD-ALS type 3 (MIM: 616437). There isn't positive finding of EMG/NCV at present, but it still needs time to follow up the patient. The mutation is novel, not appearing in the dbSNP, 1000G, HGMD, ExAC database, and 200 normal Chinese individuals. The pathogenicity prediction by the Mutation-Taster application was disease causing, with a probability equal to 1. To determine the pathogenicity of this mutation, we overexpressed *SQSTM1* S224X mutant comparable to that of wild type *SQSTM1* in cell culture. Western blot of SQSTM1 recognized by Gly 410 and Gly 162 antibodies showed significant decrease of fully intact protein and truncated protein of SQSTM1. There

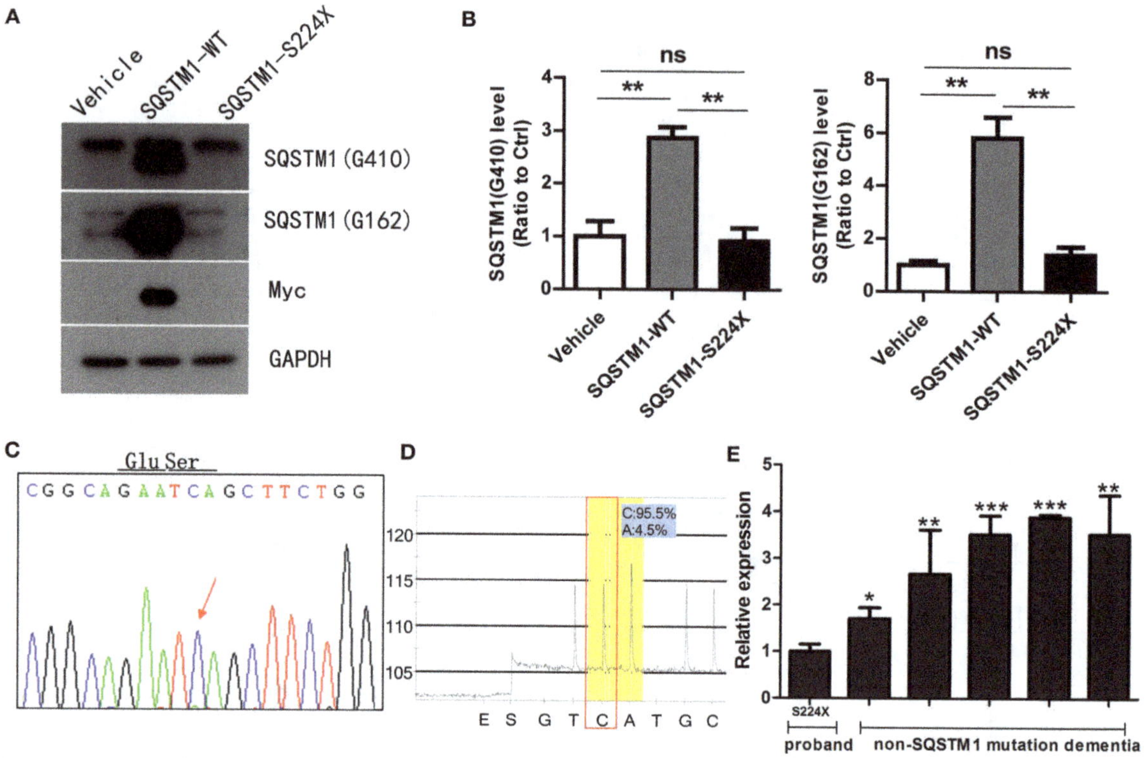

FIGURE 3 | Mutant SQSTM1 protein and cDNA levels. **(A)** HEK 293T cells were transfected with an empty vector or plasmids encoding either wild type or mutant Myc-His-tagged *SQSTM1* (S224X) for 24 h. Intact and truncated SQSTM1 proteins were recognized by western blotting with SQSTM1 (G410) and SQSTM1 (G162) antibodies, respectively. **(B)** The protein levels of SQSTM1 were quantified by densitometry and expressed as ratios to GAPDH. There were significantly reduced levels of intact or truncated SQSTM1 proteins in the S224X mutation group compared to wild type, similar to the vehicle. There was no expression of Myc protein in the vehicle or S224X mutation group, only in wild type. Data were plotted as mean ± SEM ($n = 3$). $^{**}p < 0.01$, One-way ANOVA. **(C,D)** *SQSTM1* cDNA from peripheral blood leucocytes of the patient was analyzed by Sanger sequencing and pyrosequencing. The mutation was not detected in *SQSTM1* cDNA through Sanger sequencing, and only 4% of mutation was detected through pyrosequencing. The arrow indicates the mutant site. **(E)** *SQSTM1* gene expression, measured by quantitative real-time PCR, normalized to β-actin, in peripheral blood leucocytes from the patient and five dementia controls without *SQSTM1* mutation. The expression of *SQSTM1* mRNA from the patient was significantly reduced compared to controls. Data were plotted as mean ± SEM ($n = 3$). $^{*}p < 0.05$; $^{**}p < 0.01$; $^{***}p < 0.001$, one-way ANOVA.

was no expressional difference between mutant protein and vehicle. Western blotting of the Myc tag demonstrated that the S224X mutation led to loss of SQSTM1 protein expression after eliminating the effect of endogenous SQSTM1 protein from HEK 293T cells. Furthermore, in *SQSTM1* cDNA from peripheral blood leucocytes of the patient, we didn't detect the mutation (S224X) by Sanger sequencing and pyrosequencing, and found significantly decreased level of *SQSTM1* mRNA compared to five dementia controls without SQSTM1 mutation. The above results suggested absent expression of SQSTM1/p62 protein in the S224X mutant overexpressing HEK-293T cells and significant decrease of *SQSTM1* mRNA level in the patient, which was possibly caused by nonsense-mediated mRNA decay (NMD), an mRNA degradation pathway regulating gene expression and mRNA quantity (Lopez-Perrote et al., 2016).

The *SQSTM1* gene encodes SQSTM1/p62 protein, a scaffolding protein, which regulates a variety of biological processes, including nuclear factor kappa B (NF-κB) signaling, apoptosis, transcription regulation, and ubiquitin-mediated autophagy (Rea et al., 2014). Collet et al. demonstrated that PDB patients with *SQSTM1* mutation (P392L, A381V, A390X, and L413F) had an increased level of SQSTM1/p62, and overproduction of the protein probably was involved in the pathophysiology of PDB (Collet et al., 2007). In FTD patients, *SQSTM1* mutations (E396X and R212C) are reportedly associated with p62 and TDP43 inclusions in brain (Kovacs et al., 2016). However, in the present study, we demonstrated that a novel *SQSTM1* mutation (S224X) causing loss of SQSTM1/p62 protein expression, not protein overproduction. Haack et al. identified three different biallelic loss-of-function variants (c.2T>A, p.?; R96X; E104Vfs*48) in *SQSTM1* gene in nine patients with neurodegenerative disorder, and confirmed absence of SQSTM1/p62 protein in these patients (Haack et al., 2016). In mice, the knock out of *SQSTM1* led to obesity and impaired glucose tolerance (Rodriguez et al., 2006). Furthermore, the chronic absence of SQSTM1/p62 promotes neurodegeneration with neurofibrillary tangles in hippocampal and cortical neurons manifesting with depression and short-term memory decline (Haack et al., 2016), which is similar to the clinical presentations of the present patient. There are multiple variants of *SQSTM1* gene that cause diverse patterns of protein expression. Generally speaking, the imbalance of SQSTM1/p62 expression induced by *SQSTM1* mutations is probably involved in the pathological mechanisms of FTD.

SQSTM1/p62 plays a key role in a variety of vital cellular processes, but it is unexpected that its absence is compatible with survival above age of 40 years (Haack et al., 2016), and mice lacking SQSTM1/p62 were fertile and lived more than 1 year inspite of adult-onset obesity and diabetes (Komatsu et al., 2007). This phenomenon probably argues for a redundancy of involved pathways or effective compensatory mechanisms (Haack et al., 2016). The present patient likely reflected SQSTM1 gene haploinsufficiency due to a combination of protein instability and NMD. Meanwhile, the patient displayed the *APOE ε3/ε4* genotype, which confers an increased risk of developing Alzheimer's disease (AD). Whether APOE ε4 is a risk factor for FTD remains controversial. Ji et al. examined 432 patients with AD, 62 with FTD, and 381 controls. *APOE ε4* allele frequency was significantly increased in late-onset AD (24.86), early-onset AD (18.02), and FTD (16.13) patients compared with controls (7.34), which suggested that the ApoE ε4 genotype is a risk factor for AD and FTD (Ji et al., 2013). However, Gustafson et al. and Verpillat et al. reported no correlation between the ε4 allele and FTD, but a larger increase in the ε2 allele in FTD compared with controls (Gustafson et al., 1997; Verpillat et al., 2002). Whether the *APOE ε3/ε4* genotype in this case is promoting FTD requires further scrutiny.

In summary, we firstly identified a novel *SQSTM1* mutation (S224X) in an atypical bvFTD patient, and the mutation caused absence of SQSTM1/p62 protein, which was consistent with a reduced level of *SQSTM1* mRNA from peripheral leucocytes of the patient. The mechanisms underlying these observations are possibly associated with *SQSTM1* gene haploinsufficiency. Different variants of the *SQSTM1* gene result in diverse expression patterns, and imbalance of SQSTM1/p62 protein induces different pathogenic processes. In addition, there was a factor that limited the findings of the present study. Without a large family showing dementia and enough gene samples from family members, it is difficult to demonstrate that *SQSTM1* S224X was fully responsible for FTD. However, we have provided a clue for discussing the pathogenicity significance of *SQSTM1* S224X mutation in FTD, which should foster an understanding of the effect of *SQSTM1* mutation on FTD when the mutation can be verified in a large family showing dementia.

ETHICS STATEMENT

This study was carried out in accordance with the recommendations of "Shanghai Mental Health Center ethical standards committee on human experimentation" with written informed consent from all subjects. All subjects gave written informed consent in accordance with the Declaration of Helsinki. The protocol was approved by the "Shanghai Mental Health Center ethical standards committee". All subjects also gave written informed consent for the publication of this case report.

AUTHOR CONTRIBUTIONS

LS and ZR: performed the experiments; LS: wrote the paper; WL: collected the samples; XL, SX, and HZ: supervised the experiments.

ACKNOWLEDGMENTS

This study was supported by grants of National Key R&D Program of China (2017YFC1310501500), Western medical guidance project of Shanghai science and Technology Commission (17411970100), Natural Science Foundation of China (81301139 and 81771164), Precision medical research project of Shanghai Jiaotong University School of Medicine (15ZH4010), Natural Science Foundation of Guangdong Province of China (2016A030313821 and 2017A030313604), and the Educational Department of Fujian Province of China (JZ160403).

REFERENCES

Boutoleau-Bretonnière, C., Camuzat, A., Le Ber, I., Bouya-Ahmed, K., Guerreiro, R., Deruet, A., et al. (2015). A phenotype of atypical apraxia of speech in a family carrying SQSTM1 mutation. *J. Alzheimers. Dis.* 43, 625–630. doi: 10.3233/JAD-141512

Collet, C., Michou, L., Audran, M., Chasseigneaux, S., Hilliquin, P., Bardin, T., et al. (2007). Paget's disease of bone in the French population: novel SQSTM1 mutations, functional analysis, and genotype-phenotype correlations. *J. Bone Miner. Res.* 22, 310–317. doi: 10.1359/jbmr.061106

Fecto, F., Yan, J., Vemula, S. P., Liu, E., Yang, Y., Chen, W., et al. (2011). SQSTM1 mutations in familial and sporadic amyotrophic lateral sclerosis. *Arch. Neurol.* 68, 1440–1446. doi: 10.1001/archneurol.2011250

Gustafson, L., Abrahamson, M., Grubb, A., Nilsson, K., and Fex, G. (1997). Apolipoprotein-E genotyping in Alzheimer's disease and frontotemporal dementia. *Dement. Geriatr. Cogn. Disord.* 8, 240–243. doi: 10.1159/000106637

Haack, T. B., Ignatius, E., Calvo-Garrido, J., Iuso, A., Isohanni, P., Maffezzini, C., et al. (2016). Absence of the autophagy adaptor SQSTM1/p62 causes childhood-onset neurodegeneration with ataxia, dystonia, and gaze palsy. *Am. J. Hum. Genet.* 99, 735–743. doi: 10.1016/j.ajhg.2016.06.026

Ji, Y., Liu, M., Huo, Y. R., Liu, S., Shi, Z., Liu, S., et al. (2013). Apolipoprotein Epsilon epsilon4 frequency is increased among Chinese patients with frontotemporal dementia and Alzheimer's disease. *Dement. Geriatr. Cogn. Disord.* 36, 163–170. doi: 10.1159/000350872

Komatsu, M., Waguri, S., Koike, M., Sou, Y. S., Ueno, T., and Hara, T. (2007). Homeostatic levels of p62 control cytoplasmic inclusion body formation in autophagy-deficient mice. *Cell* 131, 1149–1163. doi: 10.1016/j.cell.2007.10.035

Kovacs, G. G., van der Zee, J., Hort, J., Kristoferitsch, W., Leitha, T., Höftberger, R., et al. (2016). Clinicopathological description of two cases with SQSTM1 gene mutation associated with frontotemporal dementia. *Neuropathology* 36, 27–38. doi: 10.1111/neup.12233

Laurin, N., Brown, J. P., Morissette, J., and Raymond, V. (2002). Recurrent mutation of the gene encoding sequestosome 1 (SQSTM1/p62) in Paget disease of bone. *Am. J. Hum. Genet.* 70, 1582–1588. doi: 10.1086/340731

López-Perrote, A., Castaño, R., Melero, R., Zamarro, T., Kurosawa, H., Ohnishi, T., et al. (2016). Human nonsense-mediated mRNA decay factor UPF2 interacts directly with eRF3 and the SURF complex. *Nucleic Acids Res.* 44, 1909–1923. doi: 10.1093/nar/gkv1527

Luis, E., Ortiz, A., Eudave, L., Ortega-Cubero, S., Borroni, B., van der Zee, J., et al. (2016). Neuroimaging correlates of frontotemporal dementia associated with SQSTM1 mutations. *J. Alzheimers. Dis.* 53, 303–313. doi: 10.3233/JAD-160006

Miller, L., Rollinson, S., Callister, J. B., Young, K., Harris, J., Mann, D. M., et al. (2015). Pickering-brown: p62/SQSTM1 analysis in frontotemporal lobar degeneration. *Neurobiol. Aging* 36, 1603.e5-1603.e9. doi: 10.1016/j.neurobiolaging.2014.08.035

O'Connor, C. M., Clemson, L., Hornberger, M., Leyton, C. E., Hodges, E., Mioshi, J. R., et al. (2016). Longitudinal change in everyday function and behavioral symptoms in frontotemporal dementia. *Neurol. Clin. Pract.* 6, 419–428. doi: 10.1212/CPJ.0000000000000264

Pottier, C., Ravenscroft, T. A., Sanchez-Contreras, M., and Rademakers, R. (2016). Genetics of FTLD: overview and what else we can expect from genetic studies. *J. Neurochem.* 138(Suppl. 1), 32–53. doi: 10.1111/jnc.13622

Rea, S. L., Majcher, V., Searle, M. S., and Layfield, R. (2014). SQSTM1 mutations–bridging Paget disease of bone and ALS/FTLD. *Exp. Cell Res.* 325, 27–37. doi: 10.1016/j.yexcr.2014.01.020

Rodriguez, A., Durán, A., Selloum, M., Champy, M. F., Diez-Guerra, F., Moscat, J., et al. (2006). Mature-onset obesity and insulin resistance in mice deficient in the signaling adapter p62. *Cell Metab.* 3, 211–222. doi: 10.1016/j.cmet.2006.01.011

Rubino, E., Rainero, I., Chiò, A., Rogaeva, E., Galimberti, D., Fenoglio, P., et al. (2012). SQSTM1 mutations in frontotemporal lobar degeneration and amyotrophic lateral sclerosis. *Neurology* 79, 1556–1562. doi: 10.1212/WNL.0b013e31826e25df

Sun, L., Chen, K., Li, X., and Xiao S. (2017). Rapidly progressive frontotemporal dementia associated with MAPT Mutation G389R. *J. Alzheimers Dis.* 55, 777–785. doi: 10.3233/JAD-160802

Tosun, D., Schuff, N., Rabinovici, G. D., Ayakta, N., Miller, B. L., Rosen, L., et al. (2016). Diagnostic utility of ASL-MRI and FDG-PET in the behavioral variant of FTD and AD. *Ann. Clin. Transl. Neurol.* 3, 740–751. doi: 10.1002/acn3.330

van der Zee, J., Van Langenhove, T., Kovacs, G. G., Dillen, L., Deschamps, W., Van Broeckhoven, C., et al. (2014). Rare mutations in SQSTM1 modify susceptibility to frontotemporal lobar degeneration. *Acta Neuropathol.* 128, 397–410. doi: 10.1007/s00401-014-1298-7

Verpillat, P., Camuzat, A., Hannequin, D., Thomas-Anterion, C., Puel, M., Belliard, S., et al. (2002). Apolipoprotein E gene in frontotemporal dementia: an association study and meta-analysis. *Eur. J. Hum. Genet.* 10, 399–405. doi: 10.1038/sj.ejhg.5200820

16

Analysis of Alzheimer's Disease Based on the Random Neural Network Cluster in fMRI

Xia-an Bi*, Qin Jiang, Qi Sun, Qing Shu and Yingchao Liu

College of Information Science and Engineering, Hunan Normal University, Changsha, China

***Correspondence:**
Xia-an Bi
bixiaan@hnu.edu.cn

As Alzheimer's disease (AD) is featured with degeneration and irreversibility, the diagnosis of AD at early stage is important. In recent years, some researchers have tried to apply neural network (NN) to classify AD patients from healthy controls (HC) based on functional MRI (fMRI) data. But most study focus on a single NN and the classification accuracy was not high. Therefore, this paper used the random neural network cluster which was composed of multiple NNs to improve classification performance. Sixty one subjects (25 AD and 36 HC) were acquired from the Alzheimer's Disease Neuroimaging Initiative (ADNI) dataset. This method not only could be used in the classification, but also could be used for feature selection. Firstly, we chose Elman NN from five types of NNs as the optimal base classifier of random neural network cluster based on the results of feature selection, and the accuracies of the random Elman neural network cluster could reach to 92.31% which was the highest and stable. Then we used the random Elman neural network cluster to select significant features and these features could be used to find out the abnormal regions. Finally, we found out 23 abnormal regions such as the precentral gyrus, the frontal gyrus and supplementary motor area. These results fully show that the random neural network cluster is worthwhile and meaningful for the diagnosis of AD.

Keywords: random neural network cluster, fMRI, classification, Alzheimer's disease, functional connectivity

INTRODUCTION

Alzheimer's disease (AD) is degenerative and irreversible which results from the cognitive decline. The progress of AD increases with age and the disease easily triggers the other psychiatric diseases, and eventually causing dementia. In 2006, the number of AD patients is 26.6 million all around the world and the number would be quadruple by 2050. Therefore, it is meaningful for clinician to track its progression and diagnose the disease. Currently, there have been many different neuroimaging techniques which can be applied to diagnose AD, such as ElectroEncephaloGram (EEG) (Engels et al., 2015), Single Photon Emission Computed Tomography (SPECT) (Prosser et al., 2015), Positron Emission Tomography (PET) (Pagani et al., 2017), Magnetoencephalographic (MEG) (Engels et al., 2016), and functional magnetic resonance imaging (fMRI) (Griffanti et al., 2015). Among these techniques, fMRI is widely used in the diagnosis of AD, because it adopts a non-invasive way and could be used to find the differences of brain regions between AD and healthy controls (HC) (Challis et al., 2015).

Machine learning is a method of pattern recognition and has been used for the study of AD in recent years (Moradi et al., 2015; Khazaee et al., 2016). Among many machine learning methods, artificial neural network (ANN) is a useful classification method which evolves from human brain (Er et al., 2016). Several previous studies showed that neural network (NN) was able to be applied to diagnose neurological disease. Suk et al. (2016) proposed a method that combined deep learning and state-space model to classify Mild Cognitive Impairment (MCI) patients from HC, and the accuracy was 72.58%. Gao et al. (2017) employed an advanced convolution neural network (CNN) with 2D and 3D to diagnose AD, and the average accuracy reached to 87.6%. Ortiz et al. (2016) used deep learning architectures to classify AD patients from HC, and the accuracy approximately reached to 90%. Ortiz et al. (2013) used Learning Vector Quantization (LVQ) algorithm to classify AD patients from HC, and the accuracy was close to 90%. Luo et al. (2017) applied CNN to classify AD patients from HC, and the sensitivity and specificity of classification was 1 and 0.93 respectively. Suk et al. (2014) used deep learning to classify AD patients from HC, and the accuracy was close to 93.35%.

In existing studies, a single NN is often used to classify patients with neurological diseases and HC, and the accuracy of classification is considerable which indicates that NN is a powerful classification model (Hirschauer et al., 2015; Anthimopoulos et al., 2016). As the features of neuroimaging data are characterized by high dimension, significant information of original variables would be lost in the process of dimensionality reduction in traditional methods such as principal component analysis, local linear embedding and linear discriminate analysis (Mattioni and Jurs, 2003; McKeown et al., 2007; Mannfolk et al., 2010). In this paper, the method of the random neural network cluster is proposed to classify AD from HC. This method not only could be used in the classification, but also could be used for feature selection. The procedure of this method is as follows. Firstly, we chose Elman NN as the optimal base classifier from five types of neural networks [Back Propagation (BP) NN, Elman NN, PNN, Learning Vector Quantization (LVQ) NN and Competitive NN] based on the results of feature selection, and the accuracies of the random Elman neural network cluster could reach to 92.31% which is the highest and stable. Then we used the random Elman neural network cluster to select significant features and these features could be used to find out the abnormal regions. Finally, we found out 23 abnormal regions, such as the precentral gyrus, the frontal gyrus and supplementary motor area. These results fully show that the random neural network cluster is worthwhile and meaningful for the diagnosis of AD.

MATERIALS AND METHODS

Subjects

The experimental data was collected from the Alzheimer's Disease Neuroimaging Initiative (ADNI)[1] dataset which includes a variety of neuroimaging data. The ADNI study was approved by Institutional Review Board (IRB) of each participating site. All ADNI subjects together with their legal representatives should have written informed consent before collecting clinical, genetic and imaging data. The following two criteria need to meet when selecting data. One criterion is that the selected data should be resting-state fMRI data. Another criterion is that the selected data should have mini-mental state examination (MMSE) and clinical dementia rating (CDR) scores, and this criterion ensures that the selected data is homologous. Finally, 61 subjects were selected which consisted of 25 AD patients and 36 HC.

Data Collection and Preprocessing

Scanning images were acquired on a Philips Medical Systems 3 Tesla MRI scanner. Acquisition parameters included: pulse sequence = GR, *TR* = 3,000 ms, *TE* = 30 ms, matrix = 64*64, slice thickness = 3.3 mm, slice number = 48, flip angle = 80°.

To decrease the influence of signal-to-noise ratio of the fMRI images, the selected data should be preprocessed. The data was preprocessed based on the Data Processing Assistant for Resting-State fMRI (DPARSF) software (Chao-Gan and Yu-Feng, 2010; Wang et al., 2013). The process of the data preprocessing included: converting DICOM format into NIFTI format; removing first 10 time points; slicing timing (Sarraf et al., 2016); realigning (Jenkinson et al., 2002); normalizating images into the echo planar imaging (EPI) template (Misaki et al., 2010); temporal smoothing; removing the effect of low-level ($<$0.01 HZ) and high-level ($>$0.08 HZ) noise by a high-pass temporal filtering (Challis et al., 2015); removing covariates such as the whole brain signal and cerebrospinal fluid signal.

Functional Connectivity of Brain

After the preprocessing steps, the analysis of the functional connectivity of brain was followed. In this paper, we chose functional connectivity as the sample feature. The extraction of the functional connectivity is as follows. Firstly, the images of brain were divided into 90 regions defined by Automated Anatomical Labeling (AAL) brain atlas (Rolls et al., 2015). Secondly, the time series of each region were extracted. Thirdly, the Pearson correlation coefficient between two separated brain regions could be defined as the functional connectivity (Friston et al., 1993). Finally, 4,005 ($90 \times 89/2$) functional connectivity of each subject were taken as their features.

The Random Neural Network Cluster

The 4,005 functional connectivity belongs to the high-dimensional feature which causes the problems of computation difficulty and dimensions of disaster. Moreover, the high-dimensional features are likely to result in numerous redundant and irrelevant features which may decrease the classification performance. Therefore, the irrelevant features are needed to be removed by feature selection (Azar and Hassanien, 2015).

There are many methods of feature selection, such as principal component analysis, local linear embedding and linear discriminate analysis. However, in these methods, the process of selecting features may cause the loss of the original information, and the classification performance may be unsatisfactory (Zhou et al., 2015; Jolliffe and Cadima, 2016; Alam and Kwon, 2017).

To solve the problem above, this paper proposes the random neural network cluster by randomly selecting samples and features. The random neural network cluster could be used

[1] http://adni.loni.usc.edu/

to classify AD patients from HC and select features. In addition, the new method could achieve the purpose of reducing dimensionality, avoid losing significant information and improve classification performance.

The Design and Classification Accuracy of the Random Neural Network Cluster

The basic thought of the random neural network cluster is ensemble learning whose basic classifier is neural network. The detailed process of establishing the random neural network cluster is as follows. Firstly, the sample dataset D is randomly divided into a training set N_1 and a test set N_2, where $D = N_1 + N_2$. The real label of HC and AD is +1 and −1 respectively. Secondly, we randomly select n samples from the training set and m features from the 4,005 features. Thirdly, the selected samples and features are used to establish a single NN and the process of the second and third step is repeated for k times. Thus, k NNs are obtained which construct the random neural network cluster. It can be seen from this process that the method and the conventional process are essentially not the same in essence. **Figure 1** shows the formation of the random neural network cluster.

When a new sample enters the random neural network cluster, we could obtain k class labels from k NNs and the majority of class label is made as the predicted label of the new sample. Similarly, we could get the label of each sample in the test set N_2. Then the predicted label is compared with the real label to judge whether they are consistent, and we assume C as the number of consistent situations. The accuracy of the random neural network cluster equals to C/N_2.

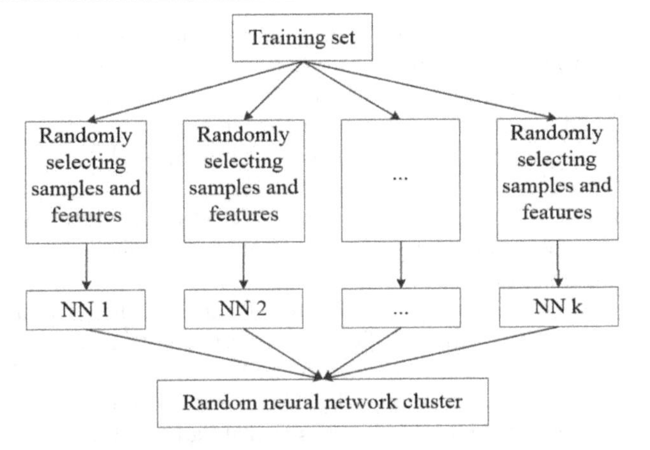

FIGURE 1 | The formation of the random neural network cluster.

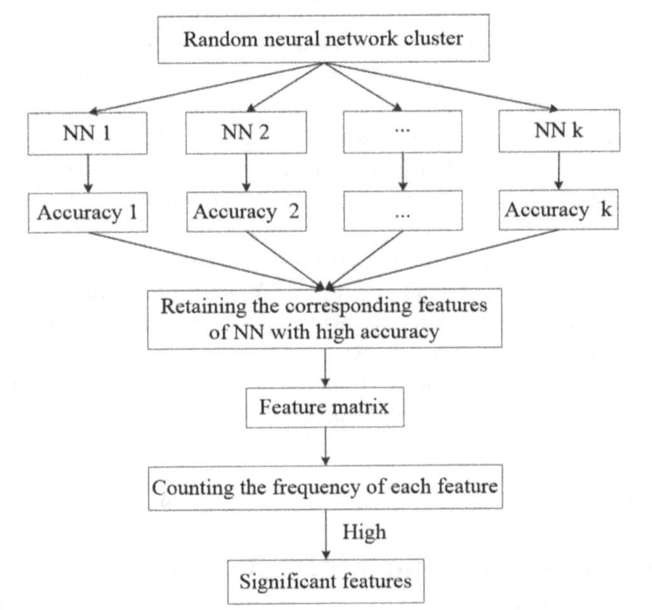

FIGURE 2 | The flow of significant feature extraction.

Extracting Features From the Random Neural Network Cluster

As the features are randomly selected, the NNs constructed by these features have different characteristics. In this paper, the accuracy of each NN is used to evaluate the significance of selected features. The features that make significant contributions to the accuracy of the NN are called the "significant features". The process of extracting significant features is as follows.

Firstly, the test samples are used to obtain the accuracy of each NN in the random neural network cluster. If the accuracy of a NN is high, the corresponding features are significant. Next, the features in each NN with high accuracy are extracted to form a feature matrix. Finally, we count the frequency of each feature in the feature matrix, and extract the features with high frequency which are called as "significant features." **Figure 2** shows the process of selecting "significant features." The significant features tremendously contribute to the accuracy of a NN, thus they also make great contributions to the accuracy of the random neural network cluster. In this paper, we use the significant features to find the difference between AD patients and HC.

The Abnormal Brain Regions

As mentioned above, the significant features make great contributions to the accuracy of the random neural network cluster, thus we could find the difference between AD and HC through these significant features. In this paper, the significant features are regarded as the abnormal functional connectivity. As the functional connectivity is defined as the relationship of two brain regions, the extracted significant features could be used to find the abnormal brain regions between AD and HC. In order to estimate the abnormal degree of a brain region, the number of features related to a certain region is considered as the weight. When there is no functional connectivity related to a certain brain region, the weight of the region is 0. When the weight is greater, the abnormal degree of the brain region is higher.

Experiment Design

The process of the experiment involves six steps in this paper.

Step 1. Building the random neural network cluster. Firstly, 61 subjects are divided into a training set and a test set according to the proportion of 8:2. Thus, the number of training samples and test samples is 48 and 13 respectively. Then, 45 subjects are randomly selected from 48 training samples and 120 features are randomly selected from 4,005 features to build a NN. Similarly, we build 1,000 NNs to construct the random neural network cluster. The result of the random neural network cluster is calculated by using neural network toolbox.

Step 2. Selecting significant NNs. We select the NNs whose accuracy is >0.6 from the 1,000 NNs and call these NNs as significant NNs.

Step 3. Selecting significant features. The features corresponding to the significant NNs form the feature matrix. Then we count the frequency of each feature, and sort the features with a descending order. Finally, we retain the first 240 features which are regarded as the original significant features.

Step 4. Determining the optimal number of the significant features. We change the number of original significant features from 140 to 240 features with a step of 10 as the new significant features, thus there are 11 types of numbers of new significant features. Then we select 120 features from the new significant features to construct a NN. We select 120 features from the original significant features, and change the number of significant features from 140 to 240 features with a step of 10. Thus, we could obtain 11 random neural network clusters. The number of the significant features corresponding to the random neural network cluster with highest accuracy is the optimal number.

Step 5. We repeat the step1-step 4 by using five types of NNs. They are BP NN, Elman NN, PNN, LVQ NN, and Competitive NN. Then we choose one of them as the best base classifier who has the highest accuracy in step 4.

Step 6. Finding abnormal brain regions through the significant features in step 4 based on the best base classifier.

RESULTS

The Demographic Information of Participants

In this study, the selected 61 subjects include 25 AD patients and 36 HC. The gender and age difference between the AD group and HC group data are examined by two-sample *t*-test and chi-square test respectively. The result is shown in **Table 1**. It is referred that the two groups have no statistical significance in the gender and the age.

Classification Results

In this study, five different types of NNs are applied to construct five different types of random neural network clusters. The number of significant features in each random neural network cluster changes from 140 to 240 and the step is 10. Therefore, we can obtain 11 results for each type of random neural network cluster, and their parameters have been made appropriate adjustments to get better results. The accuracies of five types of random neural network clusters are shown in **Figure 3**. It is referred that the accuracies of random Competitive neural network cluster are not stable; the accuracies of random Elman neural network cluster and random Probabilistic neural network cluster are high, and their highest accuracy reaches to 92.31%; the accuracies of random BP neural network cluster and random LVQ neural network cluster are lower than the random Elman neural network cluster. The accuracies of the random neural network cluster changes when the number of features changes. As the highest accuracies of the random Elman neural network cluster are relatively stable and high, this paper chooses Elman neural network as the best base classifier. From **Figure 3** we can learn that when the number of significant features is 180, the accuracy is the highest. Therefore, 180 is the optimal number of significant features.

In order to better compare the performances of the random neural network cluster and a single NN, we display the corresponding 1,000 NNs' accuracies of five types of random neural network clusters in the **Figure 4**. From **Figures 3, 4** we could learn that the accuracy of random neural network cluster is higher and more stable than a single NN except for the random Competitive neural network cluster. In addition, we also show the training errors, test errors and running time of five types of random neural network clusters in **Table 2**.

The Abnormal Brain Regions

The first 180 features constitute the optimal feature set which is used to find the abnormal brain regions between AD patients and HC. **Table 3** shows the abnormal brain regions with higher weight, their abbreviation and volume. **Figure 5** shows the abnormal degree of brain regions by using the Brain-NetViewer[2].

[2]http://www.nitrc.org/projects/bnv/

TABLE 1 | The information of participants.

Variables (Mean ± *SD*)	AD (*n* = 25)	HC (*n* = 36)	*P*-value
Gender(male/female)	12/13	20/16	0.784
Age	74.59 ± 7.03	77.00 ± 6.61	0.177

AD, Alzheimer's disease; HC, Healthy Control.

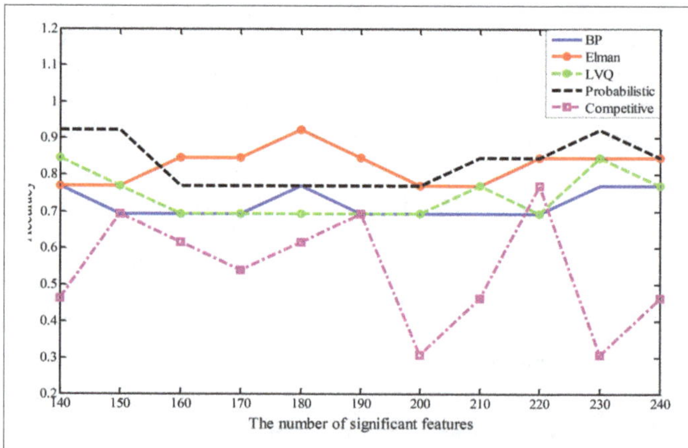

FIGURE 3 | The accuracies of five different types of random neural network clusters.

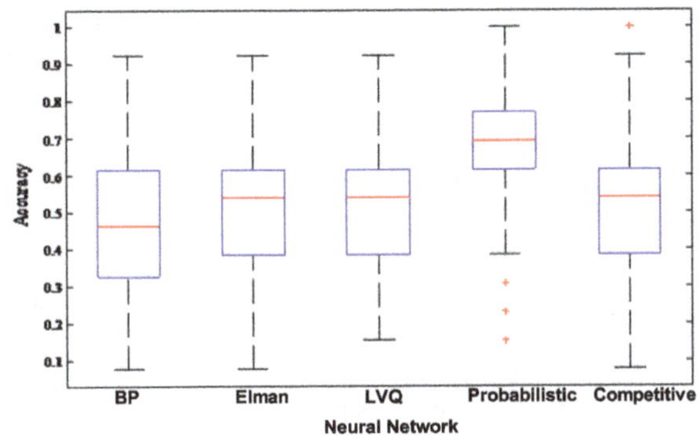

FIGURE 4 | The corresponding 1,000 NNs' accuracies of five types of random neural network clusters.

The node represents the brain region. The size of a node represents the weight of the brain region and it also indicates the abnormal degree of the brain region.

In this paper, we focus on the brain region whose weight is >17. **Figure 6** shows the functional connectivity between the 23 brain regions in the optimal feature set. **Figure 7** shows the functional connectivity between PreCG and other brain regions. The node in **Figures 6, 7** also represents the brain region and the size of a node represents the weight of the brain region. Besides, the line represents the functional connectivity between two brain regions.

DISCUSSION

Classification Performance

A number of researchers have tried to classify and diagnose AD patients from HC in the past few years. For instance, Khazaee et al. (2016) applied machine learning methods to classify MCI patients, AD patients and HC, and the accuracy of AD and HC is 72%. Kim et al. (2016) applied DNN to classify schizophrenia (SZ) patients and HC based on fMRI image, and the accuracy is 85.8%. Zhang et al. (2014) proposed a kernel support vector machine decision tree (kSVM-DT) to classify MCI patients, AD patients and HC based on the MRI data, and the accuracy of AD and HC is 96%. However, there were several disadvantages in these studies. For instance, as the features of neuroimaging data are characterized by high dimension, significant information of original variables would be lost in the process of dimensionality reduction in traditional methods.

TABLE 2 | The errors and running time of five types of random neural network clusters.

Base classifier (Mean ± *SD*)	Training errors	Test errors	Time (hour)
BP NN	0.2764 ± 0.0375	0.2797 ± 0.0388	2
Probabilistic NN	0.1709 ± 0.0712	0.1678 ± 0.0672	10
Elman NN	0.1782 ± 0.0519	0.1748 ± 0.0497	12
LVQ NN	0.2645 ± 0.0604	0.2587 ± 0.0622	48
Competitive NN	0.4627 ± 0.1532	0.4615 ± 0.1538	18

In this paper, the new method was proposed to avoid the loss of information and improve classification performance. We used five different types of NNs as the base classifier to build five different types of random neural network clusters. In the five types of random neural network clusters, the classification accuracies of the random Elman neural network cluster and the random PNN cluster could reach to 92.3%. As the resting-state fMRI data dynamically changes in a period of time and the Elman NN is able to deal with the time and spatial domain data, the Elman NN is more suitable for the fMRI data. The accuracies of the random Probabilistic neural network cluster could also reach to 92.3%, but the running time of the PNN is long which makes it not suitable for the base classifier of the random neural network cluster. Thus, we finally choose the random Elman neural network cluster as the best base classifier. To solve the problems caused by the high-dimensional data, the traditional methods suffer from the loss of some information in the process of reducing dimensionality. In this paper, we proposed a random neural network cluster which could be a good solution in dealing with the calculation of large samples and high-dimensional data. Moreover, the highest accuracies of the random Elman neural network cluster could reach to 92.3%. Therefore, this method could process high-dimensional data without information loss and improve classification performance.

The basic classifier used in this paper is the neural network. This classifier is indeed an existing classifier, and it is not the innovation point of this paper. The innovation of this article is the integrated cluster, which is the innovation in structure.

This paper researches on fMRI image, there is no innovation in the classification indicators of this article. But the classification indicators have been used in research. We used the random neural network cluster to classify the subjects and feature selection, and we got good results. That is the innovation in application.

The Additional Details of the Random Neural Network Cluster

In the part of method, we have introduced many elementary details in our method and in this part we would introduce some additional details.

In order to make the random neural network cluster less complex, each NN occupies the same weight in the random neural network cluster. When determining the label of a new sample, each NN in the random neural network cluster predicts the label of the sample. The majority of class label is made as the predicted label of the sample which is equivalent to that the weight of each NN is the same. From **Figures 3, 4** we could learn that the accuracy of a single NN is lower than the accuracy of the random neural network cluster. Moreover, when the number of significant features changes, the accuracies of five types of random neural network clusters are high and stable except for the random Competitive neural network cluster. This fully demonstrates that the robustness of the random neural network cluster is good.

TABLE 3 | Abnormal brain regions.

Regions	Abbreviation	Volume	Weight
The precentral gyrus	PreCG.L	[−39 −6 51]	19
The middle frontal gyrus	MFG.L	[−33 33 35]	
The olfactory cortex	OLF.L	[−8 15 −11]	
The orbital part of superior frontal gyrus	ORBsup.R	[18 48 −14]	18
The triangular part of inferior frontal gyrus	IFGtriang.L	[−46 30 14]	
The supplementary motor area	SMA.L	(−5 5 61)	
The orbital part of superior frontal gyrus	ORBsup.L	[−17 47 −13]	17
The orbital part of middle frontal gyrus	ORBmid.L	[−31 50 −10]	
The precentral gyrus	PreCG.R	[41 −8 52]	16
The dorsolateral of superior frontal gyrus	SFGdor.R	[22 31 44]	
The orbital part of middle frontal gyrus	ORBmid.R	[33 53 −11]	
The orbital part of Inferior frontal gyrus	ORBinf.L	[−36 31 −12]	
The orbital part of Inferior frontal gyrus	ORBinf.R	[41 32 −12]	
The olfactory cortex	OLF.R	[10 16 −11]	
The middle frontal gyrus	MFG.R	[38 33 34]	15
The rolandic operculum	ROL.L	[−47 −8 14]	
The rolandic operculum	ROL.R	[53 −6 15]	
The dorsolateral of superior frontal gyrus	SFGdor.L	[−18 35 42]	14
The opercular part of inferior frontal gyrus	IFGoperc.L	[−48 1319]	
The opercular part of inferior frontal gyrus	IFGoperc.R	[50 15 21]	
The triangular part of inferior frontal gyrus	IFGtriang.R	[50 30 14]	
The supplementary motor area	SMA.R	[9 0 62]	
The medial of superior frontal gyrus	SFGmed.L	[−549 31]	

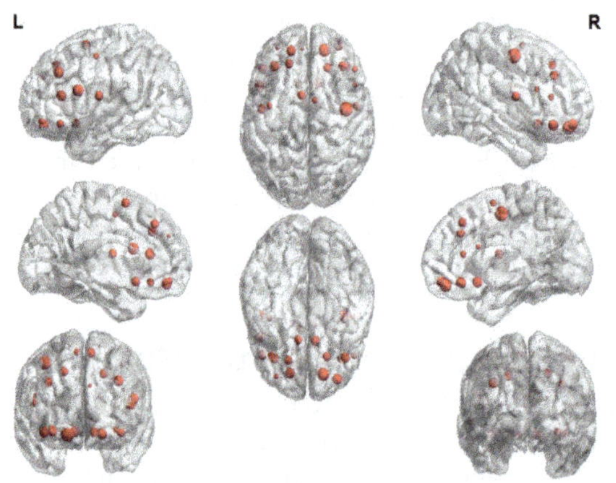

FIGURE 5 | The weight of brain regions.

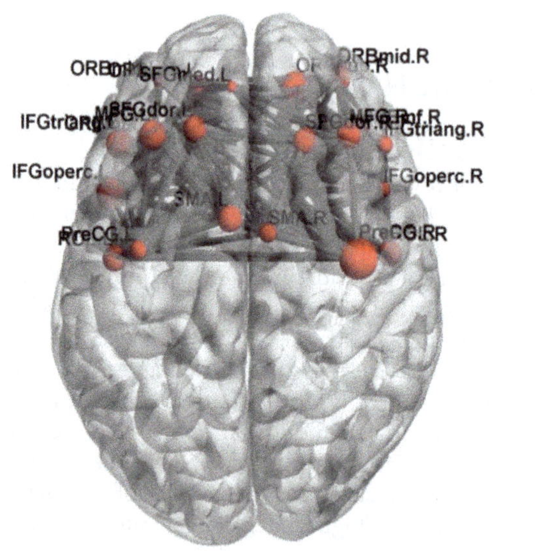

FIGURE 6 | The functional connectivity between the 23 brain regions.

In terms of the complexity of random neural network cluster, it is mainly reflected in the following two aspects. One aspect is that the number of base classifiers is large which makes the process of constructing a random neural network cluster complex. Another aspect is that we need to construct multiple random neural network clusters during finding the optimal feature set which also makes the method complex.

There are two types of parameters in our method. One type is the parameters of the random neural network cluster which are decided by the accuracy of the random neural network cluster through hundreds of experiments. Another type is the parameters of the NN which are decided by the neural network toolbox that automatically selects the optimal parameters.

The random neural network cluster is constructed by the training set and the performance is tested by the test set. The experimental results show that the random neural network cluster not only performs well on the training set, but also performs well on the test set. This fully demonstrates that

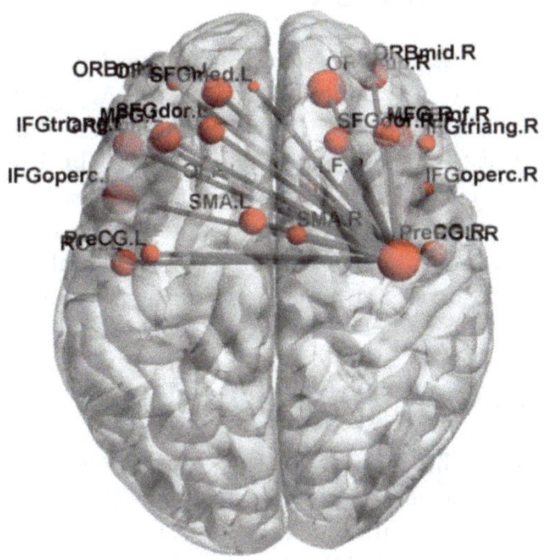

FIGURE 7 | The functional connectivity between PreCG and other brain regions.

the overfitting does not exist in the random neural network cluster.

Abnormal Brain Region Analysis

The functional connectivity differences between AD and HC could be used to find out the abnormal brain regions and we finally detected 23 abnormal brain regions between AD and HC. They are the PreCG, the OLF, the ORBsup, the IFGtriang, SMA, the SFGdor, the ORBmid, the ORBinf, the SFGmed.L, the IFGoperc, the ROL, and the MFG.

Previous studies have concluded that these abnormal brain regions are associated with AD patients. Khazaee et al. (2015) found that the lingual gyrus, the occipital gyrus and the superior frontal gyrus are abnormal brain regions in AD patients. Agosta et al. (2012) pointed out that the functional connectivity changed in the default mode network (DMN) and frontal networks in AD patients. Wang et al. (2007) discovered the decreased abnormal functional connectivity in the prefrontal and parietal lobes, meanwhile the increased abnormal functional connectivity in the occipital lobe in AD patients. Greicius et al. (2004) found that AD patients showed less deactivation in the anterior frontal, precuneus and posterior cingulate cortex. He et al. (2007) concluded that regional coherence of AD patients significantly decreased in the posterior cingulate cortex/precuneus. Binnewijzend et al. (2012) declared that the abnormal brain regions of AD patients located in the precuneus and posterior cingulate cortex. Golby et al. (2005) concluded that impaired activation changed in the temporal lobe and fusiform regions in AD patients. Grossman et al. (2003) found the activation of AD patients in the left poster lateral temporal and inferior parietal cortex. It is referred that our results are consistent with previous studies. In this paper, we focus on the precentral gyrus and the frontal gyrus which have larger weights.

Precentral Gyrus (PreCG)

The PreCG has the greatest weight in the abnormal brain regions. It is referred that the PreCG makes a great contribution to classify AD and HC in the random Elman neural network cluster. The PreCG locates in the primary motor area (Hopkins et al., 2017), and the superior part of PreCG is responsible for motor hand function (Yousry et al., 1997; Nebel et al., 2014).

Existing studies have found that the PreCG is abnormal in AD patients. Kang et al. (2013) showed that AD patients performed significant cortical thinning in superior and medial frontal gyrus, left precentral gyrus, postcentral gyrus, paracentral lobule, precuneus and superior parietal lobule. Bi et al. (2018) proposed a method of random support vector machine cluster to diagnose AD, and found out several disorder regions including inferior frontal gyrus, superior frontal gyrus, precentral gyrus and cingulate cortex. Zhang et al. (2015) pointed out that the middle occipital gyrus, the postcentral gyrus, the PreCG and precuneus were important in diagnosing AD. Brickman et al. (2015) discovered that the PreCG and right middle frontal gyrus were abnormal in AD patients based on T2-weighted MRI. Dani et al. (2017) used white matter hypointensity (WMH) volume to diagnose AD based on MRI and PET data, and they found out the difference between the PreCG, and the right medial and anterior part of orbital gyrus.

The abnormal functional connectivity between PreCG and other brain regions may lead to the physical movement dysfunction in AD patients. The above results revealed that PreCG may be a clinical diagnosis of AD in future.

Frontal Gyrus (FG)

The FG had a relatively higher weight in the abnormal regions. It is referred that the FG makes a great contribution to classify AD and HC in the random Elman neural network cluster. The left of inferior frontal gyrus is associated with language (Costafreda et al., 2006). The superior frontal gyrus contributes to higher cognitive functions and particularly the learning and working memory (WM) (Boisgueheneuc et al., 2006; Carter et al., 2006). Eliasova et al. (2014) explored that the improvement of attention and psychomotor speed resulted from the abnormity of the right IFG in AD patients.

Existing studies have found that the FG is abnormal in AD patients. Schultz et al. (2015) found out several abnormal brain regions in AD patients including the hippocampus, the posterior cingulate, the anterior cingulate and the middle frontal gyrus. Griffanti et al. (2016) pointed out that there was difference in orbito frontal network between AD patient and HC. Yetkin et al. (2006) evaluated brain activation in AD patients and HC based on fMRI while performing a WM task and found that AD group showed more activation in the right superior frontal gyrus, bilateral middle temporal, middle frontal, anterior cingulate and fusiform gyri. Karas et al. (2007) used voxel-based morphometry (VBM) to examine AD patients, and they found out several disorder regions including the left superior and inferior temporal gyrus, and the left superior frontal gyrus. Our experiment results are consistent with the existing studies.

The abnormal functional connectivity between FG and other brain regions may lead to the memory dysfunction in

AD patients. This abnormal brain region has significant effect on the identification of potentially effective biomarkers for the diagnosis of AD.

In this paper, the random neural network cluster is proposed to classify AD patients and HC and the abnormal brain regions are found out on the basis of fMRI data. Moreover, these findings suggest that the random neural network cluster might be an appropriate approach for diagnosing AD. This new method has some advantages. Firstly, the NNs make different contributions to the random neural network cluster which could make full use of each NN's characteristics, thus it could avoid losing information. Secondly, it is able to effectively deal with a large dataset even when there is many missing data. Finally, it is also able to select significant features from high-dimensional features. The new method presents a good classification performance with accuracy of 92.3% and detects several abnormal brain regions which would have influence in diagnosing AD. However, it has several limitations. Firstly, this paper only used the fMRI data and the future studies could integrate other imaging data to obtain comprehensive brain activity. Secondly, this paper only studied the brain activity, and the future studies could combine the brain and cerebellum activity. Thirdly, this paper only studies the brain difference between AD patients and HC, and the future studies could focus on the brain relationship in AD patients. Finally, the functional connectivity was regarded as feature in this paper, and the future studies could choose other attributions of the brain as feature such as clustering coefficient, degree and shortest path.

ETHICS STATEMENT

This study was carried out in accordance with the recommendations of National Institute of Aging-Alzheimer's Association (NIA-AA) workgroup guidelines, Institutional Review Board (IRB). The study was approved by Institutional Review Board (IRB) of each participating site, including the Banner Alzheimer's Institute, and was conducted in accordance with Federal Regulations, the Internal Conference on Harmonization (ICH), and Good Clinical Practices (GCP).

AUTHOR CONTRIBUTIONS

X-aB proposed the design of the work and revised it critically for important intellectual content. QSu and QJ carried out the experiment for the work and drafted part of the work. YL and QSh collected, interpreted the data, and drafted part of the work. All the authors approved the final version to be published and agreed to be accountable for all aspects of the work in ensuring that questions related to the accuracy or integrity of any part of the work are appropriately investigated and resolved.

FUNDING

This work was supported by the National Science Foundation of China (Nos. 61502167 and 61473259).

REFERENCES

Agosta, F., Pievani, M., Geroldi, C., Copetti, M., Frisoni, G. B., and Filippi, M. (2012). Resting state fMRI in Alzheimer's disease: beyond the default mode network. *Neurobiol. Aging* 33, 1564–1578. doi: 10.1016/j.neurobiolaging.2011.06.007

Alam, S., and Kwon, G. R. (2017). Alzheimer disease classification using KPCA, LDA, and multi-kernel learning SVM. *Int. J. Imaging Syst. Technol.* 27, 133–143. doi: 10.1002/ima.22217

Anthimopoulos, M., Christodoulidis, S., Ebner, L., Christe, A., and Mougiakakou, S. (2016). Lung pattern classification for interstitial lung diseases using a deep convolutional neural network. *IEEE Trans. Med. Imaging* 35, 1207–1216. doi: 10.1109/TMI.2016.2535865

Azar, A. T., and Hassanien, A. E. (2015). Dimensionality reduction of medical big data using neural-fuzzy classifier. *Soft Comput.* 19, 1115–1127. doi: 10.1007/s00500-014-1327-4

Bi, X.-A., Shu, Q., Sun, Q., and Xu, Q. (2018). Random support vector machine cluster analysis of resting-state fMRI in Alzheimer's disease. *PLoS One* 13:e0194479. doi: 10.1371/journal.pone.0194479

Binnewijzend, M. A. A., Schoonheim, M. M., Sanz-Arigita, E., Wink, A. M., van der Flier, W. M., Tolboom, N., et al. (2012). Resting-state fMRI changes in Alzheimer's disease and mild cognitive impairment. *Neurobiol. Aging* 33, 2018–2028. doi: 10.1016/j.neurobiolaging.2011.07.003

Boisgueheneuc, F. D., Levy, R., Volle, E., Seassau, M., Duffau, H., Kinkingnehun, S., et al. (2006). Functions of the left superior frontal gyrus in humans: a lesion study. *Brain* 129, 3315–3328. doi: 10.1093/brain/awl244

Brickman, A. M., Zahodne, L. B., Guzman, V. A., Narkhede, A., Meier, I. B., Griffith, E. Y., et al. (2015). Reconsidering harbingers of dementia: progression of parietal lobe white matter hyperintensities predicts Alzheimer's disease incidence. *Neurobiol. Aging* 36, 27–32. doi: 10.1016/j.neurobiolaging.2014.07.019

Carter, R. M., O'Doherty, J. P., Seymour, B., Koch, C., and Dolan, R. J. (2006). Contingency awareness in human aversive conditioning involves the middle frontal gyrus. *NeuroImage* 29, 1007–1012. doi: 10.1016/j.neuroimage.2005.09.011

Challis, E., Hurley, P., Serra, L., Bozzali, M., Oliver, S., and Cercignani, M. (2015). Gaussian process classification of Alzheimer's disease and mild cognitive impairment from resting-state fMRI. *NeuroImage* 112, 232–243. doi: 10.1016/j.neuroimage.2015.02.037

Chao-Gan, Y., and Yu-Feng, Z. (2010). DPARSF: A MATLAB toolbox for "Pipeline" data analysis of resting-state fMRI. *Front. Syst. Neurosci.* 4:13. doi: 10.3389/fnsys.2010.00013

Costafreda, S. G., Fu, C. H. Y., Lee, L., Everitt, B., Brammer, M. J., and David, A. S. (2006). A systematic review and quantitative appraisal of fMRI studies of verbal fluency: role of the left inferior frontal gyrus. *Hum. Brain Mapp.* 27, 799–810. doi: 10.1002/hbm.20221

Dani, M., Fan, Z., Wood, M., Mizoguchi, R., Morgan, R., Walker, Z., et al. (2017). amyloid deposition, tau aggregation and microglial activation correlate with vascular burden in vivo in Alzheimer's disease, Alzheimer's & Dementia. *J. Alzheimer's Assoc.* 13, 681–682. doi: 10.1016/j.jalz.2017.06.848

Eliasova, I., Anderkova, L., Marecek, R., and Rektorova, I. (2014). Non-invasive brain stimulation of the right inferior frontal gyrus may improve attention in early Alzheimer's disease: a pilot study. *J. Neurol. Sci.* 346, 318–322. doi: 10.1016/j.jns.2014.08.036

Engels, M. M., Stam, C. J., van der Flier, W. M., Scheltens, P., de Waal, H., and van Straaten, E. C. (2015). Declining functional connectivity and changing hub locations in Alzheimer's disease: an EEG study. *BMC Neurol.* 15:145. doi: 10.1186/s12883-015-0400-7

Engels, M. M. A., Hillebrand, A., van der Flier, W. M., Stam, C. J., Scheltens, P., and van Straaten, E. C. W. (2016). Slowing of hippocampal activity correlates with cognitive decline in early onset alzheimer's disease, an MEG study with virtual electrodes. *Front. Hum. Neurosci.* 10:238. doi: 10.3389/fnhum.2016.00238

Er, O., Cetin, O., Bascil, M. S., and Temurtas, F. (2016). A comparative study on parkinson's disease diagnosis using neural networks and artificial immune system. *J. Med. Imaging Health Inf.* 6, 264–268. doi: 10.1166/jmihi.2016.1606

Friston, K. J., Frith, C. D., Liddle, P. F., and Frackowiak, R. S. J. (1993). Functional connectivity: the principal-component analysis of large (PET) data sets. *J. Cereb. Blood Flow & Metab.* 13, 5–14. doi: 10.1038/jcbfm.1993.4

Gao, X. W., Hui, R., and Tian, Z. (2017). Classification of CT brain images based on deep learning networks. *Comput. Methods Programs* 138, 49–56. doi: 10.1016/j.cmpb.2016.10.007

Golby, A., Silverberg, G., Race, E., Gabrieli, S., O'Shea, J., Knierim, K., et al. (2005). Memory encoding in Alzheimer's disease: an fMRI study of explicit and implicit memory. *Brain* 128, 773–787. doi: 10.1093/brain/awh400

Greicius, M. D., Srivastava, G., Reiss, A. L., and Menon, V. (2004). Default-mode network activity distinguishes Alzheimer's disease from healthy aging: evidence from functional MRI. *Proc. Natl. Acad. Sci. U.S.A.* 101, 4637–4642. doi: 10.1073/pnas.0308627101

Griffanti, L., Dipasquale, O., Laganà, M. M., Nemni, R., Clerici, M., Smith, S. M., et al. (2015). Effective artifact removal in resting state fMRI data improves detection of DMN functional connectivity alteration in Alzheimer's disease. *Front. Hum. Neurosci.* 9:449. doi: 10.3389/fnhum.2015.00449

Griffanti, L., Wilcock, G. K., Voets, N., Bonifacio, G., Mackay, C. E., Jenkinson, M., et al. (2016). Donepezil enhances frontal functional connectivity in Alzheimer's disease: a pilot study. *Dementia Geriatric Cogn. Disord. Extra* 6, 518–528. doi: 10.1159/000450546

Grossman, M., Koenig, P., Glosser, G., DeVita, C., Moore, P., Rhee, J., et al. (2003). Neural basis for semantic memory difficulty in Alzheimer's disease: an fMRI study. *Brain* 126, 292–311. doi: 10.1093/brain/awg027

He, Y., Wang, L., Zang, Y., Tian, L., Zhang, X., Li, K., et al. (2007). Regional coherence changes in the early stages of Alzheimer's disease: a combined structural and resting-state functional MRI study. *NeuroImage* 35, 488–500. doi: 10.1016/j.neuroimage.2006.11.042

Hirschauer, T. J., Adeli, H., and Buford, J. A. (2015). Computer-aided diagnosis of Parkinson's disease using enhanced probabilistic neural network. *J. Med. Syst.* 39:179. doi: 10.1007/s10916-015-0353-9

Hopkins, W. D., Meguerditchian, A., Coulon, O., Misiura, M., Pope, S., Mareno, M. C., et al. (2017). Motor skill for tool-use is associated with asymmetries in Broca's area and the motor hand area of the precentral gyrus in chimpanzees (Pan troglodytes). *Behav. Brain Res.* 318, 71–81. doi: 10.1016/j.bbr.2016.10.048

Jenkinson, M., Bannister, P., Brady, M., and Smith, S. (2002). Improved optimization for the robust and accurate linear registration and motion correction of brain images. *NeuroImage* 17, 825–841. doi: 10.1006/nimg.2002.1132

Jolliffe, I. T., and Cadima, J. (2016). Principal component analysis: a review and recent developments. *Philos. Trans. R. Soc. A Mathemat. Phys. Eng. Sci.* 374:20150202. doi: 10.1098/rsta.2015.0202

Kang, K., Yoon, U., Lee, J.-M., and Lee, H.-W. (2013). Idiopathic normal-pressure hydrocephalus, cortical thinning, and the cerebrospinal fluid tap test. *J. Neurol. Sci.* 334, 55–62. doi: 10.1016/j.jns.2013.07.014

Karas, G., Scheltens, P., Rombouts, S., van Schijndel, R., Klein, M., Jones, B., et al. (2007). Precuneus atrophy in early-onset Alzheimer's disease: a morphometric structural MRI study. *Neuroradiology* 49, 967–976. doi: 10.1007/s00234-007-0269-2

Khazaee, A., Ebrahimzadeh, A., and Babajani-Feremi, A. (2015). Identifying patients with Alzheimer's disease using resting-state fMRI and graph theory. *Clin. Neurophysiol.* 126, 2132–2141. doi: 10.1016/j.clinph.2015.02.060

Khazaee, A., Ebrahimzadeh, A., and Babajani-Feremi, A. (2016). Application of advanced machine learning methods on resting-state fMRI network for identification of mild cognitive impairment and Alzheimer's disease. *Brain Imaging Behav.* 10, 799–817. doi: 10.1007/s11682-015-9448-7

Kim, J., Calhoun, V. D., Shim, E., and Lee, J.-H. (2016). Deep neural network with weight sparsity control and pre-training extracts hierarchical features and enhances classification performance: evidence from whole-brain resting-state functional connectivity patterns of schizophrenia. *NeuroImage* 124, 127–146. doi: 10.1016/j.neuroimage.2015.05.018

Luo, S., Li, X., and Li, J. (2017). Automatic Alzheimer's disease recognition from MRI data using deep learning method. *J. Appl. Mathemat. Phys.* 5, 1892–1898. doi: 10.4236/jamp.2017.59159

Mannfolk, P., Wirestam, R., Nilsson, M., Ståhlberg, F., and Olsrud, J. (2010). Dimensionality reduction of fMRI time series data using locally linear embedding. *MAGMA* 23, 327–338. doi: 10.1007/s10334-010-0204-0

Mattioni, B. E., and Jurs, P. C. (2003). Prediction of dihydrofolate reductase inhibition and selectivity using computational neural networks and linear discriminant analysis. *J. Mol. Graph. Model.* 21, 391–419. doi: 10.1016/S1093-3263(02)00187-0

McKeown, M. J., Li, J., Huang, X., Lewis, M. M., Rhee, S., Young Truong, K. N., et al. (2007). Local linear discriminant analysis (LLDA) for group and region of interest (ROI)-based fMRI analysis. *NeuroImage* 37, 855–865. doi: 10.1016/j.neuroimage.2007.04.072

Misaki, M., Kim, Y., Bandettini, P. A., and Kriegeskorte, N. (2010). Comparison of multivariate classifiers and response normalizations for pattern-information fMRI. *NeuroImage* 53, 103–118. doi: 10.1016/j.neuroimage.2010.05.051

Moradi, E., Pepe, A., Gaser, C., Huttunen, H., and Tohka, J. (2015). Machine learning framework for early MRI-based Alzheimer's conversion prediction in MCI subjects. *NeuroImage* 104, 398–412. doi: 10.1016/j.neuroimage.2014.10.002

Nebel, M. B., Joel, S. E., Muschelli, J., Barber, A. D., Caffo, B. S., Pekar, J. J., et al. (2014). Disruption of functional organization within the primary motor cortex in children with autism. *Hum. Brain Mapp.* 35, 567–580. doi: 10.1002/hbm.22188

Ortiz, A., Górriz, J. M., Ramírez, J., and Martínez-Murcia, F. J. (2013). LVQ-SVM based CAD tool applied to structural MRI for the diagnosis of the Alzheimer's disease. *Pattern Recognit. Lett.* 34, 1725–1733. doi: 10.1016/j.patrec.2013.04.014

Ortiz, A., Munilla, J., Górriz, J. M., and Ramírez, J. (2016). Ensembles of deep learning architectures for the early diagnosis of the Alzheimer's disease. *Int. J. Neural Syst.* 26:1650025. doi: 10.1142/S0129065716500258

Pagani, M., Nobili, F., Morbelli, S., Arnaldi, D., Giuliani, A., Öberg, J., et al. (2017). Early identification of MCI converting to AD: a FDG PET study. *Eur. J. Nucl. Med. Mol. Imaging* 44, 2042–2052. doi: 10.1007/s00259-017-3761-x

Prosser, A., Bolt, L., and Kipps, C. (2015). (99M)TC-HMPAO spect perfusion imaging predicts Alzheimer's disease cerebrospinal fluid biomarker status. *Alzheimer's & Dementia* 11, 407–408. doi: 10.1016/j.jalz.2015.06.363

Rolls, E. T., Joliot, M., and Tzourio-Mazoyer, N. (2015). Implementation of a new parcellation of the orbitofrontal cortex in the automated anatomical labeling atlas. *NeuroImage* 122, 1–5. doi: 10.1016/j.neuroimage.2015.07.075

Sarraf, S., DeSouza, D. D., Anderson, J., and Tofighi, G. (2016). DeepAD: Alzheimer's disease classification via deep convolutional neural networks using MRI and fMRI. *bioRxiv* [Preprint]. doi: 10.1101/070441

Schultz, S. A., Larson, J., Oh, J., Koscik, R., Dowling, M. N., Gallagher, C. L., et al. (2015). Participation in cognitively-stimulating activities is associated with brain structure and cognitive function in preclinical Alzheimer's disease. *Brain Imaging Behav.* 9, 729–736. doi: 10.1007/s11682-014-9329-5

Suk, H.-I., Lee, S.-W., and Shen, D. (2014). Hierarchical feature representation and multimodal fusion with deep learning for AD/MCI diagnosis. *NeuroImage* 101, 569–582. doi: 10.1016/j.neuroimage.2014.06.077

Suk, H.-I., Wee, C.-Y., Lee, S.-W., and Shen, D. (2016). State-space model with deep learning for functional dynamics estimation in resting-state fMRI. *Neuroimage* 129, 292–307. doi: 10.1016/j.neuroimage.2016.01.005

Wang, K., Liang, M., Wang, L., Tian, L., Zhang, X., Li, K., et al. (2007). Altered functional connectivity in early Alzheimer's disease: a resting-state fMRI study. *Hum. Brain Mapp.* 28, 967–978. doi: 10.1002/hbm.20324

Wang, L., Li, K., Zhang, Q.-E., Zeng, Y.-W., Jin, Z., Dai, W.-J., et al. (2013). Interhemispheric functional connectivity and its relationships with clinical characteristics in major depressive disorder: a resting state fMRI study. *PLoS One* 8:e60191. doi: 10.1371/journal.pone.0060191

Yetkin, F. Z., Rosenberg, R. N., Weiner, M. F., Purdy, P. D., and Cullum, C. M. (2006). FMRI of working memory in patients with mild cognitive impairment and probable Alzheimer's disease. *Eur. Radiol.* 16, 193–206. doi: 10.1007/s00330-005-2794-x

Yousry, T. A., Schmid, U. D., Alkadhi, H., Schmidt, D., Peraud, A., Buettner, A., et al. (1997). Localization of the motor hand area to a knob on the precentral gyrus, a new landmark. *Brain* 120, 141–157. doi: 10.1093/brain/120.1.141

Zhang, Y., Dong, Z., Phillips, P., Wang, S., Ji, G., Yang, J., et al. (2015). Detection of subjects and brain regions related to Alzheimer's disease using 3D MRI scans based on eigenbrain and machine learning. *Front. Comput. Neurosci.* 9:66. doi: 10.3389/fncom.2015.00066

Zhang, Y., Wang, S., and Dong, Z. (2014). Classification of Alzheimer disease based on structural magnetic resonance imaging by kernel support vector machine decision tree. *Progr. Electromagn. Res.* 144, 171–184. doi: 10.2528/PIER13121310

Zhou, Y., Peng, J., and Chen, C. L. P. (2015). Dimension reduction using spatial and spectral regularized local discriminant embedding for hyperspectral image classification. *IEEE Trans. Geosci. Remote Sens.* 53, 1082–1095. doi: 10.1109/TGRS.2014.2333539

17

Royal Jelly Reduces Cholesterol Levels, Ameliorates Aβ Pathology and Enhances Neuronal Metabolic Activities in a Rabbit Model of Alzheimer's Disease

Yongming Pan[1,2], Jianqin Xu[2], Cheng Chen[2], Fangming Chen[2], Ping Jin[3], Keyan Zhu[2], Chenyue W. Hu[4], Mengmeng You[1], Minli Chen[2] and Fuliang Hu[1]**

[1]College of Animal Sciences, Zhejiang University, Hangzhou, China, [2]Comparative Medical Research Center, Experimental Animal Research Center, Zhejiang Chinese Medical University, Hangzhou, China, [3]The First Affiliated Hospital, Zhejiang Chinese Medical University, Hangzhou, China, [4]Department of Bioengineering, Rice University, Houston, TX, United States

***Correspondence:**
Fuliang Hu
flhu@zju.edu.cn
Minli Chen
cmli991@zcmu.edu.cn

Alzheimer's disease (AD) is the most common form of dementia characterized by aggregation of amyloid β (Aβ) and neuronal loss. One of the risk factors for AD is high cholesterol levels, which are known to promote Aβ deposition. Previous studies have shown that royal jelly (RJ), a product of worker bees, has potential neuroprotective effects and can attenuate Aβ toxicity. However, little is known about how RJ regulates Aβ formation and its effects on cholesterol levels and neuronal metabolic activities. Here, we investigated whether RJ can reduce cholesterol levels, regulate Aβ levels and enhance neuronal metabolic activities in an AD rabbit model induced by 2% cholesterol diet plus copper drinking water. Our results suggest that RJ significantly reduced the levels of plasma total cholesterol (TC) and low density lipoprotein-cholesterol (LDL-C), and decreased the level of Aβ in rabbit brains. RJ was also shown to markedly ameliorate amyloid deposition in AD rabbits from Aβ immunohistochemistry and thioflavin-T staining. Furthermore, our study suggests that RJ can reduce the expression levels of β-site APP cleaving enzyme-1 (BACE1) and receptor for advanced glycation end products (RAGE), and increase the expression levels of low density lipoprotein receptor-related protein 1 (LRP-1) and insulin degrading enzyme (IDE). In addition, we found that RJ remarkably increased the number of neurons, enhanced antioxidant capacities, inhibited activated-capase-3 protein expression, and enhanced neuronal metabolic activities by increasing N-acetyl aspartate (NAA) and glutamate and by reducing choline and myo-inositol in AD rabbits. Taken together, our data demonstrated that RJ could reduce cholesterol levels, regulate Aβ levels and enhance neuronal metabolic activities in AD rabbits, providing preclinical evidence that RJ treatment has the potential to protect neurons and prevent AD.

Keywords: royal jelly, Alzheimer's disease, hypercholesterolemia, amyloid plaques, neuronal metabolism activity

INTRODUCTION

Alzheimer's disease (AD), the most common type of dementia, is a primary degenerative disease that occurs in the central nervous system (CNS). About 44 million people are currently suffering from AD worldwide, and this population is estimated to exceed 131 million by 2050 (Comas Herrera et al., 2016). Except for 5% of AD cases that are familial, most of the cases are sporadic AD (SAD), the onset of which is largely influenced by both environmental and genetic factors (Selkoe, 2001; Lacher et al., 2018). Though no cure has been found for AD, medications such as cholinesterase inhibitors and N-methyl D-aspartate (NMDA) receptor antagonists are widely used to treat its symptoms. However, the long-term use of these drugs are known to cause serious side-effects (Fereshtehnejad et al., 2014), therefore mandating the development of alternative treatment options.

Since AD is characterized by amyloid β (Aβ) deposition and neuronal loss in the brain (Li et al., 2015), a growing number of studies have been trying to control AD by inhibiting the formation and deposition of Aβ. It was recently found that active ingredients of certain functional foods have anti-aging effects, indicating that dietary intervention may have the potential to prevent or delay the onset of AD (Celik and Sanlier, 2017). One functional food of particular interest is royal jelly (RJ; Ramadan and Al-Ghamdi, 2012), a secretion produced from the hypopharyngeal and mandibular glands of worker bees for feeding to and developing queen bees. Consumed worldwide as a functional food, RJ consists of proteins, carbohydrates, lipids, free amino acids, vitamins (Takenaka, 1982; Nagai and Inoue, 2004; Pourmoradian et al., 2012), as well as a variety of bioactive compounds, including peptides (Fontana et al., 2004), adenosine monophosphate (AMP) N1-oxide (Hattori et al., 2010), acetylcholine (Wei et al., 2010) and fatty acids such as 10-hydroxy-2-decenoic acid (10-HAD; Butenandt and Rembold, 1957; Ramadan and Al-Ghamdi, 2012). RJ has been shown in multiple studies to have anti-aging (Honda et al., 2011), anti-oxidative (Nagai et al., 2006), lipid-lowering (Vittek, 1995) and anti-inflammatory (Kohno et al., 2004) effects. Furthermore, it was recently reported that RJ significantly improves spatial learning and memory in rats with streptozotocin-induced SAD (Zamani et al., 2012), and that RJ attenuates Aβ toxicity in a *C. elegans* model of AD (Wang et al., 2016). Despite these latest research developments in RJ's potential treatment effects related to AD, the mechanism of how RJ regulates Aβ formation and delays the development of AD remains elusive.

One hypothesis is that RJ regulates the formation of Aβ via reducing cholesterol levels. Hypercholesterolemia, a known risk factor for AD, has been shown to promote Aβ neurotoxicity, Aβ accumulation and local neuronal loss across epidemiological (Kivipelto et al., 2001; Gonzalo-Ruiz et al., 2006), animal (Sparks and Schreurs, 2003) and cellular (Galbete et al., 2000) studies. It is thought that hypercholesterolemia can enhance the activities of γ-secretase and β-secretase, facilitate the metabolism of amyloid precursor protein (APP), aggravate Aβ deposition, promote the formation of senile plaques and then lead to AD (Kuo et al., 2015; Loke et al., 2017). The potential mechanism by which hypercholesterolemia causes Aβ formation was revealed by Jaya Prasanthi et al. (2008) in which they found that the hypercholesterolemia-induced production of Aβ was correlated with an increased level of β-site APP cleaving enzyme 1 (BACE1) and receptor for advanced glycation end products (RAGE), as well as a decreased level of insulin degrading enzyme (IDE) and low density lipoprotein receptor-related protein 1 (LRP-1).

In this study, we first investigate whether RJ has an effect on cholesterol and Aβ levels using an AD rabbit model. Though transgenic rodents have been used as the main animal model for AD (e.g., APPswe/PS1dE9 double transgenic mice), this model is unsuitable for SAD due to a lack of correct APP protein sequence and a lack of cleavage enzymes to trigger Aβ peptide formation (Liu et al., 2014). In contrast, rabbits naturally produce cleavage enzymes for Aβ peptides, and their Aβ peptide sequence is identical to that of humans (Johnstone et al., 1991). Notably, the connection between cholesterol levels and Aβ plaques was first reported in rabbits (Sparks et al., 1994), in which rabbits showed a marked response to high cholesterol diets and exhibited Aβ deposition in plaques. Furthermore, Sparks and Schreurs (2003) found that after adding copper to the diet of cholesterol-fed rabbits, the rabbits developed cortical amyloid deposits and exhibited at least 12 other pathological features that are observed in the brain of human AD patients, such as learning deficits. These findings together highlight the usefulness of the rabbit model, and demonstrate the potential of using rabbits for preclinical drug evaluations (Woodruff-Pak et al., 2007).

To provide potential mechanisms of how RJ regulates Aβ deposition and potentially improves AD in rabbit models, we assess the effects of RJ on a variety of biological factors, including the expression of proteins involved in the production, translocation and clearance of Aβ, anti-oxidative capacities, neuronal loss, and neuronal metabolic activities. In particular, the effects of RJ on neuronal metabolic activities are measured using high-field proton magnetic resonance spectroscopy (^{1}H-MRS), which is a non-invasive neuroimaging technique extensively used to quantify metabolic changes in AD pathology (Chen et al., 2012). We use ^{1}H-MRS to evaluate the levels of four main metabolites of AD (i.e., N-acetyl aspartate (NAA), choline (Cho), glutamate (Glu) and myo-inositol (mI)), since numerous studies have shown that NAA and glutamate are decreased in AD, whereas Cho and mI are increased in the early stage of AD (Ackl et al., 2005; Zhang et al., 2014).

MATERIALS AND METHODS

Animals

A total of 24 male White Hair and Black Eyes (WHBE) rabbits (3–4 months old, 1.8–2.0 kg) were purchased from Xin Jian rabbit field (Certificate No. SCXK, Zhejiang, 2015-0004, China), Dashiqu town, Xinchang City (Zhejiang, China). They were housed individually under a 12-h light/dark cycle and were provided with food and water *ad libitum*. All experiments were approved by the Institutional Animal Care and Use Committee of Zhejiang Chinese Medical University (IACUC Approval No. ZSLL-2016-115), and were performed according to the guidelines from the Laboratory Animal Research Center of Zhejiang Chinese Medical University (Certificate No. SYXK, Zhejiang, 2013-0184, China).

After adaptation to the environment for 14 days, the rabbits were randomly divided into three groups (n = 8 rabbits per group): normal control (NC) group, AD model group and RJ intervention (RJ) group. The NC group rabbits were fed with a regular chow and distilled water (DW), whereas the AD model group was fed with chow plus 2% cholesterol and DW plus cooper (0.12 ppm cooper ion as sulfate) as used by Sparks and Schreurs (2003). The RJ group was fed with chow plus 2% cholesterol and DW plus cooper, and received 200 mg/kg of RJ (Jiangshan, Zhejiang, China) via oral administration twice a day (a total dose of 400 mg/kg RJ daily) in the morning and the afternoon for 12 weeks. This dose was selected based on the previous report that an oral administration of 6 g RJ per day can significantly reduce cholesterol levels in human clinic therapy (Guo et al., 2007). The duration of the experiment procedure was 12 weeks. The experimental designs of biochemical analysis, ^{1}H-MRS assessment and histological examinations are shown in **Figure 1**. After 12 weeks of administration, ^{1}H-MRS assessment, a set of biochemical index in the serum and brain, as well as all AD pathological indices were investigated.

Serum Total Cholesterol (TC), Triglycerides (TG), Low-Density Lipoprotein Cholesterol (LDL-C) and High-Density Lipoprotein Cholesterol (HDL-C) Levels Measurements

After 12-week administration, rabbits (eight per group) would first fast for 12 h, and then blood samples were drawn from their middle auricular artery. Automatic biochemical analyzer (7020, HITACHI, Japan) was used to analyze total cholesterol (TC), triglycerides (TG), low-density lipoprotein cholesterol (LDL-C) and high-density lipoprotein cholesterol (HDL-C) in blood samples by kits corresponding to each component (Shanghai Shenneng-DiaSys Diagnostic Technology Co., Ltd., China).

Quantification of Aβ Levels by ELISA

For ELISA test of Aβ1–40 and Aβ1–42 levels in the rabbit brain (six cortex and hippocampus per group), the wet mass of 100 mg cortex and the hippocampus tissues were sequentially homogenized in a 8× mass of cold 5 M guanidine hydrochloride/50 mM Tris HCl buffer using an IKA ULTRA-TURRAX homogenizer (IKA®-werke Gmbh and Co., KG, German). The homogenates were mixed for 4 h at room temperature. Samples were diluted with Dulbecco phosphate buffered saline with 5% BSA and 0.03% Tween-20 supplemented with 1× protease inhibitor mixture, and were centrifuged at 10,000 rpm for 20 min at 4°C (Jaya Prasanthi et al., 2008). The supernatants were then decanted and stored at −80°C until used. The samples were diluted with at least 1:2 standard dilution buffer, and the ELISA kits (Jiancheng Bioengineering Institute, Nanjing, China) were used to measure Aβ1–40 and Aβ1–42 levels according to the manufacturer's instructions[1]. The protein concentrations of all samples were determined by standard bicinchoninic acid (BCA) assay (Pierce, Rockford, IL, USA; Baptiste et al., 2004). The Aβ levels were normalized to the total protein content in the samples.

Determination of Superoxide Dismutase (SOD) Activities, Malonaldehyde (MDA) Contents and Reactive Oxygen Species (ROS)/Reactive Nitrogen Species (RNS) Levels

The superoxide dismutase (SOD) and malonaldehyde (MDA) contents in the brain (eight per group) were measured using colorimetric commercial kit (Jiancheng Bioengineering Institute,

[1]http://www.njjcbio.com

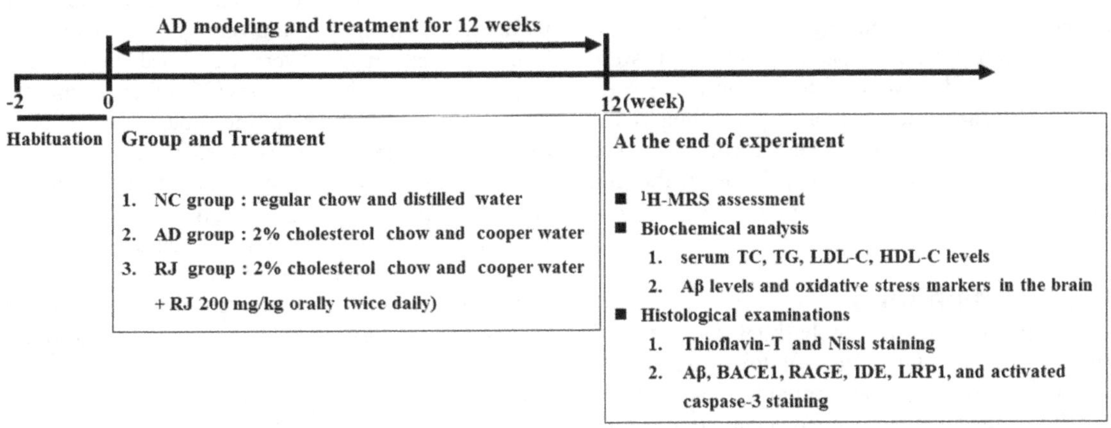

FIGURE 1 | A flowchart of the experimental design in this study.

Nanjing, China). The SOD activity was examined with xanthine oxidase method, and the MDA content was examined with sulfur barbituric acid method (Wang et al., 2005). In addition, reactive oxygen species (ROS)/reactive nitrogen species (RNS) levels in the brain (six per group) were detected with a commercially available ELISA kit (Yuanye Biotech Co., Ltd., Shanghai, China) following the procedure described by the manufacture. Briefly, a 5% w/v cortex and hippocampus homogenates were made in pre-chilled saline using an IKA ULTRA-TURRAX homogenizer (IKA®-werke Gmbh and Co., KG, German). The obtained homogenate was centrifuged at 3000 rpm for 20 min at 4°C. The supernatants were stored at −80°C until used. The protein concentration of all samples was determined by Coomassie brilliant blue method. SOD activities, MDA contents, and ROS/RNS levels were then normalized to the total protein content in the samples.

^{1}H-MRS Assessment

^{1}H-MRS was conducted using a 3.0 T MRI scanner (GE Discovery MR 750, GE, USA) coupled with an 8-channel rabbit dedicated coil (Shanghai Chenguang Medical Technology Co., Ltd., China). All rabbits (six per group) were examined by MRI at 12 weeks. Rabbits were anesthetized by intramuscular injection of 30 mg/kg ketamine and 4 mg/kg xylazine 15 min before imaging. Animals were fixed in prone position in the experiment. During examination, the body temperature was maintained at 36–37°C, and their breathing was kept smooth. T2-weighted fast spin-echo sequence (FSE) was used with the following parameters: TR = 5500 ms, TFE = 100 ms, slice thickness = 3 mm, field of view (FOV) = 100 mm × 100 mm, matrix = 352 × 256, NEX = 2. Images were used to guide MRS subsequent location checks. ^{1}H-MRS scanning used point-resolved water suppression plus sequence (PRESS) with the following parameters: TR = 2000 ms, TE = 35 ms, voxel = 9 mm × 9 mm × 9 mm, total number of scans = 128, NEX = 8. The region of interest (ROI) was positioned in the hippocampus and part of frontal cortex in the brain (**Figure 7A**). Pre-scan, automatic shimming and moisture suppression were performed prior to ^{1}H-MRS. The shimming effect was expressed as full width at half maximum (FWHM). If the FWHM was higher than 20 Hz, a manual shimming was used to obtain good magnetic field uniformity. The spectra of all rabbits were analyzed using an LC Model (version 6.3, Provencher SW; Provencher, 1993). The chemical metabolites, including NAA, glutamate, Cho, mI and creatine (Cr) were identified. Since Cr is consistent in various diseases, it was used as an internal standard to calculate the ratio of NAA/Cr, glutamate/Cr, Cho/Cr and mI/Cr.

Histological Examinations

All rabbits were euthanized with pentobarbital sodium, and were then perfused with 300 ml 4°C PBS solution after cardiac perfusion. The brain was removed, segmented into 5 mm thick parallel coronal slices, and then fixed in formalin solution for at least 24 h. The selected slices were dehydrated with gradient ethanol, embedded in paraffin and cut into 6 μm coronal sections. They were then stained immunohistochemically with Aβ, beta-site APP cleaving enzyme 1 (BACE1), receptor for advanced glycation end products (RAGE), LDL receptor related protein 1(LRP1), insulin-degrading enzyme (IDE), activated caspase-3, thioflavin-T and Nissl.

1. Thioflavin-T staining was used to evaluate the amount of amyloid-β protein (Zhang et al., 2013), with eight samples in each group. Briefly, slides were deparaffinized and rehydrated in descending grades of ethanol, placed in Mayer hematoxylin for 5 min, rinsed twice in double DW, incubated with 1% thioflavin-T (Dalian Meilun Biological Technology Co. Ltd., China) for 10 min and three changes of DW washes, cover-slipped in a neutral glycerol, and examined with the Hg-Lamp for fluorescence excitation by a Zeiss inverted microscope (Axiovert 200, Carl Zeiss, USA).
2. Nissl staining was used to evaluate neuronal loss (Chen et al., 2009), with six samples in each group. Briefly, slides were hydrated and incubated in 1% toluidine blue solution at 56°C for 30 min, washed with PBS, decolorized with 95% ethanol, dehydrated, dried and cover-slipped.
3. Aβ, BACE1, RAGE, IDE, LRP1 and activated caspase-3 staining, with six to eight samples in each group. Briefly, sections were blocked with 3% hydrogen peroxide solution for 10 min, and were then incubated with primary antibodies overnight at 4°C, including BACE1 (1:100, Santa Cruz Biotechnology, USA), RAGE (1:100, Santa Cruz Biotechnology, USA), IDE (1:100, Santa Cruz Biotechnology, USA), LRP1(1:300, Diage Biological Technology co. Ltd., China), activated caspase-3 (1:200, Biosynthesis Biological Technology co. Ltd., China) and β-amyloid (B-4, 1:100, Santa Cruz Biotechnology, USA, which recognizes APP and Aβ). PBS was used as negative control instead of the primary antibody. Subsequently, the sections were washed with PBS three times and were incubated with secondary antibody for 1 h at room temperature. Sections were visualized with DAB (ZSJQ, Beijing, China) and counterstained with hematoxylin.

All sections were scanned using a Hamamatsu Skeleton Scanner (Nanozoomer S210, Hamamatsu, Japan). Since the main pathological feature of early AD is cortical atrophy, especially in the hippocampus and the medial temporal lobe, we examined the pathological changes in the cerebral cortex and hippocampus. The captured images were examined in a blinded manner by an observer who was unware of experimental condition, and were analyzed using the Image pro plus 6.0 software (Media Cybernetics, Rockville, MD, USA). On Nissl-stained sections, five microscopic fields of the hippocampal CA1, CA3 and DG regions, the cortical cone (pyramidal cellular layer, PCL) and the polymorphic cell layer (multiform cellular layers, MCL) were selected. The neuronal counts in each view were calculated at 40× magnification. We counted Aβ and activated caspase-3 immunolabeled positive cells under 40× magnification in three random fields from the cerebral cortex and hippocampal CA1 areas in the three groups and used the averaged value. For quantification, we calculated Aβ, BACE1, RAGE, IDE, LRP1 or activated caspase-3-postive area under 40× magnification in three random fields from the cerebral cortex and hippocampal CA1 areas, and the staining was quantified as the percent positive staining area as the fraction of immunopositive staining to total area measured. In addition, plaque load was categorized based on the percentage area of tissues positive for deposits labeled by thioflavin-T immunoreactivity.

Statistical Analysis

Data were expressed as means ± SEM. Statistical analyses were performed using GraphPad Prism 6.0 (GraphPad Software, Inc., La Jolla, CA, USA). All quantitative results were analyzed by one-way ANOVA with *post hoc* Tukey's test (*$p < 0.05$, **$p < 0.01$).

RESULTS

RJ Reduced Plasma TC and LDL-C Levels

We first assessed the effects of RJ on blood liquid levels (i.e., TC, HDL-C, LDL-C and TG) in AD rabbits. As shown in **Table 1**, the levels of TC, HDL-C and LDL-C in the AD model group were higher than those in the NC group (ANOVA with *post hoc* Tukey's test, all $p < 0.01$). Compared with the AD model group, plasma TC and LDL-C levels in the RJ group were significantly reduced by 28% and 23% respectively (all $p < 0.05$), while there was no significant difference in plasma HDL-C levels between the RJ group and the AD model group ($p = 0.07$). In addition, there was no significant difference in body weight and TG levels among the three groups (ANOVA, $F = 0.08$, $p = 0.925$; $F = 2.555$, $p = 0.103$, respectively).

RJ Decreased Aβ Levels and Amyloid Burden in the Cortex and the Hippocampus of AD Rabbits

To observe the effects of RJ on Aβ pathology in the brain of AD rabbits, the Aβ level and amyloid burden were assessed in the three groups of rabbits. As shown in **Figure 2A**, the Aβ1–40 and Aβ1–42 levels were significantly increased in the cortex area (ANOVA with *post hoc* Tukey's test, $p < 0.05$ and $p < 0.01$, respectively) and the hippocampus area (ANOVA with *post hoc* Tukey's test, $p < 0.01$ and $p < 0.05$, respectively) in the AD model group compared with the NC group. In contrast, compared with the AD model group, the RJ group showed a 17%–54% reduction in both Aβ1–40 and Aβ1–42 levels in the cortex area ($p < 0.05$ and $p < 0.01$, respectively) and the hippocampus area (all $p < 0.05$).

Next, the Aβ plaque was evaluated using immunohistochemical analysis (**Figure 2B**) and thioflavin-T staining. In the frontal cortex and the hippocampus regions, we found that the expression of Aβ-positive proteins was low in the NC group, upregulated in the AD model group, and suppressed in the RJ group. Quantification analysis showed that the number of Aβ immunolabeled cells were significantly reduced in the cortex and the hippocampus of the RJ group compared to the AD model group (ANOVA with *post hoc* Tukey's test, $p < 0.01$ and $p < 0.05$, respectively). Similarly, the Aβ covered areas were reduced by approximately 45% in the cortex and by 40% in the hippocampus of the RJ group compared to the AD model group (ANOVA with *post hoc* Tukey's test, all $p < 0.01$; **Figure 2C**).

Using thioflavin-T staining, a fluorescein that specifically binds to amyloid deposits and can be excited to produce green fluorescence, we found that the RJ group significantly reduced the amount of thioflavin-T positive plaques in both the cortex and the hippocampus areas compared to the AD model group (**Figure 2D**). Quantitatively, the RJ group reduced the plaques load by 37% in the cortex area (ANOVA with *post hoc* Tukey's test, $p < 0.05$) and by 60% in the hippocampus area relative to the AD model group ($p < 0.01$; **Figure 2E**), demonstrating that RJ could greatly decrease Aβ deposition in AD brains.

RJ Reduced Aβ Accumulation by Decreasing BACE1 and RAGE Expression, and by Increasing IDE and LRP1 Expression

To investigate how RJ reduces Aβ accumulation, the expression of BACE1, RAGE, LRP1 and IDE were measured in the rabbit brains of each group by immunohistochemistry. As shown in **Figure 3**, compared with the NC group, the expression levels of BACE1 and RAGE were significantly increased in the cortex and the hippocampus of the AD model group (ANOVA with *post hoc* Tukey's test, all $p < 0.01$). In specific, the BACE1 covered area in the RJ group was significantly decreased by 65% in the cortex and by 59% in the hippocampus compared with the AD model group (all $p < 0.05$). Similarly, the RAGE covered area in the RJ group was markedly reduced by 68% in the cortex ($p < 0.01$) and by 59% in the hippocampus ($p < 0.05$) relative to the AD model rabbits. In contrast, LRP1 and IDE expression levels were markedly decreased in the AD model group (ANOVA with *post hoc* Tukey's test, all $p < 0.01$). The LRP1 covered area in the RJ group was dramatically increased

TABLE 1 | Effect of royal jelly (RJ) on weight and blood liquid levels in Alzheimer's disease (AD) rabbits at 12 weeks.

Parameters	NC group	AD model group	RJ group
Weight (kg)	2.80 ± 0.07	2.83 ± 0.09	2.85 ± 0.07
TC (mmol/L)	0.62 ± 0.09**	45.79 ± 2.97	33.04 ± 4.07*
HDL-C (mmol/L)	0.28 ± 0.05**	2.91 ± 0.10	2.51 ± 0.17
LDL-C (mmol/L)	0.32 ± 0.04**	32.29 ± 1.97	24.86 ± 2.76*
TG (mmol/L)	0.69 ± 0.04	1.91 ± 0.64	0.95 ± 0.25

*TC, total cholesterol; HDL-C, high-density lipoprotein cholesterol; LDL-C, low-density lipoprotein cholesterol; TG, triglycerides. Data are presented as mean ± SEM from eight rabbits in each group. ANOVA with post hoc Tukey's test was used. *P < 0.05, **P < 0.01 vs. the AD model group.*

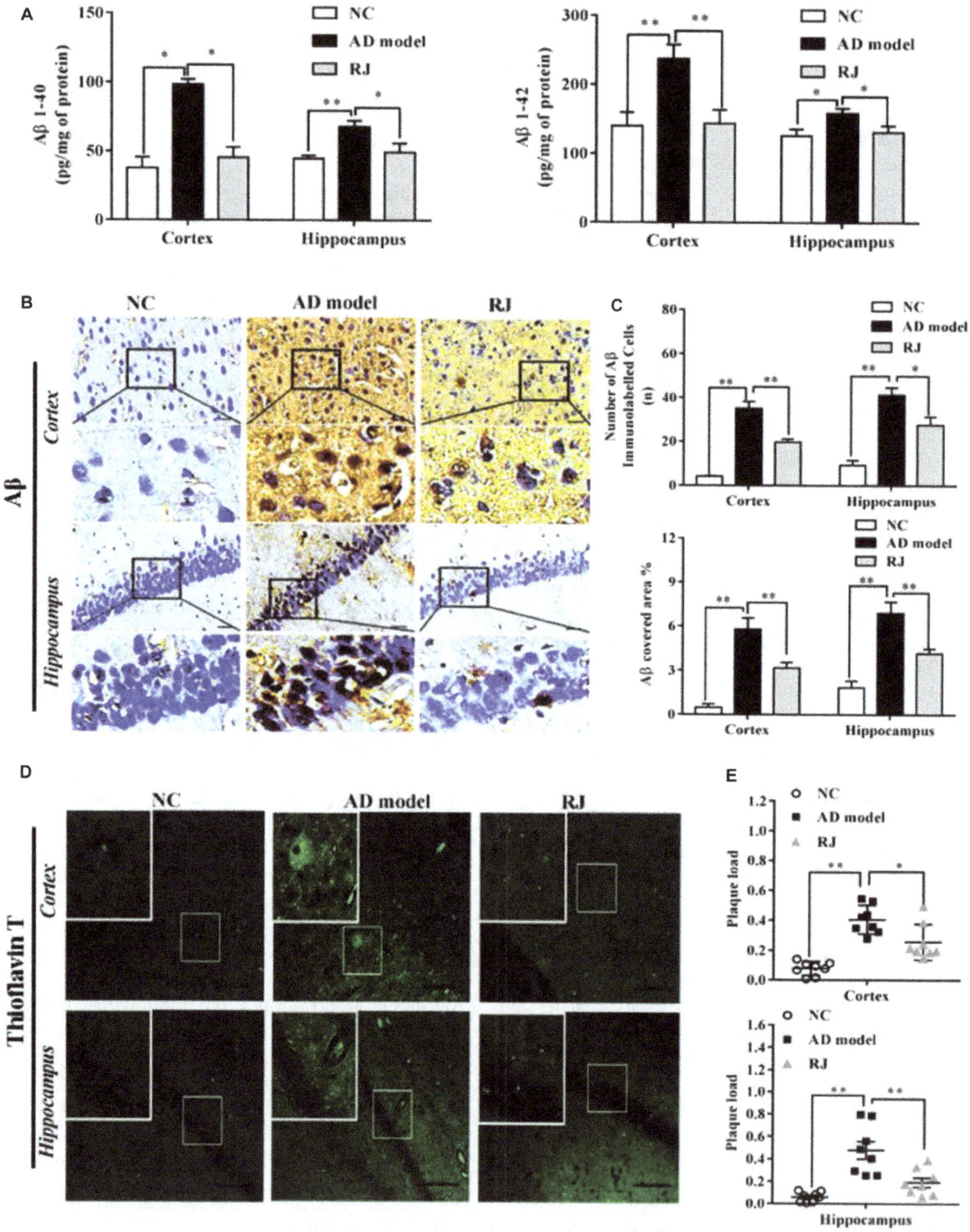

FIGURE 2 | Royal jelly (RJ) decreased brain amyloid β (Aβ) levels and alleviated Aβ pathology in Alzheimer's disease (AD) rabbits. **(A)** The levels of Aβ1–40 and Aβ1–42 in the cortex and the hippocampus of each group measured by ELISA, $n = 6$ rabbits per group. **(B)** Representative Aβ-staining images in the cortex and the hippocampus of each group. Scale bar = 50 μm. Black squares indicate images with higher-magnification. Aβ positive (brown-colored) was detected mainly in the cytoplasm of neuronal cells and the cytoplasm and membranes of endothelia cells. **(C)** The number of Aβ immunolabeled cells per view (40×) and the covered area of Aβ staining in the brain of each group, $n = 6–8$ rabbits per group. **(D)** An example image of Aβ plaque immunoreactivity in the cortex and the hippocampus of each group by thioflavin-T staining. Scale bar = 50 μm. White squares indicate images with higher-magnification. **(E)** Quantification of thioflavin-T positive deposits in the cortex and the hippocampus of the three groups, $n = 8$ rabbits per group. Data are presented as mean ± SEM. ANOVA with *post hoc* Tukey's test was used **(A,C,E)**. $^{*}P < 0.05$, $^{**}P < 0.01$ vs. the AD model group.

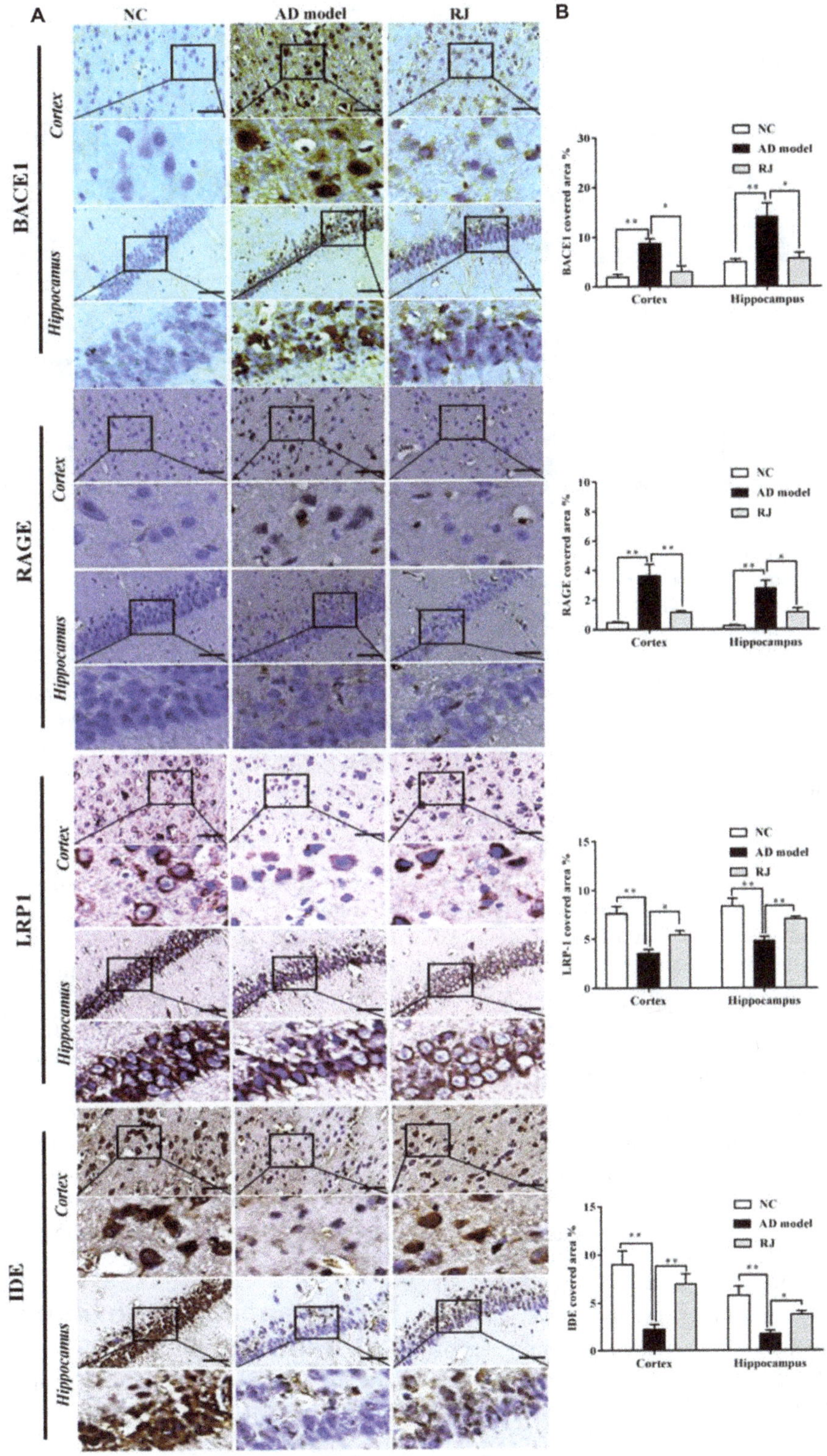

FIGURE 3 | RJ inhibited β-site APP cleaving enzyme-1 (BACE1) and receptor for advanced glycation end products (RAGE) expression levels, and increased lipoprotein receptor-related protein 1 (LRP1) and insulin degrading enzyme (IDE) expression levels, demonstrated by immunohistochemistry. **(A)** Staining for BACE1, RAGE, LRP1 and IDE using specific antibodies in the brain of the AD model, RJ and normal control (NC) group. Scale bar = 50 μm. Black squares indicate images with higher-magnification. **(B)** Quantification of the covered areas of BACE1, RAGE, LRP1 and IDE staining in the frontal cortex and the hippocampus of the three groups, n = 6–8 rabbits per group. Data are presented as mean ± SEM. ANOVA with *post hoc* Tukey's test was used. $^{*}P < 0.05$, $^{**}P < 0.01$ vs. the AD model group.

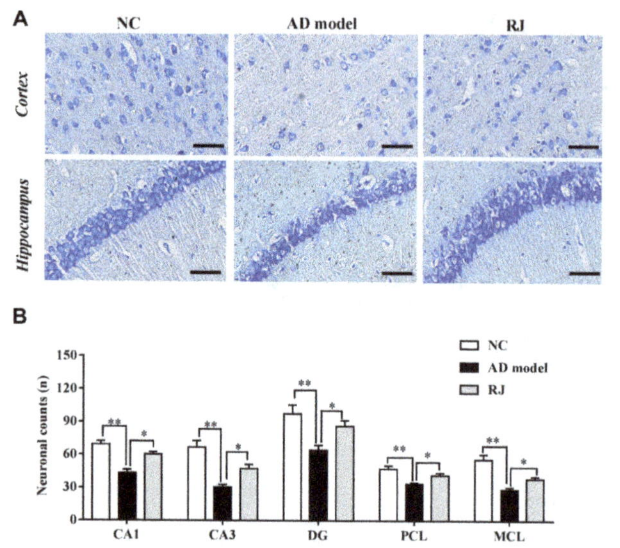

FIGURE 4 | RJ rescued neuronal loss in the brain of AD rabbits. **(A)** Nissl-staining images in the frontal cortex and the hippocampus of the AD model, RJ and NC group. Scale bar = 50 μm. **(B)** Neuronal counts per view (40×) in the hippocampal CA1, CA3, DG regions and cortical pyramidal cellular layer (PCL) and multiform cellular layers (MCL) areas among the three groups, $n = 6$ rabbits per group. Data are presented as mean ± SEM. ANOVA with *post hoc* Tukey's test was used. $^{*}P < 0.05$, $^{**}P < 0.01$ vs. the AD model group.

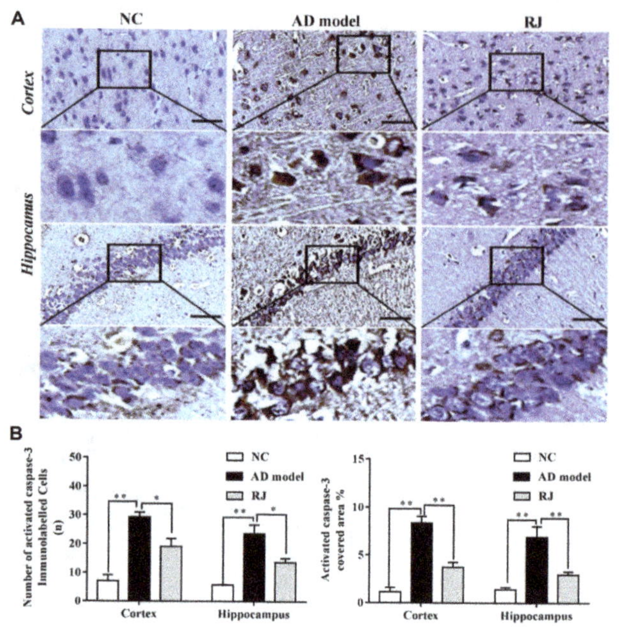

FIGURE 5 | RJ reduced activated caspase-3 expression levels in the brain of AD rabbits. **(A)** Representative activated caspase-3 staining sections in the brain of the AD model, RJ and NC group. Scale bar = 50 μm. Black squares indicate images with higher-magnification. **(B)** The number of activated caspase-3 immunolabeled cells per view (40×) and the covered area of activated caspase-3 staining in the frontal cortex and the hippocampus of the three groups, $n = 6$ rabbits per group. Data are presented as mean ± SEM. ANOVA with *post hoc* Tukey's test was used. $^{*}P < 0.05$, $^{**}P < 0.01$ vs. the AD model group.

by 53% in the cortex and by 67% in the hippocampus relative to the AD model group (all $p < 0.05$). Moreover, the IDE covered area in the RJ group was significantly increased by 2.15 folds in the cortex ($p < 0.01$) and by 1.19 folds in the hippocampus relative to the AD model group ($p < 0.05$). Taken together, these results indicate that RJ may reduce Aβ accumulation in AD brains by inhibiting the expression of BACE1 and RAGE as well as by promoting the expression of LRP1 and IDE.

RJ Reduced Neuronal Loss and Inhibited Apoptosis in AD Rabbit Brains

Nissl staining was performed to evaluate the effects of RJ on neuronal loss in the AD brain. As shown in **Figure 4**, when compared with the NC group, the AD rabbits showed a typical Alzheimer's pathology, including nucleus shrinkage, neuronal loss and disappearance of Nissl bodies in the cortex and the hippocampus (**Figure 4A**). The cell organization was notably improved in the RJ group, in which RJ treatment significantly increased the number of neurons in the hippocampal CA1, CA3, DG regions and cortical PCL and MCL areas by 40%, 56%, 34%, 23% and 34% respectively compared to the AD model group (ANOVA with *post hoc* Tukey's test, all $p < 0.05$; **Figure 4B**). These results suggest that RJ treatment can potentially increase the number of neurons and improve neuronal structures in the AD brain.

To confirm the results above, we assessed the expression level of activated caspase-3 in the brain of each group by immunohistochemistry. As shown in **Figure 5**, the number of activated caspase-3 immunolabeled cells as well as the covered areas of activated caspase-3 were both significantly increased in the cortex and the hippocampus of the AD model group compared to the NC group (ANOVA with *post hoc* Tukey's test, all $p < 0.01$). In contrast, the number of activated caspase-3 immunolabeled cells were notably decreased in the cortex and the hippocampus of the RJ group compared to the AD model group (all $p < 0.05$). Meanwhile, the covered areas of activated caspase-3 were significantly reduced by approximately 55% in the cortex and by 57% in the hippocampus of the RJ group compared to the AD model group (all $p < 0.01$), indicating that RJ can inhibit neuronal apoptosis.

RJ Enhanced Anti-oxidative Capacities in AD Rabbit Brains

The effects of RJ on anti-oxidative capacities of AD rabbit brains were measured. As shown in **Figure 6**, the SOD level was markedly reduced in the cortex and the hippocampus of the AD model group compared to the NC group (ANOVA with *post hoc* Tukey's test, all $p < 0.05$). In contrast, the SOD level in the RJ group was significantly increased by approximately 27% in the cortex and by 13% in the hippocampus relative to the AD model group (all $p < 0.05$). On the other hand, the MDA content was increased in the cortex and the hippocampus of the AD model

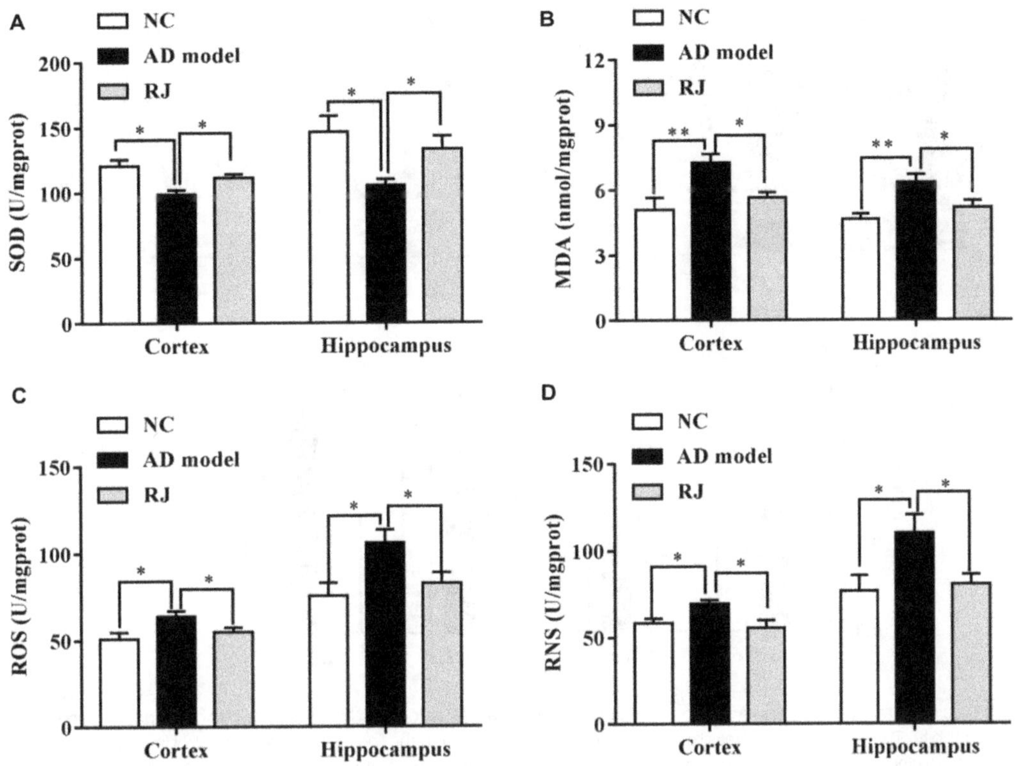

FIGURE 6 | RJ enhanced the anti-oxidative capacities in the brain of AD rabbits. **(A)** Changes of superoxide dismutase (SOD) activities in the cortex and the hippocampus of the three groups, *n* = 8 rabbits per group. **(B)** Changes of malonaldehyde (MDA) contents in the cortex and the hippocampus of the three groups, *n* = 8 rabbits per group. **(C)** Changes of reactive oxygen species (ROS) levels in the cortex and the hippocampus of the three groups, *n* = 6 rabbits per group. **(D)** Changes of reactive nitrogen species (RNS) levels in the cortex and the hippocampus of the three groups, *n* = 6 rabbits per group. Data are presented as mean ± SEM. ANOVA with *post hoc* Tukey's test was used **(A–D)**. *$P < 0.05$, **$P < 0.01$ vs. the AD group.

group compared to that of the NC group (ANOVA with *post hoc* Tukey's test, all $p < 0.01$), and it was significantly reduced by approximately 18% in the cortex and by 22% in the hippocampus of the RJ group relative to the AD model group (all $p < 0.05$). In addition, the ROS/RNS levels were increased in the cortex and the hippocampus of the AD group compared to those of the NC group (ANOVA with *post hoc* Tukey's test, all $p < 0.05$). The ROS level in the RJ group was dramatically decreased by 14.33% in the cortex and by 21.96% in the hippocampus relative to the AD model group (all $p < 0.05$). Moreover, the RNS level in the RJ group was also significantly decreased by 19.79% in the cortex and by 27.17% in the hippocampus relative to the AD group (all $p < 0.05$). These results suggest that RJ treatment can enhance anti-oxidative capacities in the AD rabbit brain.

RJ Improved Neuronal Metabolic Activities in AD Rabbit Brains

We then used ^{1}H-MRS to evaluate the changes of neruonal metabolic activities in rabbit brains, the results from which are presented in **Figure 7**. Compared with the NC group, the AD model group presented with decreased peaks of NAA and glutamate and increased peaks of Cho and mI, while RJ treatment reveresed these changes. Quantification analysis demonstrated that the levels of NAA/Cr and glutamate/Cr were significantly reduced in the brain of the AD model group when compared with the NC group (ANOVA with *post hoc* Tukey's test, $p < 0.05$ and $p < 0.01$, respectively), while the levels of Cho/Cr and mI/Cr were significantly increased (ANOVA with *post hoc* Tukey's test, $p < 0.01$ and $p < 0.05$, respectively). In specific, the levels of NAA/Cr and glutamate/Cr in the RJ group were increased by 18% and 25% respectively, relative to the AD model group (all $p < 0.05$). On the other hand, the levels of Cho/Cr and mI/Cr were markedly decreased by 16% and 26% respectively in the RJ group compared with the AD model group (all $p < 0.05$). These results indicate that RJ can elevate the levels of NAA and glutamate, and can reduce the levels of mI and Cho in the brain of AD rabbits with potential effects of improving neuronal metabolic activities in the AD brain.

DISCUSSION

Our study confirmed in a rabbit AD model that hypercholesterolemia promotes Aβ deposition and leads to neuronal loss, whereas RJ has the effects of reducing plasma TC and LDL-C levels, enhancing anti-oxidative capacities,

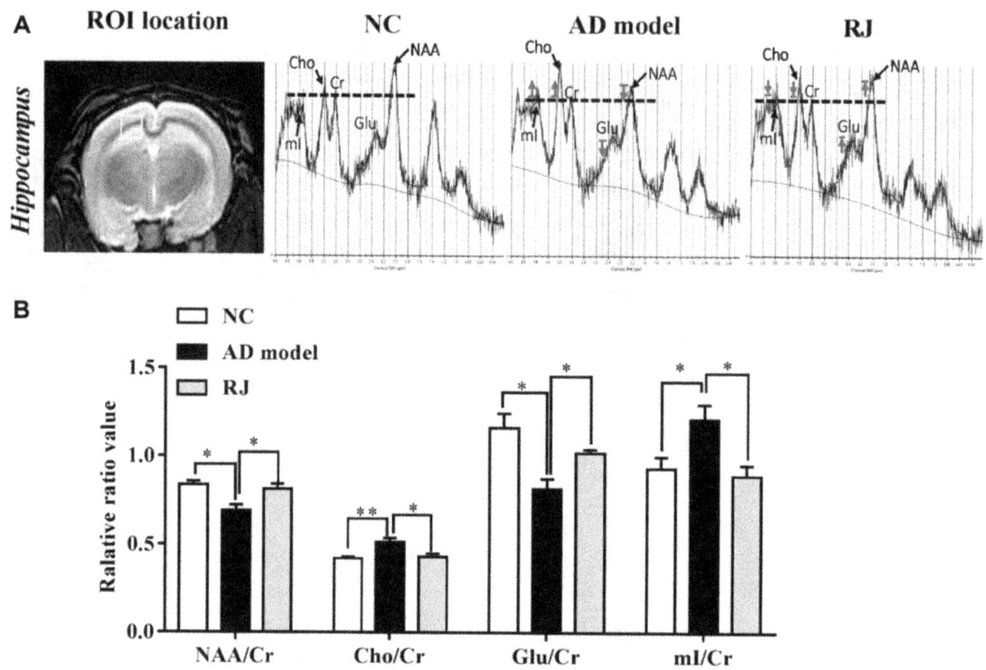

FIGURE 7 | RJ improved brain metabolic activities in AD rabbits. **(A)** Regions of interest (ROI) location in the brain (white box) and representative spectra from the AD model, RJ and NC group rabbits. The red arrow indicates direction of metabolic changes, and the line represents the control level of each metabolite. **(B)** The relative ratios of each metabolite to creatine (Cr) in the brain of the three groups, $n = 6$ rabbits per group. Data are presented as mean ± SEM. ANOVA with *post hoc* Tukey's test was used. $^{*}P < 0.05$, $^{**}P < 0.01$ vs. the AD model group.

ameliorating Aβ pathology and protecting neurons from damage. High cholesterol dietaries are known to promote Aβ generation in human brains, thereby increasing the risk of AD (Panza et al., 2006). Numerous studies have shown that rabbits fed with 1% or 2% cholesterol diet alone or plus trace amounts of copper in drinking water would develop AD pathology, including senile plaques, cognitive impairment and neuronal loss (Larry Sparks, 2004). In this study, we showed that rabbits receiving high cholesterol diets plus copper in drinking water resulted in elevated TC, LDL-C and Aβ (such as Aβ1–40 and Aβ1–42) levels, neuronal loss, and nuclear contraction or disappearance of Nissl bodies, confirming the crucial role of hypercholesterolemia in the development of AD as well as successfully establishing a rabbit AD model. In addition, we observed from an MRI analysis that there was an increase in ventricular volumes in rabbits following 12 weeks on a diet of 2% cholesterol plus copper in drinking water (data not shown), consistent with previous reports (Deci et al., 2012; Schreurs et al., 2013). Furthermore, we showed that RJ significantly reduced the levels of TC and LDL-C in AD rabbits, confirming the previously reported effects of RJ on lowering cholesterol and Aβ levels (Guo et al., 2007).

The effects of RJ on AD rabbits may be explained by its regulatory capabilities of proteins involved in Aβ production, transport, degradation and clearance, such as BACE1, RAGE, LRP1 and IDE. Regarding the regulatory role of RJ in Aβ production, BACE1 is a protease that initiates Aβ production and is mainly located on lipid rafts. Higher BACE1 protein levels were observed in the brain of AD patients (Fukumoto et al., 2002; Holsinger et al., 2002), while *BACE1* gene knocked-out mice were found not to produce Aβ (Vassar et al., 2014; Neumann et al., 2015). The activities of BACE1 are greatly influenced by the metabolism of cholesterol. The increase in Aβ levels caused by high cholesterol diets was found to associate with the up-regulation of BACE1 expression (Jaya Prasanthi et al., 2008). On the other hand, the reduction of cholesterol levels was found to inhibit the BACE1 enzyme activity and reduce Aβ production (Cui et al., 2011). In particular, cholesterol depletion has been shown to reduce the partitioning of APP into lipid rafts, precluding the interaction of BACE1 with lipid rafts and thus lowering Aβ production (Guardia-Laguarta et al., 2009). In this study, we found that BACE1 expression levels as well as cholesterol levels were significantly decreased by RJ, indicating a possible molecular mechanism underlying RJ-mediated decrease of amyloid plaques: RJ inhibits the APP cleavage of amyloid via lowering cholesterol levels and reducing the contact between BACE1 and lipid rafts.

The ability of RJ to reduce the Aβ deposition in the brain may also come from its ability to regulate the transport of Aβ through blood-brain barrier (BBB). Abnormal translocation of Aβ across BBB is considered to be a central link of AD pathogenesis. Recent studies have revealed RAGE and LRP1 as two key Aβ transporters on the BBB: RAGE mediates the transport of Aβ from the peripheral blood to the brain, whereas LRP1 mediates the transport of Aβ from the brain to the blood (Xi et al., 2013;

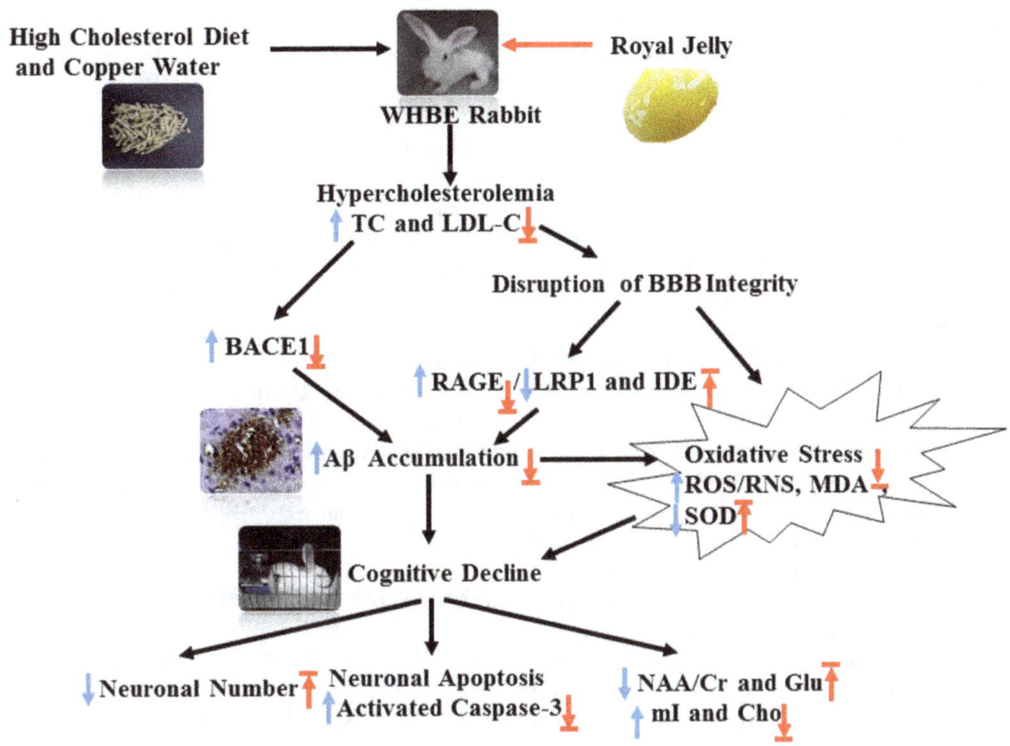

FIGURE 8 | Schematic showing the possible mechanisms by which RJ improves hypercholesterolemia-induced rabbits with AD. AD conditions were induced by feeding rabbits with a high cholesterol diet plus copper in drinking water. RJ can reduce cholesterol levels, down-regulate BACE1 and RAGE expression, increase the expression levels of LRP1 and IDE, promote the degradation and clearance of Aβ, and finally reduce Aβ. Moreover, RJ also has anti-oxidative effects, and it enhances neuronal metabolic activities and prevents neuronal loss. TC, total cholesterol; LDL-C, low-density lipoprotein cholesterol; BACE1, β-site APP cleaving enzyme 1; BBB, Blood-brain barrier; RAGE, receptor for advanced glycation end products; LRP1, LDL receptor related protein 1; IDE, insulin-degrading enzyme; Aβ, amyloid β-protein; ROS, reactive oxygen species; RNS, reactive nitrogen species; MDA, malondialdehyde; SOD, superoxide dismutase; activated caspase-3, activated cysteinyl aspartate specific proteinases 3; NAA, N-acetylaspartata; Glu, glutamate; ml, myo-inositol; Cho, choline. Arrows pointing up or down indicate statistically significant increases or decreases ($p < 0.05$). Blue arrows indicate the changes in AD rabbits, while red arrows indicate the treatment effects of RJ.

Cirillo et al., 2015). In AD patients, the expression of LRP1 was down-regulated, while the expression of RAGE was up-regulated (Shibata et al., 2000; Deane et al., 2004), consistent with what we observed in AD rabbits. Furthermore, we found that RJ could increase the expression levels of LRP1 and inhibit the expression levels of RAGE in the brain of AD rabbits. This effect may be attributed to 10-hydroxy-trans-2-decanoic acid (HDEA), a compound in RJ that can pass through BBB. HDEA has similar effects as brain-derived neurotrophic factor (BDNF), and could potentially promote neurogenesis in mature brains (Hattori et al., 2007). These results suggest that RJ can regulate the translocation of Aβ via RAGE/LRP1 and therefore potentially reduce the Aβ deposition in the brain.

As for the degradation and clearance of Aβ, RJ plays a role in this as well and thereby further reduces the deposition of Aβ. IDE is one of the main enzymes for degrading Aβ in the brain. Increased amyloid plaque and Aβ levels, along with decreased IDE activity, were found in diet-induced insulin resistance APP transgenic mice (Farris et al., 2004). Meanwhile, increased levels of IDE can activate serine/threonine protein kinase B pathway, inhibit the activity of GSK-3β, and decrease abnormal phosphorylation levels of Tau protein (Wang et al., 2006). In addition, the clearance of IDE is related to the BBB transport, and it may contribute to the pathogenesis of AD by influencing insulin signal transduction (Del Campo et al., 2015). We found in this study that the expression levels of IDE were increased by RJ treatment, indicating yet another regulatory path for RJ to reduce Aβ levels.

Apart from Aβ pathology, AD may also benefit from the anti-oxidative effects of RJ. AD is associated with neuronal loss in the brains (Zou et al., 2015), of which apoptosis is a main factor. Oxidative stress was found to promote Aβ aggregation and cause damage to neurons through apoptotic pathways, whereas antioxidant enzymes and vitamin E could antagonize these effects (Mecocci et al., 1994). Known for its anti-oxidative and anti-aging effects, RJ contains rich antioxidant enzymes and vitamins, such as SOD (Min et al., 2004) and vitamin C. In this study, we examined the changes in apoptotic activities and oxidative stress in RJ treated rabbits using five markers: activated caspase-3, a protease involved in apoptosis that has been shown to participate in the pathological process of AD neuronal damage (Zhang et al., 2017); SOD, a free radical scavenging agent for evaluating free radical production; and MDA, which serves as a sensitive index for evaluating the oxidative stress response (Mancini et al., 2017); ROS/RNS play an important role in the survival and cell death signaling cascades that are essential for neurodegenerative disorders, and an increase in ROS/RNS levels (often associated with AD) will result in lipid and protein oxidation (Limongi and Baldelli, 2016). Studying the neurons in the cortex and the hippocampus of AD rabbits, we found that the number of neurons was significantly increased and that activated caspase-3 expression was markedly inhibited by RJ treatment. Moreover, the SOD level was significantly increased and the MDA content and ROS/RNS were decreased in the brain of AD rabbits after RJ intervention, indicating that RJ has the potential to prevent neuronal loss in AD by enhancing anti-oxidative capacities.

Our assessment of neuronal metabolic activities using ^{1}H-MRS further revealed other potential mechanisms of how RJ may improve AD. First, we found that the levels of NAA and glutamate were notably increased in the brains of RJ-treated rabbits. NAA, a specific marker for neuronal viability and integrity (Chen et al., 2013), was reported to be at markedly reduced levels in AD patients (Moon et al., 2016). Glutamate, a major excitatory neurotransmitter that regulates learning, memory and movement, is a marker for neuronal survival and synaptic plasticity (Alvarez and Ruarte, 2004). The increased levels of NAA and glutamate found in RJ-treated rabbits indicate that RJ treatment can enhance neuronal metabolic activities in the brain of AD rabbits and may ultimately improve the cognitive abilities of AD. Furthermore, we found that RJ also increases the level of Cho and mI in the brain of AD rabbits. Cho, related to phospholipid metabolism of cell membranes, participates in the formation of cell membranes and myelin. Meanwhile, mI is a cell marker of glial since it is associated with the activation or proliferation of astrocytes (Zhang et al., 2014). In AD patients, Cho and mI levels were both reported to have increased due to the damage of brain cell membrane and the reactive proliferation of glial cells (Zhang et al., 2014). Our results confirmed that Cho and mI levels are increased in AD rabbits, and showed that these levels can be decreased by RJ treatment. This suggests that RJ treatment can potentially increase the stability of neural cell membrane and promote the activation of glial cells in the AD brain.

In summary, this study showed that RJ can reduce cholesterol levels, down-regulate BACE1 and RAGE expression, increase the expression levels of LRP1 and IDE, promote the degradation and clearance of Aβ, and finally reduce Aβ (**Figure 8**). Moreover, we found that RJ has anti-oxidative effects and that it enhances neuronal metabolic activities and prevents neuronal loss. These results together suggest possible mechanisms by which RJ reduces Aβ deposition and prevents neuronal loss, providing preclinical evidence of the utility of RJ as a natural product for potentially preventing and treating AD.

AUTHOR CONTRIBUTIONS

FH, MC, YP designed the research project; YP, JX, CC, FC, PJ, MY and KZ performed the experiment; YP and MC analyzed the data; YP, CWH and FH wrote the article.

ACKNOWLEDGMENTS

This work was supported by the earmarked fund for Modern Agro-industry Technology Research System from the Ministry of Agriculture of China (CARS-44), public projects of Zhejiang Province Science and Technology Department (No. 2016C37092) and Zhejiang Chinese Medical University Comparative Medical Innovation Team (No. XTD201301).

REFERENCES

Ackl, N., Ising, M., Schreiber, Y. A., Atiya, M., Sonntag, A., and Auer, D. P. (2005). Hippocampal metabolic abnormalities in mild cognitive impairment and Alzheimer's disease. *Neurosci. Lett.* 384, 23–28. doi: 10.1016/j.neulet.2005.04.035

Alvarez, E. O., and Ruarte, M. B. (2004). Glutamic acid and histamine-sensitive neurons in the ventral hippocampus and the basolateral amygdala of the rat: functional interaction on memory and learning processes. *Behav. Brain Res.* 152, 209–219. doi: 10.1016/j.bbr.2003.10.012

Baptiste, D. C., Hartwick, A. T., Jollimore, C. A., Baldridge, W. H., Seigel, G. M., and Kelly, M. E. (2004). An investigation of the neuroprotective effects of tetracycline derivatives in experimental models of retinal cell death. *Mol. Pharmacol.* 66, 1113–1122. doi: 10.1124/mol.104.001081

Butenandt, A., and Rembold, H. (1957). Royal jelly of the honeybee. I. Isolation, constitution analysis and incidence of 10-hydroxy-Δ^2-decenoi acid. *Hoppe Seylers Z. Physiol. Chem.* 308, 284–289. doi: 10.1515/bchm2.1957.308.1.284

Celik, E., and Sanlier, N. (2017). Effects of nutrient and bioactive food components on Alzheimer's disease and epigenetic. *Crit. Rev. Food Sci. Nutr.* doi: 10.1080/10408398.2017.1359488 [Epub ahead of print].

Chen, S. Q., Cai, Q., Shen, Y. Y., Wang, P. J., Teng, G. J., Li, M. H., et al. (2012). ^{1}H-MRS evaluation of therapeutic effect of neural stem cell transplantation on Alzheimer's disease in AβPP/PS1 double transgenic mice. *J. Alzheimers Dis.* 28, 71–80. doi: 10.3233/JAD-2010-110893

Chen, S. M., Fan, C. C., Chiue, M. S., Chou, C., Chen, J. H., and Hseu, R. S. (2013). Hemodynamic and neuropathological analysis in rats with aluminum trichloride-induced Alzheimer's disease. *PLoS One* 8:e82561. doi: 10.1371/journal.pone.0082561

Chen, S. Q., Wang, P. J., Ten, G. J., Zhan, W., Li, M. H., and Zang, F. C. (2009). Role of myo-inositol by magnetic resonance spectroscopy in early diagnosis of Alzheimer's disease in APP/PS1 transgenic mice. *Dement. Geriatr. Cogn. Disord.* 28, 558–566. doi: 10.1159/000261646

Cirillo, C., Capoccia, E., Iuvone, T., Cuomo, R., Sarnelli, G., Steardo, L., et al. (2015). S100B inhibitor pentamidine attenuates reactive gliosis and reduces neuronal loss in a mouse model of Alzheimer's disease. *Biomed Res. Int.* 2015:508342. doi: 10.1155/2015/508342

Comas Herrera, A., Prince, M., Knapp, M., Karagiannidou, M., and Guerchet, M. (2016). *World Alzheimer Report 2016: Improving Healthcare for People with Dementia. Coverage, Quality and Costs Now and in the Future.* London: Alzheimer's Disease International.

Cui, W., Sun, Y., Wang, Z., Xu, C., Xu, L., Wang, F., et al. (2011). Activation of liver X receptor decreases BACE1 expression and activity by reducing membrane cholesterol levels. *Neurochem. Res.* 36, 1910–1921. doi: 10.1007/s11064-011-0513-3

Deane, R., Wu, Z., and Zlokovic, B. V. (2004). RAGE (yin) versus LRP (yang) balance regulates alzheimer amyloid β-peptide clearance through transport across the blood-brain barrier. *Stroke* 35, 2628–2631. doi: 10.1161/01.str.0000143452.85382.d1

Deci, S., Lemieux, S. K., Smith-Bell, C. A., Sparks, D. L., and Schreurs, B. G. (2012). Cholesterol increases ventricular volume in a rabbit model of Alzheimer's disease. *J. Alzheimers Dis.* 29, 283–292. doi: 10.3233/JAD-2011-111415

Del Campo, M., Stargardt, A., Veerhuis, R., Reits, E., and Teunissen, C. E. (2015). Accumulation of BRI2-BRICHOS ectodomain correlates with a decreased clearance of Aβ by insulin degrading enzyme (IDE) in Alzheimer's disease. *Neurosci. Lett.* 589, 47–51. doi: 10.1016/j.neulet.2015.01.036

Farris, W., Mansourian, S., Leissring, M. A., Eckman, E. A., Bertram, L., Eckman, C. B., et al. (2004). Partial loss-of-function mutations in insulin-degrading enzyme that induce diabetes also impair degradation of amyloid β-protein. *Am. J. Pathol.* 164, 1425–1434. doi: 10.1016/s0002-9440(10)63229-4

Fereshtehnejad, S. M., Johnell, K., and Eriksdotter, M. (2014). Anti-dementia drugs and co-medication among patients with Alzheimer's disease: investigating real-world drug use in clinical practice using the Swedish Dementia Quality Registry (SveDem). *Drugs Aging* 31, 215–224. doi: 10.1007/s40266-014-0154-8

Fontana, R., Mendes, M. A., de Souza, B. M., Konno, K., César, L. L. M. M., Malaspina, O., et al. (2004). Jelleines: a family of antimicrobial peptides from the Royal Jelly of honeybees (*Apis mellifera*). *Peptides* 25, 919–928. doi: 10.1016/j.peptides.2004.03.016

Fukumoto, H., Cheung, B. S., Hyman, B. T., and Irizarry, M. C. (2002). β-secretase protein and activity are increased in the neocortex in Alzheimer disease. *Arch. Neurol.* 59, 1381–1389. doi: 10.1001/archneur.59.9.1381

Galbete, J. L., Martin, T. R., Peressini, E., Modena, P., Bianchi, R., and Forloni, G. (2000). Cholesterol decreases secretion of the secreted form of amyloid precursor protein by interfering with glycosylation in the protein secretory pathway. *Biochem. J.* 348, 307–313. doi: 10.1042/0264-6021:3480307

Gonzalo-Ruiz, A., Pérez, J. L., Sanz, J. M., Geula, C., and Arévalo, J. (2006). Effects of lipids and aging on the neurotoxicity and neuronal loss caused by intracerebral injections of the amyloid-β peptide in the rat. *Exp. Neurol.* 197, 41–55. doi: 10.1016/j.expneurol.2005.06.008

Guardia-Laguarta, C., Coma, M., Pera, M., Clarimãn, J., Sereno, L., Agulló, J. M., et al. (2009). Mild cholesterol depletion reduces amyloid-β production by impairing APP trafficking to the cell surface. *J. Neurochem.* 110, 220–230. doi: 10.1111/j.1471-4159.2009.06126.x

Guo, H., Saiga, A., Sato, M., Miyazawa, I., Shibata, M., Takahata, Y., et al. (2007). Royal jelly supplementation improves lipoprotein metabolism in humans. *J. Nutr. Sci. Vitaminol.* 53, 345–348. doi: 10.3177/jnsv.53.345

Hattori, N., Nomoto, H., Fukumitsu, H., Mishima, S., and Furukawa, S. (2007). Royal jelly and its unique fatty acid, 10-hydroxy-trans-2-decenoic acid, promote neurogenesis by neural stem/progenitor cells *in vitro*. *Biomed. Res.* 28, 261–266. doi: 10.2220/biomedres.28.261

Hattori, N., Nomoto, H., Fukumitsu, H., Mishima, S., and Furukawa, S. (2010). AMP N_1-oxide, a unique compound of royal jelly, induces neurite outgrowth from PC12 cells via signaling by protein kinase A independent of that by mitogen-activated protein kinase. *Evid. Based Complement. Alternat. Med.* 7, 63–68. doi: 10.1093/ecam/nem146

Holsinger, R. M., McLean, C. A., Beyreuther, K., Masters, C. L., and Evin, G. (2002). Increased expression of the amyloid precursor β-secretase in Alzheimer's disease. *Ann. Neurol.* 51, 783–786. doi: 10.1002/ana.10208

Honda, Y., Fujita, Y., Maruyama, H., Araki, Y., Ichihara, K., Sato, A., et al. (2011). Lifespan-extending effects of royal jelly and its related substances on the nematode *Caenorhabditis elegans*. *PLoS One* 6:e23527. doi: 10.1371/journal.pone.0023527

Jaya Prasanthi, R. P., Schommer, E., Thomasson, S., Thompson, A., Feist, G., and Ghribi, O. (2008). Regulation of β-amyloid levels in the brain of cholesterol-fed rabbit, a model system for sporadic Alzheimer's disease. *Mech. Ageing Dev.* 129, 649–655. doi: 10.1016/j.mad.2008.09.002

Johnstone, E. M., Chaney, M. O., Norris, F. H., Pascual, R., and Little, S. P. (1991). Conservation of the sequence of the Alzheimer's disease amyloid peptide in dog, polar bear and five other mammals by cross-species polymerase chain reaction analysis. *Mol. Brain Res.* 10, 299–305. doi: 10.1016/0169-328x(91)90088-f

Kivipelto, M., Helkala, E. L., Laakso, M. P., Hänninen, T., Hallikainen, M., Alhainen, K., et al. (2001). Midlife vascular risk factors and Alzheimer's disease in later life: longitudinal, population based study. *BMJ* 322, 1447–1451. doi: 10.1136/bmj.322.7300.1447

Kohno, K., Okamoto, I., Sano, O., Arai, N., Iwaki, K., Ikeda, M., et al. (2004). Royal jelly inhibits the production of proinflammatory cytokines by activated macrophages. *Biosci. Biotechnol. Biochem.* 68, 138–145. doi: 10.1271/bbb.68.138

Kuo, P. H., Lin, C. I., Chen, Y. H., Chiu, W. C., and Lin, S. H. (2015). A high-cholesterol diet enriched with polyphenols from Oriental plums (*Prunus salicina*) improves cognitive function and lowers brain cholesterol levels and neurodegenerative-related protein expression in mice. *Br. J. Nutr.* 113, 1550–1557. doi: 10.1017/s0007114515000732

Lacher, S. E., Alazizi, A., Wang, X., Bell, D. A., Pique-Regi, R., Luca, F., et al. (2018). A hypermorphic antioxidant response element is associated with increased MS4A6A expression and Alzheimer's disease. *Redox Biol.* 14, 686–693. doi: 10.1016/j.redox.2017.10.018

Larry Sparks, D. (2004). Cholesterol, copper, and accumulation of thioflavine S-reactive Alzheimer's-like amyloid β in rabbit brain. *J. Mol. Neurosci.* 24, 97–104. doi: 10.1385/jmn:24:1:097

Li, X. Y., Bao, X. J., and Wang, R. Z. (2015). Potential of neural stem cell-based therapies for Alzheimer's disease. *J. Neurosci. Res.* 93, 1313–1324. doi: 10.1002/jnr.23555

Limongi, D., and Baldelli, S. (2016). Redox imbalance and viral infections in neurodegenerative diseases. *Oxid. Med. Cell. Longev.* 2016:6547248. doi: 10.1155/2016/6547248

Liu, Q. Y., Chang, M. N., Lei, J. X., Koukiekolo, R., Smith, B., Zhang, D., et al. (2014). Identification of microRNAs involved in Alzheimer's progression using a rabbit model of the disease. *Am. J. Neurodegener. Dis.* 3, 33–44.

Loke, S. Y., Wong, T. H., and Ong, W. Y. (2017). Global gene expression changes in the prefrontal cortex of rabbits with hypercholesterolemia and/or hypertension. *Neurochem. Int.* 102, 33–56. doi: 10.1016/j.neuint.2016.11.010

Mancini, S., Balducci, C., Micotti, E., Tolomeo, D., Forloni, G., Masserini, M., et al. (2017). Multifunctional liposomes delay phenotype progression and prevent memory impairment in a presymptomatic stage mouse model of Alzheimer disease. *J. Control. Release* 258, 121–129. doi: 10.1016/j.jconrel.2017.05.013

Mecocci, P., MacGarvey, U., and Beal, M. F. (1994). Oxidative damage to mitochondrial DNA is increased in Alzheimer's disease. *Ann. Neurol.* 36, 747–751. doi: 10.1002/ana.410360510

Min, L., Li, J., Liu, K., Jiang, Y., Liu, X., and Liu, X. (2004). Isolation, purification and characterization of superoxide dismutase from royal jelly of the Italian worker bee, *Apis mellifera*. *Acta Entomol. Sin.* 47, 171–177.

Moon, C. M., Kim, B. C., and Jeong, G. W. (2016). Effects of donepezil on brain morphometric and metabolic changes in patients with Alzheimer's disease: a DARTEL-based VBM and ^{1}H-MRS. *Magn. Reson. Imaging* 34, 1008–1016. doi: 10.1016/j.mri.2016.04.025

Nagai, T., and Inoue, R. (2004). Preparation and the functional properties of water extract and alkaline extract of royal jelly. *Food Chem.* 84, 181–186. doi: 10.1016/s0308-8146(03)00198-5

Nagai, T., Inoue, R., Suzuki, N., and Nagashima, T. (2006). Antioxidant properties of enzymatic hydrolysates from royal jelly. *J. Med. Food* 9, 363–367. doi: 10.1089/jmf.2006.9.363

Neumann, U., Rueeger, H., Machauer, R., Veenstra, S. J., Lueoend, R. M., Tintelnot-Blomley, M., et al. (2015). A novel BACE inhibitor NB-360 shows a superior pharmacological profile and robust reduction of amyloid-β and neuroinflammation in APP transgenic mice. *Mol. Neurodegener.* 10:44. doi: 10.1186/s13024-015-0033-8

Panza, F., Capurso, C., D'Introno, A., Colacicco, A. M., Vasquez, F., Pistoia, G., et al. (2006). Serum total cholesterol as a biomarker for Alzheimer's disease: mid-life or late-life determinations? *Exp. Gerontol.* 41, 805–806. doi: 10.1016/j.exger.2006.06.005

Pourmoradian, S., Mahdavi, R., Mobasseri, M., Faramarzi, E., and Mobasseri, M. (2012). Effects of royal jelly supplementation on body weight and dietary intake in type 2 diabetic females. *Health Promot. Perspect.* 2, 231–235. doi: 10.5681/hpp.2012.028

Provencher, S. W. (1993). Estimation of metabolite concentrations from localized *in vivo* proton NMR spectra. *Magn. Reson. Med.* 30, 672–679. doi: 10.1002/mrm.1910300604

Ramadan, M. F., and Al-Ghamdi, A. (2012). Bioactive compounds and health-promoting properties of royal jelly: a review. *J. Funct. Foods* 4, 39–52. doi: 10.1016/j.jff.2011.12.007

Schreurs, B. G., Smith-Bell, C. A., and Lemieux, S. K. (2013). Dietary cholesterol increases ventricular volume and narrows cerebrovascular diameter in a rabbit model of Alzheimer's disease. *Neuroscience* 254, 61–69. doi: 10.1016/j.neuroscience.2013.09.015

Selkoe, D. J. (2001). Alzheimer's disease: genes, proteins, and therapy. *Physiol. Rev.* 81, 741–766. doi: 10.1152/physrev.2001.81.2.741

Shibata, M., Yamada, S., Kumar, S. R., Calero, M., Bading, J., Frangione, B., et al. (2000). Clearance of Alzheimer's amyloid-$ß_{(1-40)}$ peptide from brain by LDL receptor-related protein-1 at the blood-brain barrier. *J. Clin. Invest.* 106, 1489–1499. doi: 10.1172/jci10498

Sparks, D. L., and Schreurs, B. G. (2003). Trace amounts of copper in water induce β-amyloid plaques and learning deficits in a rabbit model of Alzheimer's disease. *Proc. Natl. Acad. Sci. U S A* 100, 11065–11069. doi: 10.1073/pnas.1832769100

Sparks, D. L., Scheff, S. W., Hunsaker, J. C. III., Liu, H., Landers, T., and Gross, D. R. (1994). Induction of Alzheimer-like β-amyloid immunoreactivity in the brains of rabbits with dietary cholesterol. *Exp. Neurol.* 126, 88–94. doi: 10.1006/exnr.1994.1044

Takenaka, T. (1982). Chemical compositions of royal jelly. *Honeybee Sci.* 3, 69–74.

Vassar, R., Kuhn, P. H., Haass, C., Kennedy, M. E., Rajendran, L., Wong, P. C., et al. (2014). Function, therapeutic potential and cell biology of BACE proteases: current status and future prospects. *J. Neurochem.* 130, 4–28. doi: 10.1111/jnc.12715

Vittek, J. (1995). Effect of Royal Jelly on serum lipids in experimental animals and humans with atherosclerosis. *Experientia* 51, 927–935. doi: 10.1007/bf01921742

Wang, Z. F., Li, H. L., Li, X. C., Zhang, Q., Tian, Q., Wang, Q., et al. (2006). Effects of endogenous β-amyloid overproduction on tau phosphorylation in cell culture. *J. Neurochem.* 98, 1167–1175. doi: 10.1111/j.1471-4159.2006.03956.x

Wang, X., Min, C., and Dong, Y. (2016). Royal jelly promotes DAF-16-mediated proteostasis to tolerate β-amyloid toxicity in *C. elegans* model of Alzheimer's disease. *Oncotarget* 7, 54183–54193. doi: 10.18632/oncotarget.10857

Wang, S. H., Wang, Y. Z., Zhang, K. Y., Shen, J. H., Zhou, H. Q., and Qiu, X. Y. (2005). Effect of superoxide dismutase and malondialdehyde metabolic changes on carcinogenesis of gastric carcinoma. *World J. Gastroenterol.* 11, 4305–4310. doi: 10.3748/wjg.v11.i28.4305

Wei, W., Wei, M., Kang, X., Deng, H., and Lu, Z. (2010). A novel method developed for acetylcholine detection in royal jelly by using capillary electrophoresis coupled with electrogenerated chemiluminescence based on a simple reaction. *Electrophoresis* 30, 1949–1952. doi: 10.1002/elps.200800721

Woodruff-Pak, D. S., Agelan, A., and Del Valle, L. (2007). A rabbit model of Alzheimer's disease: valid at neuropathological, cognitive, and therapeutic levels. *J. Alzheimers Dis.* 11, 371–383. doi: 10.3233/jad-2007-11313

Xi, Y. D., Li, X. Y., Ding, J., Yu, H. L., Ma, W. W., Yuan, L. H., et al. (2013). Soy isoflavone alleviates Aβ1–42-induced impairment of learning and memory ability through the regulation of RAGE/LRP-1 in neuronal and vascular tissue. *Curr. Neurovasc. Res.* 10, 144–156. doi: 10.2174/1567202611310020007

Zamani, Z., Reisi, P., Alaei, H., and Pilehvarian, A. A. (2012). Effect of Royal Jelly on spatial learning and memory in rat model of streptozotocin-induced sporadic Alzheimer's disease. *Adv. Biomed. Res.* 1:26. doi: 10.4103/2277-9175.98150

Zhang, Y. P., Brown, R. E., Zhang, P. C., Zhao, Y. T., Ju, X. H., and Song, C. (2017). DHA, EPA and their combination at various ratios differently modulated Aβ25–35-induced neurotoxicity in SH-SY5Y cells. *Prostaglandins Leukot. Essent. Fatty Acids* doi: 10.1016/j.plefa.2017.07.003 [Epub ahead of print].

Zhang, Q. Q., Shi, J. Q., Xu, J., Cheng, X. X., Zhu, H. Q., and Chen, J. (2013). Application of thioflavin T staining in detection of β-amyloid. *Zhonghua Bing Li Xue Za Zhi* 42, 764–765. doi: 10.3760/cma.j.issn.0529-5807.2013.11.011

Zhang, N., Song, X., Bartha, R., Beyea, S., D'Arcy, R., Zhang, Y., et al. (2014). Advances in high-field magnetic resonance spectroscopy in Alzheimer's disease. *Curr. Alzheimer Res.* 11, 367–388. doi: 10.2174/1567205011666140302200312

Zou, C., Montagna, E., Shi, Y., Peters, F., Blazquez-Llorca, L., Shi, S., et al. (2015). Intraneuronal APP and extracellular Aβ independently cause dendritic spine pathology in transgenic mouse models of Alzheimer's disease. *Acta Neuropathol.* 129, 909–920. doi: 10.1007/s00401-015-1421-4

Permissions

All chapters in this book were first published by Frontiers; hereby published with permission under the Creative Commons Attribution License or equivalent. Every chapter published in this book has been scrutinized by our experts. Their significance has been extensively debated. The topics covered herein carry significant findings which will fuel the growth of the discipline. They may even be implemented as practical applications or may be referred to as a beginning point for another development.

The contributors of this book come from diverse backgrounds, making this book a truly international effort. This book will bring forth new frontiers with its revolutionizing research information and detailed analysis of the nascent developments around the world.

We would like to thank all the contributing authors for lending their expertise to make the book truly unique. They have played a crucial role in the development of this book. Without their invaluable contributions this book wouldn't have been possible. They have made vital efforts to compile up to date information on the varied aspects of this subject to make this book a valuable addition to the collection of many professionals and students.

This book was conceptualized with the vision of imparting up-to-date information and advanced data in this field. To ensure the same, a matchless editorial board was set up. Every individual on the board went through rigorous rounds of assessment to prove their worth. After which they invested a large part of their time researching and compiling the most relevant data for our readers.

The editorial board has been involved in producing this book since its inception. They have spent rigorous hours researching and exploring the diverse topics which have resulted in the successful publishing of this book. They have passed on their knowledge of decades through this book. To expedite this challenging task, the publisher supported the team at every step. A small team of assistant editors was also appointed to further simplify the editing procedure and attain best results for the readers.

Apart from the editorial board, the designing team has also invested a significant amount of their time in understanding the subject and creating the most relevant covers. They scrutinized every image to scout for the most suitable representation of the subject and create an appropriate cover for the book.

The publishing team has been an ardent support to the editorial, designing and production team. Their endless efforts to recruit the best for this project, has resulted in the accomplishment of this book. They are a veteran in the field of academics and their pool of knowledge is as vast as their experience in printing. Their expertise and guidance has proved useful at every step. Their uncompromising quality standards have made this book an exceptional effort. Their encouragement from time to time has been an inspiration for everyone.

The publisher and the editorial board hope that this book will prove to be a valuable piece of knowledge for researchers, students, practitioners and scholars across the globe.

List of Contributors

Diling Chen, Jian Yang, Tianqiao Yong, Xiaocui Tang and Qingping Wu
State Key Laboratory of Applied Microbiology Southern China, Guangdong Provincial Key Laboratory of Microbial Culture Collection and Application, Guangdong Open Laboratory of Applied Microbiology, Guangdong Institute of Microbiology, Chinese Academy of Sciences, Guangzhou, China

Xin Yang
Department of Pharmacy, The Fifth Affiliated Hospital of Guangzhou Medical University, Guangzhou, China

Gailian Zhou
Guangxi University of Chinese Medicine, Nanning, China

Guoxiao Lai
State Key Laboratory of Applied Microbiology Southern China, Guangdong Provincial Key Laboratory of Microbial Culture Collection and Application, Guangdong Open Laboratory of Applied Microbiology, Guangdong Institute of Microbiology, Chinese Academy of Sciences, Guangzhou, China Guangxi University of Chinese Medicine, Nanning, China

Ou Shuai and Yizhen Xie
State Key Laboratory of Applied Microbiology Southern China, Guangdong Provincial Key Laboratory of Microbial Culture Collection and Application, Guangdong Open Laboratory of Applied Microbiology, Guangdong Institute of Microbiology, Chinese Academy of Sciences, Guangzhou, China
Guangdong Yuewei Edible Fungi Technology Co., Ltd., Guangzhou, China

Vladimir V. Salmin and Konstantin A. Shapovalov
Department of Medical and Biological Physics, Krasnoyarsk State Medical University named after Prof. V.F. Voino-Yasenetsky, Krasnoyarsk, Russia

Yulia K. Komleva, Natalia V. Kuvacheva, Elena D. Khilazheva, Olga L. Lopatina, Elena A. Pozhilenkova and Alla B. Salmina
Department of Biochemistry, Medical, Pharmaceutical and Toxicological Chemistry, Krasnoyarsk State Medical University named after Prof. V.F. Voino-Yasenetsky, Krasnoyarsk, Russia
Research Institute of Molecular Medicine and Pathobiochemistry, Krasnoyarsk State Medical University named after Prof. V.F. Voino-Yasenetsky, Krasnoyarsk, Russia

Andrey V. Morgun
Department of Pediatrics, Krasnoyarsk State Medical University named after Prof. V.F. Voino-Yasenetsky, Krasnoyarsk, Russia

Yulia A. Uspenskaya
Research Institute of Molecular Medicine and Pathobiochemistry, Krasnoyarsk State Medical University named after Prof. V.F. Voino-Yasenetsky, Krasnoyarsk, Russia

Ken-ichi Tabei
Department of Dementia Prevention and Therapeutics, Graduate School of Medicine, Mie University, Tsu, Japan
Department of Neurology, Graduate School of Medicine, Mie University, Tsu, Japan

Jun-ichi Ogawa
Yamaha Music Foundation, Tokyo, Japan

Tomoko Tokita
Department of Health and Welfare, Mihama Town Hall, Mihama, Japan

Noriko Nakaguchi
Department of Health and Welfare, Kiho Town Hall, Kiho, Japan

Masayuki Satoh and Hirotaka Kida
Department of Dementia Prevention and Therapeutics, Graduate School of Medicine, Mie University, Tsu, Japan

Hidekazu Tomimoto
Department of Neurology, Graduate School of Medicine, Mie University, Tsu, Japan

Koji Nakao
Department of Neurosurgery, Kinan Hospital, Mihama, Japan

Rudimar L. Frozza
Oswaldo Cruz Institute, Fundação Oswaldo Cruz (FIOCRUZ), Rio de Janeiro, Brazil

Mychael V. Lourenco
Institute of Medical Biochemistry Leopoldo de Meis, Rio de Janeiro, Brazil
Institute of Biophysics Carlos Chagas Filho, Federal University of Rio de Janeiro, Rio de Janeiro, Brazil

Fernanda G. De Felice
Institute of Medical Biochemistry Leopoldo de Meis, Rio de Janeiro, Brazil
Department of Biomedical and Molecular Sciences, Centre for Neuroscience Studies, Queen's University, Kingston, ON, Canada

Claudia Bachmann
Institute of Neuroscience and Medicine (INM-6), Institute for Advanced Simulation (IAS-6), JARA BRAIN Institute I, Jülich Research Centre, Jülich, Germany

Heidi I. L. Jacobs
Faculty of Health, Medicine and Life Science, School for Mental Health and Neuroscience, Alzheimer Centre Limburg, Maastricht University, Maastricht, Netherlands
Division of Nuclear Medicine and Molecular Imaging, Department of Radiology, Harvard Medical School, Massachusetts General Hospital, Boston, MA, United States
Department of Cognitive Neuroscience, Faculty of Psychology and Neuroscience, Maastricht University, Maastricht, Netherlands

PierGianLuca Porta Mana
Kavli Institute for Systems Neuroscience, Norwegian University of Science and Technology (NTNU), Trondheim, Norway

Kim Dillen
Cognitive Neuroscience, Institute of Neuroscience and Medicine (INM-3), Jülich Research Centre, Jülich, Germany

Nils Richter, Boris von Reutern, Julian Dronse, Oezguer A . Onur and Gereon R . Fink
Cognitive Neuroscience, Institute of Neuroscience and Medicine (INM-3), Jülich Research Centre, Jülich, Germany
Department of Neurology, University Hospital of Cologne, Cologne, Germany

Karl-Josef Langen
Cognitive Neuroscience, Institute of Neuroscience and Medicine (INM-4), Jülich Research Centre, Jülich, Germany

Juraj Kukolja
Cognitive Neuroscience, Institute of Neuroscience and Medicine (INM-3), Jülich Research Centre, Jülich, Germany
Department of Neurology, University Hospital of Cologne, Colo gne, Germany
Department of Neurology, Helios University Hospital Wuppertal, Wuppertal, Germany

Abigail Morrison
Institute of Neuroscience and Medicine (INM-6), Institute for Advanced Simulation (IAS-6), JARA BRAIN Institute I, Jülich Research Centre, Jülich, Germany
Faculty of Psychology, Institute of Cognitive Neuroscience, Ruhr-University Bochum, Bochum, Germany

Mohammad H. Baig, Khurshid Ahmad, Gulam Rabbani and Inho Choi
Department of Medical Biotechnology, Yeungnam University, Gyeongsan, South Korea

Javaria Ashraf and Jamil Ahmad
Research Center for Modeling and Simulation, National University of Sciences and Technology, Islamabad, Pakistan

Amjad Ali
Atta-Ur-Rahman School of Applied Biosciences, National University of Sciences and Technology, Islamabad, Pakistan

Zaheer Ul-Haq
Dr. Panjwani Center for Molecular Medicine and Drug Research, International Center for Chemical Sciences, University of Karachi, Karachi, Pakistan

Min Huang, Binchu Xu, Cuicui Chai and Pengfei Xing
Department of Neurology, The Seventh Affiliated Hospital, Sun Yat-sen University, Shenzhen, China

Yubin Liang
Department of Neurology, The First Affiliated Hospital of Jinan University, Guangzhou, China

Hongda Chen
Department of Traditional Chinese Medicine, The Seventh Affiliated Hospital, Sun Yat-sen University, Shenzhen, China

Fatma E. A. El-Gamal and Mohammed M. Elmogy
Faculty of Computers and Information, Information Technology Department, Mansoura University, Mansoura, Egypt
BioImaging Laboratory, Department of Bioengineering, University of Louisville, Louisville, KY, United States

Mohammed Ghazal
BioImaging Laboratory, Department of Bioengineering, University of Louisville, Louisville, KY, United States
Department of Electrical and Computer Engineering, College of Engineering, Abu Dhabi University, Abu Dhabi, United Arab Emirates

Manuel F. Casanova
School of Medicine, University of South Carolina, Greenville, SC, United States

Gregory N. Barnes
University of Louisville Autism Center, Department of Neurology, University of Louisville, Louisville

Robert Keynton
Department of Bioengineering, University of Louisville, Louisville, KY, United States

Ashraf Khalil
Department of Computer Science and Information Technology, College of Engineering, Abu Dhabi University, Abu Dhabi, United Arab Emirates

Ahmed Atwan
Faculty of Computers and Information, Information Technology Department, Mansoura University, Mansoura, Egypt

Ayman S. El-Baz
BioImaging Laboratory, Department of Bioengineering, University of Louisville, Louisville, KY, United States

Xiao Luo, Kaicheng Li, Qingze Zeng, Peiyu Huang, Yeerfan Jiaerken, Tiantian Qiu, Xiaojun Xu, Jingjing Xu and Minming Zhang
Department of Radiology, The Second Affiliated Hospital of Zhejiang University School of Medicine, Hangzhou, China

Jiong Zhou
Department of Neurology, The Second Affiliated Hospital of Zhejiang University School of Medicine, Hangzhou, China

Ghulam M. Ashraf
King Fahd Medical Research Center, King Abdulaziz University, Jeddah, Saudi Arabia

Saleh S. Baeesa
Division of Neurosurgery, College of Medicine, King Abdulaziz University, Jeddah, Saudi Arabia

Zhuqing Long, Feiyi Cui, Tingting Wang and Hongwen Chen
Medical Apparatus and Equipment Deployment, Nanfang Hospital, Southern Medical University, Guangzhou, China

Bin Jing
School of Biomedical Engineering, Capital Medical University, Beijing, China

Ru Guo
Department of Tuberculosis, Beijing Chest Hospital Capital Medical University, Beijing, China

Bo Li
Department of Traditional Chinese Medicine, Beijing Chest Hospital, Capital Medical University, Beijing Tuberculosis and Thoracic Tumor Research Institute, Beijing, China

Nermin Eissa, Nadia Khan, Shreesh K. Ojha and Bassem Sadek
Department of Pharmacology & Therapeutics, College of Medicine & Health Sciences, United Arab Emirates University, Al Ain, United Arab Emirates

Dorota Łazewska and Katarzyna Kieć-Kononowicz
Department of Technology and Biotechnology of Drugs, Faculty of Pharmacy, Jagiellonian University-Medical College, Kraków, Poland

Tapan K. Khan
Center for Neurodegenerative Diseases, Blanchette Rockefeller Neurosciences Institute, West Virginia University, Morgantown, WV, United States

Lin Sun, Wei Li, Shifu Xiao and Xia Li
Shanghai Mental Health Center, Alzheimer's Disease and Related Disorders Center, Shanghai Jiao Tong University School of Medicine, Shanghai, China

Zhouyi Rong
Fujian Provincial Key Laboratory of Neurodegenerative Disease and Aging Research, Institute of Neuroscience, College of Medicine, Xiamen University, Xiamen, China

Honghua Zheng
Fujian Provincial Key Laboratory of Neurodegenerative Disease and Aging Research, Institute of Neuroscience, College of Medicine, Xiamen University, Xiamen, China
Department of Neuroscience, Shenzhen Research Institute of Xiamen University, Shenzhen, China

Xia-an Bi, Qin Jiang, Qi Sun, Qing Shu and Yingchao Liu
College of Information Science and Engineering, Hunan Normal University, Changsha, China

Yongming Pan
College of Animal Sciences, Zhejiang University, Hangzhou, China
Comparative Medical Research Center, Experimental Animal Research Center, Zhejiang Chinese Medical University, Hangzhou, China

Jianqin Xu, Cheng Chen, Fangming Chen, Keyan Zhu and Minli Chen
Comparative Medical Research Center, Experimental Animal Research Center, Zhejiang Chinese Medical University, Hangzhou, China

Ping Jin
The First Affiliated Hospital, Zhejiang Chinese Medical University, Hangzhou, China

Chenyue W. Hu
Department of Bioengineering, Rice University, Houston, TX, United States

Mengmeng You and Fuliang Hu
College of Animal Sciences, Zhejiang University, Hangzhou, China

Index

A

Acetylcholine, 4, 21, 58, 88, 169, 175-178, 210

Akkermansia, 6, 17, 20-21, 26-28

Alzheimer's Disease, 1-2, 26-29, 38-39, 41, 43, 46-48, 50, 52, 55-63, 65, 73, 76, 81-86, 88-91, 112-116, 127-129, 131, 137-141, 144, 149-152, 155, 158-160, 166-169, 176-177, 179-183, 185-193, 197, 199, 202, 206-210, 213-214, 220

Amnesia, 170, 175-177

Amygdala, 84, 160, 164-165, 176, 220

Amyloid Beta, 39, 56, 58, 73, 85, 91-92, 127, 130, 182-183, 186-187

Amyloid Precursor Protein, 2, 49, 56, 85, 87, 91-93, 112-114, 117, 128, 210, 221

Amyloidosis, 25, 27, 116, 180-181, 184-185

Antibiotics, 1-3, 9, 11-13, 15, 17, 21, 25-26

Antidepressant, 2, 26, 117, 128, 194

Anxiety, 2, 17, 26, 116-117, 166, 168-169, 171, 174-177, 188

Apolipoprotein E, 198

Apoptosis, 1-2, 15, 30, 53, 114, 116, 121, 123, 126-128, 153, 157-159, 184, 193, 196, 216, 219

Arterial Spin Labeling, 179-180, 183, 188, 191

Astrocytes, 21, 49, 51, 58, 153, 220

Autism, 21, 129, 149, 161, 167, 207

B

Bacteroides, 6, 9, 21

Basal Ganglia, 160, 164-166, 184

Bifidobacteria, 17, 19-21, 25, 27

Biomarkers, 49-50, 53-56, 59, 62, 86, 89-90, 113, 130, 137-141, 143-144, 150, 158, 179-191, 206

Blood-brain Barrier, 30, 49, 159, 218-220, 222

Brain Atrophy, 41-42, 45-46, 181, 183

Brain Injury, 30, 38, 115, 127, 152, 159

Brain Plasticity, 2, 27, 30

C

Calpain-calpastatin, 91, 93, 113

Cell Death, 31, 39, 87, 90-92, 113-115, 119, 126, 220

Cell Proliferation, 29, 31, 33-34, 37-38, 158

Central Nervous System, 1, 21, 52, 54-55, 58, 127, 152, 158-159, 169, 177-178, 190

Cerebrospinal Fluid, 43, 55, 57, 62, 73, 77, 87, 130, 144, 149-152, 159, 179-180, 187, 189-191, 200, 207

Cognitive Impairment, 31, 42, 47, 56, 59, 61, 63, 65-66, 84, 91, 110, 116-118, 128-132, 137-141, 146, 148-151, 160, 163, 166-167, 179, 189-191, 200, 206-207, 218, 220

Cognitive Stimulation, 41-45

Computer-aided Diagnosis, 129-130, 207

Cortical Atrophy, 41, 46, 212

Cytokines, 1-4, 6, 8-9, 11, 21, 28, 51-53, 59, 93, 221

D

Depression, 2, 26, 38, 49, 53, 56-60, 116-117, 127, 131, 141, 158, 188, 194, 196

Diffusion Tensor Imaging, 146, 150-151, 179-180, 182-183, 186, 189-190

Dopamine, 6, 21, 52-53, 55, 57-58, 88, 169, 175

E

Endoplasmic Reticulum, 51-52, 56, 89, 92, 113-114

F

Fluoxetine, 116-128

Frontotemporal Dementia, 183-184, 192, 197-198

Fructooligosaccharides, 1-2, 15, 19, 21, 23, 25

G

Gene Haploinsufficiency, 192, 197

Glycation, 2, 152, 158-159, 209-210, 212, 215, 219

Gray Matter, 41, 44, 77, 140, 142, 144, 149, 151, 165-166

Gut Microbiota, 1-2, 6-7, 9-10, 12, 14-15, 17, 21, 24-28

H

Hallucinations, 130, 224

Hippocampus, 3, 6-7, 12, 25, 29-31, 33, 35-36, 38-40, 46, 51-53, 55, 57, 62, 83, 88, 116-117, 119-121, 123-127, 153, 158, 160-161, 164-165, 167, 178, 180, 182, 205, 211-217, 220

Histamine, 168-169, 174-178, 220

Hypercholesterolemia, 209-210, 217-219, 221

Hypometabolism, 139-140, 143-146, 180, 184, 188-190

I

Immunohistochemistry, 3, 8-9, 12, 31, 209, 213, 215-216

Inflammatory Bowel Disease, 1, 11

L

Logical Memory, 41, 44, 131-132, 141, 144

Long-term Memory, 58, 118-120, 168-169, 177

M

Magnetic Resonance Imaging, 61, 82, 149, 160-161, 167, 179, 182-183, 186, 189, 192, 199, 208

Major Depressive Disorder, 161, 166-167, 207

Memory Decline, 56, 116, 167, 175, 181, 192, 194-196
Metabolic Derangement, 52
Microbial Community, 1, 9, 15
Microglia, 21, 49, 51, 53, 57-59, 90, 128, 153, 157-159
Morinda Officinalis, 1-2, 23, 26-27

N

Neuritic Plaques, 129, 190
Neurodegenerative Disease, 2, 58, 85, 116, 184, 192-193
Neurodevelopment, 1
Neurofibrillary Tangles, 2, 58, 85, 92, 116, 129-131, 189-190, 196
Neurogenesis, 15, 29-33, 36-40, 127, 219, 221
Neuroimaging Studies, 135, 140, 179
Neuroinflammation, 30, 54-58, 60, 153, 158-159, 169, 190, 221
Neurologists, 161
Neuronal Loss, 6-7, 49, 53, 55, 58, 85, 116, 130, 146, 209-210, 212, 216-221
Neurons, 6, 15, 29, 31, 33, 36-39, 53, 56-58, 85, 88, 92-94, 103, 108, 111-113, 118-119, 121, 123-126, 169, 178, 196, 209, 216, 218-220
Neuropeptides, 21, 30, 89
Neuropsychopharmacology, 2, 127, 176-177
Neuroscientists, 160-161, 188
Neurotransmitters, 3, 6, 8, 21, 30, 59, 168-169, 175
Norepinephrine, 6, 21, 169

P

Parkinson's Disease, 2, 26, 86, 114, 152, 161, 207
Pathogenesis, 2, 27, 37, 48-49, 51-56, 58-59, 85, 92-93, 108, 114, 117, 126, 128, 153, 169, 180, 184, 192-193, 218-219
Peptide Inhibitors, 86-87, 89-90
Prebiotics, 1-2, 15, 17, 21, 25-26
Precentral Gyrus, 199, 204-205, 207-208
Probiotics, 1-2, 9, 17, 20-21

S

Senile Plaques, 2, 57, 92, 116, 210, 218
Serotonin, 28, 52-53, 57, 116-117, 127, 169
Stress Response, 2, 193, 220
Synapse, 15, 30, 50-51, 56-59, 87, 116, 126, 146
Synaptic Loss, 2, 179, 184-185, 190

T

Therapeutics, 41, 48, 54, 57, 86, 88-89, 113, 137, 149, 158, 168, 175,
Tyrosine Phosphatase, 85, 88-90

V

Vascular Dementia, 41, 43, 47, 152

www.ingramcontent.com/pod-product-compliance
Lightning Source LLC
LaVergne TN
LVHW060551210926
848485LV00005B/1299